Nursing of Autism Spectrum Disorder

Ellen Giarelli, EdD, RN, CRNP, is Associate Professor in the Doctoral Nursing Program in the College of Nursing and Health Professions at Drexel University in Philadelphia. She is Adjunct Associate Professor in the Biobehavioral Research Center of the University of Pennsylvania School of Nursing. Dr. Giarelli received bachelor's of science degrees in nursing and biology from the State University of New York at Stony Brook, a master's degree in nursing from New York University, a doctorate in education from Rutgers, the State University of New Jersey, and postdoctoral education in psychosocial oncology and HIV/AIDS from the University of Pennsylvania School of Nursing. Prior to moving to Drexel University, Dr. Giarelli was coinvestigator of the Centers for Disease Control and Prevention–funded Study of Epidemiology of Early Development (SEED) and principal investigator of an initiative funded by the Philadelphia Health Care Trust to integrate nursing into the care of people with autism spectrum disorders. She was Research Project Director of the University of Pennsylvania School of Nursing Centers for Disease Control and Prevention–funded Center for Autism and Developmental Disabilities Research and Epidemiology (CADDRE) and principal investigator and Director of the Pennsylvania Autism and Developmental Disabilities Surveillance Program (PADDSP). In addition to the awards from the Centers for Disease Control and Prevention, her funded projects have included an R21 from the National Institutes of Health/National Institute of Nursing Research to study self-management of genetic disorders. She is a certified registered nurse practitioner in Pennsylvania and Investigator on externally funded studies of autism spectrum disorders.

Marcia R. Gardner, PhD, RN, CRNP, CPN, is Associate Professor at Seton Hall University College of Nursing. She was a clinical fellow in the Leadership in Neurodevelopmental Disabilities program at Children's Hospital of Philadelphia and a fellow in the American Association of Critical-Care Nurses Academic Leadership Program. With an extensive background in high-risk neonatal care, general pediatrics, and care of families of developmentally vulnerable infants and children, she teaches pediatric and developmental concepts and continues to investigate family-related issues in the care of individuals with developmental risks and concerns. She is certified in pediatric nursing and as a primary-care pediatric nurse practitioner by the National Certification Board of Pediatric Nurse Practitioners and Nurses.

Nursing of Autism Spectrum Disorder

Evidence-Based Integrated Care Across the Lifespan

Ellen Giarelli, EdD, RN, CRNP

Marcia R. Gardner, PhD, RN, CRNP, CPN

Editors

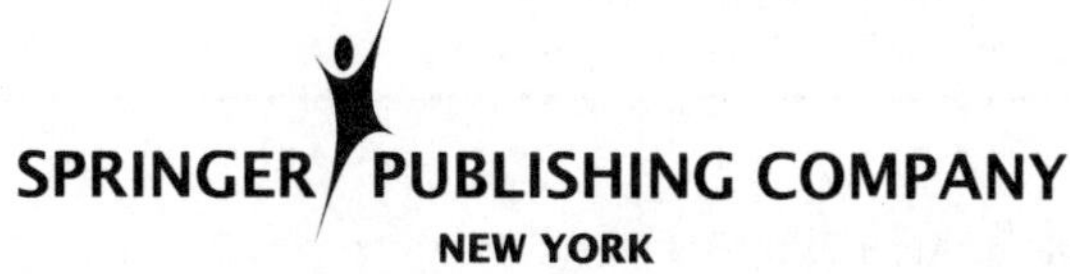

Springer Publishing Company, LLC
11 West 42nd Street
New York, NY 10036
www.springerpub.com

Acquisitions Editor: Margaret Zuccarini
Production Editor: Michael O'Connor
Composition: Techset

ISBN: 978-0-8261-0847-0
E-book ISBN: 978-0-8261-0848-7

12 13 14 15 / 5 4 3 2 1

CIP data is available from the Library of Congress

Printed in the United States of America by Bradford & Bigelow

This book is dedicated to our families.

To our spouses: James M. Giarelli and James L. Gardner provided encouragement, support, insight, and steadfast companionship during times of frustration and inspiration.

To our children: Emily Jane and James Joseph Giarelli and Michael, Jonathan, and Abby Gardner shared their sharp wits and kind hearts and demonstrated endless potential to create a crystal-clear, brilliant view of what might be.

To our parents: Grace and Bill Mounsey, Theresa and James L. Giarelli, and Dorothy and Milton Rubenstein showed through their actions the power of unconditional love.

Contents

Contributors

Karen Blake, MSN, PNP, RN
Adjunct Professor
Villanova University College of Nursing
Villanova, Pennsylvania

Lauren Blann, MSN, CPNP
Certified Pediatric Nurse Practitioner
Children's Specialized Hospital
Toms River, New Jersey

Joan Rosen Bloch, PhD, CRNP
Assistant Professor
Drexel University College of Nursing and Health Professions and School of Public Health
Philadelphia, Pennsylvania

Judith Bonaduce, RN, MSN, CRNP, PhD(c)
Widener University
School of Nursing
Chester, Pennsylvania

Marian S. Byrnes, MSN PMH CNS-BC
Vanguard School
Chadds Ford, Pennsylvania

Kathleen M. Fischer, PhD, RN, CRNP
Drexel University
Philadelphia, Pennsylvania

Marcia R. Gardner, PhD, RN, CPNP, CPN
Associate Professor
Seton Hall University College of Nursing
South Orange, New Jersey

Ellen Giarelli, EdD, RN, CRNP
Associate Professor
Drexel University College of Nursing and Health Professions
Adjunct Professor
University of Pennsylvania, School of Nursing
Philadelphia, Pennsylvania

Margaret J. Hegge, EdD, RN
Distinguished Professor of Nursing
College of Nursing
South Dakota State University
Renner, South Dakota

Brenda M. Holtzer, RN, PhD
Penn State Abington College
Abington, Pennsylvania

Lori Ioriatti, PhD(c), CPNP, RN
Pediatric Nurse Practitioner
Ambulatory Care Center Manager
Pediatric Practice Manager
Children's Specialized Hospital
Mountainside, New Jersey

Marygrace Yale Kaiser, PhD
Assistant Professor of Psychology
Eureka College
Eureka, Illinois

Karen J. Lecks, MSN, CRNP, WHNP
Clinical Research Coordinator
University of Pennsylvania
Philadelphia, Pennsylvania

Heather Marozsan, BSN, MSN, RN, CEN
Villanova University
Villanova, Pennsylvania

Kathleen Patrizzi, MSN, RN, CEN
Clinical Nurse Specialist
Emergency Department
Penn Presbyterian Medical Center
Philadelphia, Pennsylvania

Justin D. Peterson
Research Assistant
Drexel University
Philadelphia, Pennsylvania

Jennifer Pinto-Martin, PhD, MPH
Professor of Nursing
Chair, Department of Biobehavioral Health Sciences
University of Pennsylvania
Philadelphia, Pennsylvania

Adrienne P. Robertiello, BS
Autism Educator
Children's Specialized Hospital
Mountainside, New Jersey

Cordelia Robinson Rosenberg, PhD, RN
Professor,
Pediatrics, Psychiatry and Preventive Medicine; and
Director, JFK Partners, University of Colorado–Denver
School of Medicine
Aurora, Colorado

Jean Ruttenberg, MA
President
Jean Ruttenberg Consulting
Rydal, Pennsylvania

Nina Scarpinato, PMHCNS-BC, CRNP
Behavioral Health Clinical Nurse Specialist
Children's Hospital of Philadelphia
Philadelphia, Pennsylvania

Debi A. Schuhow, MSN, MH-CNS
Adult Psychiatric Mental Health Clinical Nurse Specialist/Nurse Practitioner and Case Manager
Branson Community-Based Outpatient Clinic,
Veterans Administration Medical Center
Branson, Missouri

Kathleen T. Sharp, MSN, CRNP
Pediatric Nurse Practitioner
Anesthesia Department
Children's Hospital of Philadelphia
Philadelphia, Pennsylvania

Margaret Cooney Souders, PhD, MSN, PNP
University of Pennsylvania
School of Nursing
Philadelphia, Pennsylvania

Patricia Dunphy Suplee, PhD, RNC-OB
Assistant Professor
Rutgers University–Camden
Camden, New Jersey

Kimberly K. Trout, PhD, CNM
Associate Professor and Director
Nurse-Midwifery/Women's Health Nurse Practitioner Program
Georgetown University School of Nursing & Health Studies
Washington, District of Columbia

Lorri Unumb, JD
Vice President
State Government Affairs
Autism Speaks
Lexington, South Carolina

Kristen van der Veen, AB, BSN, MSN Candidate
Pediatrics
University of Pennsylvania School of Nursing
Philadelphia, Pennsylvania

Louise Walpin, MS, APN-BC
Advanced Practice Nurse
Children's Specialized Hospital
Hamilton, New Jersey

Pamela Holtzclaw Williams, JD, PhD, RN
Assistant Professor
Medical University of South Carolina College of Nursing
Charleston, South Carolina

Tamara L. Zurakowski, PhD, GNP-BC
Practice Associate Professor
School of Nursing
Gerontological Nurse Practitioner
UPENN Living Independently for Elders Program, University of Pennsylvania
Philadelphia, Pennsylvania

Foreword

Many of us have had a time when we have struggled with an illness and trusted a nurse to guide us through tests, to provide important information, or just to offer an empathetic ear. For routine care, we trust our health care providers to check up on us and tell us whether things are going well or something about our health has gone awry. We make calls, wait for our appointments, fill out checklists, answer questions, put on the gowns, and comply when asked to "stand here," "take a deep breath," and "open up and say 'aah.'" These encounters might be routine or life-changing. Having that care is something we often take for granted when we go to the doctor's office. Most of us count on being able to report our history and symptoms and trust the people we encounter are there to help us.

Now, what if you were one of the 1% of people who has an autism spectrum disorder (ASD)? How would that change your health care encounter? From early on, your parents might have had a nagging feeling that something was different. They might have questioned whether you could hear and wonder why you did not turn around when they called your name in that sweet baby voice they used to get your attention. At a 15-month well-baby check, your mother might have kept a close eye on the nurse for any sign that something was different. She might have apologized when you cried and arched your back as you were examined. She might have been anxious and relieved at the same time when asked to answer questions about how many words you were using, whether you smiled when others smiled at you, whether you pointed out objects, and whether you pretended to talk on the phone. You might have been frustrated that you could not say you were thirsty, that people kept interrupting the way you looked at the wheels on a toy car, and that the sound of the air conditioner was scary and sharp to your ears.

From early in life, when the social, communication, and behavioral signs of autism emerge, life is different for people with an ASD. In addition to these core aspects of ASDs, people with an ASD are likely to have co-occurring conditions, such as problems with sleeping, eating, pain sensitivity, attention, and anxiety, among others. Getting routine health care can be a challenge for many reasons, such as the need to communicate and interact with other people. People with an ASD may find the unpredictability of office visits to be disconcerting. The unfamiliar people with unclear intentions in the midst of strange sights, smells, and sounds may be overwhelming. Some people with an ASD may react with outbursts that are frightening to those who do not know them, or they may just shut down and not respond. A person with an ASD may not be able to tell you where it hurts or that he or she even has pain in the first place. Even before the appointment, it may take extra steps and preparation to get ready for an office visit. Additional support and patience throughout the visit may be necessary. In these busy times, many health care professionals may not be interested in taking the time necessary to address the special needs that someone with an ASD may have.

Given the current prevalence estimates and improvements in awareness of ASDs, it is very likely that most health care offices will have patients on the spectrum at some time or other. Ideally, each person has access to a Medical Home service that provides accessible and family-centered care across the lifespan. People with ASDs may have unique developmental challenges, but they also face a range of health issues common to all people. Many of these may be compounded by autism. For too many, basic health care needs have been overshadowed by autism, with potentially treatable health issues explained away as just another part of autism. There is a need to change that standard, so that each person with ASD has access and is involved in what is needed to help him or her live a healthy life.

This volume, edited by Ellen Giarelli and Marcia R. Gardner, is a much-needed resource for nursing professionals. Nurses are a vital part of the health care team, and information and tools are essential for improving the well-being of people with ASDs. This book helps move health care forward by recognizing the range of issues across the lifespan that people with ASDs may face. In addition, the chapters address nursing care across settings, such as health care, educational, and specialized treatment facilities. This volume brings together a wealth of expertise, with information and strategies across the lifespan. The authors not only address issues of early identification but also issues of safety, nutrition, intervention, and care coordination. Although ASDs are typically lifelong conditions, little has been written about issues that affect adults with ASDs, particularly those who are elderly. The authors also address key transitions, milestones, health crises, and end-of-life issues. Each chapter provides practical illustrations and guidance to help prepare nurses for working with people with ASDs.

The editors have been dedicated to improving the information that drives health care for people with developmental disorders. This book provides much-needed information that follows reports from the Centers for Disease Control and Prevention on the prevalence of ASDs. It addresses practical issues in nursing care, such as evaluating a model for community-based pediatric screening for ASDs among toddlers. This resource will help spread important information to improve the lives of people with ASDs. Through these efforts, I hope that more people with ASDs will feel they are part of a trusted team when faced with being asked to "open up and say 'aah.'"

Catherine Rice, PhD
Behavioral Scientist
National Center on Birth Defects and Developmental Disabilities
Centers for Disease Control and Prevention

The findings and conclusions presented here are those of the author and do not necessarily represent the official position of the Centers for Disease Control and Prevention.

Preface

People with autism spectrum disorder (ASD) seek health care in pediatric primary-care offices, health-screening centers, emergency rooms, and outpatient and specialty clinics. Regardless of their work environment, nurses will inevitably encounter a patient with ASD.

At this time, ASD has no cure. There are treatments designed to mitigate the effects of symptoms and core and associated features. The core and associated features of the disorder may interfere with, or prevent, a patient's receipt of expert, quality, compassionate health care and cure for conditions that require nursing and medical treatments. This book does not discuss standard treatments for ASD; it presents issues surrounding lifelong, comprehensive care for people with ASD. Reading this book will prepare nurses to recognize the unique circumstances of providing health care to any person on the spectrum. The content assists nurses in organizing their care in ways that ensure any patient with ASD they encounter will receive expert, evidence-based care, access to appropriate medical interventions, and an equal opportunity to achieve optimal functioning and the highest possible quality of life. To accomplish this, a nurse must systematically apply, to each clinical encounter, knowledge of the typical behavioral characteristics of individuals with ASD; information on the individual's unique idiosyncrasies; and the person's stage of physical, mental, and emotional development. This will result in the delivery of intelligent, authentic, sympathetic, and deliberate care.

AN ORGANIZING PRINCIPLE

One organizing principle of this book is that of a social model of disability. In the broadest sense, a social model of disability is concerned with a clear focus on the environmental, cultural, and economic barriers encountered by people who are viewed as having some form of physical, mental, or intellectual impairment. The barriers encountered include: inaccessible educational systems and working environments; inadequate disability benefits; discriminatory health and social services; inaccessible transport, housing and public buildings, and amenities; and the devaluing of disabled people through negative images of those who are differently abled (Oliver, 2004).

Since its description over 60 years ago, autism has puzzled researchers and clinicians and generated scientific research across a wide range. Autism was under the purview of pediatric psychiatrists and other mental health professionals, who observed similarities with schizophrenia, thought disorders, and mental retardation. Psychogenetic explanations dominated the literature until a broader conceptualization of autism widened the view to include those with extremely high intelligence and unique talents and skills.

Until recently, children were the major recipients of medical and social attention. However, the increased awareness among parents, teachers, doctors, nurses, and the public has contributed to the development of a more comprehensive and integrated approach to care. Such an approach requires inclusion of a range of professionals, including nurses.

Moreover, a lifespan approach is necessary, as families have made it clear to all health care providers that ASD is not a disorder of childhood alone, but rather is a lifelong challenge for those who are affected.

Nurses are the largest group of health care professionals and will certainly provide care to many individuals with ASDs. Our case-based approach to patient care demonstrates the application of health history and physical and mental health assessments to the delivery of integrated care that is authentic, sympathetic, and deliberate. A case-study approach captures typical medical situations and demonstrates how nurses can apply care-planning strategies across communities and service settings.

The main themes are:

- ASDs is a growing public health problem and people with ASDs have special health care needs across the lifespan.
- As the largest group of health care professionals, nurses will interface with people with ASDs and their families in every health care setting.
- Nurses must integrate specialized information on ASDs into their clinical practice, across multiple practice settings.
- Setting-specific case studies illustrate "best practice" nursing care for a variety of problems experienced by people with ASDs.

The book is intended as a textbook and reference. It can serve as source of content for a continuing nursing education program or as the required text for a nursing minor in integrated ASD nursing care. It was conceived as the required textbook for a master's degree–level minor and a post-master's certificate program for master's-prepared nurses, it is therefore an excellent clinical resource for pediatric and mental health nurses, family and adult nurse practitioners, school nurses, college health nurse practitioners, and nurses in nurse-managed health care clinics. It is also suitable for post-baccalaureate education in ASD care.

The book is organized by sections and chapters. Each section begins with an overview of the section's contents and context and concludes with review questions and additional cases that will help a nurse increase his or her ability to apply knowledge to practice and generate creative solutions to clinical problems. Each chapter comprises a case study exemplar and elaboration of key problems, discussion of solutions, and a "best practice" nursing plan of care. The chapter content provides typical cases and comprehensive nursing care. Evidence-based justifications and examples apply science to nursing care in diverse settings: at the bedside, in primary and tertiary care, and in the community. Because ASD is a developmental disability, this book considers an individual's developmental needs as part of the organizing framework.

Taking a lifespan perspective, the book uses case studies that illustrate ASD scenarios across the lifespan to highlight nursing's significant role in the care of people with ASDs. To date, clinical emphasis has been placed on screening and early diagnosis of ASD. Although communication, language, and behavioral deficits may be mitigated through behavioral interventions, ASD is a pervasive disability and a chronic condition, and its core features and problems persist throughout life. Nurses will welcome this innovative and application-focused textbook and reference, which supports effective and appropriate nursing care throughout the lifespan.

TIMING

This book arrives at a most opportune point in time. Mental health and other health care professionals in the United States and globally have turned their attention to describing the trends in prevalence of ASD (Centers for Disease Control and Prevention, 2009) and its etiological factors.

This book responds to public concerns that the rise in prevalence of ASD is not sufficiently met with treatment options and responds to a call from the Obama administration and the Intra-Agency Autism Coordinating Committee to step up research and treatment for people with ASD. Taking an alternative path, this book addresses these needs by alerting nurses to the complex issues faced by people with ASDs as they struggle with this disability from diagnosis to end of life. Designed for nurses and written by nurses, it is unique among the many textbooks that elaborate on behavioral treatments and posited etiologies.

Arriving on the heels of the new statistics on the trends in prevalence of ASD in the United States (Centers for Disease Control and Prevention, in press), this nursing text affirms the profession's commitment to evidence-based care.

REFERENCES

Centers for Disease Control and Prevention. (2009). Prevalence of autism spectrum disorder—Autism and Developmental Disabilities Monitoring Network, United States, 2006. *MMWR Surveillance Summary 58*(10), 1–20. Centers for Disease Control and Prevention. (2012).

Centers for Disease Control and Prevention. (in press). Autism and Developmental Disabilities Monitoring Network Surveillance Year 2008 Principal Investigators. Prevalence of Autism Spectrum Disorders—Autism and Developmental Disabilities Monitoring Network, 14 sites, United States, 2008, MMWR.

Oliver, M. (2004). The social model in action: If I had a hammer. In C. Barnes & G. Mercer (Eds.), *Implementing the social model of disability: Theory and research* (p. 6). Leeds, UK: Disability Press.

Acknowledgments

Any text of this importance and complexity involves the help of many individuals. This text is not an exception. We gratefully acknowledge the support of the Philadelphia Health Care Trust for providing a generous grant to the University of Pennsylvania to develop ways to prepare nurses to care for the population of children and adults with autism spectrum disorder (ASD). We thank Wiley Thomas and Cathy Greenland for tirelessly advocating for a nursing presence in ASD care. With the collaboration of Jean Ruttenberg, Paula Cullinan, and Joseph Lukach and the staff from the Center for Autism in Philadelphia, we were able to observe firsthand the significant contributions nurses can make to the care of people with ASD and their families. We thank Springer for giving us the opportunity to present this unique, vital, and progressive approach to ASD care. We are indebted to Michelle Savard and Andrea Segal for their work proofreading the contents and their editorial prowess. Finally, we acknowledge our colleagues in medicine, nursing, speech-language pathology, occupational therapy, psychology, and education for helping children and adults on the spectrum find ways to be in their world.

Introduction and Background: Core Features, Autism Spectrum Disorder Prevalence, and the Role of Nursing

I

Ellen Giarelli

Since its discovery, or naming, over 65 years ago (Kanner, 1943), autism has been a curious and fascinating disorder that has engendered intense concern among parents, teachers, researchers, and communities. As a result of careful research and thoughtful observation, some once-held beliefs have been proven wrong. First, autism is not caused by poor parenting. Similar features in parents of autistic children may be due to genetic factors, as is the increased incidence among siblings of affected children (Rutter, 2001). Second, autism is not part of the childhood schizophrenia group (Kolvin, 1971). It is a neurodevelopmental disorder, not a psychosis. Third, autism is not secondary to a developmental receptive disorder (Cantwell, Baker, Rutter, & Mawhood, 1989).

AUTISM SPECTRUM DISORDER IN FAMILY CONTEXT

From the first recorded observations of a person exhibiting autistic behaviors, it has been seen as a "family matter." The earliest record of autistic-like behaviors in a patient dates back to a legal case reported in 1747 that sought an annulment of marriage of a man who had "deficits in social relationships including tactlessness and abnormal gaze, echolalia, obsessive and repetitive behaviors" and a preference for sameness (Frith, 2003; Houston & Frith, 2000; Wolff, 2004). Many decades passed before "family dynamics" became the target of health care, and many more decades passed before treatment for behavioral problems took a family-centered and integrated approach. By expanding observations of one person's problematic behaviors to encompass the effect of these behaviors on members of the extended family and the larger social network, a window opened onto the extensive impact of autism spectrum disorder (ASD) on communities. When communities are involved, nurses are involved.

Nurses assess individual, family, community, and societal health. Nurses are skilled at anticipating the impact of one individual's behaviors on others in the context of interpersonal relationships with consideration for the mental and physical health of the family and community.

Gray (1998) described becoming a family with autism as an insidious process wherein a family experiences a growing awareness of the problem and gradually adapts to the situation. Because the trajectory of the disorder varies, and there is much diversity across the group of affected persons, families have their own ways of confronting the challenges of ASD, as well as different interpretations based on cultural background. Gray (1998) noted that there is "no clear path of referral . . . no hospital emergency room to treat their child and start them on the road to recovery" (p. 23). In the past, families thought the experts had little to offer. Although this has changed with the help of teachers and therapists, autism remains a family problem. Parents are the principal advocates for their children and are often responsible for securing ongoing and consistent care. Therefore, integrated services for people with ASD must

TABLE S1.1 ■ Practice Parameters and the Clinical Encounter

Practice parameters[a]	Modified for the clinical encounter
Early identification requires training in the warning signs and symptoms of autism for individuals who work with young children.	Assessment of potential problems in the clinical encounter requires training in the warning signs and symptoms of autism for nurses who care for young children in clinical environments.
Early diagnosis requires training of professionals who can participate in the diagnostic process. Assessment requires a multidisciplinary team approach.	Assessment in the clinical encounter requires that all nurses have an understanding of the symptoms and characteristics of ASD and know when the help of a skilled, multidisciplinary team should be engaged.
With improved early identification, the availability of specialized early intervention services for young children with autism need to be enhanced.	With improved assessment of ASD characteristics in patients during a clinical encounter, the availability of specialized accommodations for patients with ASD needs to be enhanced.
Diagnostic and treatment services need to be available for older children, adolescents, and adults, regardless of the age of identification appropriate services must exist and be available and sustainable.	Assessment of the affect of ASD characteristics in the context of the clinical encounter must be applied to patients of all ages, and appropriate services must exist and be available and sustainable.

[a]Lubetsky, McGonigle, & Handen (2008).

include the family whenever possible. Nursing care of people with ASD considers the family perspective and integrates this with each clinical encounter.

Accurate diagnosis of ASD is critical to early intervention and improved outcomes for children and their families. Once ASD is diagnosed, evidence-based interventions can ameliorate the symptoms. Until recently, the traditional and consistent focus of treatment was on core features that interfered with functional ability. Now diagnostic best practice is formulated as a three-stage approach: Stage 1: first-level screening; Stage 2: second-level comprehensive developmental and medical evaluation; and Stage 3: specialized evaluation involving administration of autism-specific diagnostic tools (Filipek et al., 2000). Superimposed on these stages is a layer of assessment that considers the impact of core features, as well as characteristics and other symptoms, on other aspects of health care, such as preventive and curative medicine for conditions unrelated to ASD.

The salient points for the early identification of ASD are expanded to apply to every clinical encounter (see Table S1.1).

THE POLITICS OF DISABLEMENT

In medical sociology, the term "disable-ism" refers to the social imposition of avoidable restrictions on the life activities and well-being of people described as "impaired" by those self-described as "normal" or typical (Thomas, 2007). Disable-ism stands with sexism, ageism, and homophobia as a form of social oppression and is found both in person-to-person interactions and within the culture of institutions.

The clinical encounter between health provider and patient is one of the most purposeful of social interactions. It is guided by the expectation of the delivery of and the acceptance of care. It is also an encounter during which disable-ism may become manifest if the care is guided by unrealistic expectations by the health care provider. In other words, in the clinical encounter with a person with ASD, the nature of the patient's disability must be understood fully in order to avoid and prevent discrimination. All patients have special needs at one point or another in their lives. A patient-centered approach takes inventory of each person's abilities. This is essential for the ASD population, as one often hears in the ubiquitous phrase about ASD: "if you met one person with ASD you understand one person's ASD."

A patient-centered approach begins by thinking critically about the entire process of case management and, at minimum, communication with the individual with ASD. He or she may not look you in the eye and may seem to glance to the side if peripheral vision is better than frontal vision, but chances are he or she is listening and will respond. Idiosyncrasies can be anticipated and can be included in patient-centered treatment plans.

A study by Heidgerken and colleagues (Heidgerken, Geffken, Modi, & Frakey, 2005) of autism knowledge in health care settings reported that primary-care providers and specialists (e.g., psychiatrists, speech pathologists) had different understandings of the natural history, treatment, and prognosis of autism than autism specialists. This translates to a high potential for inconsistent health care across services, settings, and professional practice. People with special needs may have had negative, even traumatizing, experiences with the health care systems due to differences in provider knowledge and skill at interacting with these individuals. This simple fact should guide nurses to adopt a thoughtful process of caring for people with ASD, beginning at the point of screening and diagnosis and followed throughout their care by anticipating problems. Nurses should endeavor to make every patient's encounter with the health care system a positive experience that promotes wellness.

Autism was once considered incurable, but that notion has lost strength in the light of increased understanding of the disorder. Every day, individuals with ASD are showing us that they can overcome, compensate for, or manage their most challenging characteristics. The significant increase in public awareness of ASD is largely attributed to the tireless advocacy of parent support groups and national organizations, such as Autism Speaks and the Autism Society of America, which were started as early as the 1960s and are now international. Parents who are frustrated with health care services are driven to seek information and support (Baas, 2006). One important aim of Section I is to equip nurses with knowledge sufficient to help people with ASD benefit from the health care services they need and to which they are entitled.

Section I provides an overview of the public health problem of ASD and introduces the role of nurses and the contributions that the nursing profession can make to improve care for this population. Chapter 1 introduces the pervasive developmental disorder of ASD, with the description of the core features, associated features, and medical comorbidities. The features and characteristics are examined further in the context of specific clinical encounters (e.g., case studies). This chapter also presents the history of ASD, patterns of development, and the evolution of diagnostic criteria. Chapter 2 describes the natural history, etiology, rising prevalence, and risk factors of ASD. Changes in prevalence statistics and possible causes of ASD are outlined. Chapter 2 also describes the rise in public attention toward ASD, which has generated scientific inquiry on the disorder's prevalence and increased concern for the development of effective treatments and measurable outcomes. Regardless of the chief complaint or purpose for seeking medical care, the clinical management of patients with ASD may ultimately depend on the etiology. Outcomes of effective treatment for any health problem are fused, inextricably, with the behavior features of ASD. Chapter 3 addresses the purpose and value of a comprehensive, integrated approach to the clinical management of ASD, the evolving role of nurses in the care of affected people and their families, and the need for a lifespan approach to health maintenance, illness prevention, and integrated treatment protocols.

Best-practice nursing care for this population is a consequence of integrating theories of nursing with theories of ASD in the context of the clinical encounter.

REFERENCES

Baas, K. (2006). Specialty: Autism approaches need to be tailored to each person. *The Pennsylvania Nurse, 61*(1), 14–15.

Cantwell, D. P., Baker, L., Rutter, M., & Mawhood, L. (1989). Infantile autism and the developmental receptive dysphasia: A comparative follow-up into middle childhood. *Journal of Autism and Developmental Disorders, 19*, 19–30.

Filipek, P. A., Accardo, P. J., Ashwal, S., Baranek, G. T., Cook, E. H., Jr., Dawson, G., . . . Volkmar, F. R. (2000). Practice parameter: Screening and diagnosis of autism: Report of the Quality Standards Subcommittee of the American Academy of Neurology and the Child Neurology Society. *Neurology, 55*(4), 468–479.

Frith, U. (2003). *Autism: Explaining the enigma* (2 ed.). Oxford, UK: Blackwell.

Gray, D. E. (1998). *Autism and the family: Problems, prospects, and coping with the disorder*. Springfield, IL: Charles C. Thomas.

Heidgerken, A. D., Geffken, G., Modi, A., & Frakey, L. (2005). A survey of autism knowledge in a health care setting. *Journal of Autism and Developmental Disorders, 35*(3), 323–330.

Houston, R., & Frith, U. (2000). *Autism in history: The case of Hugh Blair of Borgue*. Oxford, UK: Blackwell.

Kanner, L. (1943). Autistic disturbances of affective contact. *The Nervous Child, 2*, 217–250.

Kolvin, I. (1971). Diagnostic criteria and classification of childhood psychoses. *British Journal of Psychiatry, 118*, 381–384.

Lubetsky, M. J., McGonigle, J. J., & Handen, B. L. (2008). Recognition of autism spectrum disorder. *Speaker's Journal, 8*(4), 13–23.

Rutter, M. (2001). Autism: Two-way interplay between research and clinical work. In J. Green, & W. Yule (Eds.), *Research and innovation on the road to modern child psychiatry* (Vol. I, pp. 54–80). London: Gaskell and the Association for Child Psychology and Psychiatry.

Thomas, C. (2007). *Sociologies of disability and illness: Contested ideas in disability and medical sociology*. London: Palgrave.

Wolff, S. (2004). The history of autism. *European Child & Adolescent Psychiatry, 13*(4), 201–208.

Autism Spectrum Disorder: Core Features and Medical Comorbidities

1

Cordelia Robinson Rosenberg

HISTORY

According to the Centers for Disease Control and Preventions, the condition called autism spectrum disorder (ASD) affects approximately 1 in every 88 children and has received considerable attention over the last decade (Centers for Disease Control and Prevention [CDC], 2012). Media of all types provide us almost weekly with some new piece of information about the diagnosis, prognosis, or interventions for this complex disorder. The media attention given to the prevalence of ASD, as well as its social and economic impacts, have been largely influenced by the work of parent- and grandparent-driven advocacy efforts. In addition to media attention, these advocates have influenced the U.S. Congress. The Child Health Act passed in 2000 gave considerable impetus to federal action by authorizing initiatives at the CDC, which included autism surveillance, a multisite case-cohort study (Centers for Autism and Developmental Disabilities Research and Epidemiology—Study to Explore Early Development), and a public awareness campaign around screening (Learn the Signs, Act Early [CDC, 2010]).

In 2006, the U.S. Congress passed the Combating Autism Act, which mandated the reactivation of an Interagency Autism Coordinating Committee (IACC) charged with developing and overseeing a strategic plan. This plan was organized around critical questions framed from the point of view of families: (1) When should I be concerned? (2) How can I understand what is happening? (3) What caused this to happen and can it be prevented? (4) Which treatments and interventions will help? (5) Where can I turn for services? (6) What does the future hold? (Combating Autism Act, 2006).

In December 2010, the Congressional Autism Caucus released a report on the status of the strategic plan. This level of government effort around a specific condition is unprecedented. The number of individuals and families affected by autism, the access to comprehensive care, and the predicted economic impact of a failure to attend to the issues raised by the IACC strategic plan appear to be the primary drivers of this bipartisan government action (Ganz, 2007; Kogan et al., 2008).

In this chapter, we examine the history of diagnosing conditions on the autism spectrum. We will examine the evolution of the criteria used to diagnose autism, the symptoms and behaviors considered to be core features, and the frequency of co-occurring conditions. Before considering these topics, we look at where we are now with respect to the diagnosis of ASD.

DIAGNOSING AUTISM

One of the critical aspects of the work to be done in the field concerns how a diagnosis of autism is made. It is essential to realize that there is no definitive biological test at this time to substantiate a diagnosis of autism. Autism spectrum disorders are diagnosed clinically based on three core behavioral dimensions: (1) communication delays or deficits, (2) impaired social interaction, and (3) repetitive behaviors and restricted interests (American Psychiatric Association [APA], 2000). These three domains of behavior must be looked at in the context of the individual's age and stage of development.

Individuals who meet clinical criteria for an ASD diagnosis vary greatly and can include people with extremely high IQs who lack adaptive behavior skills, as well as individuals with severe to profound impairments in intellectual development and no prospects for independence. ASD is highly heritable, and extensive research is being done to identify specific genes related to specific behaviors (Abrahams & Geschwind, 2008; see also Chapter 2, this volume). Some researchers are arguing that the effort to identify the genes responsible for autism would proceed more quickly were the triad of symptoms broken apart and careful characterization of individuals with ASD with respect to each core dimension done (Happé & Ronald, 2008).

Given the clinical nature of the diagnosis, practitioners rely on diagnostic taxonomies or conventions for making a diagnosis. In the case of ASD the systems used are the Diagnostic and Statistical Manual from the American Psychiatric Association and the International Classification of Diseases from the World Health Organization. Given these systems physicians and psychologists are the primary practitioners who are likely to make a diagnosis. Technically any licensed physician or licensed psychologist may make a diagnosis of ASD using criteria in either taxonomy. Many practitioners are reluctant to make such a diagnosis in the absence of having extensive experience with individuals with ASD. However, given the increased services and supports available, especially in the toddler and preschool years, and the long waiting lists and distances to be traveled for expert diagnostic services, some physicians and psychologists are going ahead and giving a diagnosis of autism in order to give families access to services that otherwise might not be available to them.

Currently, there is good congruence between the International Classification of Disease-10 (WHO, 1993) and the *DSM-IV Text Revision* (*DSM-IV-TR*; APA, 2000) classification systems. Both systems include three disorders in ASD: autism, Asperger's disorder, and pervasive development disorder–not otherwise specified (PDD-NOS). Both have comparable lists of criteria for the diagnosis. The development of diagnostic tools, such as the, Autism Diagnostic Observation Schedule (Lord et al., 1989), which combines knowledge of an individual's history, key informant reports, and direct observation have resulted in adequate sensitivity and specificity for the diagnosis of autism in preschool and school-age children.

Stability of the System of Diagnosis

Diagnoses of autism are generally stable. However, a number of factors are challenging the utility of the current systems. There are difficulties in reliably differentiating between autistic disorder, Asperger's disorder, and PDD-NOS. In some cases, differentiation depends on the clinician's access to an individual's history, which may be problematic, especially for adults. In light of such discrepancies, a study group in neurodevelopmental disorders has been working on a revision for the *DSM-IV-TR*, which is expected to be fully adopted in 2013 (Lord, 2011). While still being tested, there has already been extensive publicity about the proposed changes to be included in *DSM-V*. The *DSM-V* proposes the term "autism spectrum disorder," with no differentiation to be made among autistic disorder, Asperger's disorder, and PDD-NOS. Rett syndrome and childhood disintegrative disorder, which were included in *DSM-IV*, are no longer referred to within ASD. The overarching term is to be ASD, whereas in *DSM-III* and *DSM-IV* it was pervasive development disorder. Another major change in *DSM-V* for ASD is the fact that being diagnosed as meeting criteria of ASD does not exclude being identified with other diagnoses, such as attention deficit hyperactivity disorder (ADHD).

Historically, the symptoms of ASD were characterized in terms of three domains of behavior: social interaction deficits, communication delays and disorders, and behavior problems characterized by restricted and repetitive behaviors that interfere with development. In the proposed *DSM-V*, symptoms will be categorized in two domains: social communication and restricted and repetitive behaviors (RRBs). The rationale for this change is that social impairment and communication deficits are only moderately correlated in typical populations, whereas social and communication skills are highly correlated within samples of children or adults with ASD (Lord, 2011).

The *DSM-V* neurodevelopmental disorders work group has also proposed the use of specifiers and modifiers (Lord, 2011). These specifiers and modifiers address issues of intellectual disability, etiology, age of onset, and severity. With respect to intellectual disability, the recommendation is to indicate whether the person with a diagnosis of ASD also meets criteria for a diagnosis of intellectual disability (ID), which is measured intelligence and adaptive behavior of 70 or below on a valid, norm-referenced, standardized assessment tool. If a person has a genetic syndrome, such as Fragile X or Down syndrome, their diagnosis of ASD would read, for example, as ASD with Fragile X. While there are people who object to some of these changes, overall they reflect the research that has been occurring and the need expressed in the field for better documentation of the behavior of individuals and characterization of populations of people with an ASD (Agency for Healthcare Research and Quality [AHRQ], 2011).

As noted, *DSM-V* does away with a differentiation among autistic disorder, Asperger's disorder, and PDD-NOS with the rationale that accurate differentiation is not reliable among diagnosticians. When the proposed change to DSM-V was publicized in 2010, there was media attention given to the protests about this change from people who have a diagnosis of Asperger's disorder (Adams, 2010). Their concern reflected a desire on the part of people with Asperger's disorder, many of whom have a very high IQ, to not be associated diagnostically with people with autistic disorder, which they see as associated with low IQ.

Initial Identification of Autism

Autism was first described in 1943 by child psychiatrist Leo Kanner (Kanner, 1943). In his article, Kanner described 11 children he characterized as lacking the typical motivation for social interaction (Volkmar, Klin, & Cohen, 1997). One year after Kanner published his work, Hans Asperger, a medical student in Vienna, published a paper that proposed the concept of autistic psychopathology with respect to a group of boys with whom he was working (Asperger, 1944).

Kanner proposed two categories of symptoms: inadequate social responsiveness and perseverative behavior (Kanner, 1943). Kanner's descriptions of the children and their parents, particularly the mother's relationship to the child being described as "cold," led many to attribute autism to behaviors of the parents. Asperger described his cohort as having difficulties in communication, but felt as though they did not have mental retardation (Asperger, 1944). He based this distinction on the fact that many had areas of average or above average performance on some subtests of the intelligence tests administered to them (Asperger, 1944). Kanner's and Asperger's descriptions have a number of common features, but Asperger's descriptions suggested that high IQ was a feature of the disorder. Neither Kanner nor Asperger seemed aware of the other's work or their common use of the term autism (Volkmar et al., 1997).

Refining the Description and Understanding of Autism

Kanner's view that the disorder was congenital and that its expression was affected by the quality of the parent–child relationship was the predominant view of autism until the 1960s, when an alternative perspective to the psychogenic view of autism was offered. Rimland (1964) argued that autism was a biologically based disorder. Rimland's book, *Infantile Autism*, offered a view of autism as a disorder of information processing. Rimland also developed the first widely used scale focused on specific symptoms of autism (Rimland, 1968).

In 1978, Michael Rutter, a psychiatrist, published a definition of autism that included four essential features: (1) early onset by 2.5 years; (2) impaired and distinctive social development; (3) impaired and distinctive communication; and (4) unusual behaviors consistent in many ways with Kanner's concept of an "insistence on sameness" (Volkmar et al., 1997). Rutter's work, as well as that of others, laid the groundwork for the inclusion of specific criteria for the diagnosis of autism included in *DSM-III* (APA, 1980). Autism was not named specifically in the first (APA, 1952) or second (APA, 1968) editions of the *DSM*. The diagnostic option in *DSM-I* and *DSM-II* was childhood schizophrenia (Volkmar et al., 1997).

From the initial identification of autism and Asperger's disorder in 1943 and 1944 through the 1960s and 1970s, autism was still considered a rare disorder. With the work of Rutter and others and the inclusion of the disorder in *DSM-III* (APA, 1980), autism began to be identified more frequently, but still qualified as a rare disorder. Volkmar and colleagues (1997) pointed out that *DSM-III* is noteworthy, as it developed a taxonomy based upon research findings in which emphasis was placed upon assessing the reliability of descriptions of behavior consistent with a clinical diagnosis. In *DSM-III*, the term pervasive development disorder was introduced. The concept was important, because it avoided any assumptions about etiology.

The approach of looking at multiple disorders under the umbrella term of pervasive development disorder persisted through the next three iterations of the *DSM* (*DSM-III* [APA, 1980]; *DSM-III-R* [APA, 1987]; *DSM-IV* [APA, 1994]; *DSM-IV-TR* [APA, 2000]). In *DSM-IV*, five disorders were included under the term pervasive development disorder: Asperger's disorder, autistic disorder, PDD-NOS, childhood disintegrative disorder, and Rett disorder.

From 1980 to the present, work has been done within the context of the *DSM* taxonomy to refine our understanding of this complex disorder. Parallel to the work on the *DSM*, there have been refinements to the International Classification of Disease diagnostic taxonomy (WHO, 1993). Research has included comprehensive field trials involving both clinicians with extensive experience and those with less experience with the diagnosis of autism. Sensitivity and specificity of examiner's classifications of individuals were examined using *DSM-III*, *DSM-III-R*, and ICD-10 criteria (Volkmar et al., 1994). In this comparison, researchers found greater reliability using the ICD-10's more detailed criteria (Volkmar et al., 1994). Investigators also found that greater experience with autism, rather than professional discipline, was a better predictor of high reliability (Volkmar et al., 1994).

The *DSM-IV* and *DSM-IV-TR* (APA, 1994, 2000) were further refined to establish a definition "that balanced clinical and research needs, was reasonably concise and easy to use, provided reasonable coverage over the range of syndrome expression, and was applicable over the full life span, from early childhood through adulthood" (Volkmar et al., 1997, p. 25). Volkmar, Paul, and Klin (2005) argued that the convergence between systems (*DSM* and ICD) created a synergy between research and clinical practice that precipitated advances in our knowledge of the range in expression of ASD.

One of the features of the *DSM* is that it recommends that consideration be given to five axes when making a diagnosis. "The use of the multiaxial system facilitates comprehensive and systematic evaluation with attention to the various mental disorders and general medical conditions, psychosocial and environmental problems, and lack of functioning that might be overlooked if the focus were on assessing a single presenting problem" (APA, 2000, p. 27). Interestingly, mental retardation is noted on the axis that includes personality disorders. Noting the presence and severity of mental retardation, now referred to as intellectual disability, is a critical aspect of a clinical diagnosis of ASD. An individual may have one or more diagnoses or problems on any of the five axes.

ELEMENTS OF A COMPREHENSIVE ASSESSMENT

The recommended practice for diagnosing ASD includes completing multidisciplinary evaluation. The purpose of the evaluation is not simply a diagnosis, but rather a comprehensive view of the individual's strengths and weaknesses and any co-occurring conditions. Both the American Academy of Neurology (Filipek et al., 2000) and the American Academy of Pediatrics (AAP; Johnson, Myers, & the Council on Children with Disabilities, 2007) have developed guidelines for practitioners regarding this process. These guidelines are highly valued and generally viewed as the desired practice, although the AAP cautions that this guidance does not "serve as a standard of medical care" (Johnson et al., 2007, p. 183). The AAP calls for three goals to be addressed in the comprehensive evaluation of a child with suspected ASD. They are: (1) the administration of appropriate developmental or psychometric measures; (2) the presence or absence of a categorical diagnosis of ASD, made with standardized tools demonstrated to be valid and reliable for the purpose; and (3) the presence of other evaluations to determine whether there is an associated etiology for the autism, such as a genetic disorder.

Lord (2011) outlined a number of features critical to a comprehensive assessment, which is applicable for all disorders. Early history, including age of perceived onset and pattern of onset should be documented. Pattern of onset refers to whether there is a perceived or documented loss of words and social skills before 18 months or 30 months versus no clear onset and no loss of words (Lord, 2011). Assessment should also include administration of norm-referenced standardized measures of development for young children or verbal and nonverbal IQ for older individuals. Adaptive functioning should be assessed. Verbal abilities at the time of applying the diagnostic criteria should be documented. Adequacy of initiating and maintaining sleep should be evaluated. Emotional self-regulation ability for age should be evaluated. Any co-occurring developmental, medical, and psychiatric problems should be documented. It is expected that this assessment process can benefit from input from a number of disciplines, including medicine, psychology, speech and language pathology, and occupational therapy, as well as others.

Assessment Tools

As the research on autism progressed, the need for more refined diagnostic criteria became apparent. The Autism Diagnostic Observation Schedule (ADOS; Lord et al., 1989; Lord, Rutter, DiLavore, & Risi, 1999; Lord et al., 2000) and the Autism Diagnostic Interview-Revised (ADI-R; Lord, Rutter, & LeCouteur, 1994) were developed and became more commonly used for research and also for clinical purposes. Lord and Bishop (2010) point out that the current prevalence of ASD reflects a broader range of functioning referred to as the "broader autism phenotype." Given this broader range, a one-size-fits-all approach to assessment is not appropriate. However, Lord and Bishop (2010) go on to point out that there does need to be a standard protocol with steps to take depending upon specific results.

The ADOS has four modules that allow for an assessment of people with different levels of functioning. The ADI-R provides important information regarding the person's history from the parents' perspective and information as to how the person functions in a variety of situations, thus contributing unique information to the diagnosis of autism (Risi et al., 2006). When the ADOS and ADI-R are used in combination, they correlate more highly with the consensus of clinical judgments on autism and ASD than a single instrument.

Gold Standard for Assessment

Use of *DSM* criteria by an experienced clinician, plus the ADOS and ADI-R, have become the gold standard diagnostic procedure for characterizing individuals with ASD. If knowledge regarding response to intervention is to advance, it is imperative that such a standard be used in research. Yet in a recent AHRQ Comparative Effectiveness Report regarding therapies for children with ASD, the reviewers found that 125 out of 159 intervention studies failed to use or report such a standard in their study (AHRQ, 2011). The great heterogeneity in the population of individuals with ASD, the inadequate description of the participants on the core features of ASD, and the limited description of the level of functioning limit the ability of researchers to examine characteristics of the child that may modify response to treatment.

CORE SYMPTOMS OF AUTISM

Since its inclusion in *DSM-III* (APA, 1980) autism has been defined in terms of three core dimensions: impaired social interaction; impairments in communication; and restricted repetitive and stereotypical patterns of behavior, interests, and activities. These criteria were further defined and other disorders were added under the umbrella term of pervasive developmental disorders in *DSM-IV*. The diagnostic criteria for the autistic disorders, Asperger's syndrome, and PDD-NOS share many features and differ only in the number of criteria in the domains. For example, both autistic disorder and Asperger's disorder manifest qualitative impairment in social interaction, and restricted repetitive and stereotyped patterns of behavior, interests, and activities. In order for a diagnosis of autistic disorder to be applied, there must also be delays or abnormal functioning in at least one of the following areas, with onset prior to age 3 years: (1) social interaction, (2) language as used in social communication, or (3) symbolic or imaginative play. In Asperger's disorder, there are no clinically significant delays in cognitive development or in the development of age-appropriate self-help skills, adaptive behavior (other than in social interaction), and curiosity about the environment in childhood (APA, 2000).

Differentiating between autistic disorder and Asperger's disorder with regard to the triad of the core features of autism is one of the concerns that has been raised regarding the adequacy of our knowledge on the natural history of autism (First, 2008). It was felt that the *DSM-IV* criteria provided adequate information regarding how to evaluate the presentation in preschool and school-age children, but that the items do not adequately apply to toddlers, adolescents, and adults (First, 2008). Marans, Rubin, and Laurent (2005) provide detailed descriptions of core social communication challenges and emotional regulation challenges for individuals with Asperger's disorder or high-functioning autism for whom receptive and expressive language and cognitive level are in at least the average range. These challenges are presented in Table 1.1 as more detailed examples of the social communication criteria.

New Approach—Two Dimensions

In *DSM-V*, the core features have been reduced to two dimensions: (1) social communication and (2) restricted interests and repetitive behavior. One can find many individuals with an autism diagnosis who are highly verbal, with extensive vocabularies, but who do not understand the pragmatics of language. Pragmatics includes the skills that permit us to understand nonverbal communication, take another's perspective, recognize and interpret emotions, and understand jokes and double meanings.

The social communication dimension has three subdomains: (1) deficits in social–emotional reciprocity; (2) deficits in nonverbal communication behaviors used for social interaction; and (3) deficits in developing and maintaining relationships, appropriate to developmental level. Each subdomain includes a number of criteria, and an individual will need to meet criteria in all three subdomains to be diagnosed with an ASD when *DSM-V* is applied.

Within the second domain of RRB, there are four subdomains. They are: (1) stereotypical or repetitive speech, motor movements, or use of objects; (2) excessive adherence to routines, ritualized patterns of verbal or nonverbal behavior, or excessive resistance to change; (3) highly restrictive, fixated interests that are abnormal in intensity or focus; and (4) hyper- or hyporeactivity to sensory input or unusual interest in sensory aspects of environment. If a

TABLE 1.1 ■ Core Social Communication Challenges in High-Functioning Autism and Asperger's Disorder

Capacity for joint attention	Capacity for symbol use
1. Understanding the communicative intentions and emotional state of a social partner	1. Acquiring higher-level linguistic rules, grammar and syntax, that clarify one's intent (e.g., subordinate clauses and conjunctions) across social partners and environments
2. Interpreting and using nonverbal communicative signals (e.g., facial expressions, prosody, body orientation and proximity, and gestures) as they relate to one's attentional focus, affective state, and intentions	2. Understanding and using verbal conventions for initiating, exchanging turns, and terminating interactions across different social partners and social situations (e.g., rules of politeness)
3. Considering appropriate topics of conversation, maintaining information, sharing across turns, and repairing communicative breakdowns based on the social context and a listener's perspective	3. Interpreting and using language in a flexible manner by responding to language that may contain: multiple meaning words, nonliteral language, and irony
4. Modifying interpretation of more ambiguous language forms (e.g., sarcasm, humor, figurative expressions, etc.) depending upon the intentions or perspective of one's social partner	4. Using language as a tool for emotional regulation (e.g., preparing for changes in routine, preparing for the expectations of different social contexts, and using appropriate means to request assistance and comfort across social settings and social partners)

Adapted from Volkmar et al. (2005), p. 979.

person meets the behavioral criteria on at least two of the four subdomains of RRB, they qualify for a diagnosis of ASD.

Patterns and Age of Onset

One of the defining features of ASD is age of onset. Kanner (1943) argued that autism was congenital. Rutter (1978) proposed the criterion of onset before 2.5 years of age. Interest in the issue of age of onset has been investigated from multiple perspectives. Three patterns for the emergence of symptoms are described in the literature (Ozonoff, Heung, Byrd, Hansen, Hertz-Picciotto, 2008). The first pattern is that of identification of symptoms in the first year of life, labeled early-onset pattern. The second pattern, termed developmental or autistic regression, is defined as a loss of previously acquired social, communication, and motor skills prior to 36 months of age, after "near-typical" development. The third pattern involves that of near-typical milestone achievement up to 2 years, which is followed by a plateau of skill development.

Researchers have looked at these patterns in terms of the prevalence of each pattern and in terms of the relationship to child outcomes. Kokoyachi and Murata (1998; as cited in Kalb, Law, Landa, & Law, 2010) estimate the range of prevalence of the regression pattern extends from as high as 50% to a low of 15% to 18% when a strict definition of regression is used. With regard to outcomes, the data are mixed, with some studies reporting poorer outcomes in relationship to regression and others reporting minimal to no differences in outcomes (Kalb et al., 2010).

Developmental Characteristics and Outcomes

Contrary to expectations, children who were diagnosed at an early age were not found to be more severely affected than those who were diagnosed later (Landa, Holman, & Garrett-Mayer, 2007; Werner, Dawson, Munson, & Osterling, 2005). Kalb and colleagues (2010) investigated relationships among developmental characteristics and outcomes in a large sample of children assigned to groups based on the three patterns of onset of symptoms. The data for the study came from the Interactive Autism Network (IAN). Families voluntarily submit their data to the IAN registry (http://www.ianproject.org), which began in 2007 and now has data for more than 10,000 children. The sample for this study included 2,720 children of 3 to 17 years of age. Eighty three percent of the sample was male and 90% was white. Of the three patterns, 44% showed skill loss, 39% showed no loss, and 17% showed a plateau. Kalb and colleagues (2010) found that the children with regression showed milder delays in early development, but were at increased risk for poorer outcomes and more likely to have elevated autism symptom scores, which means they were more likely to have a diagnosis of autistic disorder, as opposed to Asperger's disorder or PDD-NOS.

In an effort to correct for inherent problems in parent recall regarding patterns of onset, Ozonoff and colleagues (2010) examined videotapes for the emergence of behavioral signs of autism in infants in two groups: low and high risk for autism. This longitudinal, prospective study was accomplished by rating videotapes of these children at 6, 12, 18, 24, and 36 months of age. Children were diagnosed as either ASD or typically developing by 36 months of age. The specific behaviors the researchers looked at included the frequency of gaze to face, gaze to objects, smile, nonverbal vocalizations, and word and phrase verbalizations. Raters of the videotapes were blind to child classification. The authors found no differences between the groups on the rate of the three counts of social communication behaviors, nor on the global ratings at 6 months. By 12 months, the groups differed on gaze to face and directed vocalizations. At 18, 24, and 36 months, there were significant differences between the groups on all four measures. Both groups showed linear patterns of growth, but the trajectory for the children with autism was significantly slower.

These findings have implications for both the diagnosis and the treatment of autism. Ozonoff and colleagues (2010) argued that the defined categories of early onset, regressive autism, and plateau do not accurately portray how symptoms of autism emerge and that specific probes into social development at 6-month intervals are more useful. The high correlation between the global ratings and the specific probes suggest a fruitful area for development of a screening measure. Finally, Ozonoff and colleagues (2010) suggested that the current characterization of types of onset are not useful in terms of predicting outcomes and are problematic with respect to clarity of definition and recall bias. They proposed that a more useful conceptualization is a time-based continuum. At one end are children whose loss of social interest is early, that is, between 6 and 12 months in onset. At the other end of this continuum are children whose loss of social interest and communication skills are so late that "regression" appears quite dramatic (Ozonoff et al., 2010). They further argue that identification of autism by the first birthday may not be possible in the majority of affected children. Furthermore, they argue that in addition to the recommendation for screening at 18 and 24 months, screening may need to occur later to identify these late-onset children. Finally, they make a point that any infant or toddler who demonstrates a sustained reduction in social responsiveness is a candidate for focused intervention to address social communication, whether or not the child screens positive for autism.

Severity of Presentation of Symptoms

One of the limitations of the earlier versions of the *DSM* is that the criteria are framed as simply present or absent, therefore not allowing for a systematic judgment regarding the severity of the expression of the condition. In the *DSM-IV*, severity was reflected by whether or not a person was diagnosed with autistic disorder or with the "broader phenotype" of high-functioning autism, Asperger's disorder, or PDD-NOS. In the *DSM-V* criteria, it is proposed that each of the two dimensions—deficits in social communication and restricted repetitive behavior—be rated for severity. Table 1.2 contains the proposed statements for each of these levels of severity ranging from: (1) normal variation; (2) substantial symptoms; (3) requires support; (4) requires substantial support; and (5) requires very substantial support. It is expected that this proposed system of classifying severity will contribute to a characterization of people's symptoms and a better basis for planning intervention (Lord, 2011).

Medical Diagnosis or Educational Identification

One controversy in the field of ASD is the debate as to whether or not a medical diagnosis is necessary for educational programming. Some argue that given that ASD is defined in terms of specific behaviors or absence of behaviors, identification of educational needs without an actual diagnosis is adequate. One of the potential sources of data regarding the prevalence of ASD is the annual child count data. In an educational identification context, the condition must have a "significant impact on the child's educational, emotional, or functional skills, such that specialized instruction is necessary for the child to be successful. In Colorado the official position of the Colorado Department of Education is that a medical or clinical diagnosis does not automatically qualify for special education" (Colorado Department of Education, 2008).

TABLE 1.2 ■ Proposed *DSM* Severity Rating System

Proposed dimensional ratings for ASD in *DSM-V*	Social communication	Fixated interests and repetitive behaviors
Requires very substantial support	Minimal social communication	Marked interference in daily life
Requires substantial support	Marked deficits with limited initiations and reduced or atypical responses	Obvious to the casual observer and occur across context
Requires support	Without support, some significant deficits in social communication	Significant interference in at least one context
Subclinical symptoms	Some symptoms in this or both domains; no significant impairment	Unusual or excessive but no interference
Normal variation	May be awkward or isolated but within normal limits (WNL)	WNL for developmental level and no interference

Adapted from Lord (2011).

There is considerable anecdotal evidence that schools are reluctant to identify students as having an autism educational exceptionality due to the considerable expense likely to be involved if a family demands intensive treatments using a particular methodology. However, the Individuals with Disabilities Education Act (IDEA; 1990) based definition of an educational exceptionality on the impact of educational, emotional, or functional skills. Too often we have encountered situations in which the child's speech is at age and grade level, but the pragmatics of communication are missing. Thus, the child may well meet many of the *DSM* criteria for a diagnosis on the autism spectrum, but because his or her academic work is at age level, the child is not seen as eligible for educational intervention.

There is also reason to believe that there are a number of children on the autism spectrum who are in the general education classes without a classification and therefore without an individualized educational plan (IEP). Hepburn and colleagues (2008) compared a teacher nomination strategy using a six-question checklist to the performance of the Autism Spectrum Screening Questionnaire (ASSQ; Ehlers, Gillberg, & Wing, 1999) as a strategy for identifying children with an ASD. Teachers were asked to nominate up to two children in their general education elementary classrooms (K–5) who met any of the six characteristics listed in Exhibit 1.1.

A total of 60 teachers with 1,355 students among them participated. Fifty of the 60 teachers nominated at least one child, with a total of 116 children nominated. Ninety-five children scored 17 or higher on the ASSQ, with 9.2% of boys and 5% of girls receiving scores of 17 or higher. Agreement between being nominated and scoring 17 or higher on the ASSQ was 93% to 95%. Of those nominated, 32% currently had an IEP, previously had an IEP, or had an IEP in process, and 68% were not identified as a special education student. The nomination strategy seems to have promise as a more time- and cost-efficient first-level screener for children who need assistance with the social aspects of school.

Marans, Rubin, and Laurent (2005) identified social communication skills as a critical priority for educational programming, and yet these skills, or lack thereof, are not adequately identified and attended to in educational programs. The greatest challenges in social communication for these children lies ahead, as they enter elementary, middle, and high school

EXHIBIT 1.1

Quick Screening Questions on ASD Characteristics

1. Is the person socially awkward?
2. Does the person not seem to understand the feelings of others?
3. Does the person talk a lot about own interests, but not very good at conversations?
4. Does the person not chat with peers just to be friendly?
5. Does the person demonstrate a lack of flexibility?
6. Does the person demonstrates intense interest in just a few topics or activities?

and encounter much more complex versions of joint attention skills, mastering of higher-level linguistic rules, and use of language and cognition for self-regulation and mutual regulation, (Marans et al., 2005). In theory, identification of "educationally significant needs" should be adequate to address the needs of students and a medical diagnosis of ASD should not be necessary for appropriate educational intervention. In practice, we have found reason to question such an assumption.

CO-OCCURRING CONDITIONS FOR CHILDREN WITH ASD

People with ASD may have developmental, neurological, medical, and psychiatric conditions in addition to ASD. Sometimes these conditions are referred to as comorbid conditions (Matson, LoVullo, Rivet, & Boisjoli, 2009; Volkmar and Klin, 2005) and sometimes as co-occurring or associated conditions (Levy, Giarelli, Lee, Schieve, Kriby, Cunniff, et al., 2010; Reaven, 2009). Levy and colleagues (2010) argued that the term comorbid may imply a condition that is distinct from the disorder itself or may imply causality. For this reason, the authors prefer the term co-occurring condition.

LITERATURE ON CO-OCCURRING CONDITIONS

Most of the literature documenting co-occurring conditions is based upon clinical samples and can have widely varying figures regarding prevalence, presumably due, in part, to the type of practice and the source of the sample. Levy and colleagues (2010) used population-based data to describe four groupings of co-occurring disorders. They are: (1) developmental diagnoses, (2) psychiatric, (3) neurological diagnoses, and (4) possibly causative medical diagnosis (see Table 1.3). Levy and colleagues (2010) also found that 60% of the sample of 2,568 children who meet Autism and Developmental Disabilities Monitoring (ADDM) network criteria for a case definition had one co-occurring diagnosis, while 26% had two or more diagnoses or symptoms consistent with one of the four types of conditions for a total of 86% with a co-occurring disorder. In addition, they reported that those children who were diagnosed with ASD later had a greater number of preceding co-occurring diagnoses. The authors postulated that other conditions may have a masking effect in the diagnosis of ASD. This data came from 8-year-old children born in 1994, and ADDM surveillance has continued with

TABLE 1.3 ■ Prevalence of Non-ASD Developmental, Psychiatric, and Medical Diagnoses among Study Population of ASD Cases Identified through ADDM Network, 2002

Developmental diagnoses[a]	*n* (%)	Psychiatric diagnoses[a]	*n* (%)	Neurological diagnoses[a]	*n* (%)	Possibly causative medical diagnoses[a]	*n* (%)
All cases developmental diagnosis	2,123 (82.7%)	All cases psychiatric diagnosis	258 (10.0%)	All cases neurological diagnosis	404 (15.7%)	All cases possible causative diagnosis	95 (3.7%)
Specific developmental diagnosis[a]	%	Specific psychiatric diagnosis[a]	%	Specific neurological diagnosis[a]	%	Specific causative diagnosis[a]	%
Language disorder	63.4	ODD	4.0	Epilepsy	15.5	Other genetic/ congenital[b]	1.0
ADHD	21.3	Anxiety disorder	3.4	Encephalopathy	5.9	VCF	0.9
Intellectual disability	18.3	Emotional disorder	2.4	Hearing loss	1.7	Down syndrome	0.8
Sensory integration	15.7	Mood disorder	2.3	Cerebral palsy	1.7	Chromosome disorders[c]	0.5
Learning disorder	6.3	OCD	2.0	Visual impairment	1.0	Fragile X syndrome	0.3
		Depression	1.1	TS/tics	0.5	Tuberous sclerosis	0.2
		Bipolar disorder	0.7	Brain injury	0.4		
		Mutism	0.5				
		Psychosis	0.3				
		RAD	0.3				
		Conduct disorder	0.2				
		Schizophrenia	0.1				

[a]Diagnoses are not mutually exclusive (e.g., one subject may have more than one diagnosis).

[b]Genetic or congenital syndromes or disorders (e.g., embryopathy, fetal alcohol syndrome, Cornelia DeLange syndrome, and others).

[c]Chromosomal disorders (e.g., deletion, duplication, and others). ODD, oppositional defiant disorder; OCD, obsessive–compulsive disorder; RAD, reactive attachment disorder; TS, Tourette syndrome; VCF, velocardiofacial syndrome.

Source: Reprinted with permission from Levy et al. (2010).

new birth cohorts in 4-year increments. Similar analyses with subsequent ADDM birth cohorts will provide information as to the reliability of these findings.

While coping with the diagnosis of an ASD is difficult in and of itself, the presence of one or more co-occurring conditions can complicate day-to-day care. The proposed *DSM-V* guidelines include an appraisal of all four categories noted above as essential to the recommended comprehensive approach to assessment. The *DSM-V* approach looks at the diagnosis of ASD as a factor in and of itself, with the expectation that all co-occurring conditions should be evaluated as well, not for the purpose of diagnosis, but for the purpose of prescribing effective interventions.

Co-occurring Psychiatric Disorders

As previously noted, use of the term co-occurring condition avoids any assumptions of underlying etiology for the condition. Specifically, the position is that an individual who meets diagnostic criteria for a psychiatric condition by definition has that condition. Recognition of both conditions as having independent diagnostic criteria has important implications for access to care, such that different treatments and follow-up care may be required.

Within the *DSM* system ASD and psychiatric diagnoses are Axis I disorders. This fact probably contributes to the reluctance of some clinicians to apply both an ASD diagnosis and an Axis I psychiatric diagnosis to the same person. Some argue that if a person's anxiety disorder, for example, is due to the fact that the person has autism, then from that perspective, the anxiety disorder is not amenable to treatment from the mental health system. In this example, we see the potential negative consequences of attributing symptoms to a presumed etiology. The person may not receive appropriate treatment.

THE CASE OF JAMES

Reaven (2009) offered an example of James, an 8-year-old boy with a diagnosis of Asperger's disorder with intellectual and academic abilities in the average range. His IEP was designed to address the ASD core symptoms of problems with social communication, independence, and organization. At the end of second grade, he began to express fear of making mistakes, and by third grade, his worries about making mistakes increased and he frequently asked to stay home from school. He was also bothered by loud noises to the extent that he met clinical criteria for generalized anxiety disorder and specific phobia. Reaven (2009) went on to describe how a cognitive behavioral therapy (CBT) approach can be successfully modified for use for children with ASD. Reaven (2009) recommended a variety of strategies, including extensive use of concrete supports such as video modeling and using the individual's specific interests or talents as a platform to build upon. The modification of CBT developed by Reaven and her colleagues is now available in a book, *Face Your Fears* (Reaven, Blakeley-Smith, Nichols, & Hepburn, 2011). Increasingly, investigators are developing diagnostic and treatment strategies for co-occurring psychiatric conditions for individuals with an ASD (Chalfant, Ropee, & Carroll, 2007; Sofronoff, Attwood, & Hinton, 2005; Sze & Wood, 2007).

Co-occurring Medical Conditions

In order to provide a complete assessment of the individual with ASD, it is important to look at all associated medical problems the individual may have which are relevant to his or her comprehensive clinical management (APA, 2000). These problems should be identified under Axis III of the complete clinical workup. In addition to specific neurological conditions, such as seizure disorders, there are a number of other medical problems often overlooked or undiagnosed in people with ASD. Nurses and physicians who care for people with ASD and their families have frequently cited the difficulty children have with sleep, adequate nutrition, gastrointestinal disturbance, food selectivity, and self-injury, to name just a few. Sleeping disorders and selectivity and rigidity in eating patterns can be grave issues for many families. These issues may not be satisfactorily diagnosed or treated, when in fact, treatment of such issues as sleep deprivation and hunger could ameliorate irritability, inability to concentrate, and other symptoms that intersect with those specific to ASD.

Access to medical care for co-occurring conditions can be difficult for many families. In some cases, primary-care providers may not feel capable of managing such complex problems. Parents may seek the help of a developmental behavioral pediatrician to work with their pediatric primary-care providers, but collaborative consultation can be difficult to realize. The Autism Treatment Network (ATN) consists of 17 centers, each with some funding from Autism Speaks and the Health Resource Service Administration (HRSA) under the Combating Autism Act. These centers each have a common purpose of developing our knowledge about the prevalence and range of co-occurring medical problems and assessing methods for managing these conditions (ATN, 2011). The ATN has also established a data registry composed of systematically collected and consistent information from families about common co-occurring medical conditions.

Co-occurring ASD and Specific Disorders or Syndromes

In the *Handbook of Autism and Pervasive Developmental Disorders*, Filipek (2005) makes the point that the relationship between ASD and medical conditions can be viewed from two approaches: as medical conditions associated with ASD or as ASD associated with medical conditions. One can look for conditions in a population of people with ASD or one can look for ASD in a population of individuals with a given syndrome. Some may argue "why should we have another label?" The counter-argument is that for the child who has Down syndrome (DS) and ASD, for example, it is not typical for a child with DS to not be talking, while it is an all too frequent problem for a child with autism. What is known about communication for children with ASD should inform the treatment plan for the child with DS.

Regarding the prevalence of ASD among children with DS, DiGuiseppi and colleagues (2010) recruited children with DS from a birth registry sample. All families still residing within a 10-county area, in which the children were still alive, were invited to participate in a study to look at their child's social, communication, and behavioral needs. Depending upon the age of the child, the Modified Checklist for Autism in Toddlers (M-CHAT; Robins & Dumont-Mathieu, 2001), or the Social Communication Questionnaire (SCQ; Rutter, Bailey, & Lord, 2003) was administered in a telephone interview. All of the families of children who screened positive were invited to come in for an evaluation that included the ADOS (Lord et al., 1999), ADI-R (Rutter, LeCouteur, & Lord, 2003), an age-appropriate developmental assessment, and the Vineland Adaptive Behavior Scales, Second Edition (Sparrow, Balla, & Cicchetti, 1984). In this sample, the estimated prevalence of ASD (broad phenotype) was 18.2% and that of autistic disorder was 6.4%. This estimate indicates that ASD is 17 to 20 times higher among children with DS than the estimated prevalence of ASD in the general population.

Down syndrome is just one example of a genetic syndrome that appears to have a higher than expected co-occurrence with ASD when compared to the general population (DiGuiseppi et al., 2010). Studies such as this give credence to the concerns of families with a child with a given syndrome that presents with atypical characteristics. In response to this issue, groups such as the Colorado Down Syndrome-Autism Connection have been formed (Zaborek, 2011). These families have come together in a support group in which they feel more comfortable and provide advocacy for one another.

Autism and Co-occurrence with Intellectual Disability

In Kanner's original description of infantile autism, he made a point of distinguishing autism from mental retardation (Schalock et al., 2010). In the 1940s, and for some time thereafter, the predominant view was that mental retardation was not amendable to intervention. At that time, there was not a uniformly accepted definition of mental retardation. In 1961, the American Association on Mental Deficiency (AAMD), now the American Association of Intellectual and Developmental Disabilities, proposed a definition of mental retardation that soon became the standard (Heber, 1961). This definition is relevant here due to its emphasis on measured intelligence and measured adaptive behavior, and because an underlying etiology was not part of the definition. Important elements of this definition are that the individual's scores on a norm-referenced standardized test of intelligence and test of adaptive behavior are below 70 and that these problems are apparent before 18 years of age. Once the AAMD definition became commonly adopted, the issue of etiology became irrelevant to the diagnosis of mental retardation.

In 2006, Edelson published a review of the literature on the co-occurrence of autism and mental retardation. She reviewed all reports she could find that spoke to both autism and mental retardation from 1943 through 2003, including books and book chapters, as well as journal articles. In her review, Edelson (2006) examined three questions, each of which was important to understanding the diagnosis of ASD and mental retardation. Her three questions were: (1) Do the prevalence rates (of co-occurrence of mental retardation) reported in the literature derive from empirical sources? (2) Can nonempirical sources of these statistics be traced historically to valid empirical studies? (3) When empirical studies have been conducted, are the methods by which intelligence is assessed appropriate? For the time period from 1943 to 2003, she found 145 articles that met at least one of the following three criteria: (1) level of intelligence in children with autism was investigated; (2) cognitive abilities of children with autism were discussed; or (3) cited a claim about the co-occurrence between autism and mental retardation. She found that only 26% of the claims about prevalence of mental retardation among people with ASD were derived from empirical studies. From the 53 empirical articles that spanned almost 50 years, she found an average prevalence rate of 75.20%. The lowest prevalence rate, 34.33%, was reported in three articles published prior to 1950. The highest prevalence rate, 86.78%, was reported from 9 studies conducted between 1970 and 1979. Edelson (2006) classified 165 articles as nonempirical in her total set of 215 articles. Only 25% of the nonempirical articles based their claims on empirical studies. Once she traced citations back, she found that the majority of citations were not reported accurately. She made a compelling case that the commonly quoted figure of 70% to 80% was high and not based on population-based studies.

Further compounding the potential for error in the claim that 70% to 80% of children with ASD have mental retardation, is the fact that 55% of the empirical studies were conducted prior to 1980 and 75% prior to 1990. Edelson (2006) pointed out that the claims that a majority of children with autism have mental retardation may be erroneously referenced in journal articles, child psychopathology textbooks, in abnormal psychology textbooks, and most troublesome, in the *DSM-IV-TR* criteria (Edelson, 2006).

In 2007, population-based surveillance data on ASD and associated symptoms became available from the CDC Autism and Developmental Disability Monitoring (ADDM) Network (CDC, 2009). The ADDM results for six states, published in 2009, on children who were 8 years of age in 2006 indicated that the average percent of cases of ASD with IQs below 70 was 41%, with a range of 29.3% to 51.2%. One of the cautions about the ADDM data is that it does not involve direct assessments of the children. ADDM data, however, is the source for the ubiquitous citation of the prevalence of autism as 1 in 110 children. If the field is going to accept the overall prevalence figure for autism in ADDM, then serious consideration needs to be given to the data on associated features, including the figure regarding co-occurrence of mental retardation.

Perceptions have changed regarding the previously held belief that a majority of children with autism have ID (Lord, 2011; Lord & Bishop, 2010). This change resulted in part from a review of the CDC surveillance data, and in part from the new perspective in the *DSM-V* that ID is a separate diagnosis.

SUMMARY

Autism spectrum disorder is a complex neurodevelopmental disorder with a range in expression from mild difficulties in social communication to profound difficulties with all aspects of daily living. Autism, by definition, has an onset before 3 years of age and has three core behavioral domains. Since the initial description by Kanner (1943), the criteria for a diagnosis of autism have been refined and broadened to include what is now referred to as the "broader phenotype." This broader phenotype includes people with high-functioning autism or Asperger's disorder. Autistic disorder was first included in the *DSM-III* in 1980. At that time, the superordinate category of pervasive development disorder was introduced with the subcategories of autistic disorder, Asperger's disorder, PDD-NOS, childhood disintegrative disorder, and Rett disorder.

Over the course of revisions of the *DSM* there have been refinements to the criteria for a clinical diagnosis, and on the horizon is *DSM-V*, with adoption expected in 2013. *DSM-V* includes some major changes, each of which reflects research that has been happening over the past 30 years. The recommended term will be ASD with no differentiation within the spectrum. *DSM-V* reduces the core symptom domains from three to two, with the social and communication domains combined into one domain.

Psychometric instruments are available to assist clinicians in diagnosing ASD. These tools, particularly the ADOS and the ADI-R, combined with application of the *DSM* criteria have become the gold standard for making the diagnosis of autistic disorder or the broader phenotype for research purposes. However, much of the work to date has not conformed with this standard, and studies frequently are reported in which there is inadequate detail about the characterization of the subjects (AHRQ, 2011).

From a service perspective, greater support and services are made available when a formal diagnosis of ASD is made. Therefore, clinicians may feel pressured to make a diagnosis of ASD, even when not certain. Children and adults with ASD also have a significant degree of co-occurring developmental, psychiatric, and medical problems. These problems frequently are "overshadowed" by a diagnosis of autism and are not treated as separate conditions. The reverse is also true, where other diagnoses may delay the diagnosis of an ASD. Regardless of the number of co-occurring conditions that an individual may have, each one warrants thorough assessment. Each individual should receive a comprehensive and developmentally appropriate course of treatment.

REFERENCES

Abrahams, B., & Geschwind, D. (2008). Advances in autism genetics: On the threshold of a new neurobiology. *Nature Reviews Genetics*, *9*(5), 341–355.

Adams, H. K. (2010). DSM-V: Asperger's syndrome to be eliminated; Some Aspies upset. Retrieved from http://www.associatedcontent.com/article/2695965/dsmv_aspergers_syndrome_to_be_eliminated.html?cat=5

Agency for Healthcare Research and Quality. (2011). Therapies for Children with Autism Spectrum Disorders. Executive Summary. *Comparative Effectiveness Review*, *26*. Retrieved from http://www.effectivehealthcare.ahrq.gov/ehc/products/106/651/Autism_Disorder_exec-summ.pdf

American Psychiatric Association (1952). *Diagnostic and Statistical Manual of Mental Disorders: DSM*. Washington, DC: Author.

American Psychiatric Association (1968). *Diagnostic and Statistical Manual of Mental Disorders* (2 ed.). Washington, DC: Author.

American Psychiatric Association (1980). *Diagnostic and Statistical Manual of Mental Disorders* (3 ed.). Washington, DC: Author.

American Psychiatric Association (1987). *Diagnostic and Statistical Manual of Mental Disorders* (3 ed., text revision). Washington, DC: Author.

American Psychiatric Association (1994). *Diagnostic and Statistical Manual of Mental Disorders* (4 ed.). Washington, DC: Author.

American Psychiatric Association (2000). *Diagnostic and Statistical Manual of Mental Disorders* (4 ed., text revision). Washington, DC: Author.

Asperger, H. (1944). Die "Autistischen Psychopathen" im Kindesalter. *Archiv für Psychiatrie und Nervenkrankheiten*, *117*, 76–136. [The "autistic psychopathy" in childhood. *Archive Claims Psychiatry and Nervous Disorders*]. Retrieved from http://www.dsm5.org/research/pages/autismandotherpervasivedevelopmentaldisordersconference(february3-5,2008).aspx http://www.autismcolorado.org/index.php/ds-autism-connection

Autism Treatment Network (2011). *Autism speaks*. Retrieved from http://www.autismspeaks.org/science/programs/atn/index.php

Centers for Disease Control and Prevention, National Center on Birth Defects and Developmental Disabilities, Division of Birth Defects (2010, October 1). Learn the Signs, Act Early. Retrieved from http://www.cdc.gov/ncbddd/actearly/index.html

Centers for Disease Control and Prevention. (2012). Prevalence of Autism Spectrum Disorder—Autism and Developmental Disabilities Monitoring Network, United States, 2008. *MMWR Surveillance Summaries*, *61*(ss3), 1–19.

Chalfant, A., Rapee, R., & Carroll, L. (2007). Treating anxiety disorders in children with high-functioning autism spectrum disorders: A controlled trial. *Journal of Autism and Developmental Disorders*, *37*, 1842–1857.

Children's Health Act of 2000. H.R. No. 4365, 106th Cong., 2nd Sess. (2000). Retrieved from http://frwebgate.access.gpo.gov/cgi-bin/getdoc.cgi?dbname=106_cong_bills&docid=f:h4365enr.txt.pdf

Colorado Department of Education (CDE). (2008, September). Retrieved from http://www.cde.state.co.us/cdesped/download/pdf/FF-Autism.pdf

Combating Autism Act of 2006. Public Law 109-416, 109th Cong. (2006). Retrieved from http://frwebgate.access.gpo.gov/cgi-bin/getdoc.cgi?dbname=109_cong_public_laws&docid=f:publ416.109.pdf

Congressional Autism Caucus, Interagency Autism Coordinating Committee, U.S. Department of Health and Human Services (2010). Retrieved from http://iacc.hhs.govhttp://iacc.hhs.gov

DiGuiseppi, C., Hepburn, S., Davis, J. M., Fidler, D. J., Hartway, S., Raitano Lee, N., ... Robinson, C. (2010). Screening for autism spectrum disorders in children with Down syndrome: Population prevalence and screening test characteristics. *Journal of Developmental Behavioral Pediatrics*, *31*(3), 181–191.

Edelson, M. G. (2006). Are the majority of children with autism mentally retarded? A systematic evaluation of the data. *Focus on Autism and Other Developmental Disabilities*, *21*(6), 66–83.

Ehlers, S., Gillberg, C., & Wing, L. (1999). A screening questionnaire for Asperger syndrome and other high-functioning autism spectrum disorders in school age children. *Journal of Autism and Developmental Disorders*, *29*(2), 129–141.

Filipek, P. A. (2005). Medical aspects of autism. In: F. R. Volkmar, R. Paul, A. Klin & D. Cohen (Eds.), *Handbook of Autism and Pervasive Developmental Disorders* (3 ed., pp. 534–581). Hoboken, NJ: Wiley.

Filipek, P. A., Accardo, P. J., Ashwal, S., Baranek, G. T., Cook, E. H., Jr., Dawson, G., … Volkmar, F. R. (2000). Practice parameter: Screening and diagnosis of autism: Report of the Quality Standards Subcommittee of the American Academy of Neurology and the Child Neurology Society. *Neurology, 55*, 468–479.

First, M. B. (2008, February 3–5). Autism and other Pervasive Developmental Disorders Conference. American Psychiatric Association. Retrieved from http://www.dsm5.org/Research/Pages/AutismandOtherPervasiveDevelopmentalDisordersConference(February3–5,2008).aspx

Ganz, M. (2007). The lifetime distribution of the incremental societal costs of Autism. *Archives of Pediatrics & Adolescent Medicine, 161*(4), 343–349.

Happé, F., & Ronald, A. (2008). The "Fractionable Autism Triad": A review of evidence from behavioral, genetic, cognitive and neural research. *Neuropsychology Review, 18*, 287–304.

Heber, R. (1961). Modifications in the manual on terminology and classification in mental retardation. *American Journal on Mental Deficiency, 65*, 499–500.

Hepburn, S., DiGuiseppi, C., Rosenberg, S., Kaparich, K., Robinson, C., & Miller, L. (2008). Use of a teacher nomination strategy to screen for autism spectrum disorders in general education classrooms: A pilot study. *Journal of Autism and Developmental Disorders, 38*(2), 373–382.

Individuals with Disabilities Education Act (IDEA) of 1990, Public Law 101-476, 101st Cong. (1990). Retrieved from http://idea.ed.gov/

Johnson, C., Myers, S. & the Council on Children with Disabilities. (2007). Identification and evaluation of children with autism spectrum disorders. *Pediatrics, 120*(5), 1183–1215.

Kalb, L. G., Law, J. K., Landa, R., & Law, P. A. (2010). Onset patterns prior to 36 months in autism spectrum disorders. *Journal of Autism and Developmental Disorders, 40*(11), 1389–1402.

Kanner, L. (1943). Autistic disturbances of affective contact. *Nervous Child, 2*, 217–253.

Kobayashi, R., & Murata, T. (1998). Setback phenomenon in autism and long term prognosis. *Acta Psychiatrica Scandinavia, 98*, 296–303.

Kogan, M., Strickland, B., Blumberg, S., Singh, G., Perrin, J., & van Dyck, P. (2008). A national profile of the health care experiences and family impact of autism spectrum disorder among children in the United States, 2005–2006. *Pediatrics, 122*(6), e1149–e1158.

Landa, R. J., Holman, K. C., & Garrett-Mayer, E. (2007). Social and communication development in toddlers with early and later diagnosis of autism spectrum disorders. *Archives of General Psychiatry, 64*, 853–864.

Levy, S. E., Giarelli, E., Lee, L. C., Schieve, L. A., Kriby, R. S., Cunniff, C., … Rice, C. E. (2010). Autism spectrum disorder and co-occurring developmental, psychiatric, and medical conditions among children in multiple populations of the United States. *Journal of Developmental Behavioral Pediatrics, 31*(4), 267–275.

Lord, C. (2011, March 18). What would "better" diagnosis of ASDs look like? DSM-5 and beyond. Association of University Centers on Disabilities[webinar]. Retrieved from http://www.aucd.org/resources/webinar_detail.cfm?event=2504&parent=740.

Lord, C., & Bishop, S. (2010). Autism spectrum disorders: Diagnosis, prevalence, and service for children and families. *Social Policy Report—Society for Research in Child Development, 24*(2), 1–27

Lord, C., Risi, S., Lambrecht, L., Cook, E. H., Leventhal, B. L., DiLavore, P. C., … Rutter, M. (2000). The Autism Diagnostic Observation Schedule–Generic: A standard measure of social and communication deficits associated with the spectrum of autism. *Journal of Autism and Developmental Disorders, 30*, 205–223.

Lord, C., Rutter, M. L., DiLavore, P. S., & Risi, S. (1999). *Autism Diagnostic Observation Schedule–WPS* (WPS ed). Los Angeles, CA: Western Psychological Services.

Lord, C., Rutter, M. L., Goode, S., Heemsbergen, J., Jordan, H., Mawhood, L., & Schopler, E. (1989). Autism diagnostic observation schedule: A standardized observation of communicative and social behavior. *Journal of Autism and Developmental Disorders, 19*, 185–212.

Lord, C., Rutter, M., & Le Couteur, A. (1994). Autism Diagnostic Interview–Revised: A revised version of a diagnostic interview for caregivers of individuals with possible pervasive developmental disorders. *Journal of Autism and Developmental Disorders, 24*, 659–685.

Marans, W. D., Rubin, E., & Laurent, A. (2005). Addressing social communication skills in individuals with high-functioning autism and Asperger syndrome: Critical priorities in educational programming. In F. R. Volkmar, R. Paul, A. Klin & D. Cohen (Eds.), *Handbook of autism and pervasive developmental disorders: Diagnosis, development, neurobiology, and behavior* (3 ed., pp. 977–1002). Hoboken, NJ: Wiley.

Matson, J. L., LoVullo, S. V., Rivet, T. T., & Boisjoli, J. A. (2009). Validity of the Autism Spectrum Disorder-Comorbid for Children (ASD-CC). *Research in Autism Spectrum Disorders, 3*, 345–357.

Ozonoff, S., Heung, K., Byrd, R., Hansen, R., & Hertz-Picciotto, I. (2008). The onset of autism: Patterns of symptom emergence in the first years of life. *Autism Research, 1*, 320–328.

Ozonoff, S., Losif, A. M., Baguio, F., Cook, I. C., Hill, M. M., Hutman, T., ... Young, E. S. (2010). A prospective study of the emergence of early behavioral signs of autism. *Journal of the American Academy of Child & Adolescent Psychiatry, 49*(3), 256–266.

Ozonoff, S., Young, G. S., Steinfeld, M. B., Hill, M. M., Cook, I., Hutman, T., ... Sigman, M. (2009). How early do parent concerns predict later autism diagnosis? *Journal of Developmental Behavioral Pediatrics, 30*, 367–375.

Reaven, J. (2009). Children with high-functioning autism spectrum disorders and co-occurring anxiety symptoms: Implications for assessment and treatment. *Journal for Specialists in Pediatric Nursing, 14*(3), 192–199.

Reaven, J., Blakeley-Smith, A., Nichols, S., Dasari, M., Flanigan, E., & Hepburn, S. (2005). Cognitive-behavioral group treatment for anxiety symptoms in children with high-functioning autism spectrum disorders. *Focus on Autism and Other Developmental Disabilities, 24*(1), 27–37.

Reaven, J., Blakeley-Smith, A., Nichols, S., & Hepburn, S. (2011). *Facing your fears: Group therapy for managing anxiety in children with high-functioning autism spectrum disorders.* Baltimore, MD: Brookes Publishing.

Rimland, B. (1964). *Infantile autism.* East Norwalk, CT: Appleton-Century-Crofts.

Rimland, B. (1968). On the objective diagnosis of infantile autism. *Acta Paedopsychiatrica, 35*(4), 146–161.

Risi, S., Lord, C., Gotham, K., Corsello, C., Chrysler, C., Szatmari, P., ... Pickles, A. (2006). Combining information from multiple sources in the diagnosis of autism spectrum disorders. *Journal of the American Academy of Child & Adolescent Psychiatry, 49*(9), 1094–1103.

Robins, D. L., & Dumont-Mathieu, T. M. (2001). Early screening for autism spectrum disorders: Update on the modified checklist for autism in toddlers and other measures. *Journal of Developmental Behavioral Pediatrics, 27*, 111–119.

Rutter, M. (1978). Diagnosis and definition of childhood autism. *Journal of Autism and Childhood Schizophrenia, 8*(2), 139–61.

Rutter, M., Bailey, A., & Lord, C. (2003). *SCQ: Social Communication Questionnaire.* Los Angeles, CA: Western Psychological Services.

Rutter, M., Le Couteur, A., & Lord, C. (2003). *Manual for the ADI-WPS version.* Los Angeles, CA: Western Psychological Services.

Schalock, R. L., Borthwick-Duffy, S. A., Buntinx, W., Coulter, D., & Craig, E. (2010). Intellectual disability: Definition, classification and systems of support (11 ed). Washington, DC: American Association on Intellectual and Developmental Disabilities.

Sofronoff, K., Attwood, T., & Hinton, S. (2005). A randomized controlled trial of a CBT intervention for anxiety in children with Asperger syndrome. *Journal of Child Psychology and Psychiatry, 46*, 1152–1160.

Sparrow, S. S., Balla, D. A., & Cicchetti, D. (1984) *Vineland Adaptive Behavior Scales.* Circle Pines, MN: American Guidance.

Sze, K., & Wood, J. (2007). Cognitive behavioral treatment of co-morbid anxiety disorders and social difficulties in children with high-functioning autism: A case report. *Journal of Contemporary Psychotherapy, 3*, 133–143.

Volkmar, F. R., & Klin, A. (2005). Issues in the classification of autism and related conditions. In F. R. Volkmar, R. Paul, A. Klin & D. Cohen (Eds.), *Handbook of autism and pervasive developmental disorders: Diagnosis, development, neurobiology, and behavior*, (3 ed., pp. 5–41). Hoboken, NJ: Wiley.

Volkmar, F. R., Klin, A., & Cohen, D. J. (1997). Diagnosis and classification of autism and related conditions: Consensus and issues. In F. R. Volkmar & D. J. Cohen (Eds.), *Handbook of autism and pervasive developmental disorders* (2 ed., pp. 47–59). Hoboken, NJ: Wiley.

Volkmar, F. R., Klin, A., Siegel, B., Szatmari, P., Lord, C., Campbell, M., ... Towbin, K. (1994). Field trial for autistic disorder in DSM-IV. *American Journal of Psychiatry, 151*, 1361–1367.

Volkmar, F. R., Paul, R., & Klin, A. (2005). In F. R. Volkmar, R. Paul, A. Klin & D. Cohen (Eds.), *Handbook of autism and pervasive developmental disorders: Diagnosis, development, neurobiology, and behavior* (3 ed., pp. xv–xix). Hoboken, NJ: Wiley.

Volkmar, F. R., Paul, R., Klin, A., & Cohen, D. (Eds.). (2005). *Handbook of autism and pervasive developmental disorders: diagnosis, development, neurobiology, and behavior* (3rd ed.). Hoboken, NJ: Wiley.

Werner, E., Dawson, G., Munson, J., & Osterling, J. (2005). Variation in early developmental course in autism and its relation with behavioral outcome at 3–4 years of age. *Journal of Autism and Developmental Disorders, 35*, 337–350.

World Health Organization. (1993). *The ICD-10 classification of mental and behavioral disorders: Diagnostic criteria for research.* Geneva, Switzerland: Author.

Zaborek, R. (2011, April 7). Down Syndrome–Autism connection. Autism Society of Colorado. Retrieved from http://www.autismcolorado.org/index.php/ds-autism-connection

2 Prevalence, Etiology, and Genetics

Marygrace Yale Kaiser, Ellen Giarelli, and Jennifer Pinto-Martin

In a number of studies, authors have suggested that the prevalence of diagnosed autism spectrum disorder (ASD) in the United States and elsewhere has increased substantially in the past decades. Given the reported increasing prevalence and associated impact on children and families, consistent monitoring of trends will continue to be a public health priority. The rising prevalence underscores the need for nurses to expect that more people who pass through their clinical practice will have a diagnosis or be a member of a family with an affected relative.

In this chapter we summarize the literature on the prevalence of ASD, approaches to screening for individuals who may be at risk for the diagnosis, and the leading etiological theories.

CONCEPTS IN EPIDEMIOLOGY APPLIED TO NURSING CARE OF ASD

Epidemiology is defined as the study of the distribution and determinants of disease and injuries in the human population (Mausner & Kramer, 1985). It is concerned with frequencies (prevalence) and types of disorders and whether such frequencies vary by group, geography, or other factors. Information about such frequencies in turn leads us to develop processes for screening people who may be at increased risk for the disorders and to accurately diagnose incidence. Usually referred to as a "rate," prevalence is actually a proportion and reflects the burden of disease in a population.

The epidemiology of ASD begins with the natural history of the disorder, susceptibility for risk factors, clinical manifestations, stages of disability, potential causes, and methods of prevention. Our study of the epidemiology of ASD is in the early stage of simply trying to understand how many people are affected and the possible causes. ASD is a complex disorder with many behaviorally, rather than biologically, defined symptoms. This creates a challenging problem for epidemiologists who wish to unequivocally determine cause, prevention, and treatment.

PREVALENCE OF ASD

The term "autism" referred to autistic disorder in the early decades of the twentieth century and was considered a rare disorder. In the 1990s, the diagnostic criteria were expanded by clinicians, and the disorder was placed on a spectrum of behavioral characteristics. Prior to this change, reports of the number of affected children often referred exclusively to autistic disorder, and the rate was approximately one in every 2,000 children (Fombonne, 1999, 2003, 2005; Rutter, 2005). The criteria established in the 1990s described a spectrum of disorders, such that prevalence must encompass the entire spectrum, or ASD. Autism (autistic disorder) is now one of three conditions included in the diagnostic criteria: autism, Asperger's syndrome, and pervasive developmental disability–not otherwise specified (PDD-NOS; American Psychiatric Association [APA], 1994). Using these criteria, epidemiologists estimate the prevalence of ASD as approximately 6 to 7 in 1,000 in the United States. This is 10 times greater than estimates based on earlier criteria (Newschaffer, Falb, & Gurney, 2005; Rutter, 2005).

Epidemiologists from other countries report even higher estimates of ASD. In 2011, Kim and colleagues (2011) reported a startling statistic of approximately 1 in 38 children from a population-based study in South Korea. Among a targeted sample of 55,266 children ages 7 to 12 years, the prevalence of ASD was estimated to be 2.64% (95%, confidence interval = 1.91 to 3.37), with 1.89% in the general population and 0.75% in the high-probability group (Kim et al., 2011).

There is ongoing discussion of the most appropriate method for ascertaining prevalence. The principle dispute resides between clinically diagnosed cases versus research-identified (population-based) cases (Barbaresi, Colligan, Weaver, & Katusic, 2009). Identifying all cases of ASD by using clinical diagnosis is labor intensive but highly accurate. Identifying all cases by reviewing medical and school records (administrative prevalence) is more efficient but may miss cases when all records are not available. A detailed description of the various approaches to ascertaining prevalence is not appropriate for this chapter. See Avchen and colleagues (Avchen et al., 2011), Rice and colleagues (Rice et al., 2007) and Yeargin-Allsop and colleagues (Yeargin-Allsopp, Murphy, Oakley, & Sikes, 1992) for a comparison of methodologies. The statistics on ASD prevalence, recently reported by the Centers for Disease Control and Prevention (CDC) were generated using a research-identified approach to ascertaining administrative prevalence (Avchen et al., 2011).

Systematic Monitoring of ASD

Investigators at the CDC have been systematically monitoring ASD in the United States since the 1990s through a program called the Autism and Developmental Disabilities Monitoring (ADDM) network (Rice et al., 2007). The first studies conducted by the ADDM network reported results for the year 2000 from six sites in the United States and established a baseline period prevalence of ASD by race/ethnicity and sex, along with multiple associated characteristics (CDC, 2007b). According to the CDC, in 2000, the prevalence of ASD per 1,000 children age 8 years in the six surveillance sites ranged from 4.5 to 9.9, with an overall mean of 6.7 (CDC, 2007b). Additional surveillance states were added in subsequent study years to create a larger population cohort and improve the ability to generalize to the larger U.S. population of children.

For study year 2002, 407,578 children age 8 were included. Among this cohort, ASD prevalence ranged from 5.2 to 7.6, with an overall mean of 6.6 across 14 surveillance sites. This is converted to a rate of ASD of 1 in every 152 children across the study sites (CDC, 2007a). Males were four times more likely than females to be diagnosed with ASD, and females were more likely than males to have cognitive impairment (Giarelli et al., 2010). There were differences in racial distribution depending on the state from which the data were collected. In states where prevalence varied by race, prevalence was generally higher among White children than among Black children. This may be explained by differences across sites in their access to racial subgroups. Across sites, the age of earliest diagnosis ranged from 10 months to 106 months.

Using the same methodology for case ascertainment, epidemiologists with the CDC ascertained prevalence among children age 8 years in 2006. The sample was composed of fewer states (11 surveillance sites) and 307,790 children. Prevalence ranged in a majority of sites from 7.6 to 10.4. The overall prevalence average was 9 per 1000 population (95%, confidence interval = 8.6 to 9.3; CDC, 2009). Prevalence was reported as approximately 1 in every 110. This represents a significant increase (57%) from the previous report. The increase may be explained by improved ascertainment, however, the ADDM network investigators noted that "a true increase in the risk for children to develop ASD symptoms cannot be ruled out" (CDC, 2009, p. 1).

The Rising Prevalence of ASD: Is This an Epidemic?

The prevalence of ASD is clearly on the rise, although the reasons for this rise are still hotly contested. In 1999, the autism rate was thought to be around 4 to 5 per 10,000 children; by the year 2000, estimates had climbed to a rate of 4 to 5 per 1,000 children (Bertrand et al., 2001). Reports from three large epidemiological studies show rates averaging 5 to 6 per 1,000 (Baird et al., 2000; Bertrand et al., 2001; Chakrabarti & Fombonne, 2001). The most recent data from the CDC's ADDM network indicates that the national average ASD prevalence in the United States is approximately 1 in 110 children, up from 1 in 125 from 2004, and 1 in 150 in 2002. From 2002, the prevalence of ASDs increased 57% across the country (CDC, 2009). Nationwide, the rising enrollment of children with the diagnosis of ASD in the special education classes of the public school system have been a clear indication of the increase in prevalence. Individuals with ASD are the fastest-growing special needs group in the United States, having grown by over 900% between 1992 and 2001, according to data from the U.S. Department of Education (Anonymous, 2000; Social Security Administration, 2011). The CDC reported in 2012 that the average prevalence across 14 surveillance sites rose to 1 in 88 children age 8 years (CDC, 2012).

Is this increase the result of an actual change in the risk of acquiring an ASD, or is it merely the result of increased awareness, better ascertainment, and improved diagnosis? Since 1980, the diagnostic criteria for ASD has been revised and expanded several times. In 2000, the CDC launched the Learn the Signs, Act Early campaign to improve the early identification of children with ASDs. Has the widening of the diagnostic parameters, and increased effort to diagnose children early in life increased the number of children included under the umbrella of ASD? In other words, is there an epidemic of autism in this country or simply an increase in diagnosis? We need to look at the definition of an epidemic. According to a standard epidemiology textbook, an epidemic is defined as the occurrence in a community or region of a group of illnesses of similar nature, and more than is expected (Gordis, 2000). By this definition, autism would meet the criteria of an epidemic. Parents, communities, educators, and clinicians alike would agree that there is more of this disorder around than ever before, way beyond what one might expect given the past prevalence of this disorder. However, there is an additional and critical part of the definition. The full definition says an epidemic "is the occurrence in a community or region of a group of illnesses of similar nature, clearly in excess of normal expectancy and derived from a common or propagated source" (Gordis, 2000, p. 18).

If the increase in numbers of children with ASD does not represent a change in the actual risk of acquiring the disease, then what might be an alternative explanation? It could be that we have changed the manner in which cases are identified, the diagnostic criteria for the disorder, and/or the way these criteria are applied, both in terms of who gets considered for the diagnosis and who makes the diagnosis. Clearly there have been major changes in the way autism is diagnosed, from Rutter's 1967definition (Rutter, 1967) to the criteria outlined by the *Diagnostic and Statistical Manual* (used to standardize the diagnosis of different disease entities), including the *DSM-III* criteria of 1980 and those of *DSM-III-R* in 1987 and *DSM-IV* in 1994 (APA, 1980, 1987, 1994). At each step of this evolution, the criteria to be included as a case of ASD has broadened to include PDD-NOS, Asperger's disorder, child disintegrative disorder (CDD), and Rett syndrome. In addition, the minimum number of criteria needed for the diagnosis of autism disorder has expanded from four essential criteria in Rutter's original definition to eight of 12 possible criteria under the *DSM-IV*.

Prevalence versus Incidence

Epidemiological studies conducted to date have usually monitored the prevalence of ASD (i.e., all the cases of a disorder in existence at a particular point in time) as opposed to the incidence of ASD (i.e., new cases of disease occurring in a specified time interval). Changes in prevalence can occur as the result of many factors, including:

1. Substantial migration of affected children in or out of a community;
2. Changes in age of onset or age of recognition (earlier age at diagnosis would result in an apparent increase in prevalence);
3. Large changes in the denominator (increase in population would dilute the calculated rate, resulting in an apparent decrease in prevalence);
4. Increased ascertainment of children with ASD through improved awareness, such as the CDC Learn the Signs, Act Early campaign (increases in diagnosis of ASD would result in apparent increase of prevalence);
5. Change in diagnostic criteria, such that children with milder symptoms are included under the ASD diagnosis (increase in the number of children included would result in apparent increase of prevalence); and
6. True increase in the incidence of the disorder due to increased risk.

The Example of California

The state of California can be seen as a harbinger of what is to come in terms of autism rates, because of the large annual birth population and a sophisticated and coordinated reporting system that allows for the tracking of newly identified cases of autism more reliably than elsewhere. California's Department of Developmental Services (DDS) is a statewide service-delivery system that coordinates both diagnosis and provision of services for individuals with developmental disabilities. Services are provided through a system of 21 regional centers. California was one of the first places to sound the alarm of the increasing prevalence of ASD. According to a 2002 study, the state experienced a 273% increase between 1988 and 1999 (Byrd, 2003). These data were flawed, in that they were not expressed as rates with use of an appropriate denominator but merely reflected the number of children who had accessed services for ASD. In addition, they did not account for in-migration of children seeking better services, changes in diagnostic criteria, age of entry into the system, and the differentiation of prevalence versus incidence. However, they did serve an important purpose in raising awareness about the rise in prevalence and generated further research into the issue. A later analysis (Croen, Grether, Hoogstrate, & Selvin, 2002), which carefully assessed change in prevalence over time and was limited to California-born children in the system, reported an increase in prevalence between 1987 and 1999 of 17.6% per year for 1987 to 1990 births, followed by a jump in the rate of increase for 1990 to 1992 births, and then a leveling off for the 1993 to 1994 birth cohort.

Thimerosal in Vaccines

More recently, attention has been directed at the hint of a decline in the rates in California (Geier & Geier, 2006). According to data released by the California DDS, new cases of professionally diagnosed full-syndrome autism declined 7.5% in one 3-month period of reporting, from 734 new cases entering the system during the second quarter of 2005 to 678 new cases during the third quarter. This is the first such decline that has been reported in over a decade of tracking new cases in the DDS system. The authors argued that this decline was a reflection of decreasing risk of acquiring ASD due to removal of thimerosal from vaccines, which was estimated to have been completed by 2001. Thus 3- to 5-year-olds in 2005 would be considered among the first "thimerosal-free" birth cohorts in the state. However, more recent data reported by Schechter and Grether in 2008 suggest that this decline was only transitory and that "prevalence for ages 3–5 years has increased monotonically for each birth year since 1999, during which period exposure to thimerosal has been reduced" (Schechter & Grether, 2008, p. 21).

Critics of the vaccine theory point to the fact that a sharp decline in new cases would be expected following removal of thimerosal, if vaccine injury was the cause of the increase in autism spectrum diagnoses, with an eventual decrease in total caseload or prevalence. In contrast, if the theory of better diagnostic awareness is correct, a gradual decline in new cases would be expected until caseload increase reaches population growth levels. This is consistent with the view that this decline seen in California is likely a function of a "saturation" of the diagnostic category, a phenomenon that has been seen in other diagnostic categories following their introduction into the childhood disabilities classification system.

School administrators are required by the Individual with Disabilities Education Act (IDEA) to report to the federal Department of Education an annual child count of the number of children with disabilities. Whenever a new category is introduced, an increase in its usage will ensue. This increase typically levels off over time, as children receive proper diagnostic classifications. This was apparent quite clearly with the introduction of the category of traumatic brain injury and is well described by at least two authors (Gernsbacher, Dawson, & Goldsmith, 2005; Newschaffer, 2005). Traumatic brain injury was introduced in 1992 (along with autism) and from then until 2002, the prevalence of children in this category increased steadily. The increase then leveled off, an indication that reporting had achieved a balance with actual prevalence. The same phenomenon was seen with the category of "developmental delay" introduced in 1997 to 1998. New reporting categories in the annual child count are not capitalized upon immediately. Rather, they require a certain amount of time for awareness and ascertainment to improve. Currently, few states are reporting the number of cases of ASD that would be expected based on the results of the recent large epidemiological studies (i.e., 5 to 6 per 1,000). Thus, it is likely that most state child counts for ASD will continue to rise until this number is reached. California may be the first state to show a leveling-off. Chapter 18 contains a comprehensive discussion of the legal issues associated with vaccines and ASD.

SCREENING FOR ASD

Early identification of children with developmental delays is important for generating accurate prevalence statistics, and developmental surveillance falls under the purview of health care professionals working in primary care. Clinically identifying individuals with ASD involves two levels of assessment. The first is routine developmental surveillance and screening specific for ASD. The second level is diagnosis and evaluation using an in-depth approach to differentiating ASD from other developmental disorders and other medical or psychiatric disorders. Diagnostic evaluation is essential to planning nursing interventions and treatment. For example, if a child does not respond to questions or make eye contact, the child must be screened for vision and hearing defects, as well as autism.

Screening for Developmental Disorders

According to Filipek and colleagues (Filipek et al., 2000), approximately 25% of children in any primary-care practice show developmental issues. The components of developmental screening include eliciting and attending to parental concerns, obtaining a relevant developmental history, making accurate and informative observations of children, and sharing opinions and concerns with other professionals (Dworkin, 1993). Primary-care providers may conduct developmental screening tests at well-child appointments, using such tools as the Parent's Evaluation of Developmental Status (Glascoe, 1998) and the Ages and Stages Questionnaire (Bricker & Squires, 1999). Few routinely screen for ASD, despite the availability of standardized instruments specifically suited to the pediatric population below the age of 3 years. See Chapter 5 for a discussion of screening. The American Academy of Pediatrics (AAP Committee on Children with Disabilities, 1994; Johnson, Myers, & Council on Children with Disabilities, 2007) stresses the importance of routine, sequential developmental screening at each well-child visit and also recommends collecting information from parents regarding their concerns and observations. In fact, several studies have data demonstrating that parental concerns about speech and language development, behavior, and other developmental issues were highly sensitive (75% to 83%) and specific (79% to 81%) in detecting developmental deficits (Glascoe, 1997; Glascoe & Sandler, 1995). When parental concerns are combined with standardized parent-completed instruments, such as the MCHAT (Baron-Cohen et al., 2000), screening is highly effective (Glascoe & Dworkin, 1995).

The Role of Nurses in Screening for ASD

There are behavioral and educational interventions for children with ASD that improve outcomes (Matson, Benavidez, Compton, Paclawskyj, & Baglio, 1996). Systematic screening of children by primary-care providers will result in earlier diagnosis and the selection and use of interventions at an age when maximum benefit can be achieved (Butter & Mulick, 2003). Nurses are well positioned to instruct parents on developmental milestones and may use well-child visits to solicit the parents' opinions on the child's skills, beginning at 4 months with questions that address key social, emotional, and communication milestones. For example, at 6 months, a baby should relate to the parent with genuine joy, smile often while playing, coo or babble when happy, and cry when unhappy. A nurse may ask the parent specific questions, such as "Does your baby look at you when you talk directly to him/her? Does he/she try to exchange sounds with you?" Because transient conductive hearing loss associated with otitis media with effusion can also occur in children with autism, auditory testing should be conducted, even if the child is autistic (Filipek et al., 2000; Klin, 1993). Nurses can conduct formal auditory evaluations. The Committee on Infant Hearing of the American Speech–Language–Hearing Association has guidelines for audiological assessment of children from birth through 36 months of age (American Speech–Language–Hearing Association Committee on Infant Hearing, 1991). Webb (2011) further recommends that "buy-in" by parents and staff, timing with regard to other required activities, accessing electronic health records, and choosing and administering screening tool all be considered for successful integration of ASD screening into well-child visits.

Early identification, beginning with screening by nurses, can be followed by systematic psychological support of the family and rapid implementation of treatment for the child. Pinto-Martin, Souders, Giarelli, and Levy (2005) described the barriers to standardized screening as including the reliance by pediatricians on clinical judgment rather than standardized measures. Nurses can be proactive by collaborating with physicians and advocating for the systematic and routine use of screening instruments in clinical practice, rather than reliance on clinical judgment alone (see Exhibit 2.1 for developmental milestones).

EXHIBIT 2.1

Developmental Milestones for a Child

Key Social, Emotional, and Communication Milestones for a Baby's Healthy Development

The milestones listed below are important to a child's health, learning, behavior, and development. While each child may develop differently, some differences may be signs of slight delay and others may be a cause for greater concern. These milestones can help parents keep track of a baby's development. Instruct parents to bring this milestone list to the next visit with the pediatrician to discuss with the doctor any questions or concerns they may have. If a baby does not have any skill that is listed or has LOST a skill at any age, a parent should tell this to the pediatrician.

At 4 months, a baby should. . .

- Follow and react to bright colors, movements, and objects
- Turn toward sound
- Show interest in watching people's faces
- Smile back when you smile

At 6 months, a baby should. . .

- Relate to you with real joy
- Smile often while playing with you
- Coo or babble when happy
- Cry when unhappy

At 9 months, a baby should. . .

- Smile and laugh while looking at you
- Exchange back-and-forth smiles, loving faces, and other expressions with you
- Exchange back-and-forth sounds with you
- Exchange back-and-forth gestures with you, such as giving, taking, and reaching.

(*Continued*)

EXHIBIT 2.1 (Continued)

At 12 months, a baby should…

- Use a few gestures, one after another, to get needs met, like giving, showing, reaching, waving, and pointing
- Play peek-a-boo, patty-cake, or other social games
- Make sounds, like "ma," "ba," "na," "da," and "ga"
- Turn to the person speaking when his/her name is called

At 15 months, a baby should…

- Exchange with you many back-and-forth smiles, sounds, and gestures in a row
- Use pointing or other "showing" gestures to draw attention to something
- Use different sounds to get needs met and draw attention to something of interest
- Use and understand at least three words, such as "mama," "dada," "bye-bye," and "no"

At 18 months, a baby should…

- Use lots of gestures with words to get needs met, like pointing or taking you by the hand and saying, "want milk," or "go bye-bye"
- Use at least four different consonants, such as m, n, p, b, t, d, s, and w, in babbling or words
- Use and understand at least 10 words
- Show that he or she knows the names of familiar people or body parts by pointing to or looking at them when they are named
- Do simple pretend play, like feeding a doll or stuffed animal, and attracting your attention by looking up at you

At 24 months, a baby should…

- Do pretend play with you with more than one action, like feeding the doll and then rocking the doll
- Use and understand at least 50 words
- Use at least two words together (without repeating) and in a way that makes sense, like "hold baby."
- Enjoy being next to children of the same age and show interest in playing with them
- Look for familiar objects out of sight when asked

At 36 months, a baby should…

- Enjoy pretending to play different characters with you or talking for dolls or action figures
- Enjoy playing with children of the same age, showing and telling another child about something like a toy or pet
- Use thoughts and actions together in speech and in play in a way that makes sense, like "sleepy, want nap" "like, want stay," or possibly "have pee pee, go potty"

(*Continued*)

EXHIBIT 2.1 (Continued)

- Answer "what," "where," and "who" questions easily
- Talk about interests and feelings about the past and the future

A parent should tell the doctor or family practitioner right away if the child:

- Does not have big smiles and joyful expressions by 6 months
- Does not share sounds, smiles, or other facial expression by 9 months
- Does not babble by 12 months
- Has no words by 16 months
- Has no two-word phrases that are meaningful by 24 months
- Has LOST ANY expressions, speech, babbling, or social skills at any age.

CAUSES OF ASD

Multiple causation is the canon of contemporary epidemiology, and its foundation is the belief that patterns of health and disease can be explained by a complex web of interconnected risk and protective factors. Associated with this is the corollary that this explanation imparts power to improve the public's health if factors can be isolated, and modified. This is the hypothesized web of causation (Krieger, 1994). To effect preventive measures, it is not necessary to understand the entire causal mechanism. Even knowledge of one small component may allow some degree of intervention and prevention. The notion of causal mechanisms is applied to behaviors of people with ASD in complex environments, for which the web focuses attention on those factors closest to the observed behavior.

Understanding the Cause

The approach one takes to understanding the causes of ASD depends, in part, on whether one believes that the rise represents a genuine increase in the risk or is merely an artifact of the diagnostic changes. Based on a review of the literature, it is clear that the vast majority of scientists, both physicians and epidemiologists, believe that the best explanation for the rise in prevalence is diagnostic changes and improved ascertainment. A review of 47 epidemiological studies looking at the prevalence of autism concludes that the recent increases and prevalence are very likely connected to changes in diagnostic criteria, diagnostic substitution, and increased availability of services. The rise in numbers of children diagnosed often occurred at the same time as radical shifts in the ideas, diagnostic approaches, and services for children with ASDs (Fombonne, 2009). However, it is impossible to rule out the possibility of some nongenetic risk factors contributing to the rise.

Regardless of whether one believes that the actual risk of the disorder is on the rise, no one can argue with the fact that there are many more children who carry this label now than ever before. This increase in prevalence can be used to argue for improvement in diagnostic services and treatment, including appropriate and readily available education for children with an ASD.

Speculative Etiology

The natural history of autistic symptoms must be considered by clinicians when making a diagnosis of an ASD. Understanding possible risk and contributory factors may be useful to the clinician who wishes to understand the pathophysiology of the phenotype. Multiple theories have been suggested to explain symptoms and progression. The theories address genetic and epigenetic factors, pre- and perinatal factors, hormonal and immunological factors. For a detailed explanation of the many theories of ASD causation, see Hollander, Kolevzon, and Coyle (2011). This section will address genetic factors and pre- and perinatal factors.

Genetics: Genes and Genetic Variants

Kanner's (1943) initial description of autism was that of an innate and inborn disorder involving significant behavioral disturbances from infancy. However, a genetic basis for the disorder was dismissed for the next few decades for several reasons (Rutter, 2000). First, to some researchers, there appeared to be little evidence of vertical transmission, in that there was a paucity of cases of children with autism also having a parent with autism. Second, the concordance rate between siblings was considered to be very low (estimates around 2%). Finally, there did not appear to be an identifiable chromosomal anomaly associated with autism (Rutter, Bailey, Bolton, & Le Couteur, 1993). Yet it is now generally accepted that early investigators were mistaken in taking the above as evidence against a genetic basis for the autism. Vertical transmission was very unlikely, because very few individuals with autism were married or having children. The rate of autism in siblings was actually very high when compared with the rate of autism in the general population—siblings of children with autism were 50 to 100 times more likely to also have the disorder, compared with those in the general population (Rutter, Bailey, Bolton, & Le Couteur, 1993).

Evidence now exists that there are several chromosomal disorders associated with characteristics of autism, including Fragile X syndrome (Hatton et al., 2006), Down syndrome (Ghaziuddin, Tsai, & Ghaziuddin, 1992), Prader-Willi syndrome (Demb & Papola, 1995; Dimitropoulos, & Schultz, 2007), Angelman's syndrome (Peters, Beaudet, Madduri, & Bacino, 2004; Steffenburg et al., 1996), tuberous schlerosis complex (Baker, Piven, & Sata, 1998; Bolton & Griffiths, 1997; Iznitzer, 2004), and others. See Chapter 5 for a discussion of Fragile X syndrome and tuberous sclerosis.

Anney and colleagues (2010) conducted four nonindependent genome-wide analyses of 1,558 ASD families under the Autism Genome Project Consortium. The purpose was to identify common risks by analyzing 1 million single-nucleotide polymorphisms for association with ASD. This extensive genomic study was able to identify five common alleles for ASD across the sample. They concluded that although ASDs have a substantial genetic basis, most of the known genetic risk is traced to rare variants. This report, while complicated and detailed, can be interpreted as evidence that there will not likely be a single genetic cause of ASD, but rather a constellation of genetic factors.

Complex Genetic Determinants of ASD

In complex disorders, the pattern of genetic inheritance is unclear, unlike in simple disorders, in which a single mutated gene is considered a causative gene. Alternatively, in disorders with complex gene architectures, there is evidence that multiple genes are involved and interact with the environment in different ways. In these cases, the genes involved are considered to be susceptibility genes that increase the risk of disease but are not sufficient to cause the disease (Pericak-Vance, 2003). Researchers would agree that autism falls into this latter category.

In the next section, we summarize: (1) findings from twin and non-twin sibling studies of ASD individuals, (2) evidence for candidate genes that have been positively linked to ASDs, and (3) information regarding prenatal and perinatal risk factors that are potentially associated with disorders in the autism spectrum.

Twin and Family Studies: Concordance Rates and Heritability

Results from the first twin study of autism were published by Folstein and Rutter in 1977. Eleven pairs of monozygotic (MZ) and 10 pairs of dizygotic (DZ) twins were identified in which one of the twins was diagnosed with infantile autism. After examination of the children and interviews with parents, the researchers concluded that there was a 36% concordance rate for autism in the MZ pairs, compared with a 0% concordance rate in the DZ pairs. Additionally, there was an 82% concordance rate for cognitive abnormalities in the MZ pairs and only a 10% rate in the DZ pairs (Folstein & Rutter, 1977a, 1977b). This study pointed to a heritability factor in autism that extended beyond the characteristics of basic autistic disorder. Additionally, this investigation suggested the likelihood of a broader autism phenotype, with less severe variations of the disorder in conjunction with Kanner's classic autistic disorder (Rutter, 2000).

Follow-up twin studies during the 1980s and 1990s (Bailey et al., 1995; Le Couteur et al., 1996; Steffenburg et al., 1989) used more advanced methodologies, including standardized diagnostic instruments (the Autism Diagnostic Interview [Le Couteur et al., 1989] and the Autism Diagnostic Observation Schedule [Lord et al., 1989]), widespread population screening for participants, and systematic screening for other medical conditions. These later investigations replicated the results from the Folstein and Rutter study in the late 1970s, in that the concordance rate for autism was markedly higher in MZ pairs compared with DZ pairs (60% versus 5%), with a similarly high disparity between concordance rates for broader cognitive and social impairments (90% in MZ pairs and only 10% in DZ pairs). Furthermore, a closer examination of the MZ pairs who were concordant for autism revealed how heterogeneous this group of children was in terms of symptom presentation. While one might expect children who share exact gene replicas to have similar symptom profiles, the concordant MZ pairs were no more similar with regard to symptomatology when compared with other randomly selected twin pairs (Le Couteur et al., 1996). Again, these findings are used to highlight a likely genetic basis for autism, while also suggesting the existence of a broader autism phenotype.

More recently, the largest population-based twin study was conducted by investigators in Sweden and included 7,982 twin pairs (Lichtenstein et al., 2010). Again, MZ twin pairs had higher concordance rates for autism compared with DZ twin pairs (47% for male MZ twin pairs and 14% for male DZ twin pairs); these results were in line with previous reports using smaller, more clinically based samples. Accordingly, the heritability estimate for autism in this population sample was 80% as calculated with structural equation modeling (Lichtenstein et al., 2010). These results confirm earlier assumptions of the strong hereditary component in ASDs.

Family studies also provide evidence for a genetic basis in ASDs. Such studies examine the rate of autism in siblings and parents to determine patterns of family transmission (Rutter, 2000). If one child had autism, the rates of affected siblings ranged from 3% to 6% for ASD (Bolton et al., 1994), 4.5% for autism (Jorde et al., 1991), and 12% for the broader phenotype (Bolton et al., 1994). Depending on assumptions of the prevalence of the disorder in the general population, the relative sibling recurrence risk was between 45 to 90 for ASD (Cook, 1998) and

30 to 200 for autism (Pericak-Vance, 2003; Rutter, 2000). Using latent class analysis, Pickles and colleagues (1995) estimated that several genes (anywhere from two to 10) interacting together were likely to lead to autism. They also proposed that relatives with the broader phenotype may have some susceptibility genes for autism but not enough to develop the full syndrome (Cook, 1998).

A more recent study by Constantino and colleagues (2010) examined sibling recurrence in 1,235 families with at least one child affected with an ASD. Results indicated that 10.9% of families had another child with an ASD, and an additional 20% of families had another child with a history of language delay. Interestingly, 50% of those children with a history of language delay exhibited speech qualities associated with autism and not simply language delays (Constantino et al., 2010). It was also reported that otherwise unaffected children in families with more than one child with autism displayed a wide range of subclinical autistic traits. But this was not the case among siblings in single-incidence families (Constantino et al., 2010). These results are used to argue that differences in the genetic transmission of autism and multiple genes are likely involved with the manifestation of the disorder.

Candidate Genes Associated with ASDs

Following the strong evidence from twin and family studies pointing toward a genetic basis for autism and ASDs, researchers have turned their attention toward investigations that may identify the candidate susceptibility genes that increase the likelihood of the disorder. However, even with advances in medical technology and the implementation of several studies with this goal, an indisputable "autism gene" has yet to be discovered (Losh, Sullivan, Trembath, & Piven, 2008). It has been reported that genome-wide scans have identified at least one positive link to autism on almost every chromosome (Yang & Gill, 2007) and over 100 disease genes and 40 genomic loci have been associated with individuals with ASD or autistic behaviors (Betancur, 2011). There are several candidate genes that have been extensively studied and that appear likely to be associated with the autism spectrum.

Chromosome 15: Several studies have implicated genes on chromosome 15q11–q13 region. Both deletions and duplications of genes on this area have been reported in individuals with autism (Cook, 1998). A maternal deletion results in Angelman's syndrome, which has a relatively high frequency of comorbidity with autism (Steffenburg et al., 1996). A paternal deletion results in Prader-Willi syndrome, which shares some behavioral similarities with autism, but to a lesser degree than Angelman's syndrome (Demb & Papola, 1995). Duplications of 15q11–q13 have also been identified in a large number of individuals with autism (Baker et al., 1994; Cook et al., 1997; Dykens, Sutcliffe, & Levitt, 2004). According to Cook (1998), who did a review of studies examining proximal chromosome 15q abnormalities in autism, when testing for parent of origin, all duplications of proximal 15q were maternally derived. After accounting for those cases associated with Fragile X syndrome or tuberous schlerosis, maternally derived 15q abnormalities are the most frequently observed genetic mutation in autism (Volker & Lopata, 2008) and have been reported in approximately 1% to 3% of cases (Dykens et al., 2004; Moeschler, Mohandas, Hawk, & Noll, 2002).

Serotonin transporter gene (SLC6A4): Serotonergic pathways have long been a focus of etiological inquiry in relation to autism, because reports of abnormal serotonin levels have been detected by various methods in individuals with the disorder. Elevated platelet levels of serotonin (5HTT) have been observed in approximately 25% to 30% cases of autism (Losh et al., 2008; Volker & Lopata, 2008). Medications targeting serotonin, particularly selective serotonin reuptake inhibitors (SSRIs) have also been used to treat symptoms associated with ASD. In a recent review of published studies on the use of SSRIs by individuals with ASD, three randomized, controlled trials and 10 open-label trials or retrospective chart-review studies were identified (Kolevzon, Matthewson, & Hollander, 2006). A majority of studies reported improved functioning with the use of the various SSRIs examined, particularly in symptoms associated with repetitive behaviors and anxiety. However, increased activation and agitation were also reported as common side effects, which signaled caution in SSRI use by individuals with autism (Kolevzon, Matthewson, & Hollander, 2006). The promoter region of serotonin transporter gene (*SLC6A4*) has been the focus of several investigations, with reports generally supporting its role in autism. Transmission of polymorphism was examined in 71 families with at least one child with autism (Tordjman et al., 2001). While transmission of the 5HTT promoter alleles did not differ between the children with autism and unaffected siblings, greater short-allele transmission of this gene was found in individuals with more severe social and communication impairments. The authors concluded that the 5HTT promoter alleles are more likely to modify the severity of symptoms associated with autism, rather than being the cause for the behavior themselves (Tordjman et al., 2001).

Chromosome 7-MET & RELN: Several studies have also reported a link between chromosome 7 and autism (Losh et al., 2008). Both the reelin gene (*RELN* at 7q22) and the *MET* gene (at 7q31) have both been associated with autism in genome-wide studies. What is significant about *RELN* is that it is involved with guiding the migration of neurons in children and also promotes synaptic plasticity in adults (Volker & Lopata, 2008). Skaar and colleagues (2005) examined the genetic association of *RELN* variants to autism in 371 families. The strongest association with autism was found with a large polymorphic trinucleotide repeat located in the 5′ untranslated region of the *RELN* gene (Skaar et al., 2005); this, along with findings from population-based studies, suggests an increased susceptibility to autism for individuals with a particular variation of the *RELN* gene.

The *MET* gene is also located on chromosome 7 and has also been linked to cases of autism in genome-wide studies (Losh et al., 2008). *MET* is of interest because it is involved in both brain development (particularly in the growth and organization of neurons) and in gastrointestinal (GI) functioning (many individuals with autism also have GI issues). Results from a study of 214 families with one or more ASD-affected individuals revealed that a variant of the *MET* gene was associated with co-occurring autism and GI conditions in 118 families, but was not evident in the 96 families that did not have a child with co-occurring autism and GI conditions (Campbell et al., 2009).

Tumor suppressor genes: Mutations in these genes strongly associate, statistically, with autism. One such gene is *PTEN* (phosphatase and tensin homolog) is a tumor suppressor gene responsible for making a protein that helps regulate cell division by preventing cells from growing and dividing too rapidly (Losh et al., 2008). Mutations in this gene are often associated with disorders that result in macrocephaly. Previously undetected mutations in *PTEN* were found in 17% of subjects who had both autism and head circumferences ranging between 2.5 and 8 standard deviations above the mean (Butler et al., 2005). Other studies have been performed that involve knockout mice models, in which mice are genetically engineered without *PTEN* in the cerebral cortex and the hippocampus. These data revealed that the mutant mice demonstrated abnormal social interactions with other mice, in addition to exaggerated responses to sensory stimuli similar to behaviors observed in humans with autism (Kwon et al., 2006).

Two other tumor suppressor genes, *TSC1* and *TSC2*, have also been studied extensively because of their roles in the development of tuberous sclerosis complex (TSC), which is characterized by benign tumors and lesions in many organs, including the brain (Losh et al., 2008). Autism and autism-like features have been reported in approximately 15% to 60% of cases of TSC (Curatolo, Porfirio, Manzi, & Seri, 2004; Iznitzer, 2004). The association between autism and TSC was found to be very high when lesions were localized in the temporal lobe (Bolton & Griffiths, 1997).

While the reports above are compelling as evidence for several genetic pathways leading to autism, they only scratch the surface of the issue. In a recent review of the clinical and research genetic literature, over 100 genetic and genomic disorders were reported with subjects with ASD (Betancur, 2011). It is also difficult to rigorously compare many of the research reports, as they use a variety of methodologies to identify candidate genes and different definitions of the autism phenotype. Varying study designs and small samples sizes also make it more challenging to replicate results (Losh et al., 2008). Most researchers would agree that several genes are likely involved in the etiology of autism. How these genes interact with one another and with the environment make the situation even more complicated.

Prenatal and Perinatal Risk Factors Associated with Autism

According to Bailey and colleagues (Bailey et al., 1995), most plausible neurodevelopmental theories of autism have focused recently on genetic factors. However, Bristol and colleagues (Bristol et al., 1996) noted that there is strong evidence that nonheritable pre- or perinatal events are likely to have an etiological role, including advanced maternal and paternal age, and preterm birth and growth restriction. These and other factors are discussed below.

Environmental Influences

Researchers of environmental influences have turned their attention toward exposures during the prenatal period. In an initial study of 25 children with infantile autism and 25 sex-matched and maternity clinic–matched controls, advanced maternal age (older than 30 years at time of child's birth), signs of clinical dysmaturity (a sign of intrauterine undernutrition), bleeding during pregnancy, and gestational age less than 36 weeks and greater than 41 weeks were significantly more common in the group of children with autism (Gillberg & Gillberg, 1983). The authors concluded that it was not clear whether the adverse prenatal factors were causing autism or whether there was some type of genetic factor associated with autism that led to negative events during pregnancy.

Perinatal Factors

The relationship between autism and maternal bleeding during pregnancy may be related to fetal hypoxia (Kolevson, Gross, & Reinchenberg, 2007) which involves a continual low supply of oxygen during the prenatal period. Fetal hypoxia can result in gestational bleeding and subsequent brain abnormalities. Interestingly, fetal hypoxia has also been shown to increase dopamine, which may be related to increased dopaminergic and serotonin activity in autism (Gardener, Spiegelman, & Buka, 2009).

Parental Factors

A more recent meta-analysis of the association between pregnancy-related factors and pregnancy complications and autism reviewed 40 studies published through 2007 that examined

50 different prenatal factors (Gardener et al., 2009). Factors associated with increased risk for autism included advanced parental age, use of medication during the prenatal period, bleeding during pregnancy, gestational diabetes, being firstborn versus third or later born, and having a mother born abroad. Again, advanced maternal age and gestational bleeding were identified as significant prenatal risk factors. Maternal age was examined in 13 studies. Children born to mothers ages 30 to 34 years at birth were at a 27% increased risk for developing autism, while children born to mothers over the age of 40 years at birth were at an increased risk of 106%, compared with children born to mothers below the age of 30 years. Paternal age was examined in far fewer studies ($n = 4$) but was also found to be a significant risk factor for autism, with a 5-year increase in paternal age associated with a 3.6% increase in risk. Children with fathers ages 30 to 39 years at birth were at a 24% increased risk for developing autism, while children with fathers over the age of 40 years at birth were at an increased risk of 44%, compared with children with fathers below the age of 30 years (Gardener et al., 2009).

Advanced maternal age was again identified as a significant risk factor for autism in a nested case-control study that compared birth certificate records of 8-year-old children identified with an ASD with gender-matched and birth year–matched controls (Bilder, Pinborough-Zimmerman, Miller, & McMahon, 2009). Children born to mothers ages 35 years and older were 68% more likely to have an ASD, compared with children born to mothers between 20 and 34 years of age. Similar to results from the meta-analysis described above, children with autism were significantly more likely to be firstborn, even after controlling for maternal age and gestational age (Bilder et al., 2009). The authors suggested that examining that the risk factors separately might raise more questions than answers. However, examining them collectively might highlight some type of genetic risk for autism that is shared by individuals experiencing those risk factors.

SUMMARY

Research into the genetic etiology of autism has evolved over the past 40 years from studies examining concordance rates between twins to genome-wide screening studies to knockout mutations using animal models. The heterogeneity in the behavioral expression of ASDs is likely a reflection of the complex genetic profile associated with this spectrum of disorders (Caglayan, 2010). Scientists should continue to engage in comprehensive and methodologically rigorous investigations into the genetic mechanisms associated with autism to definitively and promptly diagnose the disorder and to create promising therapies.

REFERENCES

American Academy of Pediatrics Committee on Children with Disabilities. (1994). Screening infants and young children for developmental disabilities. *Pediatrics, 93*, 863–865.

American Psychiatric Association (Ed.). (1980). *Diagnostic & statistical manual of mental disorders* (3 ed.). Washington, DC: Author.

American Psychiatric Association (Ed.). (1987). *Diagnostic & statistical manual of mental disorders* (3 ed. – Revised), Washington, DC: Author.

American Psychiatric Association (Ed.). (1994). *Diagnostic and statistical manual of mental disorders* (4 ed.). Washington, DC: Author.

American Speech–Language–Hearing Association Committee on Infant Hearing. (1991). Guidelines for the audiologic assessment of children from birth through 36 months of age. *American Speech–Language–Hearing Association, 33*(suppl 5), 37–43.

Anney, R., Klei, L., Pinto, D., Regan, R., Conroy, J., Magalhaes, T. R., ... Mallmayer, J. (2010). A genome-wide scan for common alleles affecting risk for autism. *Human Molecular Genetics, 19*(20), 4072–4082.

Anonymous. (2000). Provision of educationally-related services for children and adolescents with chronic diseases and disabling conditions. American Academy of Pediatrics. Committee on Children with Disabilities. *Pediatrics, 105*(2), 448–451.

Avchen, R. N., Wiggins, L. D., Devine, O., Van Naarden Braun, K., Rice, C., Hobson, N. C., ... Yeargin-Allsopp, M. (2011). Evaluation of a records-review surveillance system used to determine the prevalence of autism spectrum disorders. *Journal of Autism and Developmental Disorders, 41*, 227–236.

Bailey, A. J., Le Couteur, A., Gottesman, I., Bolton, P., Simonoff, E., Yuzda, E., & Rutter, M. (1995). Autism as a strongly genetic disorder: Evidence from a British twin study. *Psychological Medicine, 25*, 63–77.

Baird, G., Charman, T., Baron-Cohen, S., Cox, A., Swettenham, J., Wheelwright, S., & Drew, A. (2000). A screening instrument for autism at 18 months of age: A 6-year follow-up study. *Journal of the American Academy of Child & Adolescent Psychiatry, 39*(6), 694–702.

Baker, P., Piven, J., & Sato, Y. (1998). Autism and tuberous sclerosis complex: Prevalence and clinical features. *Journal of Autism and Developmental Disorders, 28*(4), 279–285.

Baker, P., Piven, J., Schwartz, S., & Patil, S. (1994). Brief report: Duplication of Chromosome 15q11-q13 in two individuals with autistic disorder. *Journal of Autism and Developmental Disorders, 24*(4), 529–535.

Barbaresi, W. J., Colligan, R. C., Weaver, A. L., & Katusic, S. K. (2009). The incidence of clinically diagnosed versus research-identified autism in Olmstead County, Minnesota, 1976–1997: Results from a retrospective, population-based study. *Journal of Autism and Developmental Disorders, 39*(3), 464–470.

Baron-Cohen, S. S., Wheelwright, S., Cox, A., Baird, G., Charman, T., Swettenham, J., Drew, A., & Doehring, P. (2000). Early identification of autism by the CHecklist for Autism in Toddlers (CHAT). *Journal of the Royal Society of Medicine, 93*(10), 521–525.

Bertrand, J., Mars, A., Boyle, C., Bove, F., Yeargin-Allsopp, M., & Decoufle, P. (2001). Prevalence of autism in a United States population: The Brick Township, New Jersey, investigation. *Pediatrics, 108*(5), 1155–1161.

Betancur, C. (2011). Etiological heterogeneity in autism spectrum disorders: More than 100 genetic and genomic disorders and still counting. *Brain Research, 1380*, 42–77.

Bilder, D., Pinborough-Zimmerman, J., Miller, J., & McMahon, W. (2009). Prenatal, perinatal, and neonatal factors associated with autism spectrum disorders. *Pediatrics, 123*(5), 1293–1300.

Bolton, P., Macdonald, H., Pickles, A., Rios, P., Goode, S., Crowson, M., Bailey, A., & Rutter, M. (1994). A case-control family history study of autism. *Journal of Child Psychology and Psychiatry, 35*, 877–900.

Bolton, P. F., & Griffiths, P. D. (1997). Association of tuberous sclerosis of temporal lobes with autism and atypical autism. *Lancet, 349*, 392–395.

Bricker, D., & Squires, J. (1999). *Ages and Stages Questionnaires: A parent-completed, child monitoring system.* Baltimore, MD: Paul H. Brookes.

Bristol, M. M., Cohen, D. J., Costello, E. J., Denckla, M., Eckberg, T. J., Kallen, R., ... Spence, M. A. (1996). State of the science in autism: Report to the National Institutes of Health. *Journal of Autism and Developmental Disorders, 26*, 121–154.

Butler, M. G., Dasouki, M. J., Zhou, X. P., Talebizadeh, Z., Brown, M., Takahashi, T. N., ... Eng, C. (2005). Subset of individuals with autism spectrum disorders and extreme macrocephaly associated with germline PTEN tumour suppressor gene mutations. *Journal of Medical Genetics, 42*(4), 318–321.

Butter, E. M., & Mulick, J. A. (2003). Early intervention critical to autism treatment. *Pedatric Annals, 32*, 677–684.

Byrd, R. (2003). *Autistic spectrum disorders. Changes in the California caseload. An Update: 1999–2002.* Sacramento, CA: California Health and Human Services Agency. Retrieved from http://www.mindfully.org/Health/2003/Autism-1999-2002-CA-Apr03.htm

Caglayan, A. O. (2010). Genetic causes of syndromic and non-syndromic autism. *Developmental Medicine and Child Neurology, 52*, 130–138.

Campbell, D. B., Buie, T. M., Winter, H., Bauman, M., Sutcliffe, J. S., Perrin, J. M., & Levitt, P. (2009). Distinct genetic risk based on association of *MET* in families with co-occurring autism and gastrointestinal conditions. *Pediatrics, 123*, 1018–1024.

Centers for Disease Control and Prevention. (2007a). Prevalence of autism spectrum disorders—Autism and Developmental Monitoring Network, 14 sites, United States, 2002. *Morbidity and Mortality Weekly Reports Surveillance Summaries, 58*(1), 12–28.

Centers for Disease Control and Prevention. (2007b). Prevalence of autism spectrum disorders—Autusm and Developmental Disabilities Monitoring Network, six sites, United States, 2000. *Morbidity and Mortality Weekly Report Surveillance Summaries, 56*(1), 1–11.

Centers for Disease Control and Prevention. (2009). Prevalence of autism spectrum disorders—Autism and Developmental Disabilities Monitoring Network, United States, 2006. *Morbidity and Mortality Weekly Report Surveillance Summaries, 58*(10), 1–20.

Centers for Disease Control and Prevention. (2012). Prevalence of autism spectrum disorders—Autism and Developmental Disabilities Monitoring Network, 14 sites, United States, 2008. *Morbidity and Mortality Weekly Report Summaries, 61*(3), 1–19.

Chakrabarti, S., & Fombonne, E. (2001). Pervasive developmental disorders in preschool children. *Journal of the American Medical Association, 285*(24), 3093–3099.

Constantino, J. N., Zhang, Y., Frazier, T., Abbacchi, A. M., & Law, P. (2010). Sibling recurrence and the genetic epidemiology of autism. *American Journal of Psychiatry, 167*, 1349–1356.

Cook, E. H. (1998). Genetics of autism. *Mental Retardation and Developmental Disabilities Research Reviews, 4*, 113–120.

Cook, E. H., Lindgren, V., Leventhal, B. L., Courchesne, R., Lincoln, A., Shulman, C., Lord, C., & Courchesne, E. (1997). Autism or atypical autism in maternally but not paternally derived proximal 15q duplication. *American Journal of Human Genetics, 62*, 928–934.

Croen, L. A., Grether, J. K., Hoogstrate, J., & Selvin, S. (2002). The changing prevalence of autism in California. *Journal of Autism Developmental Disorders, 32*(3), 207–215.

Curatolo, P., Porfirio, M. C., Manzi, B., & Seri, S. (2004). Autism in tuberous sclerosis. *European Journal of Paediatric Neurology, 8*, 327–332.

Demb, H., & Papola, P. (1995). PDD and Praeder-Willi syndrome. *Journal of the American Academy of Child and Adolescent Psychiatry, 34*, 539–540.

Dimitropoulos, A., & Schultz, R. T. (2007). Autistic like symptomatology in Prader-Willi syndrome: A review of recent findings. *Current Psychiatry Reports, 9*, 159–164.

Dworkin, P. H. (1993). Detection of behavioral, developmental, and psychosocial problems in pediatric primary care practice. *Current Opinions in Pediatrics, 5*, 531–536.

Dykens, E. M., Sutcliffe, J. S., & Levitt, P. (2004). Autism and 15q11–15q13 disorders: Behavioral, genetic, and pathophysiological issues. *Mental Retardation and Developmental Disabilities Research Reviews, 10*(4), 284–291.

Filipek, P. A., Accardo, P. J., Ashwal, S., Baranek, G. T., Cook, E. H., Jr., Dawson, G., & . . . Volkmar, F. R. (2000). Practice parameter: Screening and diagnosis of autism: Report of the Quality Standards Subcommittee of the American Academy of Neurology and the Child Neurology Society. *Neurology, 55*(4), 468–479.

Folstein, S., & Rutter, M. (1977a). Genetic influences and infantile autism. *Journal of Child Psychology and Psychiatry, 18*, 297–321.

Folstein, S., & Rutter, M. (1977b). Infantile autism: A genetic study of 21 twin pairs. *Journal of Child Psychology and Psychiatry, 18*, 297–321.

Fombonne, E. (1999). The epidemiology of autism: A review. *Psychosocial Medicine, 29*(4), 769–786.

Fombonne, E. (2003). Epidemiologic surveys of autism and other pervasive developmental disorders: An update. *Journal of Autism and Developmental Disorders, 33*, 365–382.

Fombonne, E. (2005). Epidemiology of autistic disorder and other pervasive developmental disorders. *Journal of Clinical Psychiatry, 66*(suppl 10), 3–8.

Fombonne, E. (2009). Epidemiology of pervasive developmental disorders. *Pediatric Research, 65*(6), 591–598.

Gardener, H., Spiegelman, D., & Buka, S. L. (2009). Prenatal risk factors for autism: Comprehensive meta-analysis. *British Journal of Psychiatry, 195*, 7–14.

Geier, D. A., & Geier, M. R. (2006). Early downward trends in neurodevelopmental disorders following removal of thimerosal containing vaccines. *Journal of American Physicians and Surgeons, II*(I), 8–13.

Gernsbacher, M. A., Dawson, D. M., & Goldsmith, H. H. (2005). Three reasons not to believe in an autism epidemic. *Current Directions in Psychological Science, 14*(2), 55–58.

Ghaziuddin, M., Tsai, L., & Ghaziuddin, N. (1992). Autism in Down's syndrome: Presentation and diagnosis. *Journal of Intellectual Disability Research, 36*, 449–456.

Giarelli, E., Lee, L.-C., Levy, S. E., Pinto-Martin, J., Kirby, R. S., & Mandell, D. (2010). Sex differences in the evaluation and diagnosis of autism spectrum disorders among children. *Disability and Health, 3*(2), 107–116.

Gillberg, C., & Gillberg, I. C. (1983). Infantile autism: A total population study of reduced optimality in the pre-, peri- and neonatal period. *Journal of Autism and Developmental Disabilities, 13*(2), 153–166.

Glascoe, F. P. (1997). Parent's concerns about children's development: Prescreening technique or screening test? *Pediatrics, 99*(4), 522–528.

Glascoe, F. P. (1998). *Collaborating with parents: Using parents' evaluation of developmental status to detect and address developmental and behavioral problems*. Nashville, TN: Ellsworth & Vandermeer.

Glascoe, F. P., & Dworkin, P. H. (1995). The role of parents in the detection of developmental and behavioral problems. *Pediatrics, 95*, 829–836.

Glascoe, F. P., & Sandler, H. (1995). Value of parent's estimates of children's developmental ages. *Journal of Pediatrics, 127*, 831–835.

Gordis, L. (2000). *Epidemiology* (2 ed.). New York: W. B. Saunders.

Gordis, L. (2004). *Epidemiology* (3 ed.). New York: W. B. Saunders.

Hatton, D. D., Sideris, J., Skinner, M., Mankowski, J., Bailey, D. B., Roberts, J., & Mirrett, P. (2006). Autistic behavior in children with fragile X syndrome: Prevalence, stability, and the impact of FMRP. *American Journal of Medical Genetics. Part A, 140*(17), 1804–1813.

Hollander, E., Kolevzon, A., & Coyle, J. T. (Eds.). (2011). *Textbook of autism spectrum disorders*. Washington, DC: American Psychiatric Publishing.

Iznitzer, M. (2004). Autism and tuberous sclerosis. *Journal of Child Neurology, 19*, 675–679.

Johnson, C. P., Myers, S. M., & Council on Children with Disabilities. (2007). Identification and evaluation of children with autism spectrum disorder. *Pediatrics, 120*, 5.

Jorde, L. B., Hasstedt, S. J., Ritvo, E. R., Mason-Brothers, A., Freeman, B. J., Pingree, C., ... Moll, A. (1991). Complex segregation analysis of autism. *American Journal of Human Genetics, 49*, 932–938.

Kanner, L. (1943). Autistic disturbances of affective contact. *Nervous Child, 2*, 217–250.

Kim, Y. S., Leventhal, B. L., Koh, Y.-J., Fombonne, E., Laska, E., Lim, E.-C., ... Grinker, R. R. (2011). Prevalence of autism spectrum disorders in a total population sample. *American Journal of Psychiatry, 168*(9), 904–912.

Klin, A. (1993). *Auditory brainstem responses in autism: Brainstem dysfunction or peripheral hearing loss? Journal of Autism and Developmental Disorders, 23*, 15–35.

Kolevzon, A., Matthewson, K. E., & Hollander, A. (2006). Selective serotonin reuptake inhibitors in autism: A review of efficacy and tolerability. *Journal of Clinical Psychiatry, 67*(3), 407–414.

Kolevzon, A., Gross, R., & Reinchenberg, A. (2007). Prenatal and perinatal risk factors for autism: A review and integration of findings. *Archives of Pediatric and Adolescent Medicine, 161*, 326–333.

Krieger, N. (1994). Epidemiology and the web of causation: Has anyone seen the spider? *Social Science & Medicine, 39*(7), 887–903.

Kwon, C.-H., Luikart, B. W., Powell, C. M., Zhou, J., Matheny, S. A., Zhang, W., ... Parada, L. F. (2006). Pten regulates neuronal arborization and social interaction in mice. *Neuron, 50*, 377–388.

Le Couteur, A., Bailey, A. J., Goode, S., Pickles, A., Robertson, S., Gottesman, I., & Rutter, M. (1996). A broader phenotype of autism: The clinical spectrum in twins. *Journal of Child Psychology and Psychiatry, 37*, 785–801.

Le Couteur, A., Rutter, M., Lord, C., Rios, P., Robertson, S., Holdgrafer, M., & McLennan, J. (1989). Autism Diagnostic Interview: A standardized investigator-based instrument. *Journal of Autism and Developmental Disorders, 19*, 363–387.

Lichenstein, P., Carlstrom, E., Rastam, M., Gillberg, C., & Anckarsater, H. (2010). The genetics of autism spectrum disorders and related neuropsychiatric disorders in childhood. *American Journal of Psychiatry, 167*, 1357–1363.

Lord, C., Rutter, M., Goode, S., Heemsbergen, J., Jordan, H., Mawhood, L., & Schopler, E. (1989). Autism Diagnostic Observation Schedule: A standardized observation of communicative and social behavior. *Journal of Autism and Developmental Disorders, 19*, 185–212.

Losh, M., Sullivan, P. F., Trembath, D., & Piven, J. (2008). Current developments in the genetics of autism: From phenome to genome. *Journal of Neuropathology and Experimental Neurology, 67*(9), 829–837.

Matson, J., Benavidez, D. A., Compton, L. S., Paclawskyj, T., & Baglio, C. (1996). Behavioral treatment of autistic persons: A review of research from 1980 to the present. *Research in Developmental Disabilities, 17*, 433–465.

Mausner, J. S., & Kramer, S. (1985). *Epidemiology: An introductory text* (2 ed.). Philadephia, PA: W. B. Saunders.

Moeschler, J. B., Mohandas, T. K., Hawk, A. B., & Noll, W. W. (2002). Estimate of prevalence of proximal 15q duplication syndrome. *American Journal of Medical Genetics, 111*, 440–442.

Newschaffer, C. J., Falb, M., & Gurney, J. G. (2005). National autism prevalence trends from United States special education data. *Pediatrics, 115*, 277–282.

Pericak-Vance, M. A. (2003). The genetics of autism. In R. Plomin, J. C. DeFries, I. W. Craig & P. McGuffin (Eds.), *Behavioral genetics in the postgenomic era* (pp. 1034–1048). Washington, DC: American Psychological Association.

Peters, S. U., Beaudet, A. L., Madduri, N., & Bacino, C. A. (2004). Autism in Angelman syndrome: Implications for autism research. *Clinical Genetics, 66*, 530–536.

Pickles, A., Bolton, P., Macdonald, H., Bailey, A., Le Couteur, A., Sim, L., & Rutter, M. (1995). Latent class analysis of recurrence risk for complex phenotypes with selection and measurement error: A twin study and family history of autism. *American Journal of Human Genetics, 57*, 717–726.

Pinto-Martin, J., Souders, M., Giarelli, E., & Levy, S. (2005). The role of nurses in screening for autistic spectrum disorder in pediatric primary care. *Journal of Pediatric Nursing, 20*(3), 163–169.

Rice, C., Baio, J., Van Naarden Braun, K., Doernberg, N., Meaney, F. J., & Kirby, R. S. (2007). A public health collaboration for the surveillance of autism spectrum disorders. *Paediatric Perinatal Epidemiology, 21*, 179–190.

Rutter, M. (1967). A children's behaviour questionnaire for completion by teachers: Preliminary findings. *Journal of Child Psychology and Psychiatry and Allied Disciplines, 8*(1), 1–11.

Rutter, M. (2000). Genetic studies of autism: From the 1970s into the millennium. *Journal of Abnormal Child Psychology, 28*(1), 3–14.

Rutter, M. (2005). Incidence of autism spectrum disorders: Changes over time and their meaning. *Acta Paediatrica, 94*, 2–15.

Rutter, M., Bailey, A., Bolton, P., & Le Couteur, A. (1993). Autism: Syndrome definition and possible genetic mechanisms. In R. Plomin & G. E. McClearn (Eds.), *Nature, nurture & psychology* (pp. 269–284). Washington, DC: American Psychological Association.

Schechter, R., & Grether, J. K. (2008). Continuing increases in autism reported to California's Developmental Services System: Mercury in retrograde. *Archives of General Psychiatry, 65*(1), 19–24.

Skaar, D. A., Shao, Y., Haines, J. L., Stenger, J. E., Jaworski, J., Martin, E. R., & ... Pericak-Vance, M. A. (2005). Analysis of the RELN gene as a genetic risk factor for autism. *Molecular Psychiatry, 10*, 563–571.

Social Security Administration, U.S. (2011). *Benefits for children with disabilities*. Washington, DC: Social Security Administration. Document #: 05-10026ICN (pp. 1–20). Retrieved from http://www.ssa.gov/pubs/10026.html

Steffenburg, S., Gillberg, C., Hellgren, L., Anderson, L., Gillberg, I., Jakobsson, G., & Bohman, M. (1989). A twin study of autism in Denmark, Finland, Iceland, Norway and Sweden. *Journal of Child Psychology and Psychiatry, 30*, 405–416.

Steffenburg, S., Gillberg, C. L., Steffenburg, U., & Kyllerman, M. (1996). Autism in Angelman syndrome: A population-based study. *Pediatric Neurology, 14*, 131–136.

Tordjman, S., Gutknecht, L., Carlier, M., Spitz, E., Antoine, C., Slama, F., ... Anderson, G. M. (2001). Role of the serotonin transporter gene in the behavioral expression of autism. *Molecular Psychiatry, 6*, 434–439.

Volker, M. A., & Lopata, C. (2008). Autism: A review of biological bases, assessment, and intervention. *School Psychology Quarterly, 23*(2), 258–270.

Webb, P. L. (2011). Screening for autism spectrum disorders during well-child visits in a primary care setting. *Journal of Nurse Practitioners, 7*(3), 229–235.

Yang, M. S., & Gill, M. (2007). A review of gene linkage, association and expression studies in autism and an assessment of convergent evidence. *International Journal of Developmental Neuroscience, 25*, 69–85.

Yeargin-Allsopp, M., Murphy, C., Oakley, G. P., & Sikes, R. K. (1992). A multi-source method for studying the prevalence of developmental disabilities in children: The Metropolitan Atlanta Developmental Disabilities Study. *Pediatrics, 89*(4), 624–630.

3 Introduction to the Integrated, Comprehensive Nursing Care of Autism Spectrum Disorder

Ellen Giarelli

The World Health Organization defines integrated care as a concept bringing together, delivery, management, and organization of services related to diagnosis, treatment, care, rehabilitation, and health promotion. Integration is a means of improving services in relation to access, quality, user satisfaction, and efficiency (Gröne & Garcia-Barbero, 2002). It is most often equated with managed care in a business model and more recently has been equated with comprehensive care and disease management.

Integrated care is also known as case management, shared care, comprehensive care, and seamless care. Integrated care is a worldwide trend in health care reform and new organizational arrangements focusing on more coordinated and integrated forms of care provision (Kodner & Spreeuwenberg, 2002). It represents a service framework with which to develop responsive and more cost-effective health systems, and is on the agenda of health care organizations and professional associations.

The word "integration" stems from the Latin verb *integer*, that is, "to complete." The adjective "integrated" means "organic part of a whole" or "reunited parts of a whole." To integrate means to bring together or merge elements or components that formerly were separate. The notion of comprehensiveness overlaps with that of integration. Similar to the original meaning of the Greek verb "diagnosis," "comprehensive" implies a full understanding of a situation. Therefore, the first aim of comprehensive and integrated care is to provide a framework for nurses to understand the relationship among elements of care that constitute the whole. This aim begins with the clinical encounter between nurse and patient and may extend to organizational design and performance.

Without integration, all aspects of health care fall short of the ideal. Patients' needs may be incorrectly identified, services are not delivered or delayed, and quality of care and patient satisfaction break down (Charns & Tewksbury, 1993; Shortell, Gillies, Anderson, Mitchell, & Morgan, 1993). Moreover, policy makers and payers in both the public and private sectors expect to save money or at least ensure that health care resources are used more wisely with integration. They look to integrated, comprehensive care as more professional and fiscally responsible.

Nursing's Place in Integrated Care

Integrated, comprehensive nursing care is the profession's response to the fragmented delivery of health and social services that characterize the care of people with ASD. The goal of integrated, comprehensive care is especially relevant for people with physical, developmental, or cognitive disabilities, who have related chronic conditions or complex illnesses. These vulnerable individuals have complicated and ongoing needs that are part medical, part physical, part psychological, and part social. Complex circumstances create difficulties in everyday living and require multiple services delivered sequentially or simultaneously by multiple providers. Patients with complex needs receive care at home and in community and institutional settings. Transitioning from one type of service or level of care to another is especially daunting when trying to maintain health and functioning. Robinson (2009) stated that it is critically important that families have the opportunity to consult with health professionals who are able to assist them in evaluating information and accessing services and continuing care at home when warranted. Nurses take a patient-centered perspective, and the Centers for Disease Control and Prevention (CDC, 2009) recognized that such a perspective is of utmost importance when the patient's health needs are complex.

Health Professional's Knowledge of Autism Spectrum Disorder

Nurses in all practice environments will encounter patients diagnosed with an autism spectrum disorder (ASD). As with any chronic disorder diagnosed in childhood, ASD has significant, lifelong health implications for those who are affected, as well as for family members and the communities in which they live. There has been sustained public attention to ASD since 2001, when the U.S. Legislature passed the Child Health Act of 2000, which mandated research into prevalence, etiology, and research on comparative effectiveness of treatment for autism. Since then, and due to concerted efforts of the CDC, reports of steadily rising prevalence of ASD have sharpened the perspective of the public and professionals. Over the last 10 years, the prevalence estimates of ASD have nearly tripled in some regions of the country (CDC, 2009). Ascertaining trends in prevalence was the essential first step toward a systematic professional response.

Even with a sustained public and professional focus, health professionals' knowledge and beliefs about ASD do not yet match the facts. In 2005, Heidgerken and colleagues (Heidgerken, Geffken, Modi, & Frakey, 2005) conducted a study of autism knowledge in the health care setting. They reported that primary health care providers differently endorsed a variety of statements regarding prognosis, course, and treatment as compared with professionals working exclusively with the ASD population. For example, a significant proportion of professionals across disciplines believed that: (a) autistic children do not show social attachments, even to parents ($F(2,150) = 21.6$, $p = .001$), (b) autistic children are deliberately negativistic and noncompliant ($F(2,152) = 12.23$, $p = .001$), (c) autistic children do not show affectionate behavior ($F(2,152) = 9.62$, $p = .001$), and (d) autistic children's withdrawal is mostly due to cold, rejecting parents ($F(2,150) = 8.8$, $p = .001$). In addition, a significant number of providers did not feel comfortable diagnosing or identifying a child as autistic. These statements are simply not supported by the evidence, and some are untrue. Such expectations and beliefs will undoubtedly affect how services can or should be delivered. These data are used to support the aim to educate all health care professionals with accurate information.

The Expanded Role of the Nurse in ASD Care

According to the Institute of Medicine (IOM, 2010) there are more than 3 million nurses practicing in the United States. Nursing is the largest profession and is the largest segment of the nation's health care workforce. As such, nurses play an important role in all aspects of health care. In 2008, the Robert Wood Johnson Foundation (RWJF) and the IOM launched a 2-year initiative to respond to the need to assess and transform the nursing profession and thereby transform health care. There are four key messages that can be readily applied to providing comprehensive nursing care of people with ASD. The key messages developed by the IOM Committee on the RWJF Initiative on the Future of Nursing are:

- Nurses should practice to the full extent of their education and training.
- Nurses should achieve higher levels of education and training through an improved education system that promotes seamless academic progression.
- Nurses should be full partners, with physicians and other health care professionals, in redesigning health care in the United States.
- Effective workforce planning and policy making require better data collection and information infrastructure.

The treatment of ASD occurs in multiple settings and is provided by a variety of health and community professionals. By applying these messages to ASD care across the lifespan, nurses have the opportunity to transform the care provided to this special population regardless of the nature of the clinical encounter. To fully endorse this opportunity, nursing must take four steps. First, nurses must expand their knowledge base to include understanding of the special needs of this population and apply this knowledge in all practice settings. Second, nurses who wish to ameliorate the health problems of people with ASD should seek higher levels of education and training about this population. Third, nurses should partner with other health care providers in all clinical environments to redesign health delivery systems to better accommodate the health needs of people with developmental disabilities. Lastly, effective nursing workforce planning and policy making require better data collection and an information infrastructure related to clinical encounters with people with ASD across the lifespan and across health care settings.

Advanced practice nurses, in particular, can oversee the work of undergraduate nurses working in any clinical setting. When working in collaboration with physicians, nurses can integrate the unique behavioral characteristics of patients with ASD with primary and tertiary medical services (see Exhibit 3.1).

EXHIBIT 3.1

List of Possible Advanced Nursing Practice Activities when Working in Collaboration with a Physician Treating a Patient with ASD

- Perform comprehensive, integrated assessments of patients with ASD and establish medical and related diagnoses.
- Order, perform, and supervise diagnostic tests for patients and, to the extent the interpretation of diagnostic tests is within the scope of the advanced practice specialty and consistent with the collaborative agreement, interpret diagnostic tests.
- Initiate referrals to and consultations with other licensed professional health care providers and consult with other licensed professional health care providers at their request.
- Develop and implement treatment plans, including issuing orders to implement treatment plans. However, only an advanced practice nurses with current prescriptive authority approval may develop and implement treatment plans for pharmaceutical treatments.

(*Continued*)

EXHIBIT 3.1 (Continued)

- Complete admission and discharge summaries for clinical units in tertiary health care centers.
- Order blood and blood components for patients.
- Order dietary plans for patients.
- Order home health and hospice care.
- Order durable medical equipment.
- Issue oral orders to the extent permitted by the health care facilities' by-laws, rules, regulations, or administrative policies and guidelines.
- Make physical therapy and dietitian referrals.
- Make respiratory and occupational therapy referrals.
- Perform disability assessments for the program providing temporary assistance to needy families.
- Issue homebound schooling certifications.
- Perform and sign the initial assessment of methadone treatment evaluations, provided that any order for methadone treatment shall be made only by a physician.

Adapted from the State Board of Nursing of the Commonwealth of Pennsylvania (1977).

Kodner and Spreeuwenberg suggested five domains in which to foster integrated care (Kodner & Spreeuwenberg, 2002). Two domains are especially germane to nursing practice: service delivery and the clinical realm. The service-delivery domain addresses how staff are trained, how they perform their responsibilities and tasks and work together, and how they relate to patients and family caregivers and their needs. The clinical domain involves a shared understanding of patient needs, common professional language and criteria, the use of agreed-upon practices and standards throughout the life cycle of a particular disease or condition, and the maintenance of ongoing patient–provider communication and feedback. These two domains are the principal targets of nursing care of people with ASD (see Exhibit 3.2).

EXHIBIT 3.2

Goals for the Establishment of Integrated, Comprehensive Care for ASD across Patient Care Settings

Level: Environment-Specific Service Delivery

- Joint and specific training of all health professionals who work in a service environment
- Ready available resources or access to information, referral, and intake protocols
- Standardized case management
- Role modeling and practice of multidisciplinary/interdisciplinary teamwork

(Continued)

EXHIBIT 3.2 (Continued)

- Around-the-clock coverage or access to consultative care
- Integrated information systems

Level: Clinical Encounter

- Standard use of diagnostic criteria (e.g., *Diagnostic and Statistical Manual of Mental Disorders, Fourth Edition*, or subsequent) and training on examining interactions of co-occurring diagnoses
- Uniform, comprehensive assessment procedures
- Joint care planning
- Shared clinical records or creation of a single patient's health history document
- Continuous, disorder-specific patient-monitoring protocols
- Shared, standardized decision support tools, such as practice guidelines, teaching aids, and protocols)
- Regular patient/family contact and ongoing support and inclusion

WAYS OF THINKING ABOUT NURSING CARE FOR ASD

To design a best-practices plan of care, nurses can integrate a patient-centered approach to care with information on developmental tasks, ASD diagnostic criteria, core features and characteristics, and observations of patients' behaviors and symptoms.

Developmental Tasks across a Lifetime

Nurses new to the field of ASD care may not know where to begin to integrate a large body of knowledge about developmental disability with an even larger body of knowledge on clinical care. The application can begin by adopting a developmental perspective on assessment. This perspective requires that the nurse evaluate different aspects of the patient's development within speech, language, social, motor, cognitive, and adaptive domains.

Developmental Assessment

Upon first encountering a patient, the nurse can compare the patient's chronological age with his or her developmental age. In other words, assess how the patient's behaviors, emotions, and communications conform to the expected behaviors, emotions, and communication of others the same age. Ask the questions: Can he or she walk and move easily and independently or does he or she have physical limitations? Does he or she use an elaborated code of language to communicate or is language truncated to "yes" and "no" and simple phrases? Does he or she avoid conversation and social gestures or is he or she withdrawn and unresponsive? Is he or she adequately groomed and clean? Factor into this assessment an allowance for the stress of the clinical encounter. The result is a profile of a patient's overall developmental accomplishments and deficits. This developmental profile can inform the approach taken by the nurse, type of communication, elaboration of speech, and expectations for compliance. Even though the comprehensiveness of the developmental profile is significantly limited by the short time frame for many nursing interactions with patients, a nurse may be able to acquire a useful image of conspicuous limitations. If necessary, developmental assessments can be conducted in a more systematic way for the purposes of creating a long-term treatment plan.

Scarpinato and colleagues (2010) supported this developmental approach and suggested that specific questions may help to begin a developmental assessment in the initial encounter. Grade level is often used as a proxy for development or cognitive ability. A nurse may ask about school or grade level for a minor child and compare the grade level to the chronological age. The simplest of questions that require abstract thinking are also useful in uncovering developmental age.

Behavioral Theories Applied to ASD Care

A theoretical assumption is that all behavior has purpose.

Behavioral interventions are treatments for ASD that are used by most clinicians. Educational researchers are familiar with behavioral techniques and apply them to helping mental health patients "relearn" healthier approaches to problems. They have been scientifically validated and are popular with family caregivers, beginning with parents, who wish to continue positive interventions outside the therapeutic environments of school and treatment centers.

There is consensus among therapists that early intervention is a predictor of better long-term outcomes for individuals with ASD. A growing body of literature over the past 25 years has suggested that children with ASD can benefit significantly from early intensive behavioral intervention based on the principles of applied behavioral analysis (Anderson, Avery, DiPietro, Edwards, & Christian, 1987; Birnbrauer & Leach, 1993; Harris, Handleman, Gordon, Kristoff, & Fuentes, 1991; Lovaas, 1987; Magiati, Charman, & Howlin, 2007; Sallows & Graupner, 2005).

While research and common wisdom support beginning behavioral interventions as early as possible, one may begin at any time across the lifespan in response to an emerging personal demand related to a health care problem. All behavioral approaches highlight the need to focus on the relationship between behavior and the environment. This type of analysis is the foundation of the case studies of ASD nursing. Nursing care and the health care environment may be adapted according to the observed or anticipated behaviors of the person with ASD, regardless of age.

Behavioral treatments have been in use for more than 45 years and were originally employed in educational programs. They were based on normal developmental sequences for instruction and included operant conditioning that selected reinforcement, extinction, and punishment procedures applied to override or supersede existing sources of reinforcement, which were often unknown (Lovaas, Newsom, & Hickman, 1987). Treatment succeeded when the selected contingency effectively prevented the unwanted behavior. The greatest appeal of behavioral techniques is that the entry point is entirely flexible.

Environmental Structuring and Facilitating

One of the earliest systematic programs of behavioral treatment, called TEACCH (Treatment and Education of Autistic and Communication-Handicapped Children), was developed by Schopler in 1972 and is the most widely used intervention for children with ASD (Lord & Schopler, 1994). The TEACCH program emphasized two basic principles: structuring the environment to promote skill acquisition and facilitating independence at all levels of functioning (Ozonoff & Cathcart, 1998). In contrast with applied behavioral analysis interventions the TEACCH program is used to help individuals with ASD to make the most of the skills they possess, rather than to teach them to enter more "typical settings," although the desired outcome might be the same. TEACCH places strong emphasis on setting up modified environments. Visual structures are used to accommodate deficits, and tasks tend to be visual–motor activities and repetitive tasks, such as sorting, matching, or sequencing. Visual cues may include boxes or envelopes labeled "start" and "finished." The environment becomes the "prosthetic" by which limitations can be circumvented with limited distress (Leader, Healy, & O'Connor, 2009).

In clinical practice, one may see the immediate value of structuring the clinical environment to promote skill acquisition when a skill is clearly identified, such as "taking medications on time" or "performing active range of motion exercises." For example, if a child or an adult must perform deep breathing exercises after surgery, a nurse may set up a visual work station that includes place mats labeled "start," "deep breath one," "deep breath two," and so on up to "finished" on which the patient places his or her incentive spirometer. A nurse is a behaviorist when he or she works with patients to adopt health-promoting behaviors.

Functional Assessment and Applied Behavioral Analysis

A related approach to initial assessment is functional analysis or functional assessment. It is used by clinicians and is part of the treatment paradigm called applied behavioral analysis or ABA. ABA is a method used by behaviorists to describe and manipulate behavior (Harris & Weiss, 2007; Lovaas, 1987; Lovaas et al., 1987). Iwata and colleagues (Iwata, Vollmer, Zarcone, & Rodgers, 1993) developed an operant methodology for identifying the specific function of unwanted behavior. This methodology was called "functional analysis" and guided clinicians, researchers, and others to identify the specific sources of reinforcement that maintained the unwanted behavior being performed by the individual.

In a clinical context, "function" refers to a reinforcer that maintains the unwanted behavior and also the information needed to develop the intervention to replace the unwanted behavior with the desired behavior. For example, a nurse may assess that a patient begins self-injurious behavior, such as pulling on intravenous lines, when bed curtains are opened abruptly and left open. This simple functional assessment of the probable cause of behavior (abrupt intrusions and exposure causes fear or insecurity) can be converted to specific instructions for staff and visitors that would remove the source of stress and eliminate reinforcers for the unwanted behavior. As a component of ABA, functional analysis was first described by Skinner (Hanley, Iwata, & McCord, 2003; Skinner, 1953) as the empirical demonstration of the causal relationship between behavior and environment.

Functional assessment provides a method for nurses to determine what variables in the environment provoke and/or maintain behaviors. The method requires direct observation and is therefore ideal for initial clinical encounters with new or returning patients. For example, a nurse may observe a patient repetitively picking and pulling on his sleeve and may first conclude that a sensation is causing the ritualistic behavior and decide to first investigate a mechanical, traumatic, or other factor. In this way, a nurse may be able to determine the function (intended effect) of a behavior in a given context. Following direct observation of the causal relationship is "experimental manipulation" or some action to interrupt causality, such as removing anything that reinforces behavior. A reinforcer can be social, such as attention or access to objects, and negative reinforcement may be an escape from negative stimuli (Iwata et al., 1994).

Self-injury is an associated feature of individuals with ASD (Aman & Farmer, 2011; Ando & Yashimura, 1979). A nurse may observe a patient performing a behavior that is self-injurious and initially assume that the intent is self-harm, when this may not be the case. Carr

(1994) posited that nearly all forms of self-injury are purposeful and are maintained by motivation for attention, escape, sensory reinforcement, or access to tangibles or events. One caveat for the nurse is to take time to assess the behavior for its underlying purpose.

Functional analysis as a component of ABA aims to eliminate problem behavior and promote desired behaviors, including appropriate purposeful communication, adaptive abilities, and, at least, situation-specific, socially acceptable behavior. In the context of the clinical encounter, behavior that interferes with a patient's receipt of required medical care or communication that does not accurately convey meaning are problematic and may be amenable to functional analysis.

Techniques of ABA

The specific strategies and techniques of ABA were developed by educators for developmentally disabled children but have a place in any learning environment, including clinical settings. A nurse may not have information right away on a co-occurring diagnosis of ASD, but a nurse may practice anticipatory nursing care and attempt to predict and prevent problems by applying approaches adapted from ABA. During a clinical encounter, a nurse should ask three questions that analyze antecedent, behavior, and consequence. The questions are: (1) What immediately preceded the behavior? (2) What precisely is the behavior itself? (3) What immediately follows the behavior? After such an assessment, the nurse may alter some aspect of the environment or interpersonal encounter. Adapting the clinical environment to accommodate the abilities and special needs of individual patients takes into account the pervasiveness of symptoms, especially behavioral atypicalities. The techniques of functional analysis are listed and described in Table 3.1. For the purpose of understanding the range of strategies, all are included, with the exception of "punishment" (aversive stimuli or aversives), which is rarely appropriate for use in any therapeutic clinical encounter (Maurice, Green, & Foxx, 2001).

ABA is hypothesis driven and data based and has the endpoint of improved behavior. Nurses may develop and test their own sets of hypotheses and assessment strategies to provide information on variables associated with a specific behavior in the context of the clinical encounter. The nurse's practical application of aspects of these techniques can be practiced with any patient. Figure 3.1 illustrates the steps in the functional assessment of a patient with ASD who arrives at an outpatient clinic for preoperative testing. A response to this situation is illustrated in Figure 3.2, which shows a discrete trial training (DTT) procedure that can easily be modified to apply to any functional assessment (Cooper, Heron, & Heward, 2007; O'Neill, Horner, Albin, Storey, & Sprague, 1997; Van Bourgondien, Reichle, & Schopler, 2003).

Professional Nursing Care for People with ASD and Families

In order to provide patients with ASD the highest standard of care throughout their lifespan, continued energies must be spent on providing better coordination of care. Nurses' unique skill sets make them the ideal coordinators of care for this population. Nurses can also provide strong family-focused advocacy and support, education, and primary-care services. Some interesting discourse on a nursing perspective on ASD is coming out of Australia. Two nursing faculty from the University of Technology, Sydney, have applied chaos theory to autism to explain the role of overregulation and have proposed different ways of looking at the health of nonlinear systems (Cashin & Waters, 2006).

TABLE 3.1 ■ Specific Strategies and Techniques of ABA

Technique	Definition
Shaping	Antecedents and consequences are systematically manipulated to increase or decrease the rate of occurrence of specific behaviors
Prompting and fading	Prompts are verbal or physical clues that increase the chance that the child will produce the desired behavior. When the person's responses begin trending in the desired direction, the prompts can be systematically decreased.
Chaining and reverse chaining	Chaining involves breaking down a complex task into smaller units that can be more easily shaped. Depending on the circumstances, the nurse may start with the first element in the sequence and work forward or the last element and work backward
Generalization	A task is not fully learned until the person can perform it regardless of the setting or the conditions. This is not an expected outcome of a brief clinical encounter. Prompts and tasks are rotated, presented in different context, and presented by different people to facilitate generalization. This technique may be more appropriate for lifelong chronic care mandates.
Discrete Trial Training (DTT)	This includes clearly defined interactions between a "trainer" and subject that follow a typical pattern: The trainer presents a stimulus (a request, task, or behavior to be imitated), the subject responds, and the trainer delivers a consequence. Consequences include:
Positive reinforcement	Providing a desired consequence, such as food, affection, verbal praise, or access to a desired object or activity.
Negative reinforcement, Extinction	Removing an undesirable consequence. For example, removing a wet, uncomfortable sheet or shirt might be used as a negative reinforcement for a patient who will not remain in bed
Punishments	Punishments are no longer recommended, and have been replaced by verbal reprimands or removal of desired objects. This technique is rarely, if ever, appropriate for a clinical encounter.
Ignoring and Time-out	Ignoring includes attempting to eliminate or "extinquish" the person's refusals of requests. As many times as the person turns away from a treatment or medication (for example), the nurse keeps presenting it. Ignoring also includes not attending to verbal complaints, demands, or leaning/threatening movements. A time-out is providing a temporary break from an activity that is difficult to complete.
Differential reinforcement	Reinforcing a socially acceptable alternative, for example, asking for help instead of yelling, or absence of behavior

Chaos Theory Applied to ASD Care

Autism is described as a construct that focuses on a way of being-in-the-world and as such justifies—or at least gives a purpose to—various behavioral characteristics. Chaos theory has some premises in existentialist philosophy (Heidegger, 1949) and is used as a framework

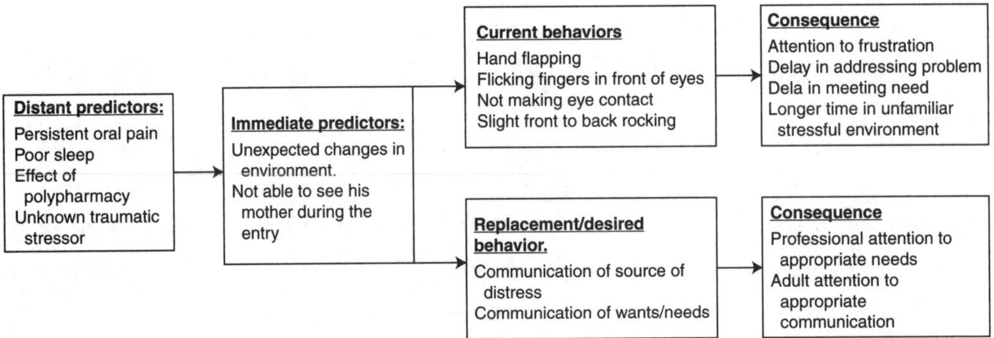

FIGURE 3.1 ■ Functional assessment of the following clinical encounter: Patient (male, age 15) arrives in a wheelchair at the outpatient clinic for preoperative testing for an oral surgical procedure scheduled for the following day.

for understanding the origin and impact of aberrant behaviors, such as restricted repetitive movements. Proponents of chaos theory believe that small changes in systems can cause unpredictable changes in the system at a later time (Barker, 1996). According to chaos theory, healthy systems are chaotic, complex, dynamic, and adaptive, and overregulation and linearity (Andrade, 1995) is unhealthy. ASD is a highly complex neurobehavioral disorder that manifests in complex collections of behaviors and symptoms.

In the case of ASD, overregulation is manifested as repetitive behaviors and restrictive interests that are deemed aberrant but also unhealthy in that they prevent adaptation. Such restrictive behaviors may be the only way a person with ASD knows how to deal with stressful situations and be-in-the-world. Applying this theoretical construct to a clinical encounter permits a nurse to understand the genesis of extreme responses to what might be considered ordinary clinical experiences. For example, an adult with ASD who must wait an hour for a medical consult may experience this wait as a major disruption to his or her pattern of

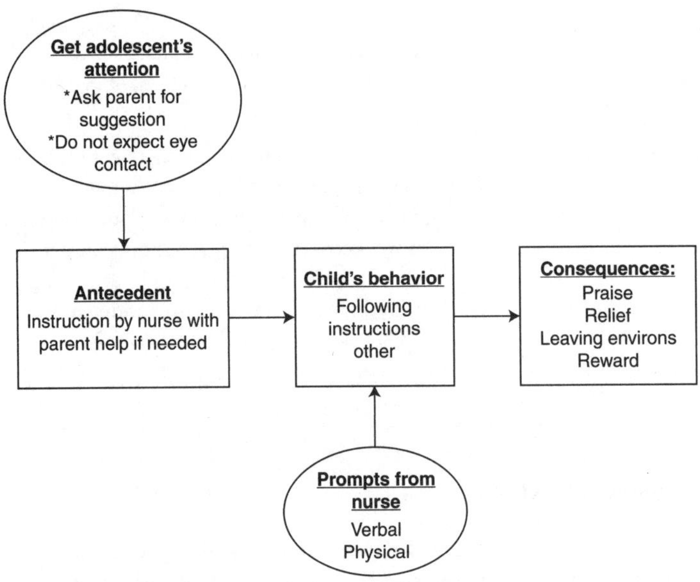

FIGURE 3.2 ■ General algorithm for a DTT.

being-in-the world and may respond by intensifying repetitious behaviors in order to "adapt" and limit the stress. The resultant behaviors may be observed as a "meltdown." A nurse who applies chaos theory to this observation will have a unique way to interpret the underlying psychological mechanisms and thereafter devise a way to assist the patient to incrementally restore balance in the need for sameness. As stated by Cashin and Waters (2006), "Exposing people with autism to new experiences even when supported is stressful . . . . Any intervention must be holistic and personalized, taking account of each aspect in the triad of impairment (communication, behavior and socialization)" (pp. 228, 229). For such a patient, the long waiting time is unacceptable and inappropriate.

Nursing Functions and Responsibilities in the Clinical Encounter

Nursing roles and professional responsibilities to a patient with ASD encompass assessments and observations, education and teaching, and interventions and treatments over time. The roles apply to any clinical environment (see Table 3.2). ASD is a long-term, chronic, pervasive condition that affects all aspects of the affected individual's life.

Historically, the purposive nature of health care had a normative focus of "doing for" the patient. Timmermas and Haas (2008) are in a long line of critics of this stance and alternatively proposed that the patient has become, and should be, a participant in the process. Over 45 years ago, Parsons (1965) advocated that patient "participation in sickness and recovery was a job to be done in cooperation with those technically qualified to help" (pp. 286–287). To be technically qualified, nurses must acquire specific knowledge about ASD that will enable them to effectively and as much as possible engage the person in their care.

Flowing from this perspective, May (2010) described the clinical encounter as consisting of socially patterned components of "work" and the organization of information about beliefs and actions related to illness and wellness. This work is organized by both the professional and the patient and is comprised of cognitive participation, collective action, and reflexive monitoring. Cognitive participation engages both the nurse and the patient in interactive work and relies on input from all participants. Collective action is the situation in which the patient is part of the "sickness" world, in which situational factors are shaped to promote engagement. In collective action, the nurse has confidence in his or her own technical ability and also has the patient's trust. Reflexive monitoring makes sense of the meaning of illness–wellness work and requires that both patient and nurse understand the work and purpose of the clinical encounter (May, 2010).

Reflexive Monitoring Examples

It is of paramount importance to superimpose consideration of the features of ASD on all clinical encounters. What does this look like in practice? In older children and adults with ASD, a lack of verbal communication may make it impossible for the person to understand subtle humor and lighthearted comments or jokes about health care or treatments. An instruction to "take deep breaths" may be taken absolutely literally and need to be followed with the instruction to stop.

Personal space is different for people with ASD, and bed curtains in the emergency department may need to be continually closed. A gentle touch on the shoulder of a person with ASD who seems distressed may be interpreted as an intrusion.

A lifetime of being told to "make eye contact" may cause a person with ASD to stare and appear to have a bizarre affect. This does not suggest an act of intimidation or opposition,

TABLE 3.2 ■ Nursing Functions and Responsibilities in ASD Care

Assessment/observation	Education/teaching	Intervention/treatment
ASD screening	Instruct parents/screening	Referral for medical evaluations
Developmental screening	Instruct parents/milestones	Referral to ophthalmologist
Hearing and vision evaluations	Instruct parents/medical monitor	Referral to audiologist
Behavioral assessments	Instruct parents/behavior therapy	Referral to psychiatrist
Physical health assessment	Instruct parents	Referral to developmental pediatrician
Monitor reactions to medications	Community education and outreach on ASD	Prescribe selected medications
Monitor side effects of medications	Instruct staff	Deliver ASD treatments
Monitor response to treatments	Consult with external care providers	Administer ASD diagnostic tools
Assess medical comorbidities	Stress management for family members	Home visits for follow-up
Environmental/home assessment	Instruct on interaction with providers	Manage medical comorbidities
Assess sleep, sensory, and activity issues	Provide sex education	Glucose monitoring and injections
Comprehensive physical exam	Collaborate with staff on health issues	Administer asthma treatments
Nutritional assessment	Conduct sibling classes	Design comprehensive plan of care
Individualize plans of care		Symptom management
Care documentation		Administer behavioral interventions
Contribute to grant preparation		Administer sensory integration therapy
Data collection for research		Establish protocols: health issues
Data entry, cleaning, and analysis		Venipuncture
Manuscript preparation		Medicate and manage medications
		Design nutritional plan of care
		Conduct screening clinics in community
		Stress management for families
		Communicate with family on medical issues
		Adolescent transition planning
		Conduct parent support groups
		Decision-making support for parents
		Coordinate elements of care
		Collaborate in team care
		Provide first aid
		Assist with hygiene

but rather a conditioned response or an attempt to fit in. Odd behaviors may be attempts at collective action (May, 2010) and engagement to control the stress of a clinical encounter.

Perseverations, tantrums, and repetitive movements may be expressions of pain. The same may also be caused by problems processing sensory stimuli. The patient with ASD may be sensory-seeking or sensory-avoiding and have an unusual reaction to light, sound, or touch. Some people with ASD have exquisite hearing and may misunderstand quiet comments made by a nurse to a colleague (Baas, 2006).

Primary Care Activities—The Medical Home Model

With additional training in ASD care, nurses are able to provide primary-care services for patients with ASD. This may include comprehensive physical and behavioral assessments, medication administration, oversight of comprehensive care plans, ASD screening and diagnostic testing, comprehensive health care and nutritional planning, and patient education. Each of these roles may be ideally served by an advanced practice nurse but can easily be provided by a professional nurse with a bachelor's degree and specialized training in ASD nursing care.

Patients with ASD may not, under current models, receive sufficient primary health care in comparison with typically developing children. A greater emphasis needs to be placed by health care practitioners on general pediatric care for this population, rather than simply focusing on the specific issues related to their ASD. However, because current pediatric service models are not developed to meet the needs of children with complicated health care conditions, additional systems of pediatric care for this population need to be developed (Brachlow, Ness, McPheeters, & Gurney, 2007).

The American Academy of Pediatrics has emphasized the role that the medical home model could have in producing the best health outcomes for the ASD population. Principally, the medical home model can be applied to ensure continuous, comprehensive care that is accessible and family-centered (Medical Home Initiatives for Children with Special Needs Project Advisory Committee, American Academy of Pediatrics, 2002).

Medical home model and nurse practitioners. The medical home model was originally proposed in 1967 by the American Academy of Pediatrics and since that time has been shown to be the most effective way to provide care for children with complex medical needs (Larson & Reid, 2010). The tenets of the medical home model are that care will be comprehensive, culturally sensitive, easily accessible, continuous, coordinated, and compassionate (Medical Home Initiatives for Children With Special Needs Project Advisory Committee, American Academy of Pediatrics, 2002). In addition, there has been a renewed effort by clinicians to create patient- and family-centered care. As patients and families experience influxes of information via the Internet and other media, it is important that care plans consider a patient's and family's knowledge base and allow for shared clinical decision making (Kilo & Wasson, 2010). Patient-centered care, especially for chronic condition such as ASD, also involves teaching patients and families about self-management methods (Kilo & Wasson, 2010).

The value of a medical home model in the care of ASD populations is further highlighted by the gaps in the health care delivery between ASD populations and other populations with complicated health conditions. For example, compared with children who have another special health care need (e.g., asthma), children with ASD received less comprehensive and coordinated care (Brachlow et al., 2007). Parents of children with ASD reported that they felt the care of their child was less family-centered when compared with reports of parents of children with other special health care needs. This lack of family focus was further associated with parents of children with ASD reporting that providers did not spend an acceptable amount of time with them during health care visits (Brachlow et al., 2007).

The results from the study above closely aligned with results from another study that was based on physicians' self-reporting. In this study, physicians were asked about the care they provided for patients with ASD in juxtaposition with patients with other neurodevelopmental and/or complex medical conditions (Golnik, Ireland, & Borowsky, 2009). Physicians reported lower feelings of competency in providing care for children with ASD and felt that key components of the medical home model were missing, mainly family trust and satisfaction. Accordingly, physicians in this study believed that the primary care for children with ASD needed more improvement than the primary care for children with other neurodevelopmental or complex disease states.

Adults with ASD face similar disparities in care. Walsh and Kastner (1999) reported general problems in the quality of health care for adults with ASD, including the lack of quality measures and patient-response system problems. They and others (Kaplan, 1991; Testa & Simonson, 1996) emphasized that quality health care for people with ASD had four domains: structure, process, health outcomes, and satisfaction. Structure and process were largely external to the patient, while health outcomes and satisfaction were derived from the recipient. Walsh and Kastner (1999) offer one perspective of quality health care that is "technically appropriate" (p. 2) and answers the question: Was the clinical intervention efficient and effective? There are no nursing studies of the domain of satisfaction among people with ASD.

Best-Practices Nursing Care

A model of nurse-managed care that is technically appropriate can help providers coordinate comprehensive services and address the unique needs of the ASD population. To be technically appropriate, such care must be flexible enough that one may integrate it with other health services, such as medication administration, diet and nutrition oversight, as well as management of comorbid and other chronic physical and mental health conditions. For example, individuals with ASD are medicated at high rates, beginning in childhood, for multiple co-occurring medical and psychiatric conditions, often with concurrent psychotropic medications (Mandell et al., 2008). These medications may cause physical sequelae and interact with medications prescribed for thyroid disorders, cardiac conditions, asthma, pain medications, and so on. The steady increase in the rates of medication, both psychotropic and nonpsychotropic, coincides with a high continuance rate. Individuals on both psychotropic and nonpsychotropic medication are 11 and five times, respectively, more likely to stay medicated than to discontinue a medication regimen (Esbensen, Greenberg, Seltzer, & Aman, 2009). See Exhibit 3.3 for general approaches to treatment.

Managing Polypharmacy

Polypharmacy is the use of a number of different drugs, possibly prescribed by different doctors and filled in different pharmacies, by a patient who may have one or several health problems. Individuals with ASD require polypharmacy and therefore more rigorous and careful management of medication. Nurse practitioners are highly qualified to manage the complex interactive dynamics of polypharmacy. Moreover, when care is comprehensive, side effects and adverse events must be monitored closely and prevented, if possible.

Lewis and Colleagues (Lewis, Lewis, Leake, King, & Lindemann, 2002) conducted a chart audit for 353 adults with developmental disabilities and reported that one-third of adults living alone or with family received psychotropic medications, yet only 24% had psychiatric consultations. Thirty-six percent of the medicated group received drugs without any identifiable diagnosis. Lubetsky and Handen (2008) surveyed 3,000 families in North Carolina and reported that 46% of respondents' affected family members were prescribed psychotropic medications for behavioral symptoms. Antidepressants were taken by 21.7%, antipsychotics were taken by 16.8%, and stimulants were taken by 13.9%. In addition, the off-label use of certain psychotropic medications was not reported but is likely highly present. See Table 3.3 for a listing of pharmaceutical agents used to treat ASD. Given that a significant number of people with ASD are prescribed psychotropic medications, it is vital that a nurse ascertain a patient's medication and dosage as soon as possible and before any treatment plans are designed.

Assuring Safety

Another health need unique to the ASD population within the framework of primary care is the need for extensive safety assessments and safety education. Basic safety skills need to be assessed on a regular basis, and subsequent interventions by behavioral specialists will often be necessary. This is because children with ASD have a much higher rate of impulsivity, which places them at high risk for wandering off, running away, jumping from heights, or attempting other actions that may pose a danger (Stull & Ladew, 2010). Some basic safety measures that are suggested by the National Autism Association include ID bracelets and home modifications (Debbaudt, 2005). These techniques to improve safety are among the list of skills taught by nurses to improve the health and safety for people in ASD families. The safety of the environment should be assessed for any person suspected of having or being diagnosed with ASD. See Table 3.4 for a list of ways to modify the environment when there is sensory impairment.

Accurate assessments of hearing and vision impairments are a vital component of safety assessment. Because this population has an equal risk of hearing and visual impairment as the general population, hearing and vision assessments are an integral part of their care. Such assessments are not confined to pediatric clients, as adults with ASD continue to have these impairments, which may exacerbate with age.

Hearing and vision evaluations, along with other assessments of safety, should be conducted during the ASD screening and diagnostic procedures to rule out alternative causes of nonattentiveness, impaired eye contact, and not answering to one's name. Both vision and hearing assessments are expeditiously accomplished by nurses, and may need to be reevaluated when signs indicate a patient may have signs of vision or hearing impairments. Moreover, hearing and vision assessments are potentially stressful experiences for any person with ASD (Davis & Stiegler, 2010). Noncompliance by the person with ASD may result in curtailed testing or inaccurate results. There are many techniques that nurses can use to best assess hearing or vision in this population, but the most important will be the nurse's willingness to understand the core features of ASD and to adapt care to individual situations.

Assuring Proper Nutrition

Nutritional assessment is important for patients, especially children or adults who have a history of feeding and sensory difficulties. While there are conflicting data regarding the nutrient levels (Herndon, DiGuiseppi, Johnson, Leiferman, & Reynolds, 2009) and relative food pickiness (Schreck, Williams, & Smith, 2004) in children with ASD compared to typically developing populations, it remains clear that nutrition in the general U.S. pediatric population is subpar. Nurses can work to educate parents of children with ASD, as well as affected adults, about nutritional requirements and food choices. At the least, nurses can help family caregivers understand the potential hazards or purported benefits of "autism diets" that are described in mass media and supported by public opinion. Nurses can assist them in providing

TABLE 3.3 Adaptations and Interventions for Sensory Impairments

Visual	• Lighting—natural, dimmers • Limit visual clutter • Consider using a picture schedule • Screens and/or curtains
Tactile	• Use firm touch • Neutral warmth • Deep pressure before procedures • Joint compression/brushing • Vibration • Fidget toys • Weighted objects • Resistance—squeezing, manipulating
Auditory	• Slow, rhythmic sounds • Steady sounds (metronome) • Quiet/monotone • Low pitch • Firm touch • Avoid multisensory input • Move slowly • Be consistent • Avoid eye contact
Proprioception	• Pushing hands together • Stretching • Chair push-ups • Standing and pushing against a wall or desk with hands or arms • Chewing on gum/blowing bubbles • Manipulating stiff putty • Eating crunchy foods/sucking on thick liquids • Pulling and chewing on a straw
Vestibular	• Linear (rocking) • Oscillation (up and down) • Inverted
Other	• Breathing—diaphragmatic, entraining

the best possible nutrition and monitoring of food intake (BMJ Group, 2010). Nurses can acknowledge and respect individual choices, while working with families to improve the long-term health of affected children and adults through rigorous nutrition education, counseling, and follow-up care.

Coordination with Other Specialists and Therapists

Meeting the health needs of people with ASD requires a multidisciplinary approach in which the nurse is an equal partner with a team of professionals, including behaviorists, physicians, and psychologists. One key component of care will be the improved use of electronic medical records to combine reports from the team. Such records will promote improved communication and better coordination of care among the core team members. Other specialists with a particular interest in working with individuals with ASD may include occupational and

TABLE 3.4 ■ Polypharmacy in ASD

Category	Symptom	Medication	Possible side effects
Stimulant (Handen, Feldman, Gosling, Breaux, & McAuliffe, 1991; D. J. Posey et al., 2004; Quintana et al., 1995)	Hyperactivity, inattention, impulsiveness	Methylphenidate (Concerta, Metadate CD, Methylin, Ritalin) Dexmethylphenidate (Focalin) Dextroamphetamine and amphetamine (Adderall)	Withdrawal Irritability Appetite loss Weight loss Weight gain Appetite gain Motor tics
Nonstimulants (Handen, Sahl, & Hardan, 2008; Jaselskis, Cook, & Fletcher, 1992; D. J. Posey et al., 2004)	Attention deficit hyperactivity disorder Hyperactivity, inattention, impulsiveness	Clonidine (Catapress, Jenloga, Kapvay, Nexiclon) Guanfacine (Tenex, Intuniv) Atomoxetine (Strattera)	Sedation Decreased activity Change in blood pressure Dry mouth Constipation Headache Dizziness Nervousness Upset stomach Vomiting Nausea Rashes
Antidepressants (Antochi, Stavrakaki, & Emery, 2003; Fukuda, Sugie, Ito, & Sugie, 2001; Hellings, Kelley, Gabrielli, Kilgore, & Shah, 1996; Hollander et al., 1998; Hollander, Kaplan, Cartwright, & Reichman, 2000; McDougle et al., 1998; McDougle et al., 1996; Steingard, Zimnitzky, DeMaso, Bauman, & Bucci, 1997)	Anxiety disorder Depressive disorder Obsessive–compulsive behavior Ritualistic and stereotypical behaviors Outbursts Bipolar disorder	SSRIs Fluoxetine (Prozac, Reconcile, Rapiflux, Sarafem, Selfemra) Fluvoxamine (Luvox) Buproprion (Wellbutrin, Budeprion, Buproban, Aplenzin, Zyban) Paroxetine (Paxil, Pexeva) Sertraline (Zoloft) Citalopram (Celexa) Venlafaxine (Effexor)	Anxiety Suicidal ideation Upset stomach Insomnia Dry mouth Drowsiness Appetite changes

(*Continued*)

TABLE 3.4 ■ *Continued*

Category	Symptom	Medication	Possible side effects
Antipsychotic Atypical neuroleptics (Aman & Langworthy, 2000; Campbell et al., 1997; Posey & McDougle, 2003)	Manias Thought disorders Aggression/agitation Stereotypy Motor tics	Chlorpromazine (Thorazine) Thioridazine (Mellaril) Haloperidol (Haldol) Risperadone (Risperdal) Olanzapine (Zyprexa) Quetiapine (Seraquel) Ziprasidone (Geodon) Aripiprazole (Abilify)	High risk for diabetes Weight gain Increased appetite Fatigue Extrapyramidal side effects Pseudoparkinsonism Akathisia Acute dystonic reactions Dizziness, drooling Drowsiness Neuroleptic malignant syndrome
Mood stabilizers (Belsito, Law, Kirk, Landa, & Zimmerman, 2001; Childs & Blair, 1997; Hollander, Dolgoff-Kasper, Cartwright, Rawitt, & Novotny, 2001; Kerbeshian, Burd, & Fisher, 1987; Steingard & Biederman, 1987)	Bipolar disorder Self-injury Aggression Depression Impulsivity Conduct disorder seizures	Topiramate (Topamax, Topiragen) Lithium (Eskalith, Lithobid) Valproic acid (Depakene, Depakote) Carbamazepine (Tegretol, Carbatrol, Epitol, Equetro) Lamotrigine (Lamictal) Oxcarbazepine (Trileptal) Levetiracetam (Keppra)	Hypothyroidism Weight gain Tremor Polydipsia Polyuria Muscle weakness Electrocardiogram changes Nephrogenic diabetes insipidus Hemorrhagic pancreatitis Possible birth defects Hepatic failure Sedation Gastrointestinal upset Alopecia Aplastic anemia Agranulocytosis Hypoglycemia Rash Swelling

EXHIBIT 3.3

Treatment Approaches

Evidence-Based Practices

- Efficacy must be established through peer-reviewed research in scientific journals using:
  - Randomized or quasi-experimental design studies
  - At least two high-quality group design studies
- Single-subject design studies
  - Three different investigators or research groups have conducted five high-quality, single-subject designs
- Combination of evidence
  - One high-quality group design and three high-quality, single-subject designs conducted by at least three different investigators or groups
- Differential reinforcement
- Discrete trial training
- Extinction
- Functional behavioral assessment
- Picture exchange communication system
- Prompting
- Reinforcement
- Self-management
- Social narratives
- Visual supports

Treatment Approaches

- Only after a comprehensive assessment should an intervention plan for the individual with ASD and family proceed. Assessments might include but not be limited to:
  - Medical and nutritional
  - Motivation (functional analysis)
  - Environmental
  - Communication levels and systems
  - Emotional regulation and developmental level
  - Behavioral functioning—disruptive or aggressive behavior
  - Social competency (interaction needs and abilities)
  - Sensory issues
  - Learning style preferences (visual, auditory)

(*Continued*)

EXHIBIT 3.3 (Continued)

- o Medical conditions and/or medication reactions will need to be addressed and stabilized
- o Core characteristic weaknesses that interfere with learning or functioning will need to be identified and treated

- Evaluators/staff/families will need training that addresses the ASD individual's strengths and needs.
- The individual with ASD will need employment and or meaningful structured day programming.
- Data collection system is necessary to monitor progress.
- Professionals and families need to partner to address the needs of the individual with ASD.

Sensory Integrative Treatment

Key Feature:

- Sensory information provides an important foundation for learning and behavior.
- The processing of sensory information is a developmental process.
- Successful integration and organization of sensory information results in and is further developed by adaptive responses.
- The "just right challenge" is the principle that the child must be able to successfully meet the challenges that are presented through playful activities.
- Children have an innate drive to seek meaningful experiences from their environment.
- As a result of neuroplasticity, enriched experiences effect change in the nervous system.
- Sensory integration is the foundation for physical and social engagement and participation in daily life activities and routines.

Outcomes of Adequate Sensory Integration

- The ability to modulate, discriminate, and integrate sensory information from the body and the environment
- Self-regulation to regulate and maintain an arousal and/or activity level needed to attend to a task or activity
- Maintaining postural control, including muscle tone, strength and balance, ocular control, and bilateral coordination and laterality
- Adequate praxis
- Organizing behavior needed for developmentally appropriate tasks and activities
- Development of self-esteem and self-efficacy

(*Continued*)

EXHIBIT 3.3 (Continued)

Treatment of Asperger's Syndrome

- Not necessarily a milder form of autism
- Greater inclusion in society but may not have the social competencies to cope with everyday experiences
- Growing number in the criminal justice system

Treatment Approaches: Older Children and Adolescents

- Communication
  - Pragmatics
- Social
  - Skills
  - Competencies
  - Expectations
- Autistic mannerisms
  - Behavior strategies
  - Coping strategies
  - Medication
- Regulation
  - Sensory
  - Emotional

Treatment Approaches: Adults

- Functionality and context
  - Current skills, attributes, and strengths
  - Safety
  - The resources and capacity of the family (emotional, cognitive, energy, financial, motivation, availability)
  - Medication-related issues
  - Health issues (weight, nutrition)
  - Sexuality issues
  - Disruptive/aggressive behaviors
  - Programming (day, recreational/leisure, evenings/weekends)

physical therapists and speech and language therapists. The ultimate goal of integrated, comprehensive care is for each professional to have access, when needed, to complete information about the patient.

Collaboration with Local School Nurses

School nurses play an important role in the lives of children with a medical problem that interferes with school attendance or performance. The school nurse can both assess communication and physical needs of children with ASD, as well provide support and education to parents and school staff about ASD. These nurses draw up individual health plans for every student with a medical need in their school (Bellando & Lopez, 2009). With this heavy workload, it is not surprising that school nurses, especially those with little advanced training in special needs, do not have a vault of comprehensive information regarding ASDs and medical comorbidities. By focusing on educating the school staff, the school nurse can create an optimal environment for healthy development for children with ASD in their school (Cade & Tidwell, 2001).

Secondary and Tertiary Health Care for Older Adolescents and Adults

The transition from pediatric to adult health services is an inefficient and difficult shift for young adults with ASD and their families (McDonough & Revell, 2010). One of the largest hurdles in transitioning is to determine what health care services are necessary for pre-adults with ASD. In some cases, school nursing care may be the only primary care available to a child. Pediatric primary care may abruptly end at age 21. Coverage on a parent's health care insurance policy may be extended. If a parent lacks health care insurance, a young adult may have no access to health care outside of emergency services. There are limited standards for services to assist with community living or finding employment (McDonough & Revell, 2010).

Extended Health Care

There is a range of issues that adolescent and adults with ASD must tackle as they access health care in the community. These include: transportation to the facility, payment for services, self-presentation, and behavior during the clinical encounter (Geller & Greenberg, 2010). Comprehensive, integrated nursing care can include counseling for transition to community, with the aim of assisting in adapting to workplace and postsecondary school environments or living in a group home.

Support for Parents and Family Caregivers

Like other diagnoses in childhood, ASD has a significant effect on the quality of life of family members, especially parents, some of whom may experience their child's diagnosis with extreme grief and a sense of loss. Added responsibilities in caring for the varied needs of this child impose personal and social burdens that may be or feel unrelenting. A challenge for nurses is to create a model of care that supports parents at all junctures in the child's health care trajectory, being mindful that some individuals with ASD will remain with their parents until the death of the elderly parent results in institutionalization.

There is a growing interest among advocates in examining the effect on patients of the interventions delivered to the individuals' caregivers. Common wisdom and studies of other populations are used by clinicians to support the notion that when the parent's stress is reduced, a reduction in the child's stress follows. The time period surrounding the ASD diagnosis is especially difficult for parents, but also may be an ideal time for nursing interventions. Giarelli and colleagues (Giarelli, Sounders, Pinto-Martin, Bloch, & Levy, 2005) found that nursing interventions delivered to the parent soon after a diagnosis was made mitigated the impact of the illness and reduced perceived stress in the parent. An important role for nurses is to help parents respond to the needs of their child with ASD, their typically developing child (if present), and their own needs. Nurses are ideally suited to teach parents effective means of handling the many responsibilities associated with having a child with ASD (Twoy, Connolly, & Novak, 2007). These may include sessions to promote honest communication, identifying constructive and unifying family rituals and outings, and providing positive feedback for efforts at joint problem solving (Twoy et al., 2007). The usefulness of these techniques can be seen by understanding the major issues that face the parents of a child with ASD.

Parent Stress and Anxiety

Stress and anxiety are common difficulties experienced by the parents of a child with ASD. Unfortunately, behavior problems in a child are associated with parental stress, and it has been shown that these two factors cyclically exacerbate each other, such that as stress on the parent increases, behavior problems of the child increase and vice versa. The levels of stress in parents who have a child with ASD are extremely high. According to a study by Dabrowska and Pisula, the stress of parents of children with ASD is significantly higher than even those levels found in parents who have a child with Down syndrome (Dabrowska & Pisula, 2010). This same study examined how three different categories of coping mechanisms (task-oriented, emotion-oriented, and avoidance-oriented) affected the parent's stress level. The researchers found that for parents who have a child with ASD, emotion-oriented coping predicted high total parental stress levels, whereas task-oriented coping predicted low levels of total parental stress among parents in general.

In light of these results, it becomes clear that parents of a child with ASD have a great need for stress-management interventions, even more so than parents of children with other complicated health conditions (Dabrowska & Pisula, 2010). Parents can significantly benefit from a task-oriented approach to managing multiple aspects of care, including health care. Furthermore, task orientation is a technique that nurse practitioners have long used to provide caregivers with an understanding of how to manage the duties of caregiving for a relative with medical needs and can be applied to the person with ASD.

Whole-family care for ASD is a complex endeavor. Rivers and Stoneman (2003) examined how increased marital stress interacted with sibling relationships to compromise these relationships when one child was typically developing and the sibling had ASD. Essentially, marital stress predicted the quality of the sibling relationship (Rivers & Stoneman, 2003). A family assessment appears to be necessary to improve family treatment outcomes, and nurses may begin by conducting an evaluation of the home environment with the aim of identifying facilitators and obstacles to a stable and nurturing home. The interpersonal relationships within each family unit are crucial for establishing long term care and support for the individual with ASD and those who care for him or her.

Support for Siblings

Comprehensive nursing care includes family support to an even greater degree than is stipulated in the medical home model. One important provision of a family intervention is sibling support. Nurses can facilitate parent and sibling group discussions and activities, as well as individual counseling sessions for siblings. Younger siblings (less than 10 years of age) are uniquely affected because they may feel left out, unsafe at home, and even victimized by a sibling with ASD if symptoms demand extensive parental attention or include aggression and destructiveness.

Siblings may be too young to understand the unique situation and may be unable to self-advocate. There is also the risk of modeling, in which an unaffected sibling may adopt aberrant behaviors that appear to be effective in garnering attention from parents and others. Younger siblings may retreat into quiet spaces, which can bring about feelings of isolation from the rest of the family (Benderix & Sivberg, 2007). This complex dynamic can be addressed through counseling by trained mental health professionals and nurse practitioners.

Both younger and older siblings of children with ASD appear to have a precocious sense of responsibility. This sense of responsibility is focused toward their family, aiming to provide relief for their parents and sibling with ASD. There are also added feelings of sadness, sorrow, and empathy for their sibling with ASD, especially in consideration of their affected sibling's long-term hopes and plans (Benderix & Sivberg, 2007). Nurses may assist siblings to develop insight and empathy for those affected with ASD, while also helping them to deal with the daily challenges that having an affected sibling presents. There is evidence that such support may ultimately unite the family (Elder & D'Alessandro, 2009).

Community Outreach and Activism

One of the fundamental challenges to living with ASD is that contemporary culture is constructed by and for individuals who are best described as neurotypical. Instead of viewing a disability as a fundamental flaw in an individual, it is more constructive and appropriate to recognize how a so-called "disability" results from incompatibility with societal norms. To make true progress within the realm of ASD, it is imperative to not simply focus on the individuals with ASD, but to also address the aspects of society that contribute to their disability.

Nurses have a long history of effective community outreach and activism. Nurses may extend this involvement through volunteer coordination, collaboration with charitable organizations, and educational outreach. An effective way to educate the community is by offering programs at community centers. Such programs can be adapted to the specific community to educate the general population about ASD or to educate community members who are affected. Programs may include descriptions of core and associated features, development milestones, services available locally, and instructions on job hunting and health-promoting strategies. Screening events can be coordinated by nurses and delivered at health fairs and in collaboration with school-based programs.

Developing Plans of Care

One difference between people who are neurotypical or neuroatypical or, who are "able" or "differently able" is the speed at which something can be accomplished, beginning with the content, leading through the process, and to completion. That is to say, any task can be done, but when? When a person is physically disabled, movement is slower, steps are labored, and positioning takes more time. Early planning and slow introduction of steps or actions are key intervention strategies. With impaired physical movement, there may be impaired language receptivity or expressivity. For the individual with ASD, their diagnosis may include language or sensory-processing delays. They may require a longer time to think of a response and may not be able to process multiple requests at once. When encountering a patient with ASD, three words will serve the nurse and the patient well when designing a plan of care at any point in the interaction: "***A***nticipated, **S**low, and ***D***eliberate."

SUMMARY

Nurses should be prepared to provide comprehensive, integrated care to people with ASD across the lifespan. Nursing care begins with an assessment of the developmental stage of the patient and a functional analysis. Best practice requires that the nurse integrate knowledge of the core characteristics and associated features of ASD with the assessment of medical problems and any comorbidities that may be present. The resulting plan of care must use a team approach, involve multiple professionals, as well as both the patient and family, and include strategies to accommodate the environment to the patient.

REFERENCES

Aman, M. G., & Farmer, C. A. (2011). Self-injury, aggression, and related problems. In E. Hollander, A. Kolevzon & J. T. Coyle (Eds.), *Textbook of autism spectrum disorder.* Washington, DC: American Psychiatric Publishing.

Aman, M., & Langworthy, K. (2000). Pharmacotherapy for hyperactivity in children with autism and other pervasive developmental disorders. *Journal of Autism and Developmental Disorders, 35*(5), 451–459.

Anderson, S. R., Avery, D. L., DiPietro, E. K., Edwards, G. L., & Christian, W. P. (1987). Intensive home-based intervention with autistic children. *Education and Treatment of Children, 10,* 352–366.

Ando, H., & Yashimura, I. (1979). Effects of age on communication skill level and prevalence of maladaptive behaviors in autistic and mentally retarded children. *Journal of Autism and Developmental Disorders, 9,* 83–93.

Andrade, C. (1995). Chaos in science, medicine and psychiatry. *Psychiatric Update, 1,* 39–41.

Antochi, R., Stavrakaki, C., & Emery, P. C. (2003). Psychopharmacological treatments in persons with dual diagnosis of psychiatric disorders and developmental disabilities. *Postgraduate Medicine Journal, 9,* 139–146.

Baas, K. (2006). Specialty: Autism approaches need to be tailored to each person. *Pennsylvania Nurse, 61*(1) 14–15.

Barker, P. (1996). Chaos and the way of Zen: Psychiatric nursing and the uncertainty principle. *Journal of Psychiatric and Mental Health Nursing, 3*(4) 235–243.

Bellando, J., & Lopez, M. (2009). The school nurse's role in treatment of the student with autism spectrum disorders. *Journal for Specialists in Pediatric Nursing, 14*(3), 173–182.

Belsito, K. M., Law, P. A., Kirk, K. S., Landa, R. J., & Zimmerman, A. W. (2001). Lamotrigine therapy for autistic disorder: A randomized, double-blind, placebo-controlled trial. *Journal of Autism and Developmental Disorders, 31,* 175–181.

Benderix, Y., & Sivberg, B. (2007). Siblings' experiences of having a brother or sister with autism and mental retardation: A case study of 14 siblings from five families. *Journal of Pediatric Nursing, 22(5),* 410–418.

Birnbrauer, J. A., & Leach, D. J. (1993). The Murdoch Early Intervention Program after 2 years. *Behavioral Change, 10,* 63–74.

BMJ Group. (2010). *Strict diets may not help children with autism.* Retrieved from http://www.guardian.co.uk/lifeandstyle/besttreatments/2010/may/20/strict-diets-may-nothelpchildren-with-autism

Brachlow, A. E., Ness, K. K., McPheeters, M. L., & Gurney, J. G. (2007). Comparison of indicators for a primary care medical home between children with autism or asthma and other special health care needs: National Survey of Children's Health. *Archives of Pediatrics & Adolescent Medicine, 161*(4), 399–405.

Cade, M., & Tidwell, S. (2001). Autism and the school nurse. *Journal of School Health, 71*(3), 96–100.

Campbell, M., Armenteros, J. L., Malone, R. P., Adams, P. B., Eisenberg, Z. W., & Overall, J. E. (1997). Neuroleptic-related dyskinesias in autistic children: A prospective, longitudinal study. *Journal of the American Academy of Child & Adolescent Psychiatry, 36*(6), 835–843.

Carr, E. (1994). Emerging themes in the functional analysis of problem behavior. *Journal of Applied Behavioral Analysis, 27*(2), 393–399.

Cashin, A., & Waters, C. (2006). The undervalued role of over-regulation in autism: Chaos theory as a metaphor and beyond. *Journal of Child and Adolescent Psychiatric Nursing, 19*(4), 224–230.

Centers for Disease Control and Prevention. (2009). Prevalence of autism spectrum disorder. Autism and Developmental Disabilities Monitoring Network, United States, 2006. *Morbidity and Mortality Weekly Review 58*(SS 10), 1–20.

Charns, M., & Tewksbury, L. (1993). *Collaborative management in health care: Implementing the integrative organization*. San Francisco, CA: Jossey-Bass.

Child Health Act. (2000). Public Law 106-310 Sec. 1004. Retrieved from http://www.samhsa.gov/legislate/Sept01/childhealth_Title31.htm

Childs, J. A., & Blair, J. L. (1997). Valproic acid treatment of epilepsy in autistic twins. *Journal of Neuroscience Nursing, 29*, 244–248.

Cooper, J. O., Heron, T. E., & Heward, W. L. (2007). *Applied behavioral analysis* (2 ed.). Upper Saddle River, NJ: Pearson Education.

Dabrowska, A., & Pisula, E. (2010). Parenting stress and coping styles in mothers and fathers of pre-school children with autism and Down syndrome. *Journal of Intellectual Disability Research, 54*, 266–280.

Davis, R., & Stiegler, L. (2010). Behavioral hearing assessment for children with autism. *ASHA Leader, 15*(5), 5–6.

Debbaudt, D. (2005). *Autism safety toolkit.* Retrieved from http://www.nationalautismassociation.org/safety toolkit.php

Elder, J. H., & D'Alessandro, T. (2009). Supporting families of children with autism spectrum disorders: Questions parents ask and what nurses need to know. *Pediatric Nursing, 35*(4), 240–245, 253.

Esbensen, A. J., Greenberg, J. S., Seltzer, M. M., & Aman, M. G. (2009). A longitudinal investigation of psychotropic and non-psychotropic medication use among adolescents and adults with autism spectrum disorders. *Journal of Autism & Developmental Disorders, 39*(9), 1339–1349.

Fukuda, T., Sugie, H., Ito, M., & Sugie, Y. (2001). Clinical evaluation of treatment with fluvoxamine, a selective serotonin reuptake inhibitor in children with autistic disorder. *No to Hattatsu [Brain & Development], 33*, 314–318.

Geller, L. L., & Greenberg, M. (2010). Managing the transition process from high school to college and beyond: Challenges for individuals, families, and society. *Social Work in Mental Health, 8*(1), 92–116.

Giarelli, E., Sounders, M., Pinto-Martin, J., Bloch, J., & Levy, S. (2005). Intervention pilot for parents of children with autistic spectrum disorder. *Pediatric Nursing, 31*(5), 389–399.

Golnik, A., Ireland, M., & Borowsky, I. W. (2009). Medical homes for children with autism: A physician survey. *Pediatrics, 123*(3), 966–971.

Gröne, O., & Garcia-Barbero, M. (2002). *Trends in integrated care: Reflections on conceptual issues.* Copenhagen, Denmark: World Health Organization.

Handen, B. L., Feldman, H., Gosling, A., Breaux, A. M., & McAuliffe, S. (1991). Adverse side effects of Ritalin among mentally retarded children with ADHD. *Journal of the American Academy of Child & Adolescent Psychiatry, 30*, 241–245.

Handen, B. L., Sahl, R., & Hardan, A. Y. (2008). Guanfacine in children with developmental disabilities. *Journal of Developmental and Behavioral Pediatrics, 29*(4), 303–308.

Hanley, G., Iwata, B. A., & McCord, B. (2003). Functional analysis of problem behavior: A review. *Journal of Applied Behavioral Analysis, 36*, 147–185.

Harris, S. L., Handleman, J. S., Gordon, R., Kristoff, B., & Fuentes, F. (1991). Changes in cognitive and language functioning of preschool children with autism. *Journal of Autism & Developmental Disorders, 21*, 281–290.

Harris, S. L., & Weiss, M. J. (2007). *Right from the start: Behavioral interventions for young children with autism* (2 ed.). Bethesda, MD: Woodbine House.

Heidegger, M. (1949). *Existence and being.* Chicago, IL: H. Regnery.

Heidgerken, A. D., Geffken, G., Modi, A., & Frakey, L. (2005). A survey of autism knowledge in a health care setting. *Journal of Autism & Developmental Disorders, 35*(3), 323–330.

Hellings, J. A., Kelley, L. A., Gabrielli, W. F., Kilgore, E., & Shah, P. (1996). Sertraline response in adults with mental retardation and autistic disorder. *Journal of Clinical Psychiatry, 57*, 333–336.

Herndon, A. C., DiGuiseppi, C., Johnson, S. L., Leiferman, J., & Reynolds, A. (2009). Does nutritional intake differ between children with autism spectrum disorders and children with typical development? *Journal of Autism and Developmental Disorders, 39*(2), 212–222.

Hollander, E., Cartwright, C., Wong, C. M., DeCaria, C. M., DelGuidice-Asch, G., Buchsbaum, M. S., … Aronowitz, B. (1998). A dimensional approach to the autism spectrum. *CNS Spectrum, 3*, 22–39.

Hollander, E., Dolgoff-Kasper, R., Cartwright, C., Rawitt, R., & Novotny, S. (2001). An open trial of divalproex sodium in autism spectrum disorders. *Journal of Clinical Psychiatry, 62*, 530–534.

Hollander, E., Kaplan, A., Cartwright, C., & Reichman, D. (2000). Venlafaxine in children, adolescents, and young adults with autism spectrum disorders: An open retrospective clinical report. *15*, 132–135.

Institute of Medicine. (2010). The future of nursing: Leading change, advancing health. Retrieved from http://www.iom.edu/Reports/2010/The-Future-of-Nursing Leading-Change-Advancing-Health.aspx

Iwata, B. A., Pace, G., Dorsey, M., Zarcone, J. R., Vollmer, T. R., Smith, R. G., . . . Willis, K. D. (1994). The functions of self-injurious behavior: An experimental-epidemiological analysis. *Journal of Applied Behavioral Analysis, 27*, 215–240.

Iwata, B. A., Vollmer, T. R., Zarcone, J. R., & Rodgers, T. A. (1993). Treatment classification and selection based on behavioral function. In R. Van Houton & S. Axelrod (Eds.), *Behavior analysis and treatment* (pp. 101–125). New York: Plenum.

Jaselskis, C. A., Cook, E. H., & Fletcher, K. E. (1992). Clonidine treatment of hyperactive and impulsive children with autistic disorder. *Journal of Clinical Psychopharmacology, 12*, 322–237.

Kaplan, R. M. (1991). Health-related quality of life in patient decision making. *Journal of Social Issues, 47*, 69–90.

Kerbeshian, J., Burd, L., & Fisher, W. (1987). Lithium carbonate in the treatment of two patients with infantile autism and atypical bipolar symptomatology. *Journal of Clinical Psychopharmacology, 7*, 401–405.

Kilo, C. M., & Wasson, J. H. (2010). Practice redesign and the patient-centered medical home: History, promises, and challenges. *Health Affairs, 29*(5), 773–778.

Kodner, D. L., & Spreeuwenberg, C. (2002). Integrated care: Meaning, logic, applications, and implications: A discussion paper. *International Journal of Integrated Care, 2*, 14.

Larson, E. B., & Reid, R. (2010). The patient-centered medical home movement: Why now? *Journal of the American Medical Association, 303*(16), 1644–1645.

Leader, G., Healy, O., & O'Connor, J. (2009). Early intensive behavioral intervention in the treatment of autistic spectrum disorder. In P. Reed (Ed.), *Behavioral theories and interventions for autism* (pp. 103–131). New York: Nova Science Publishers.

Lewis, M. A., Lewis, C. E., Leake, B., King, B. H., & Lindemann, R. (2002). The quality of health care for adults with developmental disabilities. *Public Health Reports, 117*, 174–184.

Lord, C., & Schopler, E. (1994). TEACCH services for preschool children. In S. L. Harris & J. S. Handleman (Eds.), *Preschool education programs for children with autism* (pp. 87–106). Austin, TX: PRO-ED.

Lovaas, O. J. (1987). Behavioral treatment and normal educational and intellectual functioning in young autistic children. *Journal of Consultant Clinical Psychology, 55*, 3–9.

Lovaas, O. J., Newsom, C., & Hickman, C. (1987). Self-stimulatory behavior and perceptual reinforcement. *Journal of Applied Behavioral Analysis, 20*, 45–68.

Lubetsky, M. J., & Handen, B. L. (2008). Medication treatment in autism spectrum disorder. *Speaker's Journal, 8*, 97–107.

Magiati, I., Charman, T., & Howlin, P. (2007). A two-year prospective follow-up study of community-based early intensive behavioural intervention and specialist nursery provision for children with autism spectrum disorder. *Journal of Child Psychology and Psychiatry, 48*(8), 803–812.

Mandell, D. S., Morales, K. H., Marcus, S. C., Stahmer, A. C., Doshi, J., & Polsky, D. E. (2008). Psychotropic medication use among medicaid-enrolled children with autism spectrum disorders. *Pediatrics, 121*(3), e441–e448.

Maurice, C., Green, G., & Foxx, R. M. (Eds.). (2001). *Making a difference: Behavioral intervention for autism*. Austin, TX: PRO-ED.

May, C. (2010). Retheorizing the clinical encounter: Normalization processes and the corporate ecology of care. In G. Scambler & S. Scambler (Eds.), *Assaults on the lifeworld: New directions in the sociology of chronic and disabling conditions* (pp. 129–145). New York: Palgrave Macmillan.

McDougle, C. J., Brodkin, E. S., Naylor, S. T., Carlson, D. C., Cohen, D. J., & Price, L. H. (1998). Sertraline in adults with pervasive developmental disorders: A prospective open-label investigation. *Journal of Clinical Psychopharmacology, 18*, 62–66.

McDougle, C. J., Naylor, T., Cohen, D., Volkmar, F. R., Heninger, G. R., & Price, L. H. (1996). A double-blind, placebo-controlled study of fluvoxamine in adults with autistic disorder. *Archives of General Psychiatry., 53*, 1001–1008.

McDonough, J. T., & Revell, G. (2010). Accessing employment supports in the adult system for transitioning youth with autism spectrum disorders. *Journal of Vocational Rehabilitation, 32*(2), 89–100.

Medical Home Initiatives for Children with Special Needs Project Advisory Committee. American Academy of Pediatrics. (2002). The medical home. *Pediatrics, 110*(1), 184–186.

O'Neill, R. E., Horner, R. H., Albin, R. W., Storey, D., & Sprague, J. R. (1997). *Functional assessment and program development for problem behavior: A practical handbook*. Pacific Grove, CA: Brooks/Cole.

Ozonoff, S., & Cathcart, K. (1998). Effectiveness of a home intervention program for young children with autism. *Journal of Autism and Developmental Disorders, 28*, 25–32.

Parsons, T. (1965). *Social structure and personality*. New York: Free Press.

Posey, D. J., & McDougle, C. J. (2003). Use of atypical antipsychotics in autism. In E. Hollander (Ed.), *Autism spectrum disorders* (pp. 247–264). New York: Marcel Dekker.

Posey, D. J., Puntney, J. I., Sasher, T. M., Kem, D. L., Kohn, A., & McDougle, C. J. (2004). Guanfacine treatment of hyperactivity and inattention in pervasive developmental disorders: A retrospective analysis of 80 cases. *Journal of Child and Adolescent Psychopharmacology, 14,* 233–242.

Quintana, H., Birmaher, B., Stedge, D., Lennon, S., Freed, J., Bridge, J., & Greenhill, L. (1995). Use of methylphenidate in the treatment of children with autistic disorder. *Journal of Autism and Developmental Disorders, 25,* 283–294.

Rivers, J. W., & Stoneman, Z. (2003). Sibling relationships when a child has autism: Marital stress and support coping. *Journal of Autism & Developmental Disorders, 33*(4), 383–394.

Robinson, C. (2009). What nurses need to know about the "other ASD." *Journal of Specialists in Pediatric Nursing, 14*(3), 155–156.

Sallows, G., & Graupner, G. (2005). Intensive behavioral treatment for children with autism. *American Journal of Mental Retardation, 110,* 417–438.

Scarpinato, N., Bradley, J., Batemen, X., Kurbjun, K., Holtzer, B., & Ely, B. (2010). Caring for the child with an autism spectrum disorder in the acute care setting. *Journal for Specialists in Pediatric Nursing, 15*(3), 1–11.

Schreck, K. A., Williams, K., & Smith, A. F. (2004). A comparison of eating behaviors between children with and without autism. *Journal of Autism & Developmental Disorders, 34*(4), 433–438.

Shortell, S., Gillies, R., Anderson, D., Mitchell, J., & Morgan, K. L. (1993). Creating organized delivery systems: The barriers and facilitators. *Hospital and Health Services Administration, 38*(4), 447–466.

Skinner, B. F. (1953). *Science and human behavior.* New York: Macmillan.

State Board of Nursing of the Commonwealth of Pennsylvania (1977). Pennsylvania State Board of Nursing, Nurse Practice Acts. Retrieved from http://www.samhsa.gov/legislate/Sept01/childhealth_Title31.htm

Steingard, R., & Biederman, J. (1987). Lithium responsive manic-like symptoms in two individuals with autism and mental retardation. *Journal of the American Academy of Child & Adolescent Psychiatry, 26,* 932–935.

Steingard, R. J., Zimnitzky, B., DeMaso, D. R., Bauman, M. L., & Bucci, J. P. (1997). Sertraline treatment of transition-associated anxiety and agitation in children with autistic disorder. *Journal of Child and Adolescent Psychopharmacology, 7,* 9–15.

Stull, A., & Ladew, P. (2010). Safety first for children with autism spectrum disorders. *Exceptional Parent, 40*(4), 54–57.

Testa, M. A., & Simonson, D. C. (1996). Assessment of quality-of-life outcomes. *New England Journal of Medicine, 334,* 835–840.

Timmermans, S., & Haas, S. (2008). Towards a sociology of disease. *Sociology of Health and Illness, 30,* 659–676.

Twoy, R., Connolly, P. M., & Novak, J. M. (2007). Coping strategies used by parents of children with autism. *Journal of the American Academy of Nurse Practitioners, 19*(5), 251–260.

Van Bourgondien, M. E., Reichle, N. C., & Schopler, E. (2003). Effects of a model treatment approach on adults with autism. *Journal of Autism & Developmental Disorders, 33,* 131–140.

Walsh, K. K., & Kastner, T. A. (1999). Quality of health care for people with developmental disabilities: The challenge of managed care. *Mental Retardation, 37*(1), 1–15.

Discussion Questions

I

CHAPTER 1

1. Summarize the arguments for the genetic–environment interaction as the cause of ASD.
2. Compare and contrast the core features of different types of ASDs.
3. Explain the neurobehavioral basis of ASD and give three examples of studies supporting this theory.
4. What are the medical and neurological concerns in evaluating children with ASD? Construct a set of questions to ask a parent to solicit diagnostically useful information.
5. Explain how a nurse may differentiate between focal seizures/staring spells and the absence of eye contact associated with some cases of ASD.
6. Identify a client in your practice area and apply the *DSM-IV* criteria for autism and Asperger's syndrome to determine the likelihood of a diagnosis of ASD. Does your assessment change when DSM-V criteria are applied?

CHAPTER 2

1. Design a continuing education program for staff nurses on polypharmacy in ASD care.
2. When and how often should developmental screening be performed? Recommend the sequence for evaluating a child at age: 6, 9, 12, and 24 months.
3. When and what laboratory tests are indicated for the diagnosis of autism?
4. Compare the psychometric properties of the instruments available to screen for developmental disorders.
5. Prepare an instructional program for parents that presents the causes and risk factors of ASD.
6. Evaluate your position on the role of environmental factors in the cause of ASD.

CHAPTER 3

1. Describe the changing roles for nurses in the care of people with ASD.
2. Propose your nursing philosophy with respect to the care of people with ASD.
3. Analyze safety issues for people with ASD in your practice setting.

4. Observe a clinical situation and apply the principles of TEACCH to set up a modified environment. Suggest some visual structures to accommodate the patient's deficits, visual–motor activities, repetitive tasks, and visual cues.
5. To make true progress within the realm of ASD, it is imperative to not simply focus on the individuals with ASD, but to also address the aspects of society that contribute to their disability. Identify some aspects of a clinical environment, magnetic resonance imaging or mammography suite, labor and delivery room, etc., that contribute to the view that a person with ASD is disabled.
6. Discuss the process for making a differential diagnosis between autism and childhood schizophrenia.
7. Prioritize your nursing interventions according to associated features that may be present in a patient with ASD.

ADDITIONAL CASES FOR PRACTICE

YouTube Video Clips

A Way of Explaining Autism **by Dave Spicer**

Summary:

This video uses the analogy of different types of stones to describe different characteristics of people with autism.

Length of clip: 3:37 min.
Link: http://www.youtube.com/watch?v=ic-zA4YfW-U& feature=related

Discussion questions

1. Discuss the ways that health care institutions/environments attempt to view all people as alike.
2. Describe patients you have encountered who correspond with the different characteristics of each of the stones.
3. Write your own analogy to describe different characteristics of people on the autism spectrum that you have encountered.
4. Answer the questions about the violet stone as they relate to people with autism. Think about a person on the spectrum that you know and their unique characteristics: Is a particular characteristic an asset or a liability? Can it be appreciated and enjoyed, or does it seem to just get in the way? Would the person be better off with or without it?

Thirteen-Month-Old with Facial Tics

Summary:

A 13-month-old boy shows facial tics and arm flapping behaviors when his mother opens a drawer.

Length of clip: 1:05 min.
Link: http://www.youtube.com/watch?v=MLBOZ-MgUuY& NR=1

Discussion questions

1. Describe the behaviors exhibited by this child. What evidence can you list supporting an ASD diagnosis based on this video clip?
2. What environmental factors contribute to his behaviors?
3. What further observations or tests would be helpful or necessary in making a diagnosis for this child?
4. Based on this clip, what other behaviors would you predict this child might exhibit as he develops?
5. Design a nursing staff education program about the early signs and diagnosis of ASD.

Introduction: Nursing Care in Early Childhood and Adolescence

II

Marcia R. Gardner

Autism spectrum disorders (ASD) affect individuals and families worldwide, across all ethnic and racial backgrounds, and across the lifespan. According to the Centers for Disease Control (CDC), about 1% or one in 110 children in the United States had an ASD diagnosis in 2006 (Rice, 2009). Increasing numbers of children *and adults* are being diagnosed with and living with an ASD. The prevalence of autism disorders has increased, even in the short span between 2002 and 2006 (CDC, 2010). Researchers have reported different, and sometimes surprisingly higher, prevalence statistics for autism in other countries (CDC, 2011). In a very recent study, Kim et al. (2011) reported that autism was identified, overall, in 2.64% of children ages seven through 12 living in one community in South Korea. Despite varying epidemiological data and different methodological approaches to estimations of population size, the "take-home message" from these data is that nurses, regardless of specialty, practice setting, educational preparation, or licensure level, will encounter individuals on the autism spectrum and will need to be prepared for their care, as well as for care of their family members.

The increasing numbers of children diagnosed with autism will most certainly lead to an increased number of adults, and adult or aging caregivers, who require specialized health care, along with social and supportive services. As the largest group of health care professionals in the United States and the single group of professionals found in every health care setting from acute care to long-term care to community and home care programs to schools, nurses must, and will, take the lead in developing and providing effective, comprehensive, and personalized health services for individuals with autism across the lifespan. Screening, diagnosis, referral, preventive care and health promotion, medical management, care coordination/case management, family education, counseling, and direct care are only some of the health care services needed by individuals and families affected by autism (Aylott, 2010; Carbone, Behl, Azore, & Murphy, 2009; Elder & D'Alessandro, 2009; Minnes & Steiner, 2009; Siklos & Kerns, 2006). Families of children with autism continue to have unmet needs for specialized services and have less opportunity to access individualized and family-centered health care services than do families of children with other special health care needs (Kogan et al., 2008). With knowledge of the evidence underpinnings for care of children on the autism spectrum, advanced practice nurses can effectively fill this gap.

True "personalization" of nursing care for people on the autism spectrum will take the unique characteristics, patterns, and needs of each person into account. This is not an easy task to accomplish. Individuals with autism experience the world quite differently and often do not comprehend behavior, interaction, and social conventions. They can react with responses ranging from withdrawal to confusion to violent outbursts when exposed to sensations or experiences that most of us would not find particularly confusing or distressing.

To illustrate the experience of autism, a young adult with Asperger's syndrome wrote the following comment in an email:

> Imagine that you are the only person in the world who is able to speak or understand English, and do not know any other languages. What would your life be like? How would you adapt to the outside world and learn to communicate with others? What would everyone else think of you, and how would they act towards you? This is, of course, a hypothetical scenario that is highly unlikely to occur in anyone's life. But for the ... people who have autism spectrum disorders, it is a more reflective description of reality than many people are able to appreciate. (M. J. Gardner, personal communication, April 30, 2011)

The core deficits associated with ASD: impaired communication, impaired social interaction, and a restricted set of interests and/or behaviors, in conjunction with characteristic sensory dysfunction, can make health care encounters challenging (Coplan, 2010; Johnson, Myers, & Council on Children with Disabilities, 2007; Myers, Johnson, & Council on Children with Disabilities, 2007). Many people with autism have disruptive, disturbing, or otherwise maladaptive behavior patterns that are inadvertently elicited and/or reinforced (Myers et al., 2007) by parents, teachers, caregivers, and health care professionals who are acting with good intentions but are unaware of strategies that minimize distress and mitigate difficult or self-destructive behaviors. Many experience great distress in health care settings in which providers do not use best practices for their care or do not adapt the health care environment to the needs of patients with ASD.

Nurses will be challenged to integrate the fast-growing body of research about autism. They will need to understand genetic and prenatal etiologies; early signs; environmental influences and genetic vulnerabilities; evolving pharmacotherapeutic treatments; family burdens, needs, and supports; and social imperatives. Best-practice nursing care will include integrating behavioral management strategies into systems to provide comprehensive, nontraumatic, and evidence-based but personalized health care to individuals on the autism spectrum and, importantly, to their families and caregivers.

Families have long been recognized as crucial in the health care of children with ASD. They should be considered equal team members and an essential voice in the decisions made concerning their children (Powell, Hecimovic, & Christensen, 1992)

Are you prepared to give care to a child with autism (Thorne, 2007)? Section II will introduce the use of case exemplars to study nursing care. Each chapter examines selected health care needs of children and adolescents with ASD. The chapters build on one another, begining with discussion of prenatal issues, and evaluating the ways functional deficits complicate assessment and delivery of health care across childhood and adolescence. Practice settings include the pediatrician's office, inpatient surgery, and an adolescent mental health service. The chapters expand on nursing care of individuals who have significant deficits in sensory processing and communication and focus on the prenatal period, early childhood, and the school years.

Cases illustrate the scope of advanced nursing practice with individuals on the autism spectrum in a variety of health care settings. Chapter 4 focuses on the prenatal period and offers a brief overview of evidence related to genetic etiologies for autism, along with examination of current practice standards for genetic and prenatal testing in high- and low-risk pregnancies, and best practices for prenatal management of women (and their partners) with family histories of developmental disabilities. Theories of family dynamics, health education, and supportive counseling, among others, are integrated as a framework for the care of pregnant women and families who may experience the birth of a child with a developmental disability. Chapter 5 contextualizes case findings and screening for ASD through the case example of a toddler who appears to be deaf. The chapter addresses parental empowerment, developmental surveillance, practice parameters, guidelines, tools to facilitate recognition of risks, identification of "red flags," and effective, accurate screening for ASD in primary-care settings, along with developmental, diagnostic, family, and other considerations. Chapter 6 discusses the role of the advanced practice nurse within the multidisciplinary developmental team and describes the diagnostic processes and treatment strategies used in the case of an 8-year-old child with 22q11.2 deletion syndrome, its associated complex autistic disorder with seizures, and long-standing disruptive and self-injurious behaviors. The underlying genetics, features, and morbidities associated with both autism and 22q11.2 deletion syndrome are examined. Medical and behavioral management strategies, in a best-practices framework, are outlined in the context of this highly complex and challenging case. Chapters 7 and 8 use the case-based approach to explore issues of concern for nursing care of school-aged children and adolescents. Chapter 7 further focuses on nursing strategies to facilitate high-quality care for a child in the hospital after a tonsillectomy. Chapter 8 addresses the care of children with ASD in the school setting, with a focus on the middle-school years. Legal and educational considerations grounded in the Individuals with Disabilities Education Act (Turnbull, Wilcox, & Stow, 2002); current evidence for medication use in the school setting; evidence-based, behavior-management strategies needed for school-based health care; alternative therapies; and family considerations are discussed, along with a best-practice approach.

The goal of Section II is to help the reader establish a deeper understanding of emerging autism science, diagnostic issues, manifestations of the disorder along the autism spectrum, and treatment strategies. With a broadening knowledge base related to ASD, nurses will find themselves better prepared to offer comprehensive and evidence-based care to families, children, and adolescents.

REFERENCES

Aylott, J. (2010). Improving access to health and social care for people with autism. *Nursing Standard, 24*(27), 47–56.

Carbone, P. S., Behl, D. D., Azor, V., & Murphy, N. A. (2010). The medical home for children with autism spectrum disorders: Parent and pediatrician perspectives. *Journal of Autism and Developmental Disorders, 40*(3), 317–324.

Centers for Disease Control and Prevention. (2010). Data and statistics: Prevalence. Retrieved from http://www.cdc.gov/ncbddd/autism/data.html

Centers for Disease Control and Prevention. (2011). Autism prevalence summary table. Retrieved from http://www.cdc.gov/ncbddd/autism/documents/Autism_PrevalenceSummaryTable_2011.pdf

Coplan, J. (2010). *Making sense of autistic spectrum disorders.* New York: Bantam.

Elder, J. H., & D'Alessandro, T. (2009). Supporting families of children with autism spectrum disorders: Questions parents ask and what nurses need to know. *Pediatric Nursing, 35*(4), 240–253.

Johnson, C. P., Myers, S. M., & the Council on Children with Disabilities (2007). Identification and evaluation of children with autism spectrum disorder. *Pediatrics, 120*(5), 1183–1215.

Kim, Y. S., Leventhal, B. L., Koh, Y., Fombonne, E., Laska, E., Lim, E., . . . Grinker, R. R. (2011). Prevalence of autism spectrum disorders in a total population sample. *American Journal of Psychiatry, 168*(9), 904–912. Retrieved from http://ajp.psychiatryonline.org/cgi/reprint/appi.ajp.2011.10101532v1

Kogan, M. D., Strickland, B. B., Blumberg, S. J., Singh, G. K., Perrin, J. M., & van Syk, P. C. (2008). A national profile of the health care experiences and family impact of autism spectrum disorder among children in the United States, 2005–2006. *Pediatrics, 122*(6), e1149–e1158. Retrieved from http://pediatrics.aappublications.org/content/122/6/e1149.full.html

Minnes, P., & Steiner, K. (2009). Parent views on enhancing the quality of health care for their children with fragile X syndrome, autism or Down syndrome. *Child: Care, Health and Development, 35*(2), 250–256.

Myers, S. M., Johnson, C. P., & the Council on Children with Disabilities (2007). Management of children with autism spectrum disorders. *Pediatrics, 120*(5), 1162–1182.

Powell, T. H., Hecimovic, A., & Christensen, L. (1992). Meeting the unique need of families. In D. E. Berkell (Ed.), *Autism: Identification, education, and treatment.* Hillsdale, NJ: Lawrence Erlbaum.

Rice, C. (2009). Prevalence of autism spectrum disorders—Autism and Developmental Disabilities Monitoring Network, United States, 2006. *MMWR Surveillance Summaries, 58*(SS10), 1–20. Retrieved from http://www.cdc.gov/mmwr/preview/mmwrhtml/ss5810a1.htm

Siklos, S., & Kerns, K. (2006). Assessing need for social support in parents of children with autism and Down syndrome. *Journal of Autism and Developmental Disorders, 36*(7), 931–933.

Thorne, A. (2007). Are you ready to give care to a child with autism? *Nursing, 37*(5), 59–61.

Turnbull, H. R., Wilcox, B. L., & Stowe, M. J. (2002). A brief overview of special education law with focus on autism. *Journal of Autism and Developmental Disorders, 32*(5), 479–493.

Caring for the Pregnant Woman With a Family History of Cognitive/Developmental Disabilities

4

Kimberly K. Trout, Karen Blake, and Heather Marozsan

A family history of cognitive/developmental disabilities creates special challenges for the woman who is pregnant and for her family. Whether she is expecting her first child or her fourth, there is often a great deal of anxiety and fear associated with a pregnancy when there is a positive family history of such disabilities. In some cases, genetic testing can help to alleviate fears; however, genetic testing often does not yield any conclusive results. The prenatal care provider should offer the most current information to families regarding prenatal care, genetic screening, and medical testing, as well as offering emotional support and counseling in helping parents to cope with the special challenges they face. When testing results are positive for a genetic condition, the clinician must communicate those results with care and use care in introducing and discussing any treatment options that might be available.

This chapter addresses issues related to prenatal assessment, prenatal testing, and clinical care during pregnancy for families with a history of cognitive/developmental disabilities, with a special emphasis on autism spectrum disorders (ASD), using the case of a pregnant woman with a family history of developmental disorders.

FAMILY CONSIDERATIONS

In a family that has a child who has been diagnosed with a developmental disability, such as an ASD, many of the same fears and concerns that any parents might have about pregnancy might arise. Parents will ask questions about their ability to raise a child and how they will handle the additional responsibilities. Parents might question their readiness to have a child and worry about the risks for each pregnancy, and the health and likelihood of developmental disabilities in the baby. If the new child is affected, will he or she be more or less severely affected than the existing child in the family? If this child is healthy and unaffected, how will they balance the needs of a complex child and the needs of a typical child?

Stress Associated with the Expanding Family

Major life changes for individuals with an ASD can be a source of severe stress and turmoil. In particular, the period involving the birth of a new sibling in a family can be a very stressful time and might create challenges or disrupt already established routines and family dynamics. Whether a family with a child with an ASD is exploring reproductive options or faced with a new pregnancy, nurses at all levels play a critical role helping prepare families for a variety of situations and outcomes. Nurses will refer, provide information, provide anticipatory guidance, facilitate links to information sources, educate, advocate, provide clinical care, and give support to families during this very stressful time (Cole, 2008).

Issues for Extended Family

Parents who care for children with special needs often require extra support. However, many parents report not having strong support communities, especially as related to members of their extended families (Seltzer, Krauss, Orsmond, & Vestal, 2001). Often, they feel isolated because of the sheer demands and responsibilities a child with special needs places on the family. Extended family members might be excluded, uncomfortable, uneducated, and/or misinformed. They might feel helpless and nervous or simply not know what to say or do. Extended family members also need information and resources. Studies have shown that when parents have an adequate support network, levels of stress and anxiety are decreased (Barker et al, 2010; Seltzer et al., 2001). Including, supporting, and educating extended family members through the clinical course of the pregnancy and beyond (with the permission of the pregnant woman and her partner), might enable extended families to become stronger and more supportive networks for parents and children who need them.

Cultural Issues and Prenatal Genetic Testing

Multiple studies have examined the cultural, gender-related, and socioeconomic influences on the perceptions of genetic testing. Studies have explored the use of Western-influenced genetic counseling with diverse populations, including African American, Latino, and Jewish populations (Browner, Preloran, Casado, Bass, & Walker, 2003; Ellington et al., 2006; Kinney, Gammon, Coxworth, Simonsen, & Arce-Laretta, 2010; Raz & Atar, 2003). Findings illustrate the importance of individualized counseling techniques to ensure that information is provided in a form that is understandable to participants and appropriate to their educational levels and cultural context. When providing genetic counseling to members of various ethnocultural groups, nurses must attend to social structures, communication styles, attitudes toward authority, attitudes toward expression of emotions, health care beliefs, migration patterns, and experiences of discrimination (Raz & Atar, 2003).

Kinney and colleagues (2010) noted that the decision to even *seek* genetic testing might be influenced by knowledge, cognitions, emotions, and family communication, as well as sociodemographic and clinical characteristics. The authors asserted that in order to enhance informed decision making about genetic counseling or testing among members of diverse populations, it is important to understand cultural, access, and psychosocial issues that might influence both the use of these health services and communication of genetic information. Kinney and colleagues specifically identified cultural issues surrounding genetic illness, including the stigma associated with the risk of transmitting a disease to a child and the shame associated with a genetic diagnosis. These pose barriers to seeking genetic counseling services. Additional barriers related to these genetic issues included language, fear about immigration status disclosure, fatalism, lack of interest, and lack of knowledge or information. It is very important for the clinician to provide easy-to-interpret materials that use simple words and avoid unnecessarily technical information, along with clear definitions of technical concepts, such as gene and mutation and other technical terms (Kinney et al., 2010).

CASE

Iris Martinez is a 27-year-old who is 11 weeks pregnant with her second child. She and her husband Hector are excited about this child (their first together), but they also have a great

(*Continued*)

CASE (Continued)

deal of anxiety beyond the usual concerns that affect many expectant parents. Iris's 5-year-old son Manuel and her 35-year-old brother are both affected with idiopathic autism, and Iris is aware that there are genetic implications for her unborn baby. Iris states, "I love my son, but I don't know if I can handle taking care of two kids with special needs. Manuel's father is no help at all!" She also states, "I can't go through what my mother does. Her whole life has revolved around my brother." Iris reveals that her mother suffers from many chronic medical problems (that she attributes to stress) and that her mother consistently refused social services and other supportive help for her brother once he completed school. According to Iris, "My mother says that family should take care of their own."

POTENTIAL GENETIC RISKS

This section briefly reviews genetic risks as background in the context of pregnancy care and prenatal testing. Refer to Chapter 2 for a detailed discussion of genetic and epidemiological science related to ASD.

When parents express concern that a child has or can inherit a genetic disorder, it is important to understand the possible mechanisms of inheritance. When one or both parents are identified as "affected" with a genetic disorder, the inheritance pattern might be: (a) autosomal dominant, (b) autosomal recessive, (c) sex-linked dominant, or (d) sex-linked recessive (Hartl & Jones, 2009). When a single-gene (monogenic) trait follows one of these inheritance patterns, it is fairly straightforward to predict the risk for an individual child, unless the disorder is one with variable penetrance. Penetrance refers to the extent to which there is a correlation between an individual's genotype and phenotype. For example, some disorders have very high penetrance, meaning that virtually every individual possessing that genotype manifests the disorder (such as in Huntington disease), whereas in disorders with variable penetrance, there might be other genetic or environmental modifiers that are required for the phenotype to result, such as phenylketonuria (PKU; Davidson, London & Ladewig, 2011; Zlotogora, 2003).

Many disorders do not follow classic Mendelian patterns of inheritance (Mendel, 1866, 1965) and are considered polygenic or multigenic, that is, requiring the joint effects of multiple genes that by themselves would have a relatively small effect. This might be the case with some ASD, although there are several monogenic genetic variations that are associated with an increased incidence of ASD. Only 5% to 10% of cases of ASD are the result of clearly identifiable monogenic disorders (Autism Genome Project Consortium, 2007; Johnson and Myers, 2007), such as Fragile X syndrome, tuberous sclerosis, PKU, Rett syndrome, and Smith-Lemli-Opitz syndrome (Freitag, Staal, Klauck, Duketis, & Waltes, 2010). McMahon, Baty, and Botkin (2006) note that it is important to distinguish between autism that is a component of a known syndrome (e.g., one of those noted above) and idiopathic autism. The majority of cases of ASD are idiopathic. Epidemiological evidence supporting the notion of a genetic etiology for idiopathic autism started with early studies demonstrating high autism concordance rates in monozygotic twins (Bailey et al., 1995; Folstein & Rutter, 1977). Further studies substantiating the genetic hypothesis for ASD found that siblings of individuals with ASD have a higher risk for ASD, as compared with the general population. Recurrence risks range from 2% to 8% for subsequent children of parents who have a child affected with ASD to as high as 60% to 90% for monozygotic twin pairs (Johnson & Myers, 2007; Muhle, Trentacoste, & Rapin, 2004).

Nurses should be knowledgeable about genetic risk factors prior to counseling or caring for a family with a positive history of genetic disorders. The nurse might integrate selected concepts, below, into pregnancy counseling.

Evidence from Linkage Studies

Linkage studies involve genomic analyses of families with individuals known to be affected. A few independent studies have suggested evidence for linkage with ASD on several chromosome regions (see Table 4.1; Liu, Paterson, Szatmari, & the Autism Genome Project Consortium, 2008). Karyotype analysis is usually the first-line genetic test performed in linkage studies, but karyotyping alone will miss smaller genomic deletions, duplications, or copy-number variants (CNVs; Shen et al., 2010). Chromosomal microarray analysis has the ability to detect submicroscopic CNVs. Significant CNVs have been identified in up to 10% of patients with developmental disabilities (Sagoo et al., 2009); however, at this point in time, the presence of a CNV does not predict ASD with enough accuracy to be clinically useful.

Evidence from Genome-wide Association Studies

A genome-wide association study (GWAS) involves genetic testing for multiple gene variants in large population samples (as opposed to a study that is restricted to families with a particular disorder), while looking for genomic associations with a particular disorder. With this approach, there might be less inherent bias. Ascertainment bias, a form of sampling bias,

TABLE 4.1 Selected Chromosomes Identified with ASD in Several Linkage and Genome-wide Association Studies (GWAS)*

Chromosome	Arm	Band/subbands	Common variants noted
2	q	24	*SLC25A12*: mitochondrial/glutamate carrier gene
3	p,q	24–26	*OXTR*: oxytocin receptor gene
4	p	12	GABA-A receptor gene
5	p	14.1–15	Single nucleotide polymorphism (SNP) variants
6	NS	NS	*GluR6*: glutamate receptor 6 gene
7	q	22–36	*RELN*: codes for a signaling protein important in synaptogenesis, cortical layer formation
10	q	23.3	*PTEN*: a tumor suppressor gene
15	q	11–13	GABA receptor genes; 2 deletions, 2 duplications
16	p	11.2	4 deletions, 2 duplications
17	q	NS	*SLC6A4*: serotonin-transporter gene
22	q	13.3	*SHANK3*: gene encoding a synaptic protein
X	p,q	22,13	*NLGN3, NLGN4*: neuroligin genes important in synaptogenesis
Y	NS	NS	*NLGN4Y*: SNP variant

q = indicates locus on long arm of chromosome

p = indicates locus on short arm of chromosome

NS = not specified in study results

Loci are identified by (1) Chromosome number (2) Chromosome arm (3) Band/sub-band pattern, e.g. 3p24-26 for the OXTR gene

*(Freitag et al., 2010; Shen et al., 2010)

can falsely inflate estimates of heritability when families are self-selected based on attributes (Guo, 1998; Rao, Wette, & Ewens, 1988). Two independent GWASs that investigated genomic markers for ASD found single-nucleotide polymorphisms (SNPs) on gene loci 5p14.1 (carrying a small increased risk of ASD with an odds ratio of 1.2) and 5p15 (carrying a protective effect against ASD with an odds ratio of 0.6; Freitag et al., 2010).

Refer to Table 4.1 for a summary of current information regarding selected chromosomal loci and genes that have been identified from linkage studies and GWASs.

Mitochondrial DNA

Mitochondrial DNA (different from nuclear DNA) is inherited only through maternal cells. Mitochondrial DNA inheritance is associated with several known disorders, such as mitochondrial myopathy, encephalopathy, lactic acidosis, stroke, and Leber optic atrophy (Blakely et al., 2005). Mitochondrial DNA mutations can alter the brain's ability to meet critical energy demands and have been associated with schizophrenia, bipolar disorder, and major depressive disorder (Rollins et al., 2009).

Mitochondrial DNA has recently been associated with ASD as well (Giulivi et al., 2010). In an observational study involving children ages 2 to 5 years from a subset of children involved in the Childhood Autism Risk from Genes and Environment study in California, two significant mitochondrial variations were noted in 10 children with autism versus 10 control children: (a) Reduced nicotinamide adenine dinucleotide oxidase activity in lymphocytic mitochondria was seen in children with autism when compared with controls ($p = .001$). (b) Children with autism had higher mitochondrial rates of hydrogen peroxide production when compared with controls ($p = .01$; Giulivi, et al., 2010). What is not apparent from the study is whether the mitochondrial differences found were due to genetic variations or occurred for other reasons, such as oxidative stress from environmental conditions. Further study in this area is warranted before any conclusions can be drawn.

Potential Environmental Risks

Fetal alcohol spectrum disorder, the most common preventable form of intellectual disability, can be prevented by avoidance of alcohol during pregnancy (Centers for Disease Control and Prevention, 2005). Fetal alcohol syndrome is associated with an ASD diagnosis in a small percentage of individuals (Aronson, Hagberg, & Gillberg, 1997). Since many women do not have their first prenatal appointment until well into the first trimester (i.e., after the critical period of fetal organogenesis has passed), nurses should use every opportunity to convey important information about avoidance of teratogens, such as alcohol, to all women of childbearing age.

Epidemiological studies are investigating other possible environmental risks for ASD. These include parental age, environmental toxins, and extreme prematurity, among others (Croen et al., 2008; Mercer, Creighton, Holden, & Lewis, 2006; Price et al., 2010). A recent study found an increased odds ratio (3.39) of having a child with an ASD when there were short interpregnancy intervals (<12 months) than there were with interpregnancy intervals of $\geq$36 months (Cheslack-Postava, Liu, & Bearman, 2011). The researchers suggest nutritional factor depletion as a possible mechanism to explain the increased risk for ASD when there is close pregnancy spacing, along lines similar to the association of folic acid deficiency and increased risk for neural tube defects (Blom, 2009). There is a need for additional research on this topic.

Researchers are also concerned about the interaction of genetic and environmental risks. In a large epidemiological study of twins, Hallmyer et al. (2011) found that concordance rates for ASD in dizygotic twin pairs were substantial, with 31% for male ($n = 45$) pairs and

36% for female ($n = 13$) pairs. Concordance rates were higher than those for siblings, yet lower than those for monozygotic twins. The findings suggest that factors in the shared intrauterine environment might be significant in the development of ASD. This study contributes further evidence to support the hypothesis of fetal origins for several neurodevelopmental disorders (Bale et al., 2010).

CLINICAL APPROACH

Ideally, all women who contemplate pregnancy should receive preconception counseling. For the family with a history of cognitive and developmental disabilities, preconception counseling assumes even greater importance. In addition, families at high risk for genetic disorders should meet with a genetic counselor prior to pregnancy to discuss specific genetic risks, available testing, and options for care.

Initial Prenatal Consultation and Assessment of Genetic Risks

Although preconception counseling should be provided for high-risk families, only 10% of families with a child with an ASD seek genetic counseling for a subsequent pregnancy (Selkirk, Veach, Lian, Schimmenti, & LeRoy, 2009). The initial genetic assessment often occurs with the prenatal visit after a woman first discovers that she is pregnant. The prenatal assessment should always begin with a thorough family history that accounts for the genetic pedigree. This includes asking questions about any first- or second-degree relatives on both maternal and paternal sides for any genetic disorders, birth defects, intellectual or developmental disabilities, premature deaths, or stillbirths. Constructing a three-generation family pedigree is important for identification and documentation of disorders (see Figure 4.1).

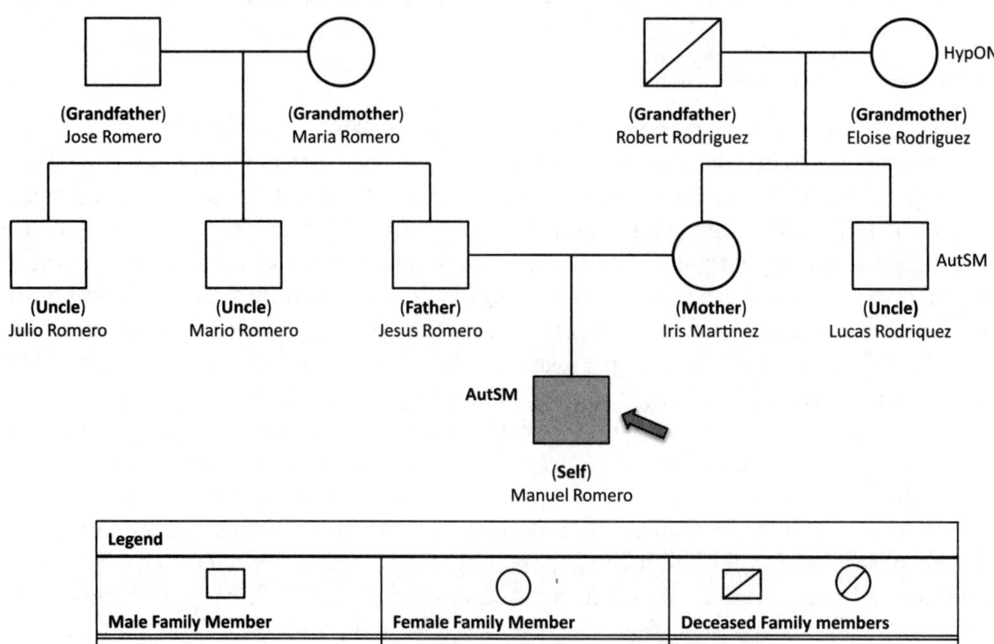

FIGURE 4.1 ■ Sample of a three-generation family pedigree.

TABLE 4.2 ■ Screening during Pregnancy

Test	Optimal timing	Results	Conditions	Association with cognitive disability/ASD
Rubella titer	Preconception or at initial prenatal visit	Positive, negative or equivocal: If nonimmune, avoid prenatal exposure; follow titers if exposure occurs; immunize prior to conception or postpartum	Fetal rubella	Yes
Sequential screen OR multiple-marker screen	10 to 13 weeks gestation	Risk for Trisomies 18, 21, neural tube defects		Yes
	15 to 20 weeks gestation	Risk for Trisomies 18/21, neural tube defects		Yes
Anatomy screen ultrasound	19 to 21 weeks gestation	Positive, negative, or inconclusive	Microcephaly neural tube defects Phenotypic features of some syndromes, (e.g., trisomies)	Yes

Genetic counselors might not be available to some clients, particularly in rural areas or resource-poor settings. Therefore, all prenatal-care nurses should be familiar with currently available genetic screening and testing options. Table 4.2 describes screening tests that are available for the general population (i.e., for individuals without a positive family history and who will be less than 35 years of age at the time of the infant's birth). Table 4.3 lists the procedures that are offered as the standard of care for individuals at high risk for genetic disorders (i.e., those with a positive family history and/or those who will be ≥35 years of age at the time of birth).

CASE–CONTINUED

Ms. Martinez was seen for preconception counseling to discuss several potential family history concerns, most notably a 5-year-old son and a 35-year-old brother with severe autism. Other areas of concern include: a maternal uncle with a history of a "bleeding problem" (not sure of exact diagnosis), paternal grandfather with type 2 diabetes, a mother with chronic hypertension, and on Hector's side of the family, a cousin with thalassemia. Ms. Martinez's ethnic background is Puerto Rican Latina (White), her husband is Mexican Latino, Italian, and African American (White and Black). No Jewish, Cajun, or French Canadian ancestry is reported.

Genetic Counseling Report

Ms. Martinez has a normal 46, XX karyotype. Her son was tested and found to have a normal 46, XY karyotype. Manuel does not have tuberous sclerosis or Fragile X

(Continued)

CASE (Continued)

syndrome and Ms. Martinez is not a carrier for Fragile X syndrome. They both also had a normal chromosome microarray analysis. Microarray analysis would have identified a 15q13.2q13.3 or 16p11.2 deletion or duplication (both associated with ASD). Microarray analysis would also have identified an Xq28 microdeletion (associated with hemophilia). Ms. Martinez screened negative for 32 common cystic fibrosis mutations. Ms. Martinez's rubella Immunoglobulin G antibody titer is 3.42, indicating rubella immunity. Complete blood count results revealed normal mean corpusular volume (MCV; 92.1); therefore, it is unlikely that she is a carrier for thalassemia.

Communicating Results of Genetic Testing

One of the most important events in genetic testing is the communication of results to patients (Daly et al., 2001; Gaff et al., 2007; Kasparian, Meiser, Butow, Job, & Mann, 2006). Effective communication is necessary for the sharing of accurate information between patients and nurses and can promote adherence with follow-up testing and potential treatment regimens. Communicating and understanding risks, or probabilities, related to genetic testing, has been an ongoing challenge for health care professionals and patients, respectively. Misunderstanding of genetic risks might lead to psychosocial harms or might significantly impact individual and family decisions (Kasparian et al., 2006). Unfamiliarity with genetic concepts and terminology, as well as preconceived perceptions of personal and familial risk, might pose barriers to understanding genetic test results. It is also important for health professionals to understand the reactions of patients during the process of communicating test results and to recognize that the personal meaning of a result is framed by many contexts, including the ethnic, cultural, and spiritual environments of the individual, family, and community.

Gettig (2010) described the need for the genetic counselor or provider to also fulfill the role of bereavement specialist when families grieve for the loss of their fantasized child. In this privileged role as a grief counselor, the provider must understand the grief process and be able to provide anticipatory guidance, as well as recognize the grieving family, the presence of unresolved grief, and when it is necessary to provide counseling or refer appropriately.

Providers must also understand that grief is a normal and natural reaction to any type of loss, including the loss of the idealized "perfect child." The processes of grief have been described in many works, but the most recognized and widely used is the "five stages of grief" outlined by Dr. Elisabeth Kübler-Ross (2005). Kübler-Ross proposed these stages of grief:

- *Denial:* "This cannot be happening to me."
- *Anger:* "Why is this happening to me?"
- *Bargaining:* "Please I will do anything to make this go away."
- *Depression:* "It doesn't matter anyway."
- *Acceptance:* "It is all going to be okay."

Understanding the stages of grieving helps providers appreciate their patients' responses when confronted with positive results for a genetic disorder. It is also important to recognize that there is no timetable or predictable pattern for the mourning process. Each person's process is unique, and it is not unusual for the active stages of grieving to last 1 or 2 years or longer

TABLE 4.3 ■ Testing for High-Risk Individuals

Procedure	Timing	Results	Conditions	Association with cognitive disability/ASD
Carrier testing (blood test)	Preconception or at initial prenatal visit	Positive or negative (If both parents are carriers, there is a 25% chance of having an affected child for autosomal-recessive disorders)	Cystic fibrosis, Tay-Sachs disease, sickle cell anemia, thalassemias, Canavan disease, Bloom syndrome, familial dysautonomia, mucolipidosis type IV, Niemann-Pick disease, Fragile X	For some of these disorders
Chorionic villus sampling	10 to 11 weeks	Positive or negative		
Amniocentesis	15 to 20 weeks	Positive or negative		
Maternal serum alpha-fetoprotein (will be needed if patient had chorionic villus sampling)	15 to 20 weeks	Risk for neural tube defects	Neural tube defects	Yes

(Kübler-Ross, 2005). Guided by such a model, providers are able to educate patients, validating their emotions and comforting them with the knowledge that they are not alone (Gettig, 2010).

Avoid Misleading Communication

Research has shown that the delivery of genetic test results to patients can significantly alter their initial reactions and levels of anxiety, as well as their ability to understand and cope with the genetic findings (La Pean & Farrell, 2005; Marteau et al., 2000; Yoshino, Takahashi, & Kai, 2008). While anxiety has been found to be associated with prenatal genetic testing and subsequent counseling, Ng, Lai, and Yeo (2004) argued that providing patients with risk stratification does not make them more anxious. In contrast, their study showed that appropriate communication and follow-up was found to reduce anxiety.

La Pean & Farrell (2005) looked at the initial report of newborn screening results delivered by medical residents to parents of newborns. The authors reported that the initial message communicated to parents was crucial to parental understanding and was in line with the ideology of "primacy effect" (p. 1499). This is the concept that the first message one hears is most effectively stored in long-term memory, because of the greater amount of time devoted to processing. In this study, the first few messages often began with unclear information and used clichéd phrases (e.g., "I have good news and bad news"; La Pean & Farrell, 2005). The authors found that the "clarifying information" usually was not provided until one-fifth of the counseling was completed. Unclear communication content and the time lag before clarification of information might complicate processes of parental understanding and heighten anxiety.

Methods of Communicating Risk

Interpretation of risk is fundamental to decision making about the use of prenatal genetic testing and relevant follow-up care. National practice standards, as articulated by the American College of Obstetricians and Gynecologists (ACOG), include offering all pregnant women screening for Down syndrome, Trisomy 18, and neural tube defects, regardless of age (ACOG, 2007). Screening test results typically provide a personalized risk estimate based on factors that include maternal age, nuchal translucency measurement, and levels of analytes, such as alpha-fetoprotein, estriol, beta-human chorionic gonadotropin, and pregnancy-associated plasma protein A (Gates, 2004).

A survey of antenatal clinics in England and Wales found that the most common and effective way of presenting negative or low-risk test results to pregnant women who had undergone serum screening for Down syndrome was as a phrase (e.g., low risk, lower risk), rather than a number (Nagle, Hodges, Wofe, & Wallace, 2009). Edwards and colleagues (2006) also asserted that there is limited evidence that the use of individualized risk estimates in screening programs promotes or achieves improvement in informed decision making. Previous studies of prenatal risk interpretation showed that less than two-thirds of women were able to correctly compare numeric results expressed similarly (Edwards et al., 2006; Nagle et al., 2009). A qualitative study of 15 women in Japan demonstrated that some women do not understand maternal serum screening, and in particular found that the ratios and statistics associated with the testing could be overwhelming and confusing to them (Yoshino, Takahashi, & Kai, 2008). Such differences, along with patients' literacy and numeracy levels, can substantially impact the effectiveness of genetic counseling. Eichmeyer and colleagues (2005) have shown that Hispanic women exhibit lower comprehension of numerical presentations of risk when compared with non-Hispanic Whites and suggest that qualitative representations could improve the effectiveness of risk communication. Graphical presentation of risk probabilities can also increase understanding of test results (Elder, Ayala, Parra-Medina, & Talavera, 2009).

Conversely, in a study examining anxiety levels in pregnant women undergoing amniocentesis, Ng and colleagues (2004) argued that risk information is necessary for patients to make informed decisions and does not cause increased or long-term anxiety. The researchers suggest that to assist a pregnant woman to make an informed decision, risk stratification and other information should be provided accurately, comprehensively, and objectively (Ng, Lai, & Yeo, 2004).

Communication Protocol

A six-step protocol for communication of distressing information (Buckman, 1992) has been modified by Daly and colleagues (2001) into an evidence-based protocol to communicate genetic test results to families. A protocol of this type can help nurses develop their own processes for communicating genetic test results effectively and compassionately. The protocol provides guidelines that focus on the patient, patient reactions, and appropriate responses and interventions. Exhibit 4.1 illustrates the protocol in the context of ASD.

The first step in any discussion of health matters is the preparatory phase of communication. The nurse makes decisions regarding environment (location, privacy, comfort), approach (face to face, presence of support persons), and length of time set aside for discussion, questions, and provision of supportive counseling. The next step is to assess the patient's background knowledge related to the issue or condition. This requires planning, concentration, and active listening by the provider. The posing of appropriate questions followed by careful listening and astute observation of patient behaviors will help the nurse appreciate the patient's understanding of the situation and current emotional status and might help guide further discussion. Nurses should then assess the amount and complexity of information the patient wishes or is able to receive. In some cases, patients might not wish to hear all of the information at once or even might not be ready to hear results of genetic tests at all. Daly and colleagues (2001) explain this as ascertaining the "level" of information the patient needs at this point. Step 4 focuses on the effective delivery of the genetic testing results in order to promote understanding of the data, as well as the relationships between results and immediate and future patient risk. This step involves educating the patient based on his or her existing knowledge. Strategies for effective delivery of information can include: using nonmedical language; offering information in small "bytes"; frequently evaluating understanding; and reinforcing, reexplaining, and clarifying information. It is also important to assess understanding by asking the individual to explain the general "drift" of what has been said and to have written or recorded material available for future reference.

Then, consider the patient's response or reaction to the information. Are there signs of excess distress? According to Daly and colleagues (2001), important criteria for assessment of such reactions include social acceptability (is the reaction within the bounds of cultural and social norms?); adaptability (does the patient's reaction increase or decrease the individual's distress?); and "fixability" (if the reaction increases the patient's distress, can the nurse intervene?). Finally, assist the patient in establishing a plan for the next steps. Ensure that the patient is aware of resources, such as genetic counselors, emotional support groups, and Internet sites, that are available once they leave the office. Evaluate the patient's own resources for further care.

EXHIBIT 4.1

Communicating Genetic Test Results

Outline of Six-Step Strategy to Better Communication

Step 1: Getting started

- Consider communication format.
- Choose appropriate setting.
- Allow adequate time for discussion and questions.

Step 2: How much does the patient know about Autism Spectrum Disorders (ASD)?

- What is your understanding of Autism?
- Do you have any questions about ASD?

Step 3: How much does the patient want to know?

- Ask for a clear invitation t disclose information.

Step 4: Sharing genetic testing information

- Explain the meaning of your test results in a sensitive but straightforward manner
- Avoid medical jargon or euphemisms
- Pause frequently and allow time for understanding and questions.
- Do not minimize the condition or situation.
- Avoid the phrase, "I am sorry."

Step 5: Responding to feelings

- Acknowledge feelings and reactions, which can be varied.
- Be supportive, remind patients that their response is normal.

Step 6: Planning and follow-through

- Refer family members to local genetic counselor.
- Establish a plan including emotional and practical support.

Adapted from Daly, M.B, Barsevick, A., Miller, S.M., Buckman, R., Costalas, J., Montgomery, S. & Bingler, R. (2001). Communicating genetic test results to the family: A six-step skills-building strategy. *Family & Community Health, 24*(3), 13–26.

ASSESSMENT OF FAMILY DYNAMICS AND SUPPORT SYSTEMS

Parenting a child on the autism spectrum is often a difficult and lifelong task. Children with ASD experience disturbances and deficits in core areas of communication and social interactions and exhibit stereotypical patterns of behaviors and interests (American Psychiatric Association, 2000). There is an extremely wide continuum of function, with countless degrees of expression and mild to severe concerns. Accepting the initial diagnosis and then coming to grips with the day-to-day needs of the child can be an agonizing journey for a family. Many children will have lifelong medical, psychological, behavioral, educational, and caregiving needs. Their needs will evolve and change as they age into adulthood (Johnson & Myers, 2007). Managing these complex needs only adds to the stress and demands of caring for these children and adults with special needs. Despite sometimes overwhelming challenges, children and adults with ASD have great strengths and can bring very unique contributions and joy to their families and communities.

Family Dynamics Related to Pregnancy

Emotional attachment to a new baby begins well before birth. From the time of seeing or hearing the fetal heartbeat, feeling the first kicks, or even earlier, families begin to attach emotionally to this new human being. The process of attachment that normally begins during pregnancy might be delayed or disrupted in the family with a history of cognitive disabilities or ASD, especially while there are prenatal diagnostic tests pending or if an abnormality is found. Hedrick (2005) noted that while increased information about a pregnancy from prenatal testing is generally viewed as positive in our Western culture, there can be many paradoxical feelings experienced if a fetal abnormality is discovered. It might be helpful for the prenatal nurse to encourage the pregnant woman and her family to discuss openly any fears and concerns that they might have during prenatal visits. Listening, maintaining a caring presence, and allowing family members to express their feelings are key elements of comprehensive nursing care.

Demands and Needs of Families

It has been speculated by some that raising a child on the spectrum is more stressful than caring for a child with other medical or developmental conditions (Bouma & Schweitzer, 1990; Myers & Johnson, 2007; Seltzer et al., 2001, 2009). The lack of reciprocal emotions, inappropriate responses, and issues in developing relationships can make parenting more difficult (Bouma & Schweitzer, 1990; Davis & Carter, 2008). If the child is medically complex and/or has difficult or disruptive behaviors, physical exhaustion can contribute to parental stress. Parents with a child or children on the spectrum have higher rates of poor mental health, anxiety, depression, and even divorce (Hartley et al., 2010; Herring, Gray, Taffe, Tonge, Sweeney, & Einfeld, 2006; Montes & Halterman, 2007; Seltzer et al., 2009). The chronic stress and demands of caring for these complex children can also affect the physical health of caretakers, especially mothers (Hartley et al., 2010; Seltzer et al., 2001, 2009). Chronic stress during pregnancy can increase the risk of several pregnancy complications, including infant prematurity and low birth weight (Schetter, 2011). Understanding family dynamics is crucial if nurses want to optimize their impact in order to help. Nurses should carefully assess the family and particularly consider issues such as:

- Was the child with special needs recently diagnosed?
- Where is the family in their journey to get help for their child?
- What have their experiences been with respect to access to specialized care?
- What supports are available for the pregnant woman, partner/spouse, and child with special needs?

We know much about the core disturbances of the spectrum disorders, yet each child is unique and might have unique autistic manifestations. The very nature of these disorders poses

EXHIBIT 4.2

PREGNANCY, GENETICS, AND FAMILY-RELATED RESOURCES FOR NURSES AND FAMILIES

- American Academy of Pediatrics: http://www.aap.org
- Autism Society of America: http://www.autism-society.org
- Autism Speaks: http://www.autismspeaks.org
- Centers for Disease Control and Prevention, Autism Information Center: http://www.cdc.govncbddd/autism/index.mtm
- First Signs: http://firstsigns.org/index.html
- Gene Tests: Website that offers information about available tests for genetic conditions, as well as a directory of certified clinical laboratories that perform the tests. www.ncbi.nlm.nih.gov/sites/GeneTests
- Genetic Science Learning Center: Website that offers educational services about many genetic conditions. http://learn.genetics.utah.edu/
- Online Mendelian Inheritance in Man (OMIM): Online catalog of human genetic disorders that is updated regularly. www.ncbi.nlm.nih.gov/omim
- March of Dimes: Website with preconception/prenatal resources. www.marchofdimes.com
- Maternal and Child Health Library, Knowledge Path: Autism Spectrum Disorders http://www.mchlibrary.info/knowledgepaths/kp_autism.html
- My Family Health Portrait: Website resource that offers advice on constructing a family pedigree. www.familyhistory.hhs.gov
- National Society of Genetic Counselors: Website provides information about how to find a genetics counselor, as well as identifying services families can expect. www.nsgc.org
- Sibling Support Project of the Arc of the United States / Sibshops http://www.thearc.org/siblingssupport

uncertainty for the future. The challenges children with ASD and their families face will evolve and change. Life circumstances, family dynamics, and age will impact on symptoms, possibly leading to exacerbations and might result in development of new concerns. It is crucial for nurses to ensure that parents receive accessible support services (see Exhibit 4.2).

Sibling Considerations

Preparing a child for the birth of a new sibling is a challenging task, even under the best of circumstances. It is inherently more difficult for a child with an ASD, not in small part because a child with an ASD will typically have problems adjusting to even the smallest environmental changes. The birth of a sibling can create an overwhelming level of stress that might require additional resources and support. Parents might also seek information about the possible influences of a developmentally challenged child on a typically developing sibling. Addressing the needs of a sibling in a family where there is a cognitively, physically, or developmentally challenged child might create additional parenting concerns, yet there can also be many rewards for family, parents, and siblings (Orsmond & Seltzer, 2007). Relationships between siblings are unique, and play an important role in promoting competency with interpersonal relationships. As children grow and develop, sibling relationships evolve, but they can be altered by family dynamics. The sibling relationship might be the longest-lasting one in a family. It is important to keep in mind that a sibling might be involved in the life of the special needs person longer than anyone else, long after parents die and extended family members pass away. Many studies have shown that siblings of children with special needs are at higher risk for developing psychosocial problems, adjustment disorders, internalization disorders, and depression (Orsmond & Seltzer, 2007). Feelings of confusion, anger, resentment, and isolation are also seen in siblings of challenged children (Bagenholm & Gillberg, 1991). However, many of these special siblings exhibit higher degrees of empathy, tolerance, and protectiveness than siblings of typical children. (Bagenholm & Gillberg, 1991). They might tend to be pleasers or overachievers and conflict-avoidant (Winter, 2006). It is important to remember that the needs, feelings, and relationships of siblings will change as they age. A young child will respond to a sibling with ASD differently than an adolescent or an adult will. Nurses should remind parents of developmental considerations, needs, and issues at various developmental stages for both the typical sibling and the sibling with an ASD. Some organizations offer programs to support families and siblings of special needs children, such as specialized sibling workshops (Sibling Support Project of the Arc of the United States, 2011). Nurses can assist parents in supporting siblings of children with autism using age-appropriate strategies such as these:

- Make sure information is honest, up-to-date, and at a developmentally appropriate level.
- Provide opportunities to meet and interact with other children or adolescents who have special needs siblings.
- Encourage family time and family outings.
- Encourage honest expression of feelings. Let the child know that it is acceptable to feel sad, resentful, or even angry with situations related to the special needs brother or sister. They do not have to hide their feelings. Their feelings matter!
- Provide opportunities for the sibling to have a voice in decision making when appropriate. Incorporate their opinions in discussions and planning.
- Ensure one-on-one time with the typically developing sibling. This time will allow for focused parental attention and can foster communication and enhance relationships in the family.
- Be careful not to expect the child or adolescent to act as a primary caregiver for the child with ASD. As siblings age, they often assist in supervising or caring for the special needs sibling or performing family chores. It is important to ensure a healthy balance of *developmentally appropriate* family responsibility, while respecting the developmental needs and concerns of the of the special sibling.
- Recognize that the needs of the special needs sibling will change as he or she ages and during times of stress or periods of family change.
- Do not be afraid to seek outside help or professional support (Winter, 2006).

BEST PRACTICES: NURSING PLAN OF CARE

CASE–CONTINUED

The obstetrics/gynecology nurse practitioner is seeing Ms. and Mr. Martinez for their first prenatal visit. They share with the advanced practice nurse that they were confused about the genetic testing results as explained by the genetic counselor. They request another explanation of those results, and want to know the steps to take for the remainder of the pregnancy.

Primary Care/Obstetrics Approach

The nurse caring for the Martinez family explained the genetic testing results. The test was negative. No genetic markers for autism were found; however, this did not rule out the possibility of this unborn child being affected, as genetic markers are often not found with idiopathic autism. Also, although tuberous sclerosis is an autosomal-dominant disorder, up to 75% of cases are the result of spontaneous mutations (Simonoff, 1998) and therefore cannot be ruled out for this pregnancy. The nurse informed Ms. Martinez of the availability of prenatal diagnosis of fetal aneuploidy by either chorionic villus sampling or amniocentesis. There was a discussion of the risks, benefits, alternatives, and limitations of CVS and amniocentesis. Because the risk of miscarriage with transabdominal CVS or amniocentesis ranges from 1 in 100 to 1 in 300 pregnancies (Cunningham et al., 2010), Ms. Martinez has elected not to have these procedures.

Additional genetic testing was offered. Ms. Martinez elected to have sequential screening for Down syndrome, Trisomy 18, and open neural tube defect risk estimates. The ultrasound for nuchal translucency and first blood draw were scheduled. The second blood draw will be scheduled between 16 to 18 weeks gestation. Also, Ms. Martinez will have a Level II ultrasound at 20 weeks for a fetal anatomy screen. She will also have hemoglobin electrophoresis done to rule out any hemoglobinopathies. If Ms. Martinez is identified as having the trait for thalassemia, her husband should also be tested, because this disorder has an autosomal-recessive inheritance pattern, and the child will have the disease only if both parents are carriers of the genetic defect.

As part of the usual plan of care, the nurse advised the parents on the avoidance of teratogens, gave them information on potential risks and exposures, and encouraged the mother-to-be to continue taking prenatal vitamins, especially if she is not able to eat a large variety of fruits and vegetables.

Other Clinical Issues

The nurse recommended additional psychotherapeutic counseling, because she had concerns about the spousal relationship, level of emotional support, and extended family issues. The parents were worried about their ability to balance the needs of a new baby with the complex needs of an older sibling who is affected with an ASD. The nurse prepared material to prepare the child for the arrival of the new sibling. Finally, the nurse gave the parents a checklist of developmental milestones to be used as a guide and advised that developmental screening is an effective way to identify problems that might be ameliorated with early intervention. It is also important to consider cultural issues that influence expectations and willingness to seek and accept help.

SUMMARY

There are many challenges related to family life to overcome when there is a family history of an ASD or other developmental disability. In families in which another child is due, these challenges will only increase. Expectant parents, or parents contemplating future children, will benefit from effective support networks that might include nurses, colleagues, friends, and extended family members, among others. Referral for genetic screening and other prenatal testing, and provision of clear information related to genetic risk is imperative. Linking families to legitimate sources of information and services will help to decrease stress and anxiety. It is also important to consider family communication patterns, extended family issues, and culture, as well as the needs of typically developing siblings and those of extended family members. Using evidence-based, clinical strategies, including standards of prenatal care, referrals, counseling, education, and effective communication, nurses can help optimize parent and family strengths as they prepare to welcome a newly born member to their family and continue to care for their special needs child.

REFERENCES

American College of Obstetricians and Gynecologists. (2007). Screening for fetal chromosomal abnormalities. In: *Practice Bulletin No.77*. Washington, DC: Author.

American Psychiatric Association. (2000). *Diagnostic and Statistical Manual of Mental Disorders* (4 ed.). Washington, DC: Author.

Aronson, M., Hagberg, B., & Gillberg, C. (1997). Attention deficits and autistic spectrum problems in children exposed to alcohol during gestation: A follow-up study. *Developmental Medicine and Child Neurology, 39*(9), 583–587.

Autism Genome Project Consortium. (2007). Mapping autism risk loci using genetic linkage and chromosomal rearrangements. *Nature Genetics, 39*(3), 319–328.

Bagenholm, A., & Gillberg, C. (1991). Psychosocial effects on siblings of children with autism and mental retardation: A population based study. *Journal of Mental Deficiency Research, 35*, 291–307.

Bailey, A., LeCouteur, A., Gottesman, I., Bolton, P., Simonoff, E., Yuzda, E., & Rutter, M. (1995). Autism is a strongly genetic disorder: Evidence from a British twin study. *Psychological Medicine, 25*, 63–77.

Bale, T. L., Baram, T. Z., Brown, A. S., Goldstein, J. M., Insel, T. R., . . . Nestler, E. J. (2010). Early life programming and neurodevelopmental disorders. *Biological Psychiatry, 68*, 314–319.

Barker, E. T., Hartley, S. L., Seltzer, M. M., Floyd, F. J., Greenberg, J. S., & Orsmond, G. I. (2010). Trajectories of emotional well-being in mothers of adolescents and adults with autism. *Developmental Psychology*, December 20 [online]. doi: 10.1037/a0021268

Blakely, E. L., de Silva, R., King, A., Schwarzer, V., Harrower, T., Dawidek, G., Turnbull, D. M., & Taylor, R. W. (2005). LHON/MELAS overlap syndrome associated with a mitochondrial MTND1 gene mutation. *European Journal of Human Genetics, 13*, 623–627.

Blom, H. J. (2009). Folic acid, methylation and neural tube closure in humans. *Birth Defects Research, 85*(4), 295–302.

Bouma, R., & Schweitzer, R. (1990). The impact of chronic childhood illness on family stress: A comparison between autism and cystic fibrosis. *Journal of Clinical Psychology, 46*(6), 722–730.

Browner, C. H., Preloran, H. M., Casado, M. C., Bass, H. N., & Walker, A. P. (2003). Genetic counseling gone awry: Miscommunication between prenatal genetic service providers and Mexican-origin clients. *Social Science & Medicine, 56*, 1933–1946.

Buckman, R. (1992). *How to break bad news: A guide for health care professionals* (pp. 65–97). Baltimore, MD: Johns Hopkins University Press.

Centers for Disease Control and Prevention. (2005). Surgeon General's advisory on alcohol use in pregnancy. *Morbidity and Mortality Weekly Report, 54*, 229.

Cheslack-Postava, K., Liu, K., & Bearman, P. S. (2011). Closely spaced pregnancies are associated with increasing odds of autism in California sibling births. *Pediatrics, 127*(2), 246–253.

Cole, L. L. (2008). Autism in school- age children. *Advance for Nurse Practitioners, 16*(3), 38–47.

Croen, L. A., Goines, P., Braunschweig, D., Yolken, C. K., Yoshida, C. K., Grether, J. K., & ...Van de Water, J. (2008). Brain-derived neurotrophic factor and autism: Maternal and infant peripheral blood levels in the Early Markers for Autism (EMA) Study. *Autism Research, 1*(2), 130–137.

Cunningham, F. G., Leveno, K. J., Bloom, S. L., Hauth, J. C., Rouse, D. J., & Spong, C. Y. (2010). Prenatal diagnosis and fetal therapy. In *Williams Obstetrics* (23 ed., chap. 13). Retrieved 05/28/11 from http://www.accessmedicine.com/content.aspx?aID=6021591

Daly, M. B., Barsevick, A., Miller, S. M., Buckman, R., Costalas, J., Montgomery, S., & Bingler, R. (2001). Communicating genetic test results to the family: A six-step, skills-building strategy. *Family & Community Health, 24*(3), 13–26.

Davidson, M. R., London, M. L., & Ladewig, P. A. (2011). Special reproductive concerns: Infertility and genetics. In M. R. Davidson, M. L. London, & P. A. Ladewig , *Olds' Maternal-Newborn Nursing & Women's Health Across the Lifespan* (9 ed., pp. 242–276). Upper Saddle River, NJ: Pearson Prentice Hall.

Davis, N. O., & Carter, A. S. (2008) Parenting stress in mothers and fathers of toddlers with autism spectrum disorders: Associations with child characteristics. *Journal of Autism and Developmental Disabilities, 38*, 1278–1291.

Edwards, A. G., Evans, R., Dundon, J., Haigh, S., Hood, K., & Elwyn, G. J. (2006). Personalised risk communication for informed decision making about entering screening programs. *Cochrane Database of Systematic Reviews, 4*, 1–8.

Eichmeyer, J. N., Northrup, H., Assel, M. A., Goka, T. J., Johnston, D. A., & Williams, A. T. (2005). An assessment of risk understanding in Hispanic genetic counseling patients. *Journal of Genetic Counseling, 14*, 319–328.

Elder, J. P., Ayala, G. X., Parra-Medina, O., & Talavera, G. A. (2009). Health communication in the Latino community: Issues and approaches. *Annual Review of Public Health, 30*, 227–251.

Ellington, L., Baty, B. J., McDonald, J., Venne, V., Musters, A., Roter, D., ... Croyle, R. T. (2006). Exploring genetic counseling communication patterns: The role of teaching and counseling approaches. *Journal of Genetic Counseling, 15*(3), 179–189.

Folstein, S., & Rutter, M. (1977). Infantile autism: A genetic study of 21 twin pairs. *Journal of Child Psychology and Psychiatry, 18*(4), 297–321.

Freitag, C. M., Staal, W., Klauck, S. M., Duketis, E., & Waltes, R. (2010). Genetics of autism disorders: Review and clinical implications. *European Child & Adolescent Psychiatry, 19*, 169–178.

Gaff, C. L., Clarke, A. J., Atkinson, P., Sivell, S., Elwyn, G., Iredale, R., Thornton, H., Dundon, J., Shaw, C., & Edwards, A. (2007). Process and outcome in communication of genetic information within families: A systematic review. *European Journal of Human Genetics, 15*(10), 999–1011.

Gates, E. A. (2004). Communicating risk in prenatal genetic testing. *Journal of Midwifery & Women's Health, 49*(3), 220–227.

Gettig, E. (2010). Grieving: An inevitable journey. In B. S. LeRoy, P. M. Veach, & D. M. Bartels (Eds.), *Genetic counseling practice: Advanced concepts and skills* (pp. 95–124). Hoboken, NJ: Wiley-Blackwell.

Giulivi, C., Zhang, Y.-F., Omanska-Klusek, A., Ross-Inta, C., Wong, S., Hertz-Picciotto, I., Tassone, F., & Pessah, I. N. (2010). Mitochondrial dysfunction in autism. *JAMA, 304*(21), 2389–2396.

Guo, S-.W. (1998). Inflation of sibling recurrence-risk ratio, due to ascertainment bias and/or overreporting. *American Journal of Human Genetics, 63*, 252–258.

Hallmyer, J., Cleveland, S., Torres, A., Phillips, J., Cohen, B., Torigoe, T., ... Risch, N. (2011). Genetic heritability and shared environmental factors among twin pairs with autism. *Archives of General Psychiatry* [Advance online publication]. doi: 10.1001/Archgenpsychitry.2011.76

Hartl, D. L., & Jones, E. W. (2009).Transmission genetic: The principle of segregation. In D. L. Hartl, & E. W. Jones , *Genetics: Analysis of genes and genomes* (7 ed., pp. 77–112). Boston, MA: Jones and Bartlett.

Hartley, S. L., Barker, E. T., Seltzer, M. M., Floyd, F., Greenberg, J., Orsmond, G., & Bolt, D. (2010). The relative risk and timing of divorce in families of children with an autism spectrum disorder. *Journal of Family Psychology, 24(4)*, 449–457.

Hedrick, J. (2005). The lived experience of pregnancy while carrying a child with a known, nonlethal congenital abnormality. *JOGNN, 34*(6),732–739.

Herring, S., Gray, K., Taffe, J., Tonge, B., Sweeney, D., & Einfeld, S. (2006). Behaviour and emotional problems in toddlers with pervasive developmental disorders and developmental delay: Associations with parental mental health and family functioning. *Journal of Intellectual Disability Research, 50*(12), 874–882.

Johnson, C. P., & Myers, S. M. (2007). Identification and evaluation of children with autism spectrum disorders. *Pediatrics, 120*(5), 1183–1215.

Kasparian, N. A., Meiser, B., Butow, P. N., Job, R. F., & Mann, G. J. (2006). Better the devil you know: High-risk individuals' anticipated psychological responses to genetic testing for melanoma susceptibility. *Journal of Genetic Counseling, 15*(6), 433–447.

Kinney, A. Y., Gammon, A., Coxworth, J., Simonsen, S. E., & Arce-Laretta, M. (2010). Exploring attitudes, beliefs, and communication preferences of Latino community members regarding *BRCA* $\frac{1}{2}$ mutation testing and preventative strategies. *Genetics in Medicine, 12*(2), 105–115.

Kübler-Ross, E. (2005). *On grief and grieving: Finding the meaning of grief through the five stages of loss.* New York: Simon & Schuster.

La Pean, A., & Farrell, M. H. (2005). Initially misleading communication of carrier results after newborn genetic screening. *Pediatrics, 116*, 1499–1505.

Liu, X.-Q., Paterson, A. D., Szatmari, P., the Autism Genome Project Consortium (2008). Genome-wide linkage analyses of quantitative and categorical autism subphenotypes. *Biological Psychiatry, 64*, 561–570.

Marteau, T. M., Saidi, G., Goodburn, S., Lawton, J., Michie, S., & Bobrow, M. (2000). Numbers or words? A randomized controlled trial of presenting screen negative results to pregnant women. *Prenatal Diagnosis, 20*, 714–718.

McMahon, W. M., Baty, B. J., & Botkin, J. (2006). Genetic counseling and ethical issues for autism. *American Journal of Medical Genetics, 142C*, 52–57.

Mendel, G. (1866). Versuche uber Pflanzen-Hybriden. *Verhandlungen des naturforschenden Vereines in Brünn, 4*(1), 3–47.

Mendel, G. (1965). *Experiments in plant hybridization. (Translation made by the Royal Horticultural Society of London).* Cambridge: Harvard University Press.

Mercer, L., Creighton, S., Holden, J. J. A., & Lewis, M. E. S. (2006). Parental perspectives on the causes of an autism spectrum disorder in their children. *Journal of Genetic Counseling, 15*(1), 41–50.

Montes, G., & Halterman, J. S. (2007). Psychological functioning and coping among mothers of children with autism: A population-based study. *Pediatrics, 119*(5), 1040–1046.

Muhle, R., Trentacoste, S. V., & Rapin, I. (2004). The genetics of autism. *Pediatrics, 113*(5), e472–e486.

Myers, S. M., & Johnson, C. P. (2007). Management of children with autism spectrum disorders. *Pediatrics, 120*(5), 1162–1182.

Nagle, C., Hodges, R., Wofe, R., & Wallace, E. M. (2009). Reporting down syndrome screening results: Women's understanding of risk. *Prenatal Diagnosis, 29*, 234–239.

Ng, C. C. M., Lai, F. M., & Yeo, G. S. H. (2004). Assessment of maternal anxiety levels before and after amniocentesis. *Singapore Medical Journal, 24*(8), 370–374.

Orsmond, G. I., & Seltzer, M. M. (2007). Siblings of individuals with autism spectrum disorders across the life course. *Mental Retardation and Developmental Disabilities Research Reviews, 13*, 313–320.

Price, C. S., Thompson, W. W., Goodson, B., Weintraub, E. S., Croen, L. A., Hinrichsen, V. L., ... DeStefano, F. (2010). Prenatal and infant exposure to thimerosal from vaccines and immunoglobulins and risk of autism. *Pediatrics, 126*(4), 656–664.

Rao, D. C., Wette, R., & Ewens, W. J. (1988). Multifactorial analysis of family data ascertained through truncation: A comparative evaluation of two methods of statistical inference. *American Journal of Human Genetics, 42*, 506–515.

Raz, A. E., & Atar, M. (2003). Nondirectiveness and its lay interpretations: The effect of counseling style, ethnicity and culture on attitudes towards genetic counseling among Jewish and Bedouin respondents in Israel. *Journal of Genetic Counseling, 12*(4), 313–332.

Rollins, B., Martin, M. V., Sequeira, A., Moon, E. A., Morgan, L. Z., Watson, S. J., ... Vawter, M. P. (2009). Mitochondrial variants in schizophrenia, bipolar disorder, and major depressive disorder. *PLoS One, 4*(3), e4913.

Sagoo, G. S., Butterworth, A. S., Sanderson, S., Shaw-Smith, C., Higgins, J. P., & Burton, H. (2009). Array CGH in patients with learning disability (mental retardation) and congenital anomalies: Updated systematic review and meta-analysis of 19 studies and 13, 926 subjects. *Genetics in Medicine, 11*(3), 139–146.

Schetter, C. D. (2011). Psychological science on pregnancy: Stress processes, biopsychosocial models, and emerging research issues. *Annual Review of Psychology, 62*, 531–538.

Selkirk, C. G., Veach, P. M., Lian, F., Schimmenti, L., & LeRoy, B. S. (2009). Parents' perceptions of autism spectrum disorder etiology and recurrence risk and effects of their perceptions on family planning: recommendations for genetic counselors. *Journal of Genetic Counseling, 18*, 507–519.

Seltzer, M. M., Greenberg, J. S., Hong, J., Smith, L. E., Almeida, D. M., Coe, C., & Stawski, R. S. (2009). Maternal cortisol levels and behavior problems in adolescents and adults with ASD. *Journal of Developmental Disorders*, November 5 [Online] doi: 10.1007/s10803-009-0887-0

Seltzer, M. M., Krauss, M. W., Orsmond, G. I., & Vestal, C. (2001). Families of adolescents and adults with autism: Uncharted territory. *International Review of Research on Mental Retardation*, *23*, 267–294.

Shen, Y., Dies, K. A., Holm, I. A., Bridgemohan, M. D., Sobeih, M. M., Caronna, M. D., . . . Autism Consortium Clinical Genetics/DNA Diagnostics Collaboration. (2010). Clinical genetic testing for patients with autism spectrum disorders. *Pediatrics*, *125*(4), e727–e735.

Sibling Support Project of the Arc of the United States. (2011). Sibshops. Retrieved from http://www.thearc.org/siblingssupport

Simonoff, E. (1998). Genetic counseling in autism and pervasive developmental disorders. *Journal of Autism and Developmental Disorders*, *28*(5), 447–456.

Winter, J. (2006). *Breakthrough parenting for children with special needs: Raising the bar of expectations.* San Francisco, CA: Jossey-Bass.

Yoshino, M. A., Takahashi, M., & Kai, I. (2008). The trick of probabilities: Pregnant women's interpretations of maternal serum screening results in Japan. *Nursing and Health Sciences*, *10*(1), 23–30.

Zlotogora, J. (2003). Penetrance and expressivity in the molecular age. *Genetics in Medicine*, *5*(5), 347–352.

Finding What We're Looking for: Evidence-Based Early Identification and Nursing Care of Young Children at Risk for Autism Spectrum Disorders

5

Marcia R. Gardner

Over the past decade, autism spectrum disorders (ASD) have commanded increasing attention in both the lay media and professional literature. Families, educators, therapists, mental health workers, and health care professionals from all disciplines, and across countries and continents, have developed greater sensitivity to the risks for autism, the crucial nature of early and accurate diagnosis in children, characteristics and comorbidities associated with autism, risks and benefits of behavioral and medical treatments, and the needs of individuals and families who "live" the diagnosis of autism every day. Autism advocacy groups have influenced health care research funding, as well as health care guidelines (Autism Speaks, 2010; Johnson & Myers, 2008; Interagency Autism Coordinating Committee, 2011). There are a growing number of instruments to assess risk for, and accurately diagnose, the spectrum of autistic disorders. Autism-tendency screens for "self-assessment" are freely available on the Internet (see, for example, the online Autism Quotient [Baron-Cohen, Wheelwright, Skinner, Martin & Clubley, 2001] at http://aq.server8.org/). Many screening and diagnostic instruments are undergoing further validation on a variety of populations and in a variety of languages. The climate of care for people with ASD has changed. Pediatric clinicians and researchers are focused increasingly on earlier diagnosis and earlier, intensive intervention. Sir John Lubbock, a nineteenth- and early twentieth-century British scientist and Member of Parliament, is often quoted. His comment, "What we do see depends mainly on what we look for" (Lubbock, 1892, p. 3), helps us to remember that we have to look for ASD. Without close attention to the subtle signs of ASD in our patients and clients, their conditions and needs can go unrecognized, and critical opportunities to promote optimal growth, development and health will be missed.

The intent of this chapter is to empower nurse clinicians in primary care and other settings to assess young children for autism risks, identify those at high likelihood of an autism diagnosis, develop familiarity with screening and diagnostic tools, and facilitate the earliest intervention possible once an autism diagnosis is made. In addition to an evidence base related to autism, nurses will certainly need a therapeutic, family-centered approach to educate, support, refer, and directly care for families and children on the autism spectrum. These processes are examined in the context of the case of Amir, a toddler who initially presents in the pediatric clinic with absence of language and maternal concerns about possible deafness.

BACKGROUND

A broad array of clinical characteristics is associated with ASD. These disorders—autistic disorder, Asperger's syndrome (AS), and pervasive developmental disorder–not otherwise specified (PDD-NOS) —represent only three of the five pervasive developmental disorders described in the *Diagnostic and Statistical Manual of Mental Disorders, Fourth Edition, Text Revision* (*DSM-IV-TR*; American Psychiatric Association [APA], 2000). The others are Rett syndrome and childhood disintegrative disorder (APA, 2000). Criteria for the diagnosis of autistic disorder are related to three core areas: disrupted social interaction; impaired, delayed, or abnormal communication; and restricted interests, activities, and behaviors. In addition, emergence of dysfunctional social interaction, language, or imaginative or pretend play must be present prior to 3 years of age. Diagnostic criteria for AS involve two core areas: social interaction and behavioral, activity, and interest patterns (APA, 2000). PDD-NOS is characterized by fewer or less severe signs (Nadel & Poss, 2007). See Section I for further discussion of characteristics of ASD.

The photograph in Figure 5.1 illustrates the lack of protodeclarative pointing as a component of joint attention. In the photo, the child does not attend to the parent who is pointing out something that should be of interest to the child.

At the turn of the twenty-first century, the American Academy of Pediatrics (AAP), the American Academy of Neurology (AAN) and the Child Neurology Society (CNS) developed and disseminated two sets of practice standards for developmental surveillance of children and autism screening of at-risk young children in primary care (AAP, 2001; Filipek et al., 2000; Johnson & Myers, 2008). The purpose was to facilitate earlier identification of autism/ASD in children. The AAP guidelines were revised in 2006 and endorsed again in 2010. The AAN guidelines recommend developmental surveillance and developmental screening, plus screening for ASD in young children at risk. The most recent set of primary-care practice standards, developed by the AAP in 2006, involve ongoing developmental surveillance for ASD and scheduled developmental screening (ages 9, 18, and 24 to 30 months), plus *universal* screening of (all) toddlers for ASD at ages 18 and 24 months (Johnson & Myers, 2008; Johnson, Myers, & the Council on Children with Disabilities, 2007). Practice standards also involve parent education and support, as well as evidence-based management of children diagnosed with ASD. The AAP, in addition, created a comprehensive toolkit for clinicians to use in order to implement this standard of care (AAP, 2007; Johnson & Myers, 2008; Johnson, Myers, & the Council on Children with Disabilities, 2007; Myers, Johnson, & the Council on Children with Disabilities, 2007).

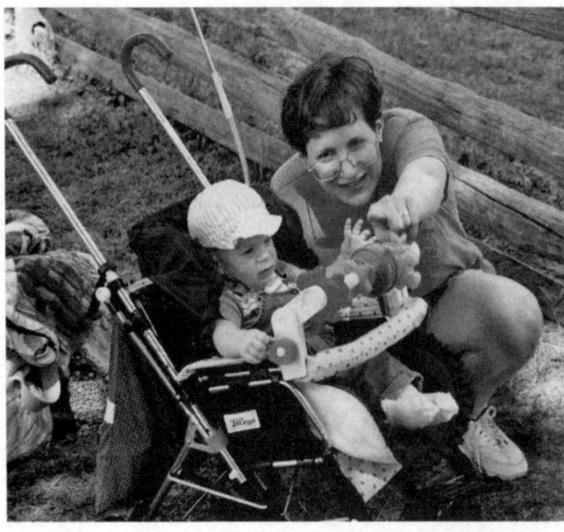

FIGURE 5.1

Universal screening of toddlers for ASD risks should promote much earlier identification of children with autism, but the full picture will emerge as evidence from full integration of the practice standard is available. Even with universal screening, considering limitations of screening tools, cross-sectional screening at only two age points, and the challenge of recognizing subtle indicators in the highest-functioning children, some children with ASD will not be identified during the screening process (Fombonne, 2009). Primary care–based surveillance for indicators of developmental problems and risk-based screening for ASD should continue throughout childhood. Teachers, school nurses, and other individuals who have close contact with older children often recognize characteristics of ASD in students, and can help to identify and refer them for diagnosis and appropriate management. Hepburn et al. (2008) reported 93% to 95% concordance between teacher identification of children with characteristics associated with ASD and respective children's ratings on an autism-screening tool after teachers received a list of manifestations of ASD.

Although universal screening is diffusing into primary care, and despite recent attention to behavioral manifestations associated with risk, it is understood that children already past the toddler years have not been monitored with the same vigilance. Diagnosis of ASD has occurred later than the most optimal time. Shattuck and colleagues (2009) studied a cohort of over 2,500 children who met criteria for the diagnosis of an ASD in 2002. The unadjusted median age for diagnosis at that time was 5.7 years (adjusted age: >6 years), and age at diagnosis varied with gender, cognitive level, and developmental regression. Slightly more than one-fourth of the cohort meeting the criteria were not identified with an ASD diagnosis through age 8 years. Researchers have reported variations in age at diagnosis and prevalence linked to other variables, including ethnicity, race, and socioeconomic status (Durkin et al., 2010; Mandell et al., 2010). Mandell et al. (2010) additionally noted a trending decrease in age of diagnosis across the course of their study.

Earlier initiation of treatment has been noted to be associated with improved outcomes in the core domains of social interaction, communication, and cognitive functioning. Therefore, it is crucial to identify and refer children with autism for intensive intervention services as early as possible (Wetherby et al., 2008). While autism is a critical focus of surveillance and screening, another benefit is that children with other developmental disabilities can also be recognized and referred for appropriate services through these improved and more structured approaches to well-child care.

CASE

Amir is an 18-month-old boy brought to the pediatric clinic by his mother for the first time. Amir and his parents relocated to the area about 6 months ago so that his father could take a new job. He had his last checkup immediately prior to the move, at approximately 12 months of age. At that time, he received the scheduled set of immunizations. His mother is able to provide maternity and birth medical records and an official immunization record, but not his pediatric chart. According to his mother, he has been well since the move. However, she tells the nurse practitioner (NP) that she is concerned because "Amir doesn't seem to hear me when I talk to him. He's not talking at all, and he doesn't pay much attention, or even look up when I call his name. I'm worried that he has a hearing problem or that he's deaf. His day care teacher told me to check on this, because he acts the same way at the day care center and she thinks he needs his hearing checked."

(*Continued*)

CASE (Continued)

Family Composition/Social History

Amir is the first child in the family. He lives with biological father, aged 39, and biological mother, aged 38. There are no other individuals in the home. Maternal and paternal grandparents, and other family members, live at a distance. Both parents speak English and use English as the primary language at home. Mother is employed part-time. Amir attends an employer-sponsored day care center. The family has health insurance and a prescription plan.

Pertinent Family History

No health problems in either parent. Mother is not aware of any maternal or paternal relatives with ASD, attention deficit hyperactivity disorder (ADHD), cognitive impairment, learning disabilities, seizures, or other neurological conditions.

Birth and Neonatal History

Amir is the product of an uncomplicated 38-week pregnancy. There was no pertinent maternal or prenatal medical history. Maternal medications by report included only vitamins and home-brewed teas as a sleep aid. Maternity records provided by the mother show that Amir was born by cesarean section due to fetal distress and meconium-stained fluid. APGAR scores were 7 at 1 minute and 9 at 5 minutes. Suctioning and blow-by oxygen were required in the delivery room. Birthweight was 3.2 kilograms (7 lb, 1 oz; 25th percentile); length and head circumference were each plotted in the 25th percentile on growth curves. He was discharged on day 4, along with his mother. His mother states that he was an "easy" baby. The rest of the neonatal history is unremarkable.

Medical History

Mother reports frequent "ear infections" in his first year, which were treated with antibiotics. She reports that he has no history of seizures, tremors, staring spells, or tics. He takes no medications or vitamins. Immunizations are up to date.

Developmental History

Amir rolled over at 4 months and sat independently at 8 months; he walked alone at 14.5 months. There is no history of babbling or use of words; he uses cries, squeals, and grunts ("unh, uhn, uhn"). He did not learn to wave "bye-bye" or play "peek-a-boo" games. Amir uses very few gestures, but will occasionally try to pull his mother in the direction of something he wants to have. He plays for long periods by himself and infrequently looks for his mother or caregiver at school. He sleeps through the night in a crib and has no "lovey" or transitional object. He frequently likes to hold one particular metal spatula from the kitchen.

Nutrition

Amir finger-feeds, and drinks from a bottle, but cannot use a spoon independently. He refuses to transition from a bottle to a cup. His diet is restricted primarily to rice,

(*Continued*)

CASE (Continued)

chicken bits, crackers, and applesauce. Foods with soft textures, including tofu, bananas, eggs, hot cereals, or yogurt, are not well tolerated. Intake of these can result in gagging, spitting, or vomiting. Although he sits well, he has refused to sit in a toddler seat at the table and will cry until placed back in his high chair.

Pertinent Physical Exam Findings

Amir's weight and height are at the 50th percentile; his head circumference plots between the 75th and 90th percentiles. A high, arched palate; very slightly posteriorly rotated ears (bilaterally); and mild cheilitis are noted. Otherwise head/ears/eyes/nose/throat findings are unremarkable. Mild diaper dermatitis is present, but no other cutaneous lesions are noted. Cardiovascular, respiratory, gastrointestinal, genitourinary, and neurological function exams are grossly normal. Significant social and communication atypicalities are observed during the exam: low affect, language delay, minimal interaction/eye contact with mother, no response to his name—although he stops and attends to the beeping sound of the automatic blood pressure cuff being used right outside his exam room. Several attempts to engage joint response attention by both his mother and the NP ("Amir, look at this!" with tapping of his arm to get his attention) fail.

KEY CLINICAL ISSUES

Currently, there are no biological or physical tests to diagnose ASD. Identification of children with any of the ASD variants is based on observed behavioral characteristics. When parents, teachers, or caregivers are astute observers, they generally recognize concerning or atypical behaviors in children and can bring these to the attention of a child's primary-care provider, even before scheduled screening occurs. Clinicians also must have a high index of suspicion when parents communicate developmental concerns or when they, themselves, note behavioral, communication, social, or other developmental deviations from normal.

Developmental Parameters

Most, if not all, clinicians working with children are quite familiar with growth and development theories, including the interplay of maturation, physiological conditions, environment, and development. Most will embrace a clinical approach that acknowledges the interactions of multiple developmental variables and their influences on developmental progress. Prenatal, genetic, health, environmental, and family factors, such as preterm birth, genetic programming, acute or chronic illnesses, nutrition, and family dysfunction can interfere with the developmental progress of a child and can provide the context for a developmental delay. Flexibility in applying developmental parameters is needed, but nurse clinicians should be aware of, and act immediately, when they notice red flags for ASD. Many conditions (e.g., cerebral palsy, neurological insult, cognitive impairment, or extreme prematurity) account for developmental deviations. On the other hand, certain conditions (e.g., tuberous sclerosis [TS], Fragile X syndrome) are associated directly with autistic disorder (see "Associated Conditions and Signs" and Chapter 6). Clinicians need to comprehensively assess young children's prenatal, birth, and health histories, consider current and past illness, look for comorbid conditions, and be cognizant of the physical, social, and family environments in which development plays out for each child. Clinicians should not automatically rule out ASD simply because other conditions that influence development or account for developmental lags are present.

Pediatric clinicians in primary-care settings should be well-versed in child development and highly skilled in the assessment of achievement of developmental milestones. An organized approach using a valid tool promotes accurate evaluation, and especially helps to avoid missing important signs of developmental or related health disorders. Glascoe and Dworkin (1993) discussed the possibility of bias and inaccuracy when informal clinical judgment, rather than a standardized tool, is used for developmental monitoring or surveillance. Developmental surveillance is addressed in more detail beginning on page 117 in the section entitled Developmental Supervision—Surveillance.

Indicators of ASD, including such signs as atypical responsiveness, abnormal postures and facial expressions, atypical play, staring, lack of gaze orientation, and aversion to affectionate touch are evident during infancy (Baranek, 1999; Clifford, Young & Williamson, 2007). Parents often recall these early signs after the child has been given an ASD diagnosis. Research has documented that many recognizable signs of ASD, including those that are more clearly perceptible to parents, emerge during the second year of life (De Giacomo & Fombonne, 1998; Ozonoff et al., 2010).

Lack of emotional reciprocity might first be noticed as a dull or low affect, as illustrated in Figure 5.2.

Whether all children with ASD, or just some, demonstrate manifestations of autism during infancy has not yet been determined. Regardless, the toddler years are crucial in terms of language and social development. Developmental tasks of toddlers include, among others, mastery of communication, consolidation of motor skills, and deepening of skills related to interpersonal interaction and emotion. Social and communication deficits of ASD interfere with these developmental processes, which are important for evolution of a theory of mind [TOM] (Broderick & Blewitt, 2010). This is a component of social-cognitive ability, allowing a child to recognize that others have different thoughts, perceptions, emotions, and experiences than they do (Korkmaz, 2011). TOM is present in normal preschoolers. Although rudimentary, TOM is believed to be active between 13 and 15 months; researchers hypothesize that between 18 and 24 months, toddlers begin to better understand that other people are separate from themselves, which they demonstrate through joint attention behaviors and beginning pretend or imaginative play (Korkmaz, 2011). In light of these findings, it is particularly important for nurses to be familiar with the developmental

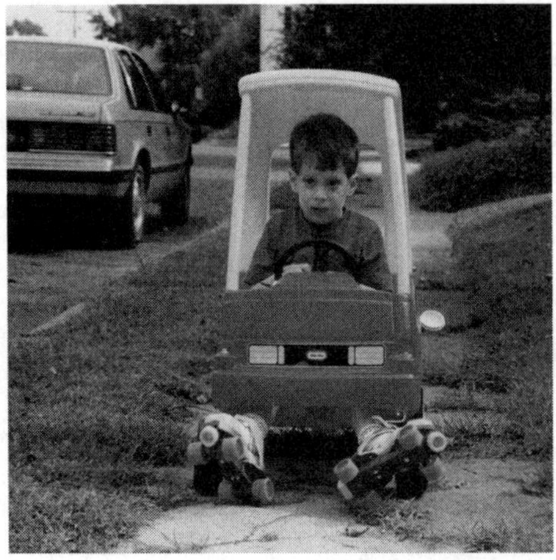

FIGURE 5.2

parameters of the toddler period. See Table 5.1 for an example of toddler developmental milestones related to core problems associated with ASD.

Critical Indicators for Autism in Young Children

Any child who has not begun to babble or gesture by 12 months of age, who has no words at 16 months, or who demonstrates developmental regression, such as losing language skill, should be considered at very high risk for a developmental disorder and immediately referred for further evaluation by the developmental team (Johnson, Myers, & the Council on Children with Disabilities, 2007; see Exhibit 5.1).

Indicators of risk for an ASD diagnosis in very young children include social unresponsiveness, absence of joint attention, delay, atypicality, or absence of language skills, including odd prosody, repetitive or odd movements, posturing, atypical motor skills, and atypical play (Exhibit 5.2). Absence of language and related questions about a child's hearing, as described by Amir's mother, are often the initial concerns that focus attention on developmental lags and risks (Chawarska et al., 2007). The Early Language Milestone Scale-2 (Coplan, 2010) can be used to assess the degree of language development in infants and toddlers up to 3

TABLE 5.1 ■ Typical Developmental Achievements at 18 and 24 Months by ASD Core Indicators

Core indicator	By 18 months	By 24 months
Social	Responds to name Has developed joint attention Follows a point and gaze ("Look at that!") Brings objects to show Acts to share pleasure/happiness Comforted by caregiver Shows affection	Plays near age-peers Tries to engage other children (giving a toy)
Communication/ language	Uses/understands eight to 10 words (receptive language > expressive) Has many gestures Indicates wants Imitates words and actions Points to object when it is named	Uses/understands 50 words (may understand more) Uses self-initiated short phrases and two-word questions Uses "mine," calls self by name Follows one- to two-step commands Knows body parts
Fine motor	Self-feeds, holds own spoon Builds 3- to 4-block tower Scribbles and looks at paper	Hand preference Builds 6- to 8-block tower Imitates line, attempts circle Throws ball overhand
Gross motor	Walks well Runs Still falls	Kicks ball Walks up stairs Better coordination, without falling
Play	Imitative Symbolic play with single-action pretend play (gives doll a bottle) Engages with caregiver in play	Symbolic, multiaction pretend play Engages with caregiver in play Aware of/enjoys playing near other children

Based on Ball, Bindler, & Cowen (2010); Boyd & Bee (2012); Kyle (2008); Wilson (2011).

EXHIBIT 5.1

Critical Indicators for Developmental Disabilities

Absence of babbling by 12 months
Lack of gestures by 12 months
Lack of words by 16 months
Absence of independently generated two-word phrases by 24 months
Language or skill regression

Based on Filipek et al. (2000); Wetherby et al. (2004).

years and can be used in older children with language delays. It is not a diagnostic tool, but was designed to assist primary-care and community providers to quickly determine progress in language development (Coplan, 2010).

The absence of joint attention is an important indicator of risk. Joint attention refers to behaviors associated with sharing interest in an object or situation with another. It is theorized to be important in the development of communication and language. Abnormal joint attention is correlated with ASD diagnoses and is associated with poorer language skills (Delinicolis

EXHIBIT 5.2

Risk Indicators for ASD in Infants and Toddlers

Absence of or atypical joint attention
Atypical gaze
Atypical or absent orientation to name
Limited manifestations of pleasure and positive affect
Decreased frequency of social smiling
Limited social responsiveness and/or social interest
Language delay or absence (receptive and expressive), language regression (also delayed or minimal babbling, absent reciprocality)
Unusual prosody
Low frequency and limited type of gestures
Lack of responsiveness to voice; might attend to other auditory stimuli (hearing seems inconsistent)
Delayed achievement of motor milestones and/or atypical motor skills (also repetitive actions; stereotypic behaviors can be present, but usually appear later)
Repetitive movements and/or posturing
Delay in or absence of imitative behaviors
Atypical play with toys; attachment to unusual objects
Sibling with ASD

Based on Esposito, Venuti, Apicella, & Muratori (2010); Johnson, Myers, & the Council on Children with Disabilities (2007); Matson, Mahan, Kozlowski, & Shoemaker (2010); Naber et al. (2008); Ozonoff et al. (2010); Sullivan et al. (2007); Weismer, Lord, & Esler (2010); Wetherby, et al. (2004); Zwaigenbaum et al. (2009).

& Young, 2007; Sullivan et al., 2007). Receptive attention or response to joint attention (RJA) is demonstrated when an infant or toddler follows a point (or gaze) initiated by a parent or other adult, looking alternately between the object and the parent's face (e.g., "Amir, look at this!" as in the case above).

At about 8 months, infants are typically able to follow a parent's gaze (gaze monitoring). The ability to follow a point is present by about 10 to 12 months of age. RJA requires an ability to understand the other person's intent (i.e., to look in that direction, to see something). Toddlers then develop expressive joint attention (initiation of joint attention [IJA]). First, they will point at things that they want. Next, at about 14 to 16 months, toddlers use protodeclarative pointing in order to share their interest or pleasure in something with another person (Johnson, Myers, & the Council on Children with Disabilities, 2007; Sullivan et al., 2007). For example, a child might be excited to see a bird at the park, and point at it, in order to direct his mother's attention to the bird, to share his pleasure, and monitor her response. This can be accompanied by verbalizations. Absence of or abnormal joint attention is an important marker of risk for autism in infants and young children (Johnson, Myers, & the Council on Children with Disabilities, 2007; Sullivan et al., 2007; Naber et al., 2008). The Modified Checklist for Autism in Toddlers, or M-CHAT (Robins, Fein, Barton, & Green, 2001), a widely used, 23-item, parent reporting risk screen for ASD in children ages 16 to 30 months contains items reflective of joint attention. (A failure on two critical items or three items total indicates the need for further evaluation for ASD).

Echolalia (repeating verbatim phrases and sentences) is often seen in children with autism. For example, a young child with echolalia could respond to the question, "Would you like a cookie?" by repeating the entire phrase or most of it, as in "You like a cookie?" Phrases or words can be repeated hours or days after being heard (delayed echolalia). Children might repeat sentences, strings of dialogue from videos or television, or songs. The absence of spontaneously generated phrasing is a sign of atypical language development associated with ASD. Some research links echolalia with lower levels of receptive language ability in children with autistic disorder (Roberts, 1989). Clinicians should be aware that echolalia occurs normally in infants and young toddlers as they are developing language and syntax, but should fade over time (Johnson, Myers, & the Council on Children with Disabilities, 2007). By 24 months, children should have clear patterns of self-initiated short phrases (see Table 5.1). Additional behavioral patterns associated with an ASD diagnosis include rigid attention to routines, motor mannerisms, self-injurious behaviors, preoccupation with moving or spinning objects, aggression and tantrums, hyper- or hyposensitivity to sensations, and hyperactivity (Johnson & Myers, 2008).

Importance of Parental Observations, Impressions, and Concerns

Parents of young children are crucially important informants, because they are very familiar with their children's developmental progress and behaviors. They are the "experts" on their own children. To help parents recognize developmental deviations associated with autism risk and take action as early as possible (and to facilitate parenting confidence and competence in general) it is important that they have a practical understanding of usual, typical, normal early childhood behaviors, beginning with developmental milestones (Bethell, Peck, & Schor, 2001; De Giacomo & Fombonne, 1998; Rowe, 2006).

Combs-Orme, Nixon, and Herrod (2011) reported that only about 11% of a convenience sample of parents/caregivers of young children from six primary-care settings recalled receiving anticipatory guidance about development. Bethell, Peck, and Schor (2001) found variations in amount and type of guidance provided to parents related to health plan, parenting experience (i.e., whether a first-time parent), and several demographic factors. They also concluded that a greater focus on such anticipatory guidance is indicated in health care settings. Parental observations of behavior and development are important in the screening process for ASD, since some screens involve parental reporting of behaviors. Health care encounters in primary care should always include anticipatory guidance about health, growth, and development, and providers should encourage parents to ask questions about child development, to include developmentally supportive activities in family life, and to observe their children's responses and behaviors. Many resources are available to help parents or other primary caregivers learn about expected developmental milestones at each phase of childhood. See Exhibit 5.3 for a list of selected parent educational resources.

Age of Recognition

Significant time lags between the age at which a parent first recognizes behaviors and patterns associated with ASD, and the age at which an ASD is diagnosed have been reported in the literature. A study of 601 children with ASD by Noterdaeme and Hutzelmeyer-Nickels (2010) found that about one-fourth of parents noted atypicalities in their children during their first

EXHIBIT 5.3

Early Childhood Development Resources for Parents

- www.cdc.gov/ncbddd/actearly/milestones/index.html
  Interactive website to educate parents about developmental milestones
- www.firstsigns.org
  Created by First Signs autism advocacy group. Has authoritative information on development, screening, and early signs of ASD for parents and health care providers.
- http://www.healthychildren.org
  American Academy of Pediatrics' website for parents
- http://www.cdc.gov/ncbddd/index.html
  National Center on Birth Defects and Developmental Disabilities
- http://www.asha.org/public/speech/development/chart.htm
  American Speech–Language–Hearing Association milestones for language development
- http://www.reachoutandread.org/parents/milestones/
  Reach Out and Read parent handouts on the development of literacy skills
- Shelov & Altman (2009). *Caring for Your Baby and Young Child.* Published by AAP.
- *What to Expect...* book series. Published by Workman Press

year of life; the mean age of recognition of atypical development was 15 months, and the mean age at diagnosis of autistic disorder was 76 months. Behaviors of concern in children with AS were noted later, and an AS diagnosis was made at an average age of 9 years. The impact of the AAP standard for universal screening on the time lag between recognition of risks and diagnosis is, as of yet, undetermined (Fombonne, 2009). In addition, as younger children are screened and referred for evaluation, centers and providers specializing in autism diagnosis may face an increased volume of patients and increase the wait time for an appointment during what is a stressful time for families (Fombonne, 2009). Johnson and Myers (2008) emphasize the fact that early intervention can begin without a finalized autism diagnosis, and clinicians should not delay referrals to these services. Many early-intervention programs also offer comprehensive assessment of hearing, vision, language, motor, and social development, along with specialized diagnostic services by psychologists and medical providers.

Findings from studies of children with ASD demonstrate that parents are acutely aware of their children's behavior and recognize concerning behavior patterns related to an ASD diagnosis during very early childhood (Fombonne, 2009). Patterns of concern most commonly identified by parents include speech and language delays, slowing of developmental progress, failure to achieve major developmental milestones, unusual social responses or interactions, and loss of skills or regression (Chawarska et al., 2007). De Giacomo and Fombonne (1998) found that a majority of parents of children with ASD recognized behaviors associated with the diagnosis at a mean age of about 19 months and first reported their concerns to a health care provider when their children were about 2 years of age. In this study, the most frequently reported concern was language related. Baghdadli and colleagues (2003) found the mean age for recognition of concerns to be 17 months, and more than one-third of the sample identified atypical behaviors before age 1 year. The presence of other medical problems, especially neurological disorders, infection and perinatal problems, and lower cognitive level, were significantly associated with earlier recognition. Chawarska et al. (2007) reported that in their study of 75 cases with autism, the mean age when parental concern about their children developed was 14.7 months.

Although much of the research on age of parent recognition of signs is retrospective, with possible recall bias, there is still a preponderance of evidence that parents recognize indicators associated with ASD and other developmental disabilities during infancy and early toddlerhood, and that the concerns they express correlate with later diagnoses (Glascoe, 1999). Their impressions are trustworthy and should be addressed carefully. During health care encounters, clinicians should emphasize the importance of the impressions that parents have of their children's development, elicit and welcome discussion of their concerns, and take the necessary follow-up actions to rule out or diagnose developmental disabilities or other problems. A brief open-ended statement, such as, "Tell me what concerns you about Amir's development or behavior right now," can facilitate communication of concerns. Some screening tools require parents to share their concerns. False reassurance ("You are just a first-time mother ...") is inappropriate. "Watch and wait" approaches are no longer the standard of care, because they can delay access to the earliest intervention. Parents and children benefit when a diagnosis is made and plans put into place for help (Noterdaeme & Hutzelmeyer-Nickels, 2010; Zwaigenbaum et al., 2009). In the case above, Amir's mother and his teacher expressed concerns about responses to others, language development, and hearing.

Associated Conditions and Signs

Autism is a genetically linked disorder, although the degree of contribution of environmental factors to the disorder continues to be debated. Families who already have a child with an ASD have a 2% to 8% risk of having another child with the disorder (Muhle, Trentacoste, & Rapin,

2004). Language delays, autistic features, ADHD, and psychiatric disorders are also more common in family members of children with ASD (Constantino et al., 2010). When ASD risk is identified, a three-generation family pedigree should be created.

Genetic testing techniques have resulted in identification of an increasing number of gene sites associated with ASD presentations, but most ASD is idiopathic. Autistic patterns are seen in several genetic syndromes, such as TS, Fragile X syndrome, CHARGE syndrome, and 22q11.2 deletion syndrome. The literature also identifies associations of autism with Angelman, Cornelia DeLange, Goldenhar, and Moebius syndromes (Cohen et al., 2005; Zafeiriou, Ververi, & Vargiami, 2007). Inborn errors of metabolism, such as untreated phenylketonuria (rare because of universal PKU screening), are found in about 5% of children with ASD (Manzi, Liozzo, Giana, & Curatolo, 2008). Children identified with genetic syndromes should be scrutinized for ASD risks, and conversely, children manifesting with ASD signs should be closely scrutinized for signs of genetic or chromosomal disorders. Unusual or atypical features can be cues to the presence of a genetic syndrome.

The prevalence of congenital anomalies is high in children with ASD. Findings from population studies demonstrate that as many as 13% of individuals with ASD and PDD and 3% of children with AS have birth defects, and that there is a significantly higher risk for these conditions than in the general population (Chen, Chen, Liu, Huang, & Lin, 2009; Dawson, Glasson, Dixon, & Bower, 2009; Ozgen et al., 2011). All body systems can be involved, but ear, face, neck, neurological, and urogenital anomalies are common (Dawson, Glasson, Dixon, & Bower, 2009). Children with ASD also have a higher rate of macrocephaly, epilepsy, and minor congenital anomalies (MCAs), which may or may not be syndromic manifestations. Commonly reported MCAs include ear anomalies, such as posterior rotation (Rodier, Bryson, & Welch, 1997).

A comprehensive physical examination should be completed, with attention to the presence of dysmorphic features, major or minor congenital anomalies, and indicators of systemic disorders. Depending on the physical presentation and associated developmental markers, a karyotype and polymerase chain reaction (PCR) analysis for Fragile X or genetic analysis for other disorders might be done (Johnson, Myers, & the Council on Children with Disabilities, 2007). See Chapter 6 for further discussion of complex and syndromic ASD and genetic considerations.

Macrocephaly

Frank macrocephaly occurs in about 25% of children with autism (AAP, 2001). Neonatal and early infancy head circumference (HC) in these children are usually normal, but an accelerated rate of head growth during the second 6 months of life has been documented to be associated with ASD (Courchesne, Carper, & Akshoomoff, 2003). A study of siblings of children with diagnosed ASD found that the siblings who demonstrated rapid head growth and macrocephaly by 12 months of age were significantly more likely to be diagnosed later with ASD (Elder, Dawson, Toth, Fein, & Munson, 2008). Head size frequently normalizes by the preschool period, as the fast rate of HC increase is not sustained past about age 2 years.

Seizures

Approximately one-third of children with ASD will have an associated seizure disorder, although a wide range of prevalence has been reported (Trevathan, 2004; Tuchman,

Alessandri, & Cuccaro, 2010). Seizures are more common in children with ASD who have concomitant cognitive impairments. An electroencephalogram is indicated when a seizure or seizure history is part of the clinical presentation but is not routinely recommended for children with ASD in general (Johnson, Myers, & the Council on Children with Disabilities, 2007). Close attention to neurological status and scrutiny for seizure activity are, however, important at each primary-care visit. Parents should be educated about the various seizure presentations, including staring, posturing, atony, and repetitive movements associated with partial, absence, and atypical seizures, in addition to the more familiar of tonic-clonic seizuric manifestations. It may be difficult for parents to differentiate between ASD-related inattentiveness to the environment and seizure manifestations.

Tuberous Sclerosis

Tuberous sclerosis is a genetic microdeletion syndrome resulting in lesions in one or more body systems, including the integumentary, cardiac, neurological, and renal systems. Ninety percent of individuals with TS have cerebral involvement, which results in seizure disorders, intellectual impairment, and a variety of psychiatric disorders. Estimates of the prevalence of autism in children with TS range from 16% to 65%; the prevalence of TS in individuals with ASD and seizure disorder is reported to be as high as 14%, and about 4% in those without epilepsy (Zafeiriou, Ververi, & Vargiami, 2007). Hypomelanotic skin lesions are frequent signs of TS. A thorough examination, along with Wood's lamp examination of the skin for TS lesions is routine, and essential, for children who demonstrate risks for ASD.

Fragile X Syndrome

Fragile X syndrome is caused by a repeat expansion error on the X chromosome and is the most common genetic cause of intellectual disability. ASD is found in 25% to 33% of children with Fragile X syndrome (Zafeiriou, Ververi, & Vargiami, 2007). Cognitive impairment is seen primarily in males with Fragile X syndrome; about 70% of females with Fragile X are normal (Bay & Steel, 2002).The physical signs of Fragile X syndrome are sometimes subtle or occult prior to puberty. The nurse should examine the child for protuberant ears, a long narrow face with wide nasal bridge, jaw prominence, hyperextensible joints, smooth "velvety" skin, and cardiac murmurs associated with mitral valve prolapse. In pubertal and postpubertal males, macroorchidism is present (Bay & Steel, 2002; Zafeiriou, Ververi, & Vargiami, 2007) . Genetic testing (polymerase chain reaction) can differentiate Fragile X from other disorders.

CHARGE

CHARGE syndrome or association is a condition manifested by a cluster of signs that include coloboma, heart defects, choanal atresia, growth and developmental restriction or retardation, genital hypoplasia, and anomalies of the ear (Bay & Steel, 2002, p. 22). Up to 45% of children with CHARGE association have ASD characteristics (Zafeiriou, Ververi, & Vargiami, 2007).

22q11.2 Deletion

The genetic disorder of 22q11.2 is also called DiGeorge syndrome and presents with a set of distinctive features. As with most genetic syndromes, not all features of the syndrome are found in every individual. On examination, children with 22q11.2 deletion syndrome can exhibit abnormal ears, wide nasal bridge, upturned nasal tip, and high arched or cleft palate. Hypoplasia of the thymus and parathyroid glands leads to abnormal immune function and hypocalcemia. Cardiac defects are seen in 75% of children with the syndrome (Gentile, Michaels, & Skoner, 2002; Park & Beerman, 2002). Between 20% and 30% of children with 22q11.2 deletion syndrome have associated ASD (Zafeiriou, Ververi, & Vargiami, 2007). See Chapter 2 for a discussion of other genetic determinants of ASD.

Other Issues

Lead poisoning is a risk associated with ASD. Lead burden might account for atypical behaviors. However, lead ingestion might be the result of pica, mouthing, and other repetitive behavioral symptoms. The initial assessment of young children with ASD should include a lead level (Johnson, Myers, & the Council on Children with Disabilities, 2007). Any child who presents with language delay should have a hearing evaluation. Hearing impairment can also lead to behavioral signs mimicking ASD.

Typical primary-care hearing-assessment measures, such as tympanometry to screen for conductive loss, or audiometry, can be difficult to accomplish with children suspected of having ASD, who are likely to be unable to cooperate. Evoked otoacoustic emission, and auditory brain stem response (ABR) tests, commonly used for neonatal screening, are other options. ABR results are most accurate when performed on a sleeping child. This mode of screening will likely require sedation, which in some children with ASD leads to paradoxical reactions, such as hyperactivity (AAP, 2009; Johnson, Myers, & the Council on Children with Disabilities, 2007). For accurate results, it may be necessary to refer to an audiologist experienced in assessing developmentally disabled children.

CLINICAL APPROACH

Comprehensive assessment for developmental disorders involves a layered process of developmental surveillance for ASD, screening, and comprehensive assessment for autism in children identified with risks. When a diagnosis is made, it should be followed by compassionate, evidence-based management of issues associated with ASD, which are described in subsequent chapters in this volume. Nurses in advanced roles are exceptionally well-suited by nature of education, practice philosophy, and scope of practice for this process, and can offer developmental supervision, screening, management, and support of young children and their families. The advanced practice nurse disciplinary focus integrates biomedicine with nursing's emphasis on partnership, holism, wellness and preventive care, patient- and family-centeredness, and promotion of adaptation to life transitions (Gardner, Posmontier, & Conti, 2011). These are also a cornerstone of pediatric nursing.

Family Considerations

Developmental concerns are worrisome to families. Hearing that a child has an ASD diagnosis can be emotionally devastating for parents and other family members, and they will need support as well as referral to a variety of services. Parents can experience grief as they hear that a beloved child has a lifelong and potentially significantly disabling condition. Others might feel relief when they understand that there is a reason for the child's behavior and see that help is available (Bloch & Gardner, 2007; Elder & D'Alessandro, 2009). Families and children benefit when a partnership between parents and health care provider is established. Parents can feel empowered when they know that their perspectives, concerns, and experiences are valued and recognized as important in the development of a plan of care for their child. The ongoing care of a child with ASD, which may require hours of behavioral management; interrupted sleep; adaptation of the home environment; medications; interfacing with multiple health care, therapy, and educational service providers; and many other activities can be highly stressful, especially over time. Parental caregiving for children, adolescents, and adults with ASD is associated with stress, depression, and poorer physical health (Boyd, 2002; Phetrasuwan & Miles, 2009; Seltzer et al., 2009; Seltzer, Krauss, Orsmond, & Vestal, 2001; Twoy, Connolly, & Novak, 2007).

Assessment of parent and family status, coping, and needs is essential, because parents are the "hub of the wheel" for their children's health and welfare. Nursing care should involve an empathetic approach, emphasize family strengths, and provide a scaffold of supports, including referrals to community programs, respite care, and counseling, where needed. Simply asking "What's it like for you right now?" can help parents communicate their needs to the nurse. Assessment of family management style (FMS) can also help clinicians to understand family patterns and select appropriate intervention strategies (Deatrick et al. 2006; Knafl, Breitmeyer, Gallo, & Zoeller, 1996; Knafl & Deatrick, 2003). Deatrick and colleagues (2006) note that families respond in a variety of ways to the life changes associated with a child's chronic illness. Some families integrate these changes into daily life and normalize their experiences more effectively than others. Some families just seem to fall apart. Their patterns of response can be categorized using the FMS "typology" (Deatrick et al., 2006, p. 20). The model specifies five patterns of family management or functioning: thriving, accommodating, enduring, struggling, or floundering (Deatrick et al., 2006; Knafl & Deatrick, 2003).

Family management style research on developmental issues is evolving. Application of the theory to families challenged as they live with ASD can help the nurse make sense of family members' actions and help him or her design the most appropriate, targeted interventions. Family management style theory is also a possible organizing framework for nursing research on family issues or effectiveness of family interventions associated with the care of a child with ASD. The Family Management Measure (2011; Knafl et al., 2011) evaluates families' success incorporating chronic disorders and conditions into routine family life. Effective care for families also involves the establishment of streamlined collaborations with specialists in neurology, psychiatry, psychology, developmental pediatrics, nutrition, genetics, occupational therapy, and speech–language pathology, along with strong liaisons with educational and school health staff.

Screening for Identification of Risk

Early and intense intervention in the social, behavioral, and communication realms is key for the best developmental, educational, and functional outcomes in children with ASD. Early identification of risk and early diagnosis is necessary for the earliest intervention to occur. As above, recognition of ASD involves developmental surveillance, universal screening for ASD risk, and ASD-specific screening and diagnosis when risk is found, along with attention to emerging parental concerns and the developmental history (Chakrabarti, Haubus, Dugmore, Orgill, & Devine, 2005; Filipek et al., 2000; Johnson, Myers, and the Council on Children with Disabilities, 2007; Johnson et al., 2008; Pinto-Martin et al., 2008). Current guidelines involve ongoing assessment of developmental progress along with use of Level 1 screening tools to assess the full population of toddlers at 18 and 24 months for ASD risks, followed by Level 2 screens for individuals who have been identified to be at risk (AAP, 2007; Johnson, et al., 2007; Robins, 2008).

Accuracy Considerations in Developmental Screening

All screening tools have their limits. Pinto-Martin et al. (2008) reported that the Parents' Evaluation of Developmental Status (PEDS; Glascoe, 2010) failed to identify a proportion of children with risks for ASD. They suggest that the PEDS likely taps domains of child development associated with other types of developmental disabilities. Miller et al. (2011) reported that neither use of the Infant–Toddler Checklist (ITC) nor the M-CHAT identified all cases of ASD in toddlers in a large pediatric practice. Sices, Stancin, Kirchner, and Bauchner (2008) found discrepancies between results of the simultaneously administered PEDS and ASQ in primary care and also surmise that they tap different dimensions of development. These findings highlight the need to understand instrument strengths and limitations, and especially to understand their targets.

An integrated approach that includes both surveillance and screening, emphasizing clinician and parent impressions of developmental patterns, is recommended. Clinicians should keep in mind that screens are intended to identify risk, not to diagnose, and that some children with positive screens will not have an ASD. Some children with an ASD can be missed. How well an instrument identifies children with and without ASD is its sensitivity and specificity. Sensitivity of a test reflects its ability to identify those with the disorder, while specificity indicates its strength in identifying those without the disorder (Kirton, 2010). The ideal instrument has both good sensitivity and good specificity. When both sensitivity and specificity are high, few people with the disorder will be missed, and few people without the disorder will be incorrectly flagged as positive. Sensitivity or specificity scores between .70 and .80 are considered acceptable in screening for ASD (Norris & Lecavalier, 2010). Predictive value is related to sensitivity and specificity, but indicates the way an instrument performs in different populations and accounts for the prevalence of a disorder. Positive predictive value (PPV) is the proportion of individuals testing positive who actually have the condition (are later diagnosed); negative predictive value (NPV) is the proportion of individuals testing negative who, in reality, do not have the condition (Kirton, 2010; Norris & Lecavalier).

Instrument accuracy in identifying cases at risk for ASD can vary with age, ASD variant, and other factors. For example, instruments can be less accurate identifying children who are high functioning or who have AS. Several screening tools, (for example, the Autism Spectrum Screening Questionnaire [ASSQ]), are targeted for this population of children. Studies of screening instruments can report conflicting findings. Some instruments have been studied less often, making it difficult to draw conclusions about accuracy.

Most screens and diagnostic tools for ASD in general use are geared to be used for children at the toddler age or older. The lower age limit of the Autism Diagnostic Observation Schedule-Toddler Module (ADOS-T) is 12 months, but the 12-month-old infant must meet motor and cognitive criteria for accurate results (Luyster et al., 2009). New ASD-specific screening and diagnostic tools designed for assessment of infants, such as the Autism Observation Scale for Infants (AOSI), for infants between 6 and 18 months of age (Bryson, Zwaigenbaum, McDermott, Rombough, & Brian, 2008), are being rapidly developed and tested. For younger toddlers and infants, screens that are not ASD focused but that include items from the communication and social domains, such as the ITC (see ASD Risk Screens section) are useful in identifying those at risk for ASD.

ASD-specific screening tools, such as the M-CHAT, are not designed to identify risks for, or the presence of, other developmental disabilities, although deficits found in ASD overlap with deficits associated with other developmental disorders (Ventola et al., 2006). Once an at-risk child is identified, the diagnostic process will include a comprehensive assessment, including evaluation of family history; genetic risks; physiological conditions; social, emotional, communication, cognitive, and behavioral manifestations associated with ASD; and structured diagnostic measures. It is difficult to make a stable ASD diagnosis in very young children, but diagnoses made at about age 2 years and up have been reported to be stable across childhood (Robins, 2008).

CASE

Since Amir is 18 months of age, his mother had completed the M-CHAT (Robins, Fein, Barton, & Green, 2001) in the clinic waiting room before being called to the examination room. Amir failed 14 items, including all critical items on the instrument: interest in other children, pointing, showing objects of interest to the mother, imitating, response to name, and RJA. A targeted autism evaluation is indicated for failure of two critical items or a total of three failed items. Amir's score is well beyond this cutoff. In addition, Amir has an algorithm risk score of 3 (parent, caregiver, and NP concerns), which indicates a need for immediate further evaluation for ASD. A thorough physical examination, focused on identification of other dysmorphic features is essential. Routine blood work, along with a lead level and karyotype and PCR for Fragile X are sent. An audiology consult is obtained to more comprehensively evaluate Amir's hearing. He is immediately referred to the comprehensive autism center and to the nearby early intervention program. With input from Amir's father, a three-generation family pedigree is constructed. The pedigree shows a pattern of hypertension and heart disease on both maternal and paternal lines, but no neurological or psychiatric conditions. Neither parent is aware of any family history of learning disabilities, ADHD, genetic disorders, or congenital anomalies. His father recalls an uncle who "acted strangely. He was always talking about sports statistics but never listened to anyone else. He had an odd way of talking." This is noted in the pedigree.

His blood work is unremarkable and no syndromic markers are found. Hearing is determined to be within normal limits. Evaluation at the autism center results in a preliminary diagnosis of autistic disorder. A follow-up appointment is scheduled with his mother to further assess needs, provide support, and make referrals to other community services.

Developmental Supervision—Surveillance

The AAP defines surveillance as an ongoing, longitudinal process of health supervision to recognize developmental patterns and developmental risks in infants and children. Surveillance also involves assessment of protective factors that support development, such as an enriched environment, invested and nurturing caregivers, and adequate nutrition (Council on Children with Disabilities, 2006). Developmental surveillance, with a focus on signs of ASD, is needed at every primary health care encounter. This supervision should include scrutiny of the family, birth and health history for factors related to developmental disability and ASD, eliciting parent's impressions of developmental progress, assessment of the family environment (protective factors), and specifically asking for their concerns. In addition, it includes observation and physical assessment, along with completion of a standardized developmental instrument or checklist so that the developmental pattern is clearly documented (Council on Children with Disabilities, 2006). General clinical impressions of a child's behavior and patterns are very important. However, accurate assessment of developmental progress and, more specifically, recognition of patterns that suggest a risk for ASD, is facilitated with the use of more formalized developmental checklists.

American Academy of Pediatrics guidelines include an array of tools that can be adopted for each level of screening. Clinicians should review the performance statistics of any tool that might be considered for surveillance or screening. Factors such as time involved in screening, language, reading level, and both financial and staff time costs for use and scoring, and population of children served, should also be considered in the decision to adopt a particular screen. One developmental checklist for surveillance is the PEDS: Developmental Milestones (PEDS:DM). Brothers, Glascoe, and Robertshaw (2008), reported that the PEDS:DM demonstrated 83% sensitivity and 84% specificity across multiple developmental domains, along with strong reliability, and has a reading level average of grade 1.8. It is designed for children from birth to 8 years of age. Completion of the instrument involves parent observation and report of developmental skills, and the authors report that the checklist takes only a few moments (Brothers, Glascoe, & Robertshaw 2008). The package provides for longitudinal documentation of developmental progress so that patterns over time can been recognized.

The Ages and Stages Questionnaire, Third Edition (ASQ-3; Squires & Bricker, 2009) is another parent reporting tool for children between 1 month and 5.5 years. The ASQ-3, like the PEDS:DM, asks parents to observe/report achievement of age-specific skills and can be completed and scored quickly. Sensitivity and specificity have been reported to be 86% percent overall and 85% overall, respectively (Squires, Twombly, Bricker, & Potter, 2009). It is considered valid and reliable with adequate sensitivity and specificity for developmental screening (AAP, 2001; Sices, Stancin, Kirchner, & Bauchner, 2009). One survey found the ASQ to be the most commonly used developmental screening tool used by community-based providers (Pizur-Barnekow et al., 2010).

ASD Risk Screens

Screening with a valid and reliable tool should take place at the 9-month, 18-month, and 24- to 30-month well-child visits, and in addition, any time there is a developmental concern identified by a parent or by the primary-care provider (Johnson, Myers, & the Council on Children with Disabilities, 2007). The ITC/Communication and Symbolic Developmental Scales—Behavior Profile (CSDS-BP), although not an ASD-specific screen, demonstrates accuracy in identifying ASD risk in infants and toddlers younger than 18 months (Luyster et al., 2009; Johnson, Myers, & the Council on Children with Disabilities, 2007; Wetherby, Brosnan-Maddox, Pearce, & Newton, 2008; Zwaigenbaum et al., 2009) The AAP recommends that all children undergo screening specifically for ASD risks at the routinely scheduled 18- and 24-month well-child visits. A detailed algorithm of approach, decision points, and action to summarize the process and to direct clinical practice has been developed (see Figure 5.3).

There are a large number of screening and diagnostic tools for ASD available and emerging. It is beyond the scope of this chapter to review all instruments. Selected instruments for clinical practice are described below. Johnson and Myers (2007, pp. 1200–1201) provide a detailed table describing various instruments recognized as appropriate for Level 1 and 2

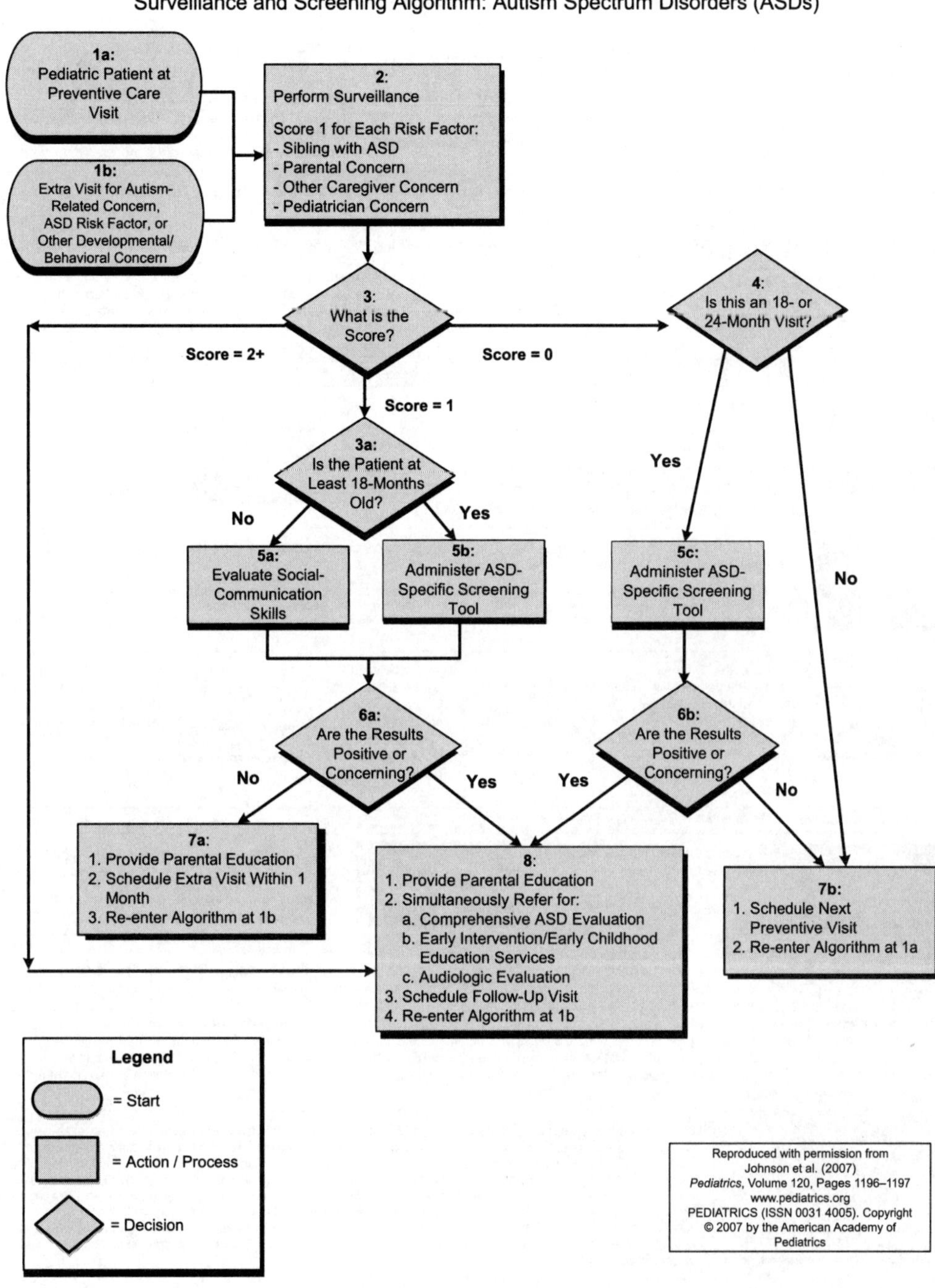

FIGURE 5.3 ■

(Continued)

screening by the AAP. Clinicians will find their summary of sensitivity and specificity data and sites for accessing instruments, along with other information, very helpful. However, it is important to remember that as instruments are used and tested in studies, new data become available (see also Tables 5.2 and 5.3).

Surveillance and Screening Algorithm: Autism Spectrum Disorders (ASDs)

1a: Pediatric Patient at Preventive Care Visit

1a - Developmental concerns, including those about social skill deficits, should be included as one of several health topics addressed at each pediatric preventive care visit through the first 5 years of life. *(Go to step 2)*

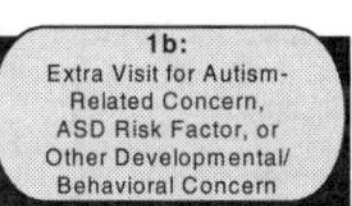

1b – At the parents' request, or when a concern is identified in a previous visit, a child may be scheduled for a "problem-targeted" clinic visit because of concerns about ASD. Parent concerns may be based on observed behaviors, social or language deficits, issues raised by other caregivers, or heightened anxiety produced by ASD coverage in the media. *(Go to step 2)*

2: Perform Surveillance

Score 1 for Each Risk Factor:
- Sibling with ASD
- Parental Concern
- Other Caregiver Concern
- Pediatrician Concern

2 - Developmental surveillance is a flexible, longitudinal, continuous, and cumulative process whereby health care professionals identify children who may have developmental problems. There are 5 components of developmental surveillance: eliciting and attending to the parents' concerns about their child's development, documenting and maintaining a developmental history, making accurate observations of the child, identifying the risk and protective factors, and maintaining an accurate record and documenting the process and findings. The concerns of parents, other caregivers, and pediatricians all should be included in determining whether surveillance suggests that the child may be at risk of an ASD. In addition, younger siblings of children with an ASD should also be considered at risk, because they are 10 times more likely to develop symptoms of an ASD than children without a sibling with an ASD. Scoring risk factors will help determine the next steps. *(Go to step 3)*

For more information on developmental surveillance, see "Identifying Infants and Young Children With Developmental Disorders in the Medical Home: An Algorithm for Developmental Surveillance and Screening" (*Pediatrics* 2006;118:405-420).

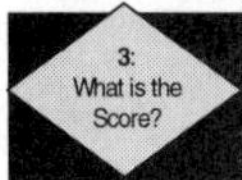

3 - Scoring risk factors:

- If the child does not have a sibling with an ASD and there are no concerns from the parents, other caregivers, or pediatrician: Score=0 *(Go to step 4)*
- If the child has only 1 risk factor, either a sibling with ASD or the concern of a parent, caregiver, or pediatrician: Score=1 *(Go to step 3a)*
- If the child has 2 or more risk factors: Score=2+ *(Go to step 8)*

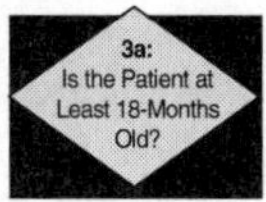

3a –

- If the child's age is <18 months, *Go to step 5a*
- If the child's age is ≥18 months, *Go to step 5b*

4: Is this an 18- or 24-Month Visit?

4 – In the absence of established risk factors and parental/provider concerns (score=0), a level-1 ASD-specific tool should be administered at the 18- and 24-month visits. *(Go to step 5c)* If this is not an 18- or 24-month visit, *(Go to step 7b).*

Note: In the AAP policy, "Identifying Infants and Young Children With Developmental Disorders in the Medical Home: An Algorithm for Developmental Surveillance and Screening", a general developmental screen is recommended at the 9-, 18-, and 24-or 30-month visits and an ASD screening is recommended at the 18-month visit. This clinical report also recommends an ASD screening at the 24-month visit to identify children who may regress after 18 months of age.

5a: Evaluate Social-Communication Skills

5a - If the child's age is <18 months, the pediatrician should use a tool that specifically addresses the clinical characteristics of ASDs, such as those that target social-communication skills. *(Go to step 6a)*

5b: Administer ASD-Specific Screening Tool

5b - If the child's age is ≥18 months, the pediatrician should use an ASD-specific screening tool. *(Go to step 6a)*

5c: Administer ASD-Specific Screening Tool

5c – For all children ages 18 or 24 months (regardless of risk factors), the pediatrician should use an ASD-specific screening tool. *(Go to step 6b)*

AAP-recommended strategies for using ASD screening tools: *"Autism: Caring for Children with Autism Spectrum Disorders: A Resource Toolkit for Clinicians" (in press)**

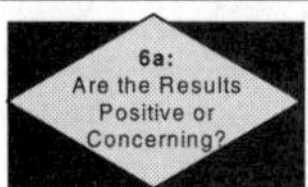

6a – When the result of the screening is *negative, Go to step 7a*

When the result of the screening is *positive, Go to step 8*

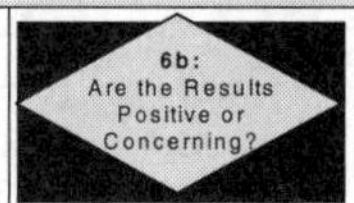

6b – When the result of the ASD screening (at 18- and 24-month visits) is *negative, Go to step 7b*

When the result of the ASD screening (at 18- and 24-month visits) is *positive, Go to step 8*

7a:
1. Provide Parental Education
2. Schedule Extra Visit Within 1 Month
3. Re-enter Algorithm at 1b

7a – If the child demonstrates risk but has a negative screening result, information about ASDs should be provided to parents. The pediatrician should schedule an extra visit within 1 month to address any residual ASD concerns or additional developmental/ behavioral concerns after a negative screening result. The child will then re-enter the algorithm at 1b. A "wait-and-see" approach is discouraged. If the only risk factor is a sibling with an ASD, the pediatrician should maintain a higher index of suspicion and address ASD symptoms at each preventive care visit, but an early follow-up within 1 month is not necessary unless a parental concern subsequently arises.

7b:
1. Schedule Next Preventive Visit
2. Re-enter Algorithm at 1a

7b – If this is not an 18- or 24-month visit, or when the result of the ASD screening is *negative*, the pediatrician can inform the parents and schedule the next routine preventive visit. The child will then re-enter the algorithm at 1a.

8:
1. Provide Parental Education
2. Simultaneously Refer for:
   a. Comprehensive ASD Evaluation
   b. Early Intervention/Early Childhood Education Services
   c. Audiologic Evaluation
3. Schedule Follow-up Visit
4. Re-enter Algorithm at 1b

8 – If the screening result is *positive* for possible ASD in step 6a or 6b, the pediatrician should provide peer reviewed and/or consensus-developed ASD materials. Because a positive screening result does not determine a diagnosis of ASD, the child should be referred for a comprehensive ASD evaluation, to early intervention/early childhood education services (depending on child's age), and an audiologic evaluation. A categorical diagnosis is not needed to access intervention services. These programs often provide evaluations and other services even before a medical evaluation is complete. A referral to intervention services or school also is indicated when other developmental/behavioral concerns exist, even though the ASD screening result is negative. The child should be scheduled for a follow-up visit and will then re-enter the algorithm at 1b. All communication between the referral sources and the pediatrician should be coordinated.

AAP information for parents about ASDs includes: *"Is Your One-Year-Old Communicating with You?*"* and *"Understanding Autism Spectrum Disorders.*"*

*Available at www.aap.org

Reproduced with permission from Johnson et al. (2007)
Pediatrics, Volume 120, Pages 1196–1197. www.pediatrics.org, Copyright © 2007 by the American Academy of Pediatrics

FIGURE 5.3 ■ *(Continued)*

Tools for Universal Screening of Toddlers

Some instruments, such as the Checklist for Autism in Toddlers (CHAT) and the M-CHAT, were designed specifically to screen for autism risk. Some, such as the PEDS (Glascoe, 2010) and ITC, were designed to screen broadly for developmental risks. Research on the PEDS

TABLE 5.2 ■ Selected Screens and Diagnostic Instruments for ASD by Age

Age range	Screens–levels 1 and 2	Diagnostic instruments
Toddler/child	CHAT (18 to 24+ months) ITC (6 to 24 months) M-CHAT (16 to 30 months) PEDS (birth to 8 years) STAT (24 to 35 months)	ADI-R ADOS-T (12 to 30 months) ADOS-G (>30 months) CARS[a]
Child/adolescent	ASSQ (7 to 16 years) AQ-Adolescent version (10 to 16 years) AQ (>16 years) CARS[a] (>24 months) ASQ (>4 years)	ADI-R ADOS-G CARS

[a]CARS used as both a screen and a diagnostic tool.

TABLE 5.3 ■ Selected Screening Instruments

Instrument	Method	Comments
CHAT (18 to 24 months)	Parent interview or parent reporting (nine items) plus clinician observation (five items) ASD-specific items	Developed for children in the United Kingdom Several modifications: CHAT with Denver modifications; CHAT-23 tested in Chinese children
M-CHAT (16 to 30 months)	Parent report Has ASD-specific items Six critical items and 23 total items	High sensitivity and false-positive rate to eliminate missed cases Structured follow-up interview to confirm findings[a] Sensitivity range: .77 to .93 PPV with follow-up interview 65% Good internal consistency of both the critical item cluster and total instrument Many language versions Reading level grade 6
PEDS (birth to 8 years)	Parent interview or parent report Also available via the Internet, integrated with other screens and decision algorithm Elicits parental concerns Not ASD-specific	Reading level grade 1.8 Reported ASD sensitivity to M-CHAT: .78 Reported ASD specificity to M-CHAT: .26
ITC (6 to 24 months)	Infant–toddler checklist component of CSDS-BP 25-item parent report Items in communication and social domains Elicits parent concerns Not ASD-specific	Has been used in children <18 months of age PPV and NPV reported >70% in sample of children 9 to 24 months

Based on Glascoe (2010); Glascoe, Macias, Wegner, & Robertshaw (2007); Kleinman et al. (2008); Pandey et al. (2008); Robins (2008); Wetherby et al. (2008); Zwaigenbaum et al. (2009).

[a]Robins (n.d.). http://www2.gsu.edu/~psydlr/DianaLRobins/Official_M-CHAT_Website_files/M-CHAT_header.pdf

compared with the M-CHAT shows that it demonstrates varying efficacy in screening for autism risk (Glascoe, Macias, Wegner, & Robertshaw, 2007; Pinto-Martin et al., 2008). PEDS is a parent reporting questionnaire that elicits concerns about specific developmental domains. The CHAT (Baron-Cohen, Allen, & Gillberg, 1992) is a 14-item ASD risk-screening tool that includes both parent reporting and clinician-interaction/observation items. The CHAT-23 is a 23-item screen developed from the CHAT and M-CHAT items for use with Chinese children (Wong et al., 2004) The M-CHAT (see Exhibit 5.4) is a 23-item parent reporting instrument to establish ASD risk (Robins, 2008; Robins et al., 2001). This tool incorporated the initial CHAT parent items along with expanded assessment items. Six of the items on the M-CHAT are considered critical. The ITC (Wetherby & Prizant, 2002) is another parent reporting instrument, not ASD-specific, which is focused on the social-communicative domains. It has 25 items, including a question eliciting parent concerns, and yields composite scores for social, speech, and symbolic functioning.

ASD Screens for Children and Adolescents

Norris and Lecavalier (2010) reviewed screening instruments for children ages 3 years and older. They examined the evidence supporting use of the Social Communication Questionnaire (SCQ), Gilliam Autism Rating Scale, Second Edition (GARS-2), ASSQ, and Asperger Syndrome Diagnostic Scale (ASDS). The SCQ is a 40-item parent reporting scale. The SCQ performed well when used with children ages 7 and older. It had less than optimal performance in identifying children with ASD when used in young children, even though the instrument was designed for use in children ages 4 and up. No studies of use of the GARS-2 could be located by the authors. However, Norris and Lecavalier (2010) note that the GARS and GARS-2 are quite similar, and that the GARS was found to have less than optimal sensitivity in all ages. The ASSQ (Ehlers, Gillberg, & Wing, 1999) is a screen for high-functioning autistic disorder and AS in children ages 6 to 17 years. It is designed to be completed by parents or caregivers. It consists of 27 items, each of which is rated on a scale from zero to two. It can be completed in about 10 minutes. In the review, the ASDS was found to have inadequate evidence to currently support its use.

The Autism Quotient (AQ)–Adolescent Version (Baron-Cohen, Wheelwright, Hoekstra, & Knickmayer, 2006) is intended for use in screening adolescents 11 to 16 years of age for autism traits. Adolescents who are older than 16 can be screened with the self-report AQ (Baron-Cohen, Wheelwright, Skinner, Martin & Clubley, 2001). The AQ is easily accessible on the Internet at many websites. The AQ–Adolescent Version is a 50-item parent reporting instrument assessing behavior across five domains associated with ASD and is reported to have good sensitivity and specificity when tested in clinical samples (Johnson, Myers, & the Council on Children with Disabilities, 2007).

Diagnostic Instruments

Differential diagnosis of ASD includes hearing and language disorders, intellectual disability, and an array of neurological disorders, all of which can also coexist with an ASD. The diagnostic process involves a comprehensive assessment of speech and language, IQ, physiological functioning, behavior, social skills, and communication (Zwaigenbaum et al., 2009). Diagnostic instruments (see Exhibit 5.2) include the Childhood Autism Rating Scale (CARS), Autism Diagnostic Interview–Revised (ADI-R) or toddler form, and Autism Diagnostic Observation Schedule–Generic (ADOS-G), which includes a specialized toddler module (ADOS-T; Luyster et al. 2009). Diagnostic instruments typically require specialized training

EXHIBIT 5.4

M-CHAT

Child's Name: ___________________ Child's Date of Birth: ________ MRN: ________________

Name of Person Completing Form: ____________________ Relationship to Child: __________________

Today's Date: ___________

M-CHAT

Please fill out the following about your child's usual behavior, and try to answer every question. If the behavior is rare (you've only seen it once or twice), please answer as if your child does *not* do it.

1. Does your child enjoy being swung, bounced on your knee, etc.? Yes No
2. Does your child take an interest in other children? Yes No
3. Does your child like climbing on things, such as up stairs? Yes No
4. Does your child enjoy playing peek-a-boo/hide-and-seek? Yes No
5. Does your child ever pretend, for example, to talk on the phone or take care of a doll or pretend other things? Yes No
6. Does your child ever use his/her index finger to point, to ask for something? Yes No
7. Does your child ever use his/her index finger to point, to indicate interest in something? Yes No
8. Can your child play properly with small toys (e.g. cars or blocks) without just mouthing, fiddling, or dropping them? Yes No
9. Does your child ever bring objects over to you (parent) to show you something? Yes No
10. Does your child look you in the eye for more than a second or two? Yes No
11. Does your child ever seem oversensitive to noise? (e.g., plugging ears) Yes No
12. Does your child smile in response to your face or your smile? Yes No
13. Does your child imitate you? (e.g., you make a face-will your child imitate it?). Yes No
14. Does your child respond to his/her name when you call? Yes No
15. If you point at a toy across the room, does your child look at it? Yes No
16. Does your child walk? Yes No
17. Does your child look at things you are looking at? Yes No
18. Does your child make unusual finger movements near his/her face? Yes No
19. Does your child try to attract your attention to his/her own activity? Yes No
20. Have you ever wondered if your child is deaf? Yes No
21. Does your child understand what people say? Yes No
22. Does your child sometimes stare at nothing or wander with no purpose? Yes No
23. Does your child look at your face to check your reaction when faced with something unfamiliar? Yes No

(*Continued*)

EXHIBIT 5.4 (Continued)

M-CHAT Instructions for Use

The M-CHAT is validated for screening toddlers between 16 and 30 months of age, to assess risk for ASD. The M-CHAT can be administered and scored as part of a well-child check-up, and also can be used by specialists or other professionals to assess risk for ASD. The primary goal of the M-CHAT was to maximize sensitivity, meaning to detect as many cases of ASD as possible. Therefore, there is a high false- positive rate, meaning that not all children who score as at risk for ASD will be diagnosed with ASD. To address this, we have developed a structured follow-up interview for use in conjunction with the M-CHAT; it is available at the two **websites listed above.** Users should be aware that even with the follow-up questions, a significant number of the children who fail the M-CHAT will not be diagnosed with an ASD; however, these children are at risk for other developmental disorders or delays, and evaluation is therefore warranted for any child who fails the screening.

The M-CHAT can be scored in less than 2 minutes. Scoring instructions can be downloaded from **http://www.mchatscreen.com** or www.firstsigns.org. We also have developed a scoring template, which is available on these websites; when printed on an overhead transparency and laid over thecompleted M-CHAT, it facilitates scoring. Please note that minor differences in printers may cause your scoring template not to line up exactly with the printed M-CHAT.

Children who fail 3 or more items total or 2 or more critical items (particularly if these scores remain elevated after the M-CHAT follow-up interview) should be referred for diagnostic evaluation by a specialist trained to evaluate ASD in very young children. In addition, children for whom there are physician, parent, or other professional's concerns about ASD should be referred for evaluation, given that it is unlikely for any screening instrument to have 100% sensitivity.

for administration, include many more items or observations than screening tools, and are more time-consuming to administer and score. Diagnostic measures are usually considered in conjunction with the rest of the comprehensive assessment.

The CARS can be used for both Level 2 screening and as a diagnostic instrument by adjusting the cutoff score (i.e., adjusting its sensitivity and specificity) for classification with ASD. Items on the CARS closely align to the *DSM-IV* criteria for autistic disorder. The instrument is comprised of items from 14 behavioral domains related to ASD, plus one item providing for general impressions, each rated on a scale from one to four. Higher scores on the CARS indicate more severe impairments. Scores can range between 15 and 60 and in typical diagnostic use, a score above 30 indicates autism (Chlebowski, Green, Barton, & Fein, 2010).

Evaluation of children for autism with the ADOS involves observation and rating of communication, social interaction, and play-related skills. The ADOS can be used in toddlers through adults. It consists of four modules, plus the toddler module. Selection of the module is determined by the individual's speech/language capabilities and age. Children are offered a series of activities to engage in, providing opportunities to observe and rate communication, social interaction, social relatedness, and symbolic play. Social and communication domains are rated, and a combined social-communication score is created. Each score is compared to the cutoff score to determine the severity of the condition: AD, ASD, or none (Lord, Rutter, DiLavore, & Risi, n.d.; Ventola et al., 2006).

The ADI-R and its companion toddler form involve structured parent interviews with over 100 questions in the domains of communication, socialization, play, and degree of restricted or stereotyped behaviors. Responses to questions are scored on a scale from 0 to 3, reflecting increasing severity of autism-related behavior. The score in each domain must exceed the cutoff score for the child to be diagnosed with autism. A child is classified as autistic or not (Rutter, Le Couteur, & Lord, n.d.; Ventola et al., 2006).

CASE

If Amir's M-CHAT had not indicated risk for ASD, follow-up screening would have occurred at his 2-year checkup. Amir and his mother returned to the clinic 6 weeks after the initial visit. By then, he had undergone a comprehensive developmental evaluation, fitting criteria for autistic disorder (idiopathic) according to results from the ADOS-T. He was additionally diagnosed with a severe speech–language delay, and intellectual disability (mental age equivalent: 13 months). He has started in the 0-3 early intervention program, which involves both center-based and home-based speech–language and occupational therapy, along with visits by the teacher/interventionist and social worker. His mother reports that she and his father were "quite shocked" by the diagnosis. His parents have not shared information about Amir's condition with their family members still in India, but his mother has told a neighbor who has a child of similar age about Amir's diagnosis. Amir's physical examination is unchanged.

BEST PRACTICES: PLAN OF CARE

Primary care can be enhanced by incorporating a social-ecological view, the long view, to enhance sensitivity to family strengths and needs as well as resources for, and barriers to, appropriate intervention. Social-ecological models take account of individuals in their family, community, and larger systems, considering factors in each of these systems, or layers, that impact a person's health status. A social-ecological perspective emphasizes the context in which individuals manage health needs and promotes consideration of health issues, needs, and resources at multiple levels, from societal through neighborhood level to family and individual (Bronfenbrenner, 1989). This perspective requires clinicians to look beyond an individual patient's medical needs and to consider the larger environmental context of care (Figure 5.4). Best practices for the identification and care of children with ASD evolve from the research-based evidence contextualized with the strengths and needs of each family, community, and the larger social systems.

SUMMARY

This chapter has emphasized the importance of early recognition of ASD, especially in the youngest children. Evidence is mounting that intensive intervention early in the developmental course of ASD can facilitate better social, communication, language, cognitive, behavioral, and functional outcomes. Social and educational services for individuals across the lifespan will likely become increasingly stressed by the volume of people with ASD and their family members. Fiscal and access-to-service repercussions will be felt at the individual, family, community, and national levels, because more funds will be required to treat more people with ASD; without additional funding, people may go without services. Decisions about the proportion of government funds directed toward treatment, research, education, and community services for people affected by an ASD will be difficult to make, because all of these services are costly, and all are important. Over time, early intervention with the youngest children might help to minimize the societal burdens by maximizing abilities in the core domains—social, communication, and behavioral. We can hypothesize that fewer services will be needed if children with ASD are able to demonstrate improved functional outcomes. It is best for children and families and best for society.

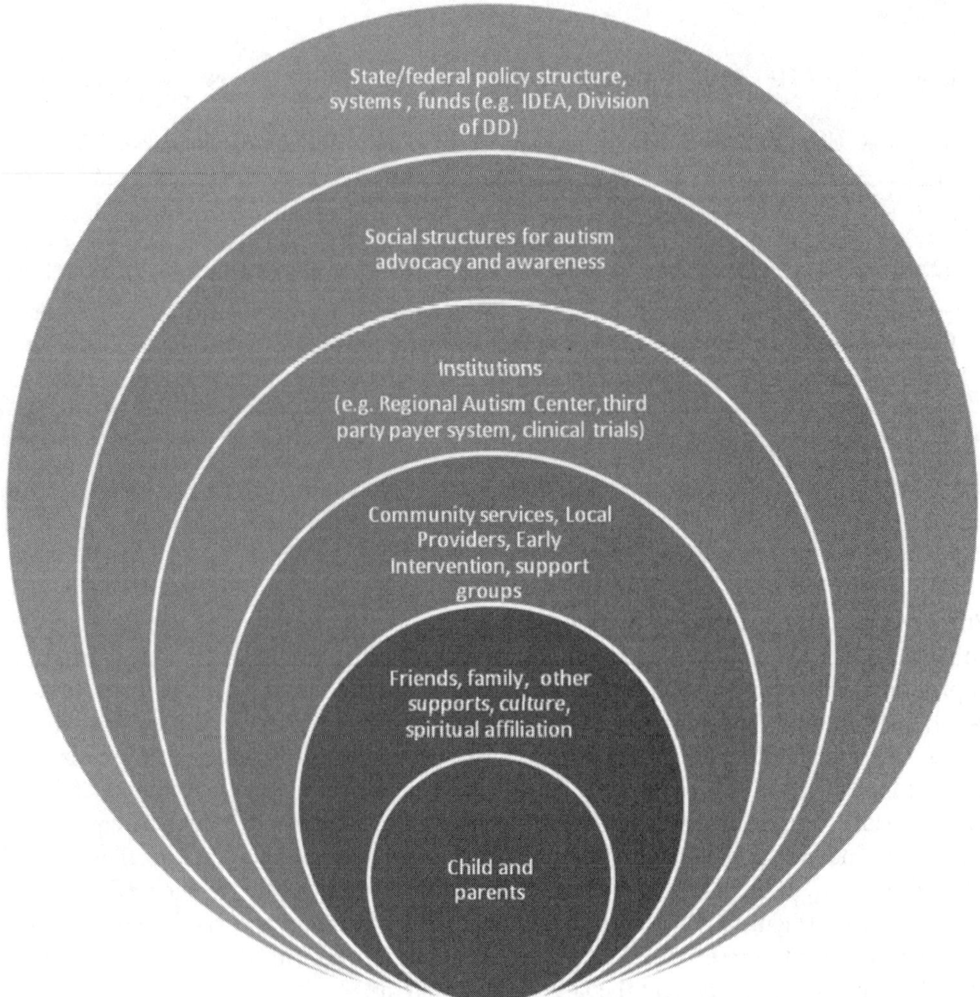

FIGURE 5.4 ■ Family, community, and system perspective of the child with autism.

To achieve the goal of the earliest possible identification of, and intervention with, all cases of ASD, nurses and other clinicians in primary care, schools, and other community settings need to use a thorough and organized approach based on evidence-based strategies of developmental surveillance, effective screening, and appropriate management. Screening and intervention need to be placed in the context of children's and families' individual patterns, styles, strengths, and needs, and considered in the context of the larger social environment, especially in relation to the availability of, and access to, family support resources and services. Close attention to all of these factors is a best-practices approach to early recognition and management of ASD. Remember that we see what we look for.

REFERENCES

American Academy of Pediatrics. (2001). Developmental surveillance and screening of infants and young children. *Pediatrics, 108*(1), 192–196.

American Academy of Pediatrics. (2007). *Autism: Caring for children with autism spectrum disorders: A resource toolkit for clinicians.* Elk Grove Village, IL: Author.

American Academy of Pediatrics. (2009). Clinical report—hearing assessment in infants and children: Recommendations beyond neonatal screening. *Pediatrics, 124*(4), 1252–1263.

American Psychiatric Association. (2000). *Diagnostic and statistical manual of mental disorders* (4 ed. text revision). Washington, DC: Author.

Autism Speaks. (2010). *Forging a Path of Progress and Hope* [Annual Report]. Retrieved from http://www.autismspeaks.org/sites/default/files/documents/as_annual_report_2010-web_01.pdf

Baghdadli, A., Picot, M. C., Pascal, C., Pry, R., & Aussilloux, C. (2003). Relationship between age of recognition of first disturbances and severity in young children with autism. *European Child & Adolescent Psychiatry, 12*(3), 122–127.

Ball, J. W., Bindler, R. C., & Cowen, K. J. (2010). *Child health nursing: Partnering with children and families* (2 ed.). New York: Pearson.

Baranek, G. T. (1999). Autism during infancy: A retrospective video analysis of sensory-motor and social behaviors at 9–12 months of age. *Journal of Autism and Developmental Disorders, 29*(3), 213–224.

Baron-Cohen, S., Allen, J., & Gillberg, C. (1992). Can autism be detected at 18 months? The needle, the haystack, and the CHAT. *British Journal of Psychiatry, 161*, 839–843.

Baron-Cohen, S., Wheelwright, S., Hoekstra, R. A., & Knickmeyer, R. (2006). The Autism Spectrum Quotient–Adolescent Version. *Journal of Autism and Developmental Disorders, 36*(3), 343–350.

Baron-Cohen, S., Wheelwright, S., Skinner, R., Martin, J., & Clubley, E. (2001). The Autism-Spectrum Quotient (AQ): Evidence from Asperger syndrome/high-functioning autism, males and females, scientists and mathematicians. *Journal of Autism and Developmental Disorders, 31*(1), 5–17.

Bay, C. A., & Steele, M. W. (2002). Genetic disorders and dysmorphic conditions. In B. J. Zitelli, & H. W. Davis (Eds.), *Atlas of Pediatric Physical Diagnosis* (4 ed., pp. 1–28). St. Louis, MO: Mosby.

Bethell, C., Peck, C., & Schor, E. (2001). Assessing health system provision of well child care: The promoting healthy development survey. *Pediatrics, 107*(5), 1084–1094.

Bloch, J., & Gardner, M. (2007). Accessing a diagnosis for a child with autism spectrum disorder: The burden is on the caregiver. *Journal for Nurse Practitioners, 11*(8), 10–17.

Boyd, B. A. (2002). Examining the relationship between stress and lack of social support in mothers of children with autism. *Focus on Autism & Other Developmental Disabilities, 17*(4), 208–216.

Boyd, D., & Bee, H. (2012). *Lifespan development* (6 ed.). Boston: Pearson-Allyn & Bacon.

Broderick, P., & Blewitt, P. (2010). The lifespan: Human development for helping professionals (3 ed.). Upper Saddle River, N.J.: Pearson.

Bronfenbrenner, U. (1989). Ecological systems theory. *Annals of Child Development* (*6*), 198–249.

Brothers, K. B., Glascoe, F. P., & Robertshaw, N. S. (2008). PEDS: Developmental Milestones—An accurate brief tool for surveillance and screening. *Clinical Pediatrics, 47*(3), 271–279.

Bryson, S. E., Zwaigenbaum, L., McDermott, C., Rambough, V., & Brain, J. (2008). The autism observation scale for infants: Scale development and reliability data. *Journal of Autism and Developmental Disorders, 38*(4), 731–738.

Cbakraharti, S., Haubus, C., Dugmore, S., Orgill, G., & Devine, F. (2005). A model of early detection and diagnosis of autism spectrum disorder in young children. *Infants and Young Children, 18*(3), 200–211.

Chawarska, K., Paul, R., Klin, A., Hannigan, S., Dichtel, L. E., & Volkmar, F. (2007). Parental recognition of developmental problems in toddlers with autism spectrum disorders. *Journal of Autism and Developmental Disorders, 37*, 62–72.

Chen, C., Chen, K., Liu, C., Huang, S., & Lin, K. (2009). Increased risks of congenital, neurologic, and endocrine disorders associated with autism in preschool children: Cognitive ability differences. *Journal of Pediatrics, 154*(3), 345–350e1.

Chlebowski, C., Green, J. A., Barton, M. L., & Fein, D. (2010). Using the Childhood Autism Rating Scale to diagnose autism spectrum disorders. *Journal of Autism and Developmental Disorders, 40*, 787–799.

Clifford, S., Young, R., & Williamson, P. (2007). Assessing the early characteristics of autistic disorder using video analysis. *Journal of Autism and Developmental Disorders, 37*(2), 301–313.

Cohen, D., Pichard, N., Tordjman, S., Baumann, C., Burglen, L., Excoffier, E., . . . Heron, D. (2005). Specific genetic disorders and autism: Clinical contribution towards their identification. *Journal of Autism and Developmental Disabilities, 35*(1), 103–116.

Combs-Orme, T., Nixon, B. H., & Herrod, H. G. (2011). Anticipatory guidance and early child development: Pediatrician advice, parent behaviors, and unmet needs as reported by parents from different backgrounds. *Clinical Pediatrics, 50*(8), 729–737.

Constantino, J., Zhang, Y., Frazier, T., Abbacchi, A., & Law, P. (2010). Sibling recurrence and the genetic epidemiology of autism. *American Journal of Psychiatry, 167*(11), 1349–1356.

Coplan, J. (2010). Early language milestone scale-2. Retrieved from http://www.drcoplan.com/early-language-milestone-scale-2

Council on Children with Disabilities. (2006). Identifying infants and young children with developmental disorders in the medical home: An algorithm for developmental surveillance and screening. *Pediatrics, 118*(1), 405–420.

Courchesne, E., Carper, R., & Akshoomoff, N. (2003). Evidence of brain overgrowth in the first year of life in autism. *Journal of the American Medical Association, 290*, 337–344.

Dawson, S., Glasson, E. J., Dixon, G., & Bower, C. (2009). Birth defects in children with autism spectrum disorders: A population-based, nested case-control study. *American Journal of Epidemiology, 169*(11), 1296–1303.

Deatrick, J. A., Thibodeaux, A., Mooney, K., Schmus, C., Pollack, R., & Davey, B. H. (2006). Family management style framework: A new tool to assess families who have children with brain tumors. *Journal of Pediatric Oncology Nursing, 23*(1), 19–27.

De Giacomo, A., & Fombonne, E. (1998). Parental recognition of developmental abnormalities in autism. *European Child and Adolescent Psychiatry, 7*, 131–136.

Delinicolas, E. K., & Young, R. L. (2007). Joint attention, language, social relating, and stereotypical behaviours in children with autistic disorder. *Autism, 11*(5), 425–436.

Durkin, M. S., Maenner, M. J., Meaney, F. J., Levy, S. E., DiGuiseppi, C., Nicholas, J. S., ... Schieve, L. A. (2010). Socioeconomic inequality in the prevalence of autism spectrum disorder: Evidence from a U.S. cross-sectional study. *PLoS One, 5*(7), 1–8. Retrieved from http://www.plosone

Ehlers, S., Gillberg, C., & Wing, L. (1999). A screening questionnaire for Asperger syndrome and other high-functioning autism spectrum disorders in school age children. *Journal of Autism and Developmental Disorders, 29*(2), 129–141.

Elder, J. H., & D'Alessandro, T. (2009). Supporting families of children with autism spectrum disorders: Questions parents ask and what nurses need to know. *Pediatric Nursing, 35*(4), 240–253.

Elder, L. M., Dawson, G., Toth, K., Fein, D., & Munson, J. (2008). Head circumference as an early predictor of autism symptoms in younger siblings of children with autism spectrum disorder. *Journal of Autism and Developmental Disorders, 38*(3), 1104–1111.

Esposito, G., Venuti, P., Apicella, F., & Muratori, F. (2010). Analysis of unsupported gait in toddlers with autism. *Brain and Development, 33*, 367–373.

Family Management Measure. (2011). Retrieved from http://nursing.unc.edu/research/rsc/resources/famm/index.htm

Filipek, P. A., Accardo, P. J., Ashwal, S., Baranek, G. T., Cook, E. H., Dawson, G., ... Volkmar, F. R. (2000). Practice parameter: Screening and diagnosis of autism. Report of the Quality Standards Subcommittee of the American Academy of Neurology and the Child Neurology Society *Neurology, 55*(4), 468–479.

Fombonne, E. (2009). A wrinkle in time: From early signs to a diagnosis of autism [Editorial]. *Journal of the American Academy of Child and Adolescent Psychiatry, 48*(5), 463–464.

Gardner, M. R., Posmontier, B., & Conti, M. (2011). The evolution of advanced practice nursing roles. In H. M. Dreher, & M. E. Glasgow (Eds.), *Role Development for Doctoral Advanced Nursing Practice* (pp. 69–90). New York: Springer.

Gentile, D. A., Michaels, M. G., & Skoner, D. P. (2002). Allergy and immunology. In B. J. Zitelli, & H. W. Davis (Eds.), *Atlas of Pediatric Physical Diagnosis* (4 ed., pp. 87–126). St. Louis, MO: Mosby

Glascoe, F. P. (1999). The value of parents' concerns to detect and address developmental and behavioural problems. *Journal of Paediatric and Child Health, 35*(1),1–8.

Glascoe, F. P. (2010). *Parents' Evaluation of Developmental Status (PEDS)*. Nolensville, TN: PEDSTest.com.

Glascoe, F. P., & Dworkin, P. H. (1993). Obstacles to effective developmental surveillance: Errors in clinical reasoning. *Journal of Developmental & Behavioral Pediatrics, 14*(5), 344–349.

Glascoe, F. P., Macias, M. M., Wegner, L. M., & Robertshaw, N. S. (2007). Can a broadband developmental-behavioral screening test identify children likely to have autism spectrum disorder? *Clinical Pediatrics, 46*(9), 801–805.

Hepburn, S. L., DiGuiseppi, C., Rosenberg, S., Kaparich, K., Robinson, C., & Miller, L. (2008). Use of a teacher nomination strategy to screen for autism spectrum disorders in general education classrooms: A pilot study. *Journal of Autism and Developmental Disorders, 38*, 373–382.

Interagency Autism Coordinating Committee. (2011). 2009 IACC autism spectrum disorder research portfolio analysis report. Retrieved from http://iacc.hhs.gov/portfolio-analysis/2009/index.shtml

Johnson, C. P., & Myers, S. M. (2008). The 2007 AAP autism spectrum guidelines and toolkit: What's the bottom line? *Contemporary Pediatrics, 25*(10), 43–67.

Johnson, C. P., Myers, S. M., & the Council on Children with Disabilities. (2007). Identification and evaluation of children with autism spectrum disorders. *Pediatrics, 120*(5), 1183–1215.

Kirton, C. A. (2010). Tools for applying evidence to practice. In G. LoBiodo-Wood, & J. Haber (Eds.), *Nursing research: Methods and critical appraisal for evidence-based practice* (7 ed., pp. 438–463). St. Louis, MO: Mosby.

Kleinman, J., Robins, D. L., Ventola, P. E., Pandey, J., Boorstein, H. C., Esser, E. L., & ...Fein, D. (2008). The modified checklist for autism in toddlers: A follow-up study investigating the early detection of autism spectrum disorder. *Journal of Autism and Developmental Disorders, 38*, 827–839.

Knafl, K., Breitmeyer, B., Gallo, A., & Zoeller, L. (1996). Family response to childhood chronic illness: Description of management styles. *Journal of Pediatric Nursing, 11*(5), 315–326.

Knafl, K., & Deatrick, J. A. (2003). Further refinement of the family management style framework. *Journal of Family Nursing, 9*(3), 252–256.

Knafl, K., Deatrick, J., Gallo, A., Dixon, J., Grey, M., Knafl, G., & O'Malley, J. (2011). Assessment of the psychometric properties of the Family Management Measure. *Journal of Pediatric Psychology, 36*(5), 494–505.

Korkmaz, B. (2011). Theory of mind and neurodevelopmental disorders of childhood. *Pediatric Research, 69*(5, part 2), 101R–108R.

Kyle, T. (2008). *Essentials of pediatric nursing*. Philadelphia, PA: Lippincott, Williams and Wilkins.

Lord, C., Rutter, M., DiLavore, P. C., & Risi, S. Autism Diagnostic Observation Schedule (ADOS). Retrieved from http://portal.wpspublish.com/portal/page?_pageid=53,70384&_dad=portal&_schema=PO RTAL

Lubbock, J. (1892). *The beauties of nature and the wonders of the world we live in*. London: McMillan & Company.

Luyster, R., Gotham, K., Whitney, G., Coffing, M., Petrak, R., Pierce, K., & ... Lord, C. (2009). The Autism Diagnostic Observation Schedule—Toddler Module: A new module of a standardized diagnostic measure for autism spectrum disorders *Journal of Autism and Developmental Disorders, 39*, 1305–1320.

Mandell, D. S., Morales, K. H., Xie, M., Lawer, L. J., & Stahmer, A. C. Age of diagnosis among Medicaid-enrolled children with autism, 2001–2004. *Psychiatric Services, 61*(8), 822–829.

Matson, J. L., Mahan, S., Kozlowski, A. M., & Shoemaker, M. (2010). Developmental milestones in toddlers with autistic disorder, pervasive developmental disorder–not otherwise specified and atypical development. *Developmental Neurorehabilitation, 13*(4), 239–247.

Manzi, B., Liozzo, A. L., Giana, G., & Curatolo, P. (2008). Autism and metabolic diseases. *Journal of Child Neurology, 23*(3), 307–314.

Miller, J. S., Gabrielsen, T., Villalobos, M., Alleman, R., Wahmhoff, M., Carbone, T., & Segura, B. (2011). The each child study: Systematic screening for autism spectrum disorders in a pediatric setting. *Pediatrics, 27*(5), 866–871.

Muhle, R., Trentacoste, S. V., & Rapin, I. (2004). The genetics of autism. *Pediatrics, 113*, e472–486. Retrieved from http://pediatrics.aappublications.org/content/113/5/e472.full.html

Myers, S. M., Johnson, C. P. the Council on Children with Disabilities. (2007). Management of children with autism spectrum disorders. *Pediatrics, 120*(5), 1162–1182.

Naber, F. B., Bakermans-Kranenburg, M. J., van Ijzendoorn, M. H., Dietz, C., van Daalen, E., Swinkels, S. H., ...van Engeland, H. (2008). Joint attention development in toddlers with autism. *European Journal of Child and Adolescent Psychiatry, 17*(8), 143–152.

Nadel, S., & Poss, J. E. (2007). Early detection of autism spectrum disorders: Screening between 12 and 24 months of age. *Journal of the American Academy of Nurse Practitioners, 19*, 408–417.

Norris, M., & Lecavalier, L. (2010). Screening accuracy of level 2 autism spectrum disorder rating scales: A review of selected instruments. *Autism, 14*(4), 263–284.

Noterdaeme, M., & Hutzelmeyer-Nickels, A. (2010). Early symptoms and recognition of pervasive developmental disorders in Germany. *Autism, 14*(6), 575–588.

Ozgen, H., Helleman, G. S., Stellato, R. K., Lahuis, B., van Daalen, E., Staal, W. G., ... van Engeland, H. (2011). Morphological features in children with autism spectrum disorders: A matched case–control study. *Journal of Autism and Developmental Disorders, 41*, 23–31.

Ozonoff, S., Iosif, A., Baguio, F., Cook, I. C., Hill, M. M., Hutman, T., ...Young, G. S. (2010). A prospective study of the emergence of early behavioral signs of autism. *Journal of the American Academy of Child and Adolescent Psychiatry, 49*(3), 256–266.

Pandey, J., Verbalis, A., Robins, D. L., Boorstein, H., Klin, A., Babitz, T., ... Fein, D. (2008). Screening for autism in older and younger toddlers with the Modified Checklist for Autism in Toddlers. *Autism, 12*(5), 513–535.

Park, S. C., & Beerman, L. B. (2002). Cardiology. In B. J. Zitelli, & H. W. Davis (Eds.), Atlas of Pediatric Physical Diagnosis (4 ed., pp. 127–153). St. Louis, MO: Mosby.

Phetrasuwan, S., & Miles, M. S. (2009). Parenting stress in mothers of children with autism spectrum disorders. *Journal for Specialists in Pediatric Nursing, 14*(3), 157–165.

Pinto-Martin, J. A., Young, L. M., Mandell, D. S., Poghosyan, L., Giarelli, E., & Levy, S. E. (2008). Screening strategies for autism spectrum disorders in pediatric primary care. *Journal of Developmental and Behavioral Pediatrics, 29*(5), 345–350.

Pizur-Barnekow, K., Erikson, S., Johnston, M., Bass, T., Lucinski, L., & Bleuel, D. (2010). Early identification of developmental delays through surveillance, screening, and diagnostic evaluation. *Infants and Young Children, 23*(4), 323–330.

Squires, J., Twombly, E., Bricker, D., & Potter, L. (2009). Psychometric properties of ASQ-third edition. Retrieved from http://www.brookespublishing.com/store/books/squires-asq/asq3-technical.pdf

Roberts, J. M. (1989). Echolalia and comprehension in autistic children. *Journal of Autism and Developmental Disorders. 19*(2), 271–81.

Robins, D. L. (n.d). *Instructions and permissions for the use of the M-Chat.* Retrieved from http://www2.gsu.edu/~psydlr/DianaLRobins/Official_M-CHAT_Website_files/M-CHAT_header.pdf

Robins, D. L. (2008). Screening for autism spectrum disorders in primary care settings. *Autism, 12*(5), 537–556.

Robins, D. L., Fein, D., Barton, M. L., & Green, J. A. (2001). The modified checklist for autism in toddlers: An initial study investigating the early detection of autism and pervasive developmental disorders. *Journal of Autism and Developmental Disorders, 31,* 131–144.

Rodier, P. M., Bryson, S. E., & Welch, J. P. (1997). Minor malformations and physical measurements in autism: Data from Nova Scotia. *Teratology, 55*(5), 319–325.

Rowe, M. L. (2006). Child-directed speech: relation to socioeconomic status, knowledge of child development and child vocabulary skill. *Journal of Child Language, 35*(1), 185–205.

Rutter, M., Le Couteur, A., & Lord, C. Autism Diagnostic Interview-Revised. Retrieved from http://portal.wpspublish.com/portal/page?_pageid=53,70436&_dad=portal&_schema=PORTAL

Seltzer, M. M., Greenberg, J. S., Hong, J., Smith, L. E., Almeida, D. M., Coe, C., & Stawski, R. S. (2009). Maternal cortisol levels and behavior problems in adolescents and adults with ASD. *Journal of Developmental Disorders, 40*(4), 457–459.

Seltzer, M. M., Krauss, M. W., Orsmond, G. I., & Vestal, C. (2001). Families of adolescents and adults with autism: Uncharted territory. *International Review of Research on Mental Retardation, 23,* 267–294.

Shattuck, P. T., Durkin, M., Maenner, M., Newschaffer, C., Mandell, D., Wiggins, L., . . . Cuniff, C. (2009). Timing of identification among children with an autism spectrum disorder: Findings from a population-based surveillance study. *Journal of the Academy of Child and Adolescent Psychiatry, 48*(5), 474–483.

Sices, L., Stancin, T., Kirchner, H. L., & Bauchner, H. (2009). PEDS and ASQ developmental screening tests may not identify the same children. *Pediatrics, 124,* e640–e647. Retrieved from http://pediatrics.aappublications.org/content/124/4/e640.full.html

Squires, J., & Bricker, D. (2009). Ages & Stages Questionnaires (3 ed.). Baltimore: Paul H. Brookes. http://www.brookespublishing.com/store/books/squires-asq/index.htm

Sullivan, M., Finelli, J., Marvin, A., Garrett-Mayer, E., Bauman, M., & Landa, R. (2007). Response to joint attention in toddlers at risk for autism spectrum disorder: A prospective study. *Journal of Autism and Developmental Disorders, 37*(1), 37–48.

Trevathan, E. (2004). Seizures and epilepsy among children with language regression and autistic spectrum disorders. *Journal of Child Neurology, 19,* S49–57.

Tuchman, R., Alessandri, M., & Cuccaro, M. (2010). Autism spectrum disorders and epilepsy: moving towards a comprehensive approach to treatment. *Brain Development, 32*(9), 719–730.

Twoy, R., Connolly, P. M., & Novak, J. (2007). Coping strategies used by parents of children with autism. *Journal of the American Academy of Nurse Practitioners, 19,* 251–260.

Ventola, P. E., Kleinman, J., Pandey, J., Barton, M., Allen, S., Green, J., . . . Fein, D. (2006). Agreement among four diagnostic instruments for autism spectrum disorders in toddlers. *Journal of Autism and Developmental Disabilities, 36,* 839–847.

Weismer, S. E., Lord, C., & Esler, A. (2010). Early language patterns of toddlers on the autism spectrum compared to toddlers with developmental delay. *Journal of Autism and Developmental Disorders, 40*(10), 1259–1273.

Wetherby, A. M., Brosnan-Maddox, S., Pearce, V., & Newton, L. (2008). Validation of the Infant-Toddler Checklist as a broadband screener for autism spectrum disorders from 9 to 24 months of age. *Autism, 12*(5), 487–511.

Wetherby, A. M., & Prizant, B. M. (2002). *CSBS DP infant-toddler checklist.* Baltimore: Paul H. Brookes.

Wetherby, A. M., Woods, J., Allen, L., Cleary, J., Dickinson, H., & Lord, C. (2004). Early indicators of autism spectrum disorders in the second year of life. *Journal of Autism and Developmental Disorders, 34*(5), 473–493.

Wilson, D. (2011). Health promotion of the toddler and family. In M. J. Hockenberry, & D. Wilson (Eds.), *Wong's nursing care of infants and children* (9 ed.). St. Louis, MO: Elsevier-Mosby.

Wong, V., Hui, L. S., Lee, W., Leung, L., Ho, P., Lau, W., . . . Chung, B. (2004). A modified screening tool for autism (Checklist for Autism in Toddlers [CHAT-23]) for Chinese children *Pediatrics, 114*(2), e166–e176. Retrieved from http://www.pediatrics.org/cgi/content/full/114/2/e166

Zafeiriou, D. I., Ververi, A., & Vargiami, E. (2007). Childhood autism and associated comorbidities. *Brain and Development 29*(5), 257–272.

Zwaigenbaum, L., Bryson, S., Lord, C., Rogers, S., Carter, A., Carver, L., . . . Yirmiya, N. (2009). Clinical assessment and management of toddlers with suspected autism spectrum disorder: Insights from studies of high-risk infants. *Pediatrics, 123*(5), 1383–1391.

Complex Autism: Is It Rare or a Family Affair? 6

Margaret Cooney Souders and Kathleen T. Sharp

Approximately 15% to 20% of children diagnosed with autism spectrum disorder (ASD) have complex autism (Miles et al., 2008). Moreover, one-third of children with complex autism have an autism-associated syndrome or genetic disorder (Miles et al., 2008). The word "syndrome" is used to describe a group of malformations, functional deficits, or behavioral differences that have been seen recurrently in a relatively constant and unique pattern (Cassidy & Allanson, 2010). Thus, a syndrome comes to be defined by the co-occurrence of "hallmark" abnormalities. However, other features may be observed at lower frequencies (Cassidy & Allanson, 2010). Fragile X syndrome, Phelan-McDermid syndrome, 22q11.2 deletion syndrome, and Kabuki syndrome are all examples of syndromes with high rates of co-occurring ASD and could be considered cases of complex autism (Farzin et al., 2006; Hagerman, Rivera, & Hagerman, 2008; Harris et al., 2008).

The definition of complex autism reflects an individual with ASD who also presents with dysmorphic features and/or microcephaly, characteristics that indicate some variation of early morphogenesis (Miles & Hillman, 2000; Miles et al., 2005, 2008). Disturbances in early morphology can alter the end modeling of our body formation and can result in dysmorphic features. The size, shape, pattern, and appearance of the face, skin, and other body parts can provide clues about the morphogenesis of other internal organs, including the brain (Cassidy & Allanson, 2010; Miles et al., 2005, 2008).

In this chapter, the key clinical and behavioral problems of a child with complex autism are presented and evidence for best practices are discussed. Ongoing family support and education is integrated with the plan of care. In addition to the nursing role, we describe family participation in the assessment, treatment development, and implementation of behavioral strategies and clinical care during hospitalization. We explore the nursing role on a multidisciplinary team in the development of a comprehensive medical and behavioral plan of care for a child with ASD, dysmorphic features, congenital cardiac defect, seizure disorder, and severe undesirable behaviors. The case study can be considered a case of complex autism.

To maintain confidentiality, we have changed the name, amended the characteristics, and changed all of the family characteristics to create the case of a boy with complex autism. We present a picture later in the chapter for educational purposes; however, this is NOT a picture of the child in the case, but rather a picture of a boy with similar facial features. We have obtained written permission from the child and mother for this picture to be published.

PROLOGUE

Joey was the first child with autism for whom I ever cared. His mother had no front teeth. I was introduced to the family on the day of his admission to the Biobehavioral Unit (BBU).

I asked the mother, "What happened to your teeth?" She replied, "My son keeps knocking them out when he head-butts me. I try to get under him and hold him tight to protect him from hitting his head on the floor. He then head-butts me in the face. I had my teeth replaced and then he knocks them out again! I love my son but we cannot go on like this any longer. We desperately need help. Can you help us?"

This mother had tremendous love for her son, despite his vicious tantrums. Her ongoing devotion and continued effort to protect him from harm, regardless of the danger to her, was heroic and I was genuinely moved. My nursing care and relationship with this family was challenging and captivating. I had just starting working on the BBU and was a new nurse practitioner. This incredible experience gave me a clear direction for my life's work as an advanced practice nurse. As my relationship with Joey and his family evolved, I was compelled to become a strong advocate for children with autism. I wanted to be a voice for children who were nonverbal and families at their "wits end." My role model and mentor in the BBU was a pediatric nurse practitioner, Kathy Sharp. Together we will take you back in time and present "Joey," a composite case of complex autism.

CASE—INTRODUCTION

Joey, an 8-year-old male with a pervasive developmental disorder, nonverbal communication, history of seizures, status-post vascular ring repair at 2 months of age, and dysmorphic features, was admitted to a BBU for treatment of his severe undesirable behaviors. Joey had self-injurious behavior (SIB) in the form of head-banging and tantrums 5 to 6 times a day. Each tantrum could last up to 45 to 60 minutes, with head-banging and head-butting, spitting, hitting, screaming, and pinching. Joey was in an autistic support classroom with a one-on-one aide. Due to his behaviors, he could no longer be accommodated in the classroom. His mother had to take a leave of absence from her job in order to be with him during the day. Joey's undesirable behaviors had created a condition of complete social isolation for his family. The school district was in the process of finding a more appropriate placement. Joey's parents were desperate and agreed to a hospitalization in the BBU. Long-term comprehensive medical and behavioral care would be needed to achieve the best outcome possible for Joey's future development and to optimize his and his family's quality of life.

CARE DELIVERY SETTING

We provided care for Joey in the BBU, an inpatient unit at a large, urban, pediatric hospital in Philadelphia. This unit provided comprehensive care for 18 individuals with severe, undesirable behaviors. The BBU's approach was based on a behavioral psychology model of intervention. The BBU team consisted of a program director, a behavioral psychologist, four behavioral psychology team leaders, eight nurses (two pediatric nurse practitioners and six registered nurses), a developmental pediatrician, four master's-prepared behavioral specialists, predoctoral psychology students, behavioral support staff, one social worker, one special education teacher, four teaching assistants, and weekly psychiatric consultations from a pediatric psychiatrist.

The BBU could accommodate 18 patients in nine double-bed rooms. Beds could retract into the walls, so that each room could be converted into a behavioral treatment room. Walls and closets were covered with a soft, washable, durable fabric, and the floor was tiled. Large gym mats were available to create a padded floor. Each room had an antechamber with a one-way mirror so behavioral sessions could be observed. The antechamber had a desk and two chairs and video technology and laptops to document and record behavioral sessions. The unit also had a large classroom, kitchen, laundry room, playroom, large outside playground, nurses' station, medication and treatment rooms, conference room, and staff offices.

The mission of the inpatient BBU was to provide behavioral and medical care for individuals with severe undesirable behaviors. The goal was to create a treatment plan to decrease undesirable behaviors and optimize development, health, daily function, and, ultimately, the quality of life for the individual and family. The multidisciplinary team offered the capacity for developing a comprehensive treatment plan that could be implemented in the home and community. The average length of stay during hospitalization was 10 to 12 weeks. On admission, each individual received an in-depth medical and developmental history and a thorough physical exam, including a dysmorphological exam by the nurse practitioner in collaboration with a developmental pediatrician. In the first week, a clinical and behavioral assessment plan was developed by the team. These plans often involved consultation with subspecialties at the hospital such as neurology, gastroenterology, genetics, and ophthalmology.

Preexisting Medication Regimens

In the United States, psychopharmacological medications are frequently used as the first line of treatment for aberrant behavior (Burgio, Page, & Capriotti, 1985; Cohen, Campbell, & Posner, 1980; Gobbi & Pulvirenti, 2001; Malone, Gratz, Delaney, & Hyman, 2005; McCracken et al., 2002); however, drug trials conducted in the ASD population often have multiple methodological limitations, such as small sample size, open-label design, and outcome measures that are inadequate to establish treatment efficacy (Burgio, Page, & Capriotti, 1985; Malone et al., 2005; McCracken et al., 2002; Scahill et al., 2001). In addition, many medications that have shown efficacy in recent randomized clinical trials have serious side effects and unknown long-term effects on developing brains of children and adolescents (Malone, Sheikh, & Zito, 1999; McCracken et al., 2002; Scahill et al., 2001). To this end, the plan for all individuals admitted to the BBU was to wean them from all psychopharmacologic agents slowly, if medically possible. Individuals on multiple psychopharmacological agents were often admitted to the BBU; it often was not clear whether or not the medications were effectively addressing targeted undesirable behaviors. The multidisciplinary team's intent was to analyze each individual's behavior without the effects of behavior-altering medication. The weaning process was implemented by the nurse practitioners in collaboration with the developmental pediatrician, registered nurses, and psychology team and in consultation with the child psychiatry subspecialty.

CASE—JOEY'S HISTORY

Pertinent Medical and Developmental History

Birth and Infancy

Joey's mother's pregnancy was complicated by polyhydramnios and headaches. She took acetaminophen for headaches and experienced relief. At 37 weeks gestation, she had a spontaneous vaginal delivery with no complications at birth. During the first months of life, Joey had feeding difficulties and frequent respiratory infections. He had a hospitalization for respiratory

(*Continued*)

CASE—JOEY'S HISTORY (Continued)

distress and pneumonia at 3 months. He was diagnosed with a cardiac vascular ring, which was repaired at 4 months of age. Subsequently, Joey's feedings improved and he began to grow and develop over the first year of life.

Early Childhood

Joey was noted to have developmental delays by his mother and pediatrician. At age 20 months he used no words nor babbling sounds. He had social regression, and stopped pointing and gesturing for help. He received early intervention, both speech and occupational therapy, weekly. He attended a specialized preschool beginning at age 3 years. Joey had frequent ear infections. His parents believed the infections were the reason for his speech delay. He required bilateral myringotomy tubes at age 4 years. A subsequent audiology evaluation revealed normal hearing; however, he continued to have no words. He was diagnosed with pervasive developmental disorder–not otherwise specified (PDD-NOS) and hypotonia at age 4 years by a neurologist.

At age 5 years, Joey had multiple episodes of questionable seizures: staring, eyes turning to the right, and questionable left arm jerks, but no loss of consciousness. These episodes occurred over the period of several weeks. Joey and his mother returned to the neurologist. However, his undesirable behaviors interfered with the ability to obtain a good-quality electroencephalogram (EEG). The neurologist diagnosed him with simple partial seizures. Valproic acid sprinkles were prescribed to address his seizures and to target his SIB and tantrums. His mother was unable to get him to take his medication, regardless of the delivery method. Furthermore, as Joey grew larger, clinicians were unable to complete a full physical examination.

Adaptive Abilities

On admission, Joey's mother reported several adaptive problems. He had poor sleep, including difficulties falling asleep and nighttime teeth grinding. He ate a highly selective diet that consisted of only chicken fingers, french fries, and potato chips. He refused to dress himself. He was toilet trained for urine only; he required disposable, diaper-like underwear for stools each evening after dinner. After defecating, he would remove his underwear and hand it to his mother.

Pertinent Social History

Joey lived with his family in a single-family home in the suburbs. His mother, age 42 years, completed two years of college and worked part-time in an accountant's office. His father, age 38 years, had a history of attention deficit hyperactivity disorder (ADHD) and gastroesophageal reflux disease (GERD). He had completed some college and worked at a restaurant. Joey's sister was 12 years old, and had been diagnosed with ADHD and a learning disability. She was in special education classes in middle school. She had a history of frequent ear infections. Paternal grandparents were killed in a car accident. Maternal grandparents lived in Florida. The family affiliated as Christian, but had stopped going to church because of Joey's disruptive behaviors. The mother voiced significant concerns about being isolated because of her children's disabilities.

BEST PRACTICES: PHYSICAL EXAMINATION

In preparation for the physical exam, we gowned, gloved, and put on protective eyewear because of Joey's spitting behaviors. It took 4 days of frequent, short assessments to complete a thorough physical exam. Each assessment required three staff members, along with his mother, to help hold and distract him. We used potato chips, a favorite food, and verbal praise as a reward throughout the exam. We reinforced each small step toward adherence to directions or requests (Souders, Freeman, DePaul, & Levy, 2002). We also modeled the requested behaviors and then asked him to perform them. For example, we asked him to hold out his arm in order to measure blood pressure (BP). The cuff was hidden. We held out our arms and said "arm out" (Souders et al., 2002). When he complied, he was rewarded with verbal praise. We shaped the behavior with verbal praise and made a game of taking turns holding out our arms. Once Joey could hold his arm out for 10 seconds, we rewarded him with a potato chip and verbal praise. We then introduced the BP cuff. He was allowed to hold and touch it, and we slowly shaped his behavior with potato chips and verbal praise.

Two days later we were able to measure his BP. The mother happily noted that this was the first thorough physical exam Joey had in quite a long time, and she cried with joy. She stated that she was comforted by our commitment to adapting to her child's behavioral and sensory needs (Souders et al., 2002). She said she did not feel compelled to apologize for her son's undesirable behaviors, as she often did elsewhere. ASD is one of the most devastating neurobiological disorders of brain development (DiCicco-Bloom et al., 2006). A child with autism often has developed alternative behaviors because he or she has severe communication, processing, and sensory differences. Difficult behaviors are not a result of a character flaw or malice. Nurses have the power to create a positive and accepting health care encounter for families with a child with autism. Findings from Joey's physical examination are included in Exhibit 6.1.

KEY CLINICAL ISSUES AND TREATMENT GOALS

Diagnosis

Joey's presenting diagnosis was PDD-NOS. However, Joey had severe deficits. He was nonverbal, with severe impairments in social interaction and multiple stereotypic behaviors, as well as a history of regression. Joey lost skills at 20 months and appeared to have severely impaired cognitive function.

Plan

The main object of the plan of care was to establish a more accurately defined diagnosis. This was achieved by using diagnostic measurements that included the *Diagnostic and Statistical Manual of Mental Disorders, Fourth Edition, Text Revision* (*DSM-IV-TR*) criteria checklist (American Psychiatric Association [APA], 2000) and the Childhood Autism Rating Scale, (CARS; Schopler, Reichler, & Renner, 1986) and by reviewing all previous developmental and newly acquired neuropsychological testing and observations during the first week of hospitalization. In addition, an immediate need was to obtain a speech–language therapy consultation. Joey was referred for a speech–language therapy consultation with an expert in alternative/augmentative devices in children with neurodevelopmental disabilities.

EXHIBIT 6.1

Results of Joey's Physical Examination

Anthropometry

Height: 1st percentile; weight: 25th percentile; head circumference: 10th percentile; interpupillary distance: 25th percentile; inner and outer canthus: 10th to 25th percentile; palpebral fissure length: 10th to 25th percentile bilateral.

Head and Face

Low hairline, two hair whorls, hooding of eyes, protuberant ears, slightly bulbous and broad nasal tip, thin upper lip.

Ear/Nose/Throat

PERRLA (pupils equal, round, reactive to light and accommodation), high arched palate, tonsils + 2, uvula midline, negative adenopathy, supple neck, thyroid palpable and normal size.

Chest

Lungs clear bilaterally, equal excursion of chest, negative retractions, lips and mucous membranes pink, no bony malformations.

Cardiac

+2 systolic ejection murmur, peripheral pulses +2 bilaterally in upper and lower extremities, capillary refill brisk, feet cool to touch, BP: 100/60, HR: 92.

Skin

Raised calloused area of hard dry skin on forehead (2 cm × 1 cm) and raised; calloused area of pink, dry skin on back of head (2 cm × 2 cm); negative Wood's lamp; red, raised rash on buttocks (diaper rash).

Musculoskeletal

Flat feet, bilateral pronation, waddle-like gait, good range of motion in all extremities, arm span normal.

Neurological

Alert, no tremors, no cog wheeling (ratcheting effect of arm or leg), Cranial nerves III-XII grossly intact, no facial asymmetry, nonverbal, no dystonia, tremor, prolonged muscle contraction, or abnormal posture, DTR + 2 bilaterally in upper and lower extremities.

Evidence for Practice: Accurately Diagnosing Severity of the ASD

Over the past decade, a greater understanding of continuity among the PDD diagnoses has led the autism community to embrace autism as a spectrum disorder. The autism community has adopted the term ASD as the favored umbrella designation. This concept, however, is not reflected in the present *DSM-IV-TR* or the *DSM-IV* (APA, 2000 and 1994, respectively). In these *DSM* editions, PDD is a category including autistic disorder (AD), Asperger's syndrome (AS), PDD-NOS, Rett disorder (RD), and childhood disintegrative disorder (CDD). For a comparison of autism diagnoses, see Table 6.1.

With a prevalence of 1 in 110 children (Centers for Disease Control and Prevention [CDC], 2009), the term ASD refers to three of the five diagnoses and excludes RD and CDD. In 2012, with the launch of the *DSM-V*, the term ASD will replace autism, PDD-NOS, and AS terminology. Clinicians and researchers will provide a diagnosis of ASD and will assign a severity of mild, moderate, or severe. Individuals previously diagnosed with autism will most likely be categorized in the moderate-to-severe level of ASD. Mild ASD most likely will be assigned to individuals with a previous diagnosis of AS or PDD-NOS.

Rett disorder and CDD, the two diagnoses not included in the autism spectrum, are rare and are associated with a severe developmental regression, acute changes in motor control, cognitive impairment, and often epilepsy. The causative gene for RD is the methyl CpG-binding protein2 gene (*MECP2*), located on the Xq28 chromosome (Amir et al., 1999). The prevalence of classic RD is 1 in 10,000; however, current understanding of RD variants suggests that the overall prevalence may be much higher (Kerr, 1992). CDD is characterized by late-onset symptoms of autism after the age of three. CDD has a prevalence of 2 in 100,000 (Burd, Fisher, & Kerbeshian, 1989; Mouridsen, Rich, & Isager, 1999; Volkmar, Cicchetti, Cohen & Bregman, 1992). CDD is often accompanied by severe regression, including a motor regression and a loss of previously acquired toileting skills. CDD and the behaviors described have commonalities to other neuropsychiatric phenomena, such as catatonia in children, and there is uncertainty about nosology of this diagnosis.

Our case, Joey, had developmental delay and a regression at 20 months. Developmental regression, a perceptible loss of skills, occurs in up to one-third of children with autism (Tuchman & Rapin, 1997). The period of regression usually appears between 15 and 24 months and can occur with those having typical development, as well as with those having noticeable developmental delays. The regression phenomenon that Joey experienced is a commonality in children with ASD and in all cases with RD and CDD (see Table 6.1). The etiology of regression in ASD, RD, and CDD is not well understood and co-occurs more frequently with seizures. (Amir et al., 1999; Burd et al., 1989; Kim et al., 2006; Mouridsen et al., 1999; Spence & Schneider, 2009; Volkmar et al., 1992). Nevertheless, we may gain insights in understanding the biological mechanisms of regression from the advances in knowledge about the RD and MECP2 mutations associated with the disorder.

In order to qualify for the diagnosis of autism with the *DSM-IV-TR* criteria checklist (APA, 2000), an individual needs a total of six or more deficits from the three core impairment categories. Specifically, at least two deficits are needed from the social interaction category and one each from the communication impairment and the behavioral impairment category. To be diagnosed with PDD-NOS, an individual must demonstrate deficits in all three core areas, but the severity is less than with a diagnosis of autism. Asperger's syndrome is characterized by relatively normal language development (including timing, grammar, and vocabulary), but requires deficits in at least two behavioral areas: social interactions and repetitive or restricted interests (Asperger, 1944; Frith, 1991). Individuals with AS have normal to above-average cognitive abilities.

TABLE 6.1 ■ Comparison of Autism Diagnoses

Diagnosis	Characteristics	Seizure prevalence	Timing of regression	Prevalence in population
ASDs	Core deficits: social, communication, behaviors		15 to 24 months	1 in 110
Autistic disorder	30% to 50% with cognitive impairments (44.6%; CDC, 2009)	Approx. 25%		
PDD-NOS			Approximately one-third of ASD	
Asperger's syndrome	Normal to above average IQ Social impairments and restricted interests	7%		
RD	Normal prenatal and perinatal period Psychomotor developmental largely normal; may have some delays Normal head circumference at birth Regression of social, communication and cognitive skills Motor skills Impaired locomotion Loss of fine motor skills and use of hands	Approximately 80%	12 to 24 months	1 in 10,000
CDD	Normal prenatal and perinatal period Normal development up to age 3 years Normal head circumference at birth Regression of social, communication and cognitive skills Regression of motor skills with impaired locomotion	100% 3 to 8 years	77%	2 in 100,000

Diagnostic Process

Diagnosing a child with ASD requires a comprehensive medical and developmental history and a physical exam that includes developmental testing, dysmorphology and cognitive assessment, and should be based on the *DSM-IV-TR* criteria. In addition, the diagnostician should incorporate at least one autism-specific diagnostic tool, such as the CARS or the "gold standard" assessment tools: Autism Diagnostic Interview or Autism Diagnostic

Observation Schedule (Filipek et al., 1999). The severity of the core deficits should be well-described for each child, along with his or her strengths. Joey's assessment and diagnosis were based on our observations, a developmental history from parental reporting, a review of school reports, and the *DSM-IV-TR* and CARS assessments.

The CARS is a behavior rating scale that was developed by Eric Schopler, Robert J. Reichler, and Barbara R. Renner (1989). The CARS is able to differentiate children with autism from those with other neurodevelopmental disorders, including intellectual disability. The CARS is a diagnostic tool intended to be completed by a clinician. It rates children on a scale from 1 to 4, for 15 items The CARS provides a composite score ranging from nonautistic to mildly autistic, moderately autistic, or severely autistic. The clinician bases the rating on observation, parental reporting, and review of past evaluations. Each of the 15 criteria is rated for the child's age with a score of: 1 = normal; 2 = mildly abnormal; 3 = moderately abnormal; 4 = severely abnormal. Midpoint scores of 1.5, 2.5, and 3.5 are also used. Total CARS scores range from 15 to 60. A minimum score of 30 is the cutoff for a diagnosis of autism on the mild end of the ASD. Previously, Joey had been diagnosed with PDD-NOS, but he met full criteria for the diagnosis of autism when the *DSM-IV-TR* criteria and the CARS were employed. His CARS score of 51 placed him in the category of severe autism (Table 6.2).

We presented the results of our comprehensive assessment, including the *DSM-IV-TR* criteria (American Psychiatric Association, 2000) and the CARS ratings to Joey's parents and explained his diagnosis of severe autism. His parents cried. They stated that they always knew that Joey had autism, but they were told by their neurologist that he had PDD-NOS. They expressed feelings of guilt, because they had attributed Joey's lack of progress to their decisions about his care. Clarification of the diagnosis was very helpful for the parents, and they stated that a huge burden had been removed from their shoulders.

TABLE 6.2 ■ Joey's Results on the CARS

CAR CATEGORY	Score
Relationship to people	4
Imitation	3
Emotional response	4
Body use	4
Object use	4
Adaptation to change	4
Visual response	3
Listening response	3
Taste–smell–touch response and use	3
Fear and nervousness	3
Verbal communication	4
Nonverbal communication	3
Activity level	3
Level and consistency of intellectual response	2
General impression	4
Total Score	51

Speech–Language Evaluation and Consultation for an Augmentative and Alternative Communication System

Difficulty in social language or delays in language development are core features of ASD. Approximately one-half of children with autism are either nonverbal or have insufficient speech and language abilities (CDC, 2007). Augmentative and alternative communication (AAC) systems can support individuals with ASD who cannot effectively use conventional speech (Mirenda, 2001, 2003). Augmentative and alternative communication includes sign language, communication boards, picture-exchange communication systems (PECS), speech-generating devices (SGDs), or voice output communication aids (VOCAS). Speech-generating devices and VOCAS are portable, electronic AAC devices that usually combine digitized or synthesized speech with static visual symbols. A recent meta-analysis showed that aided AAC interventions had the largest effect on targeted behavioral outcomes overall (Ganz et al., 2011). Of these, PECS and SGDs had the greatest effects: 0.99 for each. (Ganz et al., 2011). Joey's speech–language evaluation revealed a receptive language age of 29 months and an expressive language age of 20 months. The speech–language consultant identified an AAC—a communication switch—for Joey to incorporate into his communicative acts. Joey received speech/language therapy daily for 3 months, and learned to use the switch to ask for his favorite toys, a break, and food items. The communication switch was also utilized in his behavioral treatment plan. Joey's parents quickly learned to incorporate the switch into their interactions with him. His ability to use the switch to communicate his wants and needs was the beginning of change from the use of tantrums for communication.

Key Clinical Issues

Neurocompromise: Joey was admitted for severe SIB in the form of head-banging. Any prior attempts to have him wear a helmet had escalated his SIB. During the behavioral sessions, nurses observed Joey and performed neurological checks before and after behavioral sessions and every 10 minutes during sessions. If the head-banging had resulted in a change in level of consciousness or other neurological signs suggesting more serious injury, Joey would have been taken for an immediate CAT scan.

Epilepsy: Joey was diagnosed with simple partial seizures and trialed on valproic acid, but had refused all attempts at administration. At age 5, Joey had multiple episodes of staring spells, eye deviation, and eye blinking with left arm jerks. The past EEG was of poor quality. No further seizure activity was observed during the first week of hospitalization; however, he did stare frequently. We observed him for suspected seizure activity and start a seizure log to document frequency of staring and abnormal movements. We obtained a neurology consult and an EEG, and implemented a pill-swallowing protocol when Joey's undesirable behaviors decreased.

Evidence for Practice: Epilepsy and Regression in ASD

One of the important associations between central nervous system dysfunction and ASD is the elevated risk of epilepsy (Spence & Schneider, 2009). Epilepsy has been reported in approximately one-third of individuals with ASD, with a range from 5% to 46% (Bryson, Clark, & Smith, 1988; Hughes & Melyn, 2005; Trevathan, 2004; Tuchman, Alessandri, & Cuccaro, 2010). The high variability in prevalence is thought to be the result of the age of the subjects and the definition of epilepsy, with older children experiencing higher rate of seizures

(Trevathan, 2004; Tuchman et al., 2010; Berg et al., 2009). There are two peaks in the age of onset of epilepsy in ASD: early childhood and adolescence (Hara, 2007; Volkmar & Nelson, 1990).

Seizures are the most striking feature of epilepsy, although recent definitions of epilepsy have emphasized the cognitive, psychological, and social consequences of this group of disorders (Tuchman et al., 2010). Epilepsy is defined in most prevalence studies as occurrence of more than one unprovoked seizure (Berg et al., 2009; Tuchman et al., 2010). Still, the methods for best defining epilepsy and classifying seizures are continuing to evolve (Tuchman et al., 2010). It has been posited that intellectual disability drives the association between epilepsy and ASD. A meta-analysis of 10 studies found an epilepsy rate of 21.5% for individuals with ASD, a rate of 13% to 17% for those without co-ocurring syndromes, and a rate of 8% for individuals with normal intelligence (Amiet et al., 2008; Canitano, Luchetti, & Zapella, 2005). The general population risk is 1% to 2 %. Thus, ASD itself is associated with higher epilepsy rates.

A primary seizure type in autism has not been identified. Partial seizures (with or without secondarily generalized seizures), absence, and generalized tonic-clonic seizure types have all been reported (Hara, 2007; Parmeggiani et al., 2007; Steffenburg, Steffenburg, & Gillberg, 2003; Tuchman, Rapin, & Shinnar, 1991).

Moreover, the behavioral abnormalities associated with partial and absence seizures (for example, staring and unresponsiveness, with or without repetitive movements) can also be interpreted as features of ASD themselves (Spence & Schneider, 2009). Parents frequently state that their children appear to be "in their own world" and often stare. This makes the assessment of seizure activity and diagnosis of absence and partial seizures even more challenging for health providers. Nurses can play a significant role in helping families describe their children's behaviors and movements and in developing strategies for documenting suspicious behaviors in a seizure diary.

Autism spectrum disorder is also prevalent in the epilepsy population; up to 32% of individuals with epilepsy meet criteria for ASD (Brooks-Kayal, 2010; Spence & Schneider, 2009). Recently, the question of whether an epileptic encephalopathy plays a role in the etiology of autism has been posed (Brooks-Kayal, 2010). Currently, the associations among occurrence of regression, epilepsy, and epileptiform EEG abnormalities are unclear (Spence & Schneider, 2009). Many practitioners send children with ASD characteristics for EEGs when regression is present, in order to rule out Landau- Kleffner syndrome, but conflicting findings in the literature do not fully support this practice. Landau-Kleffner syndrome is described as rapid onset in a typically developing child of the inability to understand expressive language. It is usually accompanied by seizures. The EEG characteristically shows severe abnormality in deep sleep or electrical status epilepticus in sleep. In many cases, seizures and language impairments improve with normalization of EEG abnormalities. EEGs are considered standard for all children with clinical or suspected seizures. However, the practice of performing EEGs on all children with ASD has been questioned. More recently, attention has been drawn to possibilities of deleterious transient cognitive impairments due to the presence of background epileptiform discharges in patients with epilepsy (Binnie, 2003; Holmes & Lenck-Santini, 2006). Epileptiform discharges on EEG alone have been associated with children's academic and attention problems, which remitted after normalization of the EEGs (Kavros et al., 2008). Theoretically, treating abnormal EEG's in children with ASD may positively impact cognition and behavior with ASD. However, essential questions about relationships among the occurrence of epilepsy and the cognitive, language, and behavioral deficits seen in autism are still unanswered, Future research into the common molecular, cellular, and genetic mechanisms of action in ASD and epilepsy might provide insights into the underlying etiology and illuminate new treatments for these conditions (Brooks-Kayal, 2010).

Best practice for all children with ASD is to perform a comprehensive neurological exam and screen for seizure activity at each health care encounter. Clinicians should have a high index of suspicion for questionable behaviors that are reported by parents, teachers, and therapists. Frequent staring episodes warrant an EEG and perhaps an overnight video EEG. Any new regression or a prolonged plateau of skill acquisition also warrants an EEG.

CASE—CONTINUED

Joey's behaviors represented possible simple partial seizures. We obtained a neurology consult. The neurologist agreed with the plan of obtaining an EEG after Joey's undesirable behaviors had decreased, at which time he would be more likely to tolerate the procedure. In addition, the neurologist recommended a dose of clonidine (0.05 mg Catapres), an alpha-agonist, prior to the procedure, to induce sleepiness. This medication can be used as a sleep aid for children with neurodevlopmental disabilities, and would not interfere with the EEG results. By week 7 of hospitalization, undesirable behaviors had decreased by 60%. Joey was then able to tolerate the procedure with behavioral support and the dose of clonidine embedded in a Starburst candy. The EEG was positive for focal seizures in the left temporal area, and he was diagnosed with simple partial seizure disorder, and valproic acid was prescribed. Joey was able to take the medication (for both the staff and family members) as sprinkles on pudding during week 7 of the hospitalization.

Key Clinical Issue: Dysmorphic Features and Congenital Anomalies

Joey had short stature, low hairline, hooding of the eyes, protuberant ears, high arched palate, bulbous tipped nose, thin upper lip, a cardiac defect (vascular ring status postrepair), heart murmur, developmental delays, and ASD. No workup for this collage of characteristics had ever taken place. Our plan included a genetics consult, a cardiology consult, and tracking of vital signs every day while implementing behavior strategies.

Evidence for Practice: Dysmorphology and Congenital Anomalies

An estimated 7.9 million children worldwide are born with serious birth defects of genetic or epigenetic (combination of environment and genes) origin (Christianson, Howson, & Modell, 2006). The best way to begin the identification of a genetic syndrome is to measure and photograph potentially dysmorphic features, to document congenital abnormalities, and to obtain a thorough genealogy, along with a developmental and behavioral history of the individual (Cassidy & Allanson, 2010). A clinician's subjective impression of an abnormality can be confirmed with selected measurements and comparison to normal standards. Using anthropometry, standard photographs, and radiographic data, a clinician can identify abnormal characteristics. Common craniofacial dimensions include head circumference; inner and outer canthal distances; interpupillary distance; ear length, position, and rotation; and size and shape of the face. A dysmorphology evaluation also includes height, weight, upper and lower body segments, arm span, and hand, palm, and foot lengths. A clinician often notes a different "look" and has a general impression that a person is dysmorphic. The clinician then needs to systematically assess features from head to toe and thoroughly describe those characteristics that appear dysmorphic.

The term "syndrome" is used to describe a broad array of dysmorphology. Syndromes involve the simultaneous presence of dysmorphic features, malformations, and/or behavioral and functional differences that have been seen repeatedly in a fairly consistent and unique pattern and that are known or assumed to be a result of a single etiology. The initial definition of a syndrome occurs after the publication of several similar cases and becomes refined over time (Cassidy & Allanson, 2010).

In any individual, one or more hallmark features may be absent, although the person still presents with the syndrome (Cassidy & Allanson, 2010). Genetic testing facilitates identification of genetically derived clinical syndromes. Genetic testing has expanded rapidly in recent years. Testing demonstrates the vastness of the clinical spectrum for many disorders. Many gene mutations cause their adverse effects through altered gene expression. Subsequently, there can be either an over- or underproduction of proteins. In recent years, epigenetic mutations in the genetic apparatus have also been recognized as causes of human disorders. Epigenetic mutations are biochemical changes to DNA that modify its expression and that may result in diseases or disorders.

Genetic research has provided multiple lines of evidence for the strong genetic contribution to ASD, but the specific etiology for an individual patient can be elusive. Autism spectrum disorder also has been found to be a component of several known genetic syndromes with distinct clinical features, such as RD, Fragile X, and 22q11.2 deletion (Farzin et al., 2006; Hagerman et al., 2008; Harris et al., 2008). However, a recent twin-pair population-based study highlighted the epigenetic contribution to ASD, concluding that susceptibility to ASD had a moderate genetic heritability factor, but a substantial environmental component. The high genetic heritability rate demonstrated in prior studies had shifted the research focus away from potential environmental triggers. Future studies should seek to identify environmental influences that may enhance or suppress genetic susceptibility.

CASE—CONTINUED

Joey's physical exam was significant for short stature (height 1%), low hairline, two hair whorls, hooding of eyes, protuberant ears, slightly bulbous and broad nasal tip, thin upper lip, and cardiac defect (vascular ring). He also presented with cognitive impairment and autism. Joey's dysmorphic characteristics were confirmed by clinical geneticists. Blood work was sent for karyotyping, Fragile X evaluation, and fluorescence in situ hybridization (FISH) for 22q11.2 deletion. The FISH result was positive for the 22q 11.2 microdeletion. Joey was recognized to have 22q11.2 deletion syndrome, previously known as DiGeorge syndrome or velocardofacial syndrome. A cardiology consult was obtained during his BBU admission and his physical exam, electrocardiogram, and echocardiogram were all within normal limits.

We planned a family meeting to share the results with Joey's parents. Both parents were able to attend. They were overwhelmed by the results. The father stated that he also had dysmorphic features, as well as behavioral and learning differences, as did his daughter. All family members were referred to the genetics team and had a comprehensive evaluation with genetic testing. The father and sister also tested positive for the 22q11.2 deletion. The mother tested negative. Joey and his family members were scheduled to see multiple subspecialists to provide a comprehensive evaluation and to detect abnormalities often associated with 22q11.2 deletion.

22q11.2 Deletion—Molecular Genetics

The 22q11.2 deletion is the most frequent microdeletion syndrome in humans (Bassett et al., 2011; Cassidy & Allanson, 2010; McDonald-McGinn & Sullivan, 2011) with a prevalence estimate of 1 in 4,000. Most deletions are de novo, spontaneous, and not inherited from the parents. The cause of the high prevalence of this microdeletion rests in the structure of the chromosome 22q11.2 section (Cassidy & Allanson 2010; McDonald-McGinn & Sullivan, 2011). This section is bordered with segmental duplications, resulting in susceptibility to rearrangements during meiotic crossovers (Emanuel, Budard, Shaikh, & Driscoll, 1998). The majority of affected individuals have the same large deletion, encompassing about 30 functional genes (Cassidy & Allanson 2010; McDonald-McGinn & Sullivan, 2011). The high rate of 22q11.2 deletion supports the need to think broadly when assessing individuals with characteristics associated with 22q11.2 deletion, and to consider additional co-occurring genetic disorders (Cassidy &Allanson, 2010; McDonald-McGinn & Sullivan, 2011; McDonald-McGinn & Zachai, 2008).

FISH Genetic Testing

FISH combines chromosome analysis with the use of fluorescence-tagged molecular markers (called probes) that are applied after the chromosome preparation is produced (Fuller & Perry, 2002). Thus, to test whether there is a small deletion (called a microdeletion) that is not visible using chromosome analysis alone, fluorescence-tagged molecular probes complementary to the deleted material are applied to the chromosome preparation. If a normal amount of chromosome material is present, a fluorescent signal will be visible at that site under the fluorescence microscope. If the normal chromosome material is deleted or absent, no fluorescent signal will be present (Fuller & Perry, 2002). FISH is a powerful tool used to identify microdeletions, duplications, and structural rearrangements or translocations (Fuller & Perry, 2002).

Clinical Manifestations of 22q11.2 Deletion Syndrome

Individuals with 22q11.2 syndrome have multisystem problems involving the development and end-modeling of the brain, spinal cord and vertebrae, palate, teeth, neck glands, immune system, thorax, and heart. Approximately 90% of individuals with 22q11.2 deletion have dysmorphic features (see Figure 6.1), hypernasal speech (90%), cardiac defect (50% to 75%), recurrent infections (35% to 40%), endocrine issues (60%), dysmotility (35%), and urinary tract anomalies (31%). Moreover, 14% to 50% of individuals with 22q11.2 deletion have ASD (Benayed et al., 2005; Fine et al., 2005, Vorstman et al., 2006). Table 6.3 summarizes characteristics associated with 22q11.2 deletion syndrome, along with management strategies for care of individuals with the syndrome.

During the first months of life, Joey had feeding difficulties and frequent respiratory infections, and he developed pneumonia at age 3 months. He was diagnosed with a cardiac vascular ring at a children's hospital, and it was surgically repaired at 4 months of age. Subsequently, Joey did better with his feedings and began to grow. Joey's last visit with a cardiologist was at age 2 years. As part of Joey's treatment plan, we requested a cardiology consult as a follow-up to the vascular ring repair.

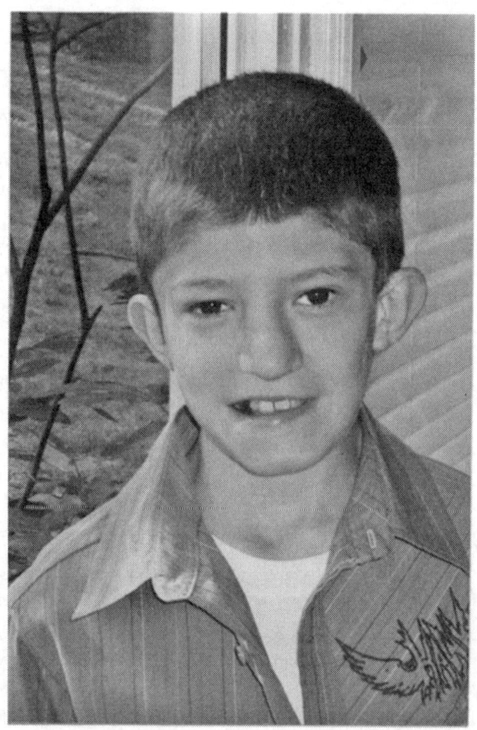

FIGURE 6.1 ■ Child with 22q11.2 deletion syndrome. Printed with parental permission.

Vascular Ring in Embryonic Development

Vascular ring occurs very early in embryonic development (Kellenberger, 2010; Weinberg, 2006). Normally, the aorta develops from one of several curved arches. The developing embryo breaks down some of the remaining arches, while others form into arteries. Some arteries that should break down do not (Kellenberger, 2010). With a vascular ring, some of the arches and vessels that should have changed into arteries or disintegrated are still present at birth. These arches form a ring, which encircles and presses down onto the trachea and/or esophagus. There are several different types of vascular rings. In some types, the vascular ring only partially encircles the trachea and esophagus, but it still may cause symptoms (Kellenberger, 2010).

Vascular rings are very rare and account for less than 1% of all congenital heart problems. The condition occurs as often in males as in females. A vascular ring may also be associated with another congenital heart problem. Some children with vascular rings never develop symptoms; however, in Joey's case and in most cases, symptoms are seen during infancy (Zackai et al., 1996). Joey experienced pressure on the trachea and esophagus that lead to his respiratory distress and feeding difficulties.

Joey also had difficulty swallowing; he frequently choked and was a very slow eater. In line with best practices for evaluation of these conditions, Joey had a chest X-ray, as well as an echocardiogram and a computed tomography scan of the heart, which was followed by surgical repair for the vascular ring. The goal of vascular ring repair surgery is to split the vascular ring and relieve pressure on the surrounding structures (Kellenberger, 2010). The surgical procedure was done through a small surgical cut in the left side of the chest between the ribs. Joey recovered well and his respiratory symptoms and feedings behaviors improved.

TABLE 6.3 ■ Common Phenotypical Features, Clinical Findings, and Management in 22q11.2 Deletion Syndrome

System/site	Diagnoses	Clinical features	Management
Craniofacial	Cleft palate Submucosal cleft palate Velopharyngeal insufficiency Midface hypoplasia	Prominent articulation problems Hypernasal speech Feeding difficulties Difficulty swallowing Failure to thrive	Plastic surgery GI, feeding team, nutrition, speech and audiology consultation Cleft palate repair Velopharyngeal insufficiency repair
Cardiac	Atrial and septal defects Pulmonary atresia or stenosis Tetralogy of Fallot Patent ductus arterious Vascular ring Raynaud phenomenon Varicose veins Rhythm abnormalities	Poor perfusion Failure to thrive Feeding difficulties	Cardiology consultation Cardiac surgery Pacemaker
Immune	Reduced T-cell populations Hypoplastic thymus	Frequent respiratory infections, pneumonia Frequent otitis media	Vaccine titers Minimize infectious exposures RSV prophylaxis
Endocrine	Hypocalcemia Hypoparathyroidism Hypothyroidism	Hypotonia Seizures Mood Lethargy Hallucinations	Endocrine consultation Replacement therapy assessment during surgeries and physiological stress Vitamin D and calcium supplementation Growth hormone
Neurological	Hypotonia Headaches Migraines Seizures Unprovoked Provoked	5% unprovoked seizures	Neurology consult EEG MRI Calcium and magnesium levels assessment
Skeletal	Scoliosis Club foot C-spine abnormalities Chronic leg pain Flat feet	Joint pain fatigue	Orthopedic consultation Radiographics Orthodontics
Learning	Borderline intellect Learning disabilities	Concrete thinking Reading and math	Pediatric psychologist IQ testing
Psychiatric	ADHD ASD Obsessive–compulsive disorder Schizophrenia Anxiety	Short attention span Difficulties with social interaction Perseverative behaviors Delusions	Pediatric psychiatrist Psychiatric nurse practitioner Screening for development at each checkup
Developmental	Global delays Social immaturity	Delayed milestones	Developmental pediatric consultation
Gastrointestinal tract	Dysmotility Hernias Imperforated anus Hirschsprung disease Diaphragmatic hernia Malrotation	Constipation GERD Cyclical vomiting	GI Consultation

(*Continued*)

TABLE 6.3 ■ *Continued*

System/site	Diagnoses	Clinical features	Management
Genitourinary tract	Urinary tract anomalies Duplex/echogenic kidney Hydronephrosis Cryptorchidism Absent uterus Nephrocalcinosis	Frequency Abdominal pain Infection	Ultrasound Urology Nephrology Gynecology
Sleep	Insomnia Parasomnias Obstructive sleep apnea	Sleepy Moody	Sleep study Sleep hygiene

MANAGING COMPLEX CLINICAL ISSUES

SIB and Tantrums

Joey's undesirable behaviors included SIBs: head-banging on hard surfaces and head-butting others; tantrums that included spitting, hitting, crying, screaming, and pinching; and medication refusal. When Joey was first admitted to the unit, he would have a tantrum when approached by staff. He would throw himself on the floor and bang his head. The related behavioral treatment goal was to decrease Joey's undesirable behaviors by 80%. Self-injurious behavior was defined as the contact of Joey's head with surfaces such as the floor, wall, furniture, and another person's face or head. Tantrums were defined as a constellation of disruptive behaviors: spitting, crying, and pinching that escalated rapidly within 1 to 3 minutes to screaming, flailing, and hitting. The duration at home on average was approximately 45 minutes. Medication refusal was defined as unwillingness to allow medication into the mouth or spitting out of medication after administration.

Evidence for Practice: Functional Analysis

All patients admitted to the BBU had functional analysis (FA) of their undesirable behaviors led by a behavioral psychologist. The purpose of FA was: 1) to describe the severe undesirable behaviors in terms of the frequency, intensity, duration, antecedents, and circadian timing; 2) to identify the relationship between the undesirable behaviors and antecedents and consequences; 3) to design behavioral strategies to decrease undesired behaviors and increase developmentally adaptive behaviors; and 4) to test and refine the behavioral strategies into a behavioral protocol that could be implemented by the family, therapists, and teachers (Lalli, Mace, Livezey, & Kates, 1998).

A key goal of the inpatient program was to facilitate generalization of skills with creation of a behavioral protocol tailored to each individual for the home and school environment. Families needed to be included in the FA from the first days of the hospitalization in order to be educated about the assessment and intervention process. Parents often needed to take off from work in order to be available during the day or early evening in order to participate in the FA and intervention development. The nursing staff often played a strong advocacy role for the families as they negotiated the training process with the psychology team.

Behavioral Data Collection and Results

Behavioral staff used a computerized data collection procedure to record each occurrence of SIB and tantrums during FA sessions. A rate of 85% interobserver agreement was needed in order to classify a behavior as SIB or tantrum. Four to five sessions of FA and treatment evaluation, lasting 10 minutes each, were conducted each day, 5 days a week. FA conditions were assessed in a multielement design, with a therapist providing attention, escape from self-care tasks, or a toy following Joey's SIB. The therapist used a variable-interval reinforcement schedule. Each of these sessions was followed by a 120-minute alone session for observation of SIB under extended conditions of low stimulation.

The descriptive and experimental analyses suggested that Joey's SIB and tantrums were maintained by attention. Analyses identified physical contact as the type of attention that maintained the SIB. We hypothesized that the presence of an adult was a discriminate stimulus for SIB. Therefore, the behavioral psychologist selected the distance between the adult and Joey as the target stimulus dimension to vary during the generalization assessment. The behavioral strategies devised by the psychology staff were effective in decreasing Joey's SIB and tantrums by 90%. He developed the ability to complete self-care tasks with a prompt from a therapist located 8 feet away. These strategies have been effective with another patient and were subsequently published (Lalli et al., 1998). The strategies were then shaped into a behavioral protocol for implementation throughout the day by his therapists. After a successful week, the team was able to transition the implementation of the behavioral protocol to family and community staff.

Family Training Program

Once Joey's family was trained and could effectively implement the behavioral protocol in the hospital setting, training continued at home. This transition was a difficult boundary to navigate. Protocols developed and implemented in the structured hospital setting by very skilled behavioral staff can be challenging to use in the home setting. Family members who will be responsible for the behavioral protocol need support to invest the energy and time required for success. Parents often face competing demands of running a household and working and caring for siblings, and need frequent reinforcement from the behavioral staff. Nurses, as witnesses to the families' hospital experiences, and with in-depth knowledge of behavioral protocols, can offer families support and encouragement, especially during extinction bursts of severe problem behaviors. Extinction bursts involve short-term, high rates of an undesirable behavior.

If behavioral protocols are not successfully implemented in the hospital or the home, nursing staff can act as family advocates, exploring the possibility of medication use in conjunction with behavioral strategies and discussing options with parents and the multidisciplinary team. For Joey, medication choices were based on the undesirable behaviors or target behaviors identified by the psychology team, and on mechanisms of drug action and side-effect profiles.

Medication Administration

Barriers to smooth administration of medication to children with ASD include difficulty swallowing pills and sensory issues related to the taste and smell of crushed or liquid preparations (Beck, Cataldo, Slifer, Pulbrook, & Guhman, 2005; Pelco, Kissel, Parrish, & Miltenberger, 1987). Some children with ASD might not have the necessary sustained attention and oral motor skills to swallow a pill or capsule. Others have significant sensory differences and/or have had many negative eating experiences. Moreover, children with ASD often demonstrate severe restrictions in food, along with a conditioned anxiety to new foods or food groups. Parents or other caregivers often resort to hiding medication in foods. This can often heighten suspicions in children with ASD and escalate refusal behaviors. A pill-swallowing protocol based on a child's behavioral program can be developed; it is best to delay pill-swallowing skill development until maladaptive behaviors, such as tantrums and SIB, are addressed. Joey was able to tolerate Valproic Acid sprinkles on pudding and ice cream, and a pill protocol was not necessary. Evidence for the use of psychoactive and other medications to manage aberrant behavior in children with ASD is evolving rapidly. Refer to Chapter 3 for a summary of pharmacotherapeutic agents used in the treatment of ASD. Deep understanding of the mechanisms of action, potential targeted behaviors, and side-effect profiles of these drugs is essential for any clinician caring for individuals with autism. Further nursing research addressing a variety of phenomena related to medication use in the population of individuals with ASD is important. During individual medication trials or as investigators, nurses need medication expertise to take lead roles during individual medication trials or as investigators in randomized, controlled drug trials (Scahill et al., 2001).

Key Clinical Issue: Health Maintenance

Children with undesirable behaviors often have health maintenance challenges (Souders et al., 2002). Joey was unable tolerate primary pediatric exams and the administration of immunizations. Joey had disruptions in self-care activities and sleeping, toileting, and eating behaviors. With regard to sleeping, we found that the consistent routines of the BBU provided the cues to establish better sleep patterns. After 3 weeks, a structured bedtime routine was established, and Joey was able to sleep 8 to 9 hours each night. He continued to grind his teeth, and a dental consult was obtained.

We developed a toileting protocol for Joey in the evening. He had an established circadian rhythm to his stooling behavior. His mother reported that Joey consistently stooled after dinner; therefore, the behavioral strategy was to have Joey sit on the toilet for 15 to 30 seconds every 15 minutes for 2 hours after dinner. He was to be rewarded for sitting on toilet for 15 to 30 seconds. If he was successful and stooled in the toilet, he received an enormous amount of verbal praise and a preferred small toy. After 2 weeks, Joey was consistently able to stool in the toilet 1 hour after dinner each evening. The speech therapist then developed a picture-exchange card for the bathroom. This was then incorporated into Joey's after-dinner routine. At week 6, Joey was able to use a picture-exchange card after dinner to request the bathroom.

Health Maintenance Protocols

Joey had problems with food selectivity. We obtained a nutritional consultation and developed a behavioral protocol to increase food choices. Joey was able to tolerate one new food group per week with a shaping protocol. We obtained a dental consult and developed a treatment plan that included tooth-brushing skills and a behavioral protocol for bath and bedtime routines. After 3 weeks, Joey was able to his brush teeth with one-on-one aide prompts. We designed a morning routine protocol that included dressing skills. After 2 weeks Joey was able to put on a T-shirt, gym shorts, socks, and Velcro sneakers

Immunization Catch-up

We evaluated immunization status and provided catch-up immunizations. The last week of hospitalization, Joey received catch-up immunizations. This procedure required 5 adults. He sat on the lap of a therapist. The therapist was able to secure his chest and one arm. The other therapist secured the other arm. Another therapist stood behind the chair and gently held his shoulders, to prevent him from standing up. Two nurses prepared all vaccines ahead of time and hid them from sight. One nurse prepared the injection site with an alcohol swab, and another nurse administered the injections.

We obtain comprehensive lab work after all consultations are complete: comprehensive metabolic panel (C) with prealbumin, lead level, heavy metal, and micronutrient screens and complete blood count (CBC) with differential and ferritin levels. All of Joey's laboratory work was within normal levels.

Finally, with respect to health maintenance, we started a daily children's multivitamin and developed behavioral protocols for health care providers to use for physical assessment, routine immunizations, and other health-related interventions.

Key Clinical Issue: Family Support—Family Education and Counseling and Estate Planning

The family of the child affected with complex autism needs support. A social work consultation involved daily meetings to review the hospitalization plan and treatment goals with the family. Nursing and the social work staff met weekly to develop a collaborative discharge plan. The team identified the key community stakeholders: teachers, therapists, and primary-care providers within the first week of hospitalization. An effort was made to include the therapeutic team in the training program in the BBU. Nursing staff and social workers played a significant role in coordinating their training sessions with the psychology staff.

Nursing and social work staff identified multiple community resources and services to which the child was entitled and for which the family must advocate. Joey should be in small class with a child-to-teacher ratio of four to one and with a one-on-one aide in a private school for children with autism. An after-school program should have the same ratio of providers to children. The parents should receive behavioral support services, with respite care for weekends. They were advised to identify stress-relieving activities and were referred to the YMCA for exercise activities 3 to 4 times a week. The family was advised that church groups can provide special needs support. They were informed that a pediatric psychologist or psychiatric nurse practitioner could be an excellent source of ongoing family therapy. Key issues to address with the family for ongoing social support are building resilience and maintaining connections to the extended family and community. Finally, the parents were referred to a local law project to begin the necessary process of estate planning. Refer to Chapter 18 for a discussion of the issue of guardianship.

SUMMARY

In this chapter, we presented a composite case of complex ASD. Joey had dysmorphic features and a cardiac birth defect, characteristics that indicate some variation of early morphogenesis. This case is an exemplar of the clinical and etiological heterogeneity within ASD. The physiological, biochemical, endocrinologic, neuroanatomical, and cognitive characteristics are biological, and perhaps more closely related to the underlying etiological processes of ASD than the behavioral symptoms (Gottesman & Gould, 2003; Miles et al., 2010). Knowing that children with complex autism often have an associated genetic disorder, the nurse practitioners pursued this line of inquiry and obtained genetics consultation.

Joey was subsequently diagnosed with 22q11.2 deletion syndrome, along with his father and sister. The new genetic knowledge empowered the family and health providers to develop a comprehensive medical, psychological, and behavioral plan, including anticipatory guidance.

Joey's severe language impairments and high frequency and intensity of undesirable behaviors prompted the nurse practitioners to utilize the *DSM-IV-TR* criteria and CARS to describe Joey's core deficits of ASD. They recognized that Joey had severe ASD or classic autism. An accurate diagnosis allowed the team to identify the appropriate level of intensity of services Joey would need on an ongoing basis to improve and maintain communication and function.

Children with autism often require an educational setting with small class sizes and one-on-one support, with a behavioral protocol implemented throughout the day. A multidisciplinary approach is best. Each child needs a strong primary nurse, special educator, speech therapist, occupational therapist, behavioral psychologist, neurologist, psychiatrist or developmental pediatrician, social worker, financial planner, and a resilient family. Joey's family (and families like his) need ongoing support from a multidisciplinary team to implement, evaluate, and revise the plan of care, to continue to maximize development, and to maximize quality of life for him and his family. Nurses are well-positioned to lead the multidisciplinary team and make a tremendous contribution to the autism community.

Nurses have the training, astute observation skills, and the work force size to make a significant contribution to describing the diverse endophenotypes and biomarkers of ASD. Nurses can lead the way in defining subgroups within the spectrum. Well-characterized subgroups offer the possibility to better predict outcomes and provide direction for treatment choices. Intensive, individualized interventions that are family oriented will then provide outcomes to improve the overall function and well-being of the individual in context of his or her family and community.

REFERENCES

American Psychiatric Association. (2000). *Diagnostic and statistical manual of mental disorders* (4 ed., text revision). Washington, DC: Author.

Amiet, C., Gourfinkel-An, I., Bouzamondo, A., Tordjman, S., Baulac, M., Lechat, P., Mottron, L., & Cohen, D. (2008). Epilepsy in autism is associated with intellectual disability and gender: Evidence from a meta-analysis. *Biological Psychiatry*, *64*(7), 577–582.

Amir, R. E., Van den Veyver, I. B., Wan, M., Tran, C. Q., Francke, U., & Zoghbi, H. Y. (1999). Rett syndrome is caused by mutations in X-linked MECP2, encoding methyl-CpG-binding protein 2. *Nature Genetics*, *23*, 185–188.

Asperger, H. (1944). *Die Autistischen Psychopathen in Kindersalter*. Cambridge, UK: Cambridge University Press.

Bassett, A., McDonald-McGinn, D. M., Devriendt, K., Digilio, M. C., Goldenberg, P., Habel, A., Marino, B., Oskarsdottir, S., Philip, N., Sullivan, K., Swillen, A., & Vorstman, J. (2011). Practical guidelines for managing patients with 22q11.2 deletion syndrome. *Journal of Pediatrics*, *159*(2), 1–8.

Beck, M. H., Cataldo, M., Slifer, K. J., Pulbrook, V., & Guhman, J. K. (2005). Teaching children with attention deficit hyperactivity disorder (ADHD) and autistic disorder (AD) how to swallow pills. *Clinical Pediatrics*, *44*(6), 515–526.

Benayed, R., Gharani, N., Rossman, I., Mancuso, V., Lazar, G., Kamdar, S., . . . Millonig, J. H. (2005). Support for the homeobox transcription factor gene ENGRAILED 2 as an autism spectrum disorder susceptibility locus. *American Journal of Human Genetics*, *77*(5), 851–868.

Berg, A., Berkovic, S. F., Brodie, M. J., Buchhalter, J., Cross, J. H., & Van Emde Boas, W. ... (2009). Revised terminology and concepts for organization of the epilepsies: Report of the Commission on Classification and Terminology. *Commission Report, 1-19.*

Binnie, C. D. (2003). Cognitive impairment during epileptiform discharges: is it ever justifiable to treat the EEG? *Lancet Neurology, 2*(12), 725–730.

Brooks-Kayal, A. (2010). Epilepsy and autism spectrum disorders: Are there common developmental mechanisms? *Brain Development, 32*(9), 731–738.

Bryson, S. E., Clark, B. S., & Smith, I. M. (1988). First Report of a Canadian epidemiological study of autistic syndromes. *Journal of Psychology and Psychiatry, and Allied Disciplines, 29*(4), 433–445.

Burd, L., Fisher, W., & Kerbeshian, J. (1989). Pervasive disintegrative disorder: Are Rett syndrome and Heller dementia infantilis subtypes? *Developmental Medicine and Child Neurology, 31*(5), 609–616.

Burgio, L. D., Page, T. J., & Capriotti, R. M. (1985). Clinical behavioral pharmacology: Methods for evaluating medications and contingency management. *Journal of Applied Behavior Analysis, 18*(2), 45–59.

Canitano, R., Luchetti, A., & Zappella, M. (2005). Epilepsy, electroencephalographic abnormalities and regression in children with autism. *Journal of Child Neurology, 20*(1), 27–31.

Cassidy, S. B., & Allanson, J. E. (2010). Introduction. *In Management of genetic syndromes* (3 ed., pp. 2). Hoboken, NJ: Wiley-Blackwell.

Centers for Disease Control and Prevention. (2009). *Facts about ASD.* Retrieved from http://cdc.gov/ncbddd/autism/facts.html

Christianson, A., Howson, C. P., & Modell, B. (2006). *Global report on birth defects.* White Plains, NY : March of Dimes Birth Defects Foundation.

Cohen, I. L., Campbell, M., & Posner, D. (1980). A study of haloperidol in young autistic children: A within-subjects design using objective rating scales. *Psychopharmacology Bulletin, 16*(3), 63–65.

DiCiccio-Bloom, E., Lord, C., Zwaigenbaum, L., ... Young, L. J. (2006). The developmental neurobiology of autism spectrum disorders. *Journal of Neuroscience, 26*, 6897–6906.

Emanuel, B. S., Budard, M. L., Shaikh, T., & Driscoll, D. (1998). Blocks of duplicated sequences define the endpoints of DGS/VCFS 22q11.2 deletion. *American Journal of Human Genetics, 63*, A11.

Farzin, F., Perry, H., Hessl, D., Loesch, D., Cohen, J., ... Hagerman, R. (2006). Autism spectrum disorders and attention-deficit/hyperactivity disorder in boys with the fragile X premutation. *Journal of Development and Behavioral Pediatrics, 27*, S137–S144.

Filipek, P. A., Accardo, P. J., Baranek, G. T., Cook, E. H., Dawson, G., Gordon, B., ... Volkmar, F. R. (1999). The screening and diagnosis of autistic spectrum disorders. *Journal of Autism and Developmental Disorders, 29*, 439–84.

Fine, S., Weissman, A., Gerdes, M., Pinto-Martin, J., Zacxkai, E., McDonald-McGinn, D., & Emanuel., B. S. (2005). Autism spectrum disorders and symptoms in children with molecularly confirmed 22q11.2. *Journal of Autism and Developmental Disability. 35*, 461–470.

Frith, U. (1991). Autistic psychopathy in childhood. In U. Frith (Ed.), *Autism and Asperger syndrome* (pp. 37–92). Cambridge, UK: Cambridge University Press.

Fuller, C. E., & Perry, A. (2002). Fluorescence in situ hybridization (FISH) in diagnostic and investigative neuropathology. *Brain Pathology, 12*(1), 67–86.

Ganz, B. J., Earles-Vollrath, T. L., Heath, A. K., Parker, R. I., Rispoli, M. J., & Duran, J. B. (2011). A meta-analysis of single case research studies on aided augmentative and alternative communication systems with individuals with autism spectrum disorders. *Journal of Autism and Developmental Disorders, 42*(1), 60–74.

Gobbi, G., & Pulvirenti, L. (2001). Long-term treatment with clozapine in an adult with autistic disorder accompanied by aggressive behaviour. *Journal of Psychiatry and Neuroscience, 26(4)*, 340–341.

Gottesman, I. I., & Gould, T. D. (2003). The endophenotype concept in psychiatry: Etymology and strategic intentions. *American Journal of Psychiatry, 160*, 636–45.

Hagerman, R. J., Rivera, S. M., & Hagerman, P. J. (2008). The Fragile X family of disorders: A model for mutism and targeted treatments. *Current Pediatric Review, 4*, 40–52.

Hara, H. (2007). Autism and epilepsy: A retrospective follow-up study. *Brain Development, 29*, 486–90.

Harris, S. W., Hessl, D., Goodlin-Jones, B., Ferranti, J., Bacalman, S., Barbato, I., & ... Hagerman, R. J. (2008). Autism profiles of males with fragile X syndrome. *American Journal of Mental Retardation, 113*, 427–438.

Holmes, G. L., & Lenck-Santini, P. P. (2006). Role of interictal epileptiform abnormalities in cognitive impairment. *Epilepsy and Behavior, 8*(3), 504–515.

Hughes, J. R., & Melyn, M. (2005). EEG and seizures in autistic children and adolescents: Further findings with therapeutic implications. *Clinical EEG and Neuroscience: Official Journal of the EEG and Clinical Neuroscience Society (ENCS), 36*(1),15–20.

Kavros, P. M., Clarke, T., Strug, L. J., Halperin, J. M., Dorta, N. J., & Pal, D. K. (2008). Attention impairment in rolandic epilepsy: Systematic review. *Epilepsia, 49*(9), 1570–1580.

Kellenberger, C. J. (2010). Aortic arch malformations. *Pediatric Radiology, 40*(6), 876–884.

Kerr, A. M. (1992). A review of the respiratory disorder in the Rett syndrome. *Brain and Development, 14,* 43–45.

Kim, H. L., Donnelly, J. H., Tournay, A. E., Book, T. M., & Filipek, P. (2006). Absence of seizures despite high prevalence of epileptiform EEG abnormalities in children with autism monitored in a tertiary care center. *Epilepsia, 47,* 394–398.

Lalli, J. S., Mace, F. C., Livezey, K., & Kates, K. (1998). Assessment of stimulus generalization gradients in the treatment of self-injurious behavior. *PubMed, 31*(3). Retrieved from http://www.ncbi.nlm.nih.gov/pubmed?term=Lalli%2C%20Mace%2C%20Livezey%2C%20%3Cates%2C%201998

Malone, R. P., Gratz, S. S., Delaney, M. A., & Hyman, S. B. (2005). Advances in drug treatments for children and adolescents with autism and other pervasive developmental disorders. *CNS Drugs, 19*(11), 923–934.

Malone, R. P., Sheikh, R., & Zito, J. M. (1999). Novel antipsychotic medications in the treatment of children and adolescents. *Psychiatric Services, 50*(2), 171–174.

McCracken, J. T., McGough, J., Shah, B., Cronin, P., Hong, D., Aman, M. G., . . . McMahon, D. (2002). Risperidone in children with autism and serious behavioral problems. *New England Journal of Medicine, 347*(5), 314–321.

McDonald-McGinn, D. M., & Sullivan, K. E. (2011). Chromosome 22q11.2 deletion syndrome (DiGeorge syndrome/velocardiofacial syndrome). *Medicine, 90*(1), 1–18.

McDonald-McGinn, D. M., & Zackai, E. H. (2008).Genetic counseling for the 22q11.2 deletion. *Developmental Disabilities Research Reviews, 14*(1), 69–74.

Miles, J. H., & Hillman, R. E. (2000). Value of a clinical morphology examination in autism. *American Journal of Medical Genetics, 91,* 245–253.

Miles, J. H., McCathren, R. B., Stichter, J., Shinawi, M., Pagon, R. A., Bird, T. D., Dolan, C. R., & Stephens, K. (Eds.). (2010). *Autism spectrum disorders.* Seattle, WA: University of Washington. [updated 2010 Apr 13]. Retrieved from http://www.ncbi.nlm.nih.gov/books/NBK1442

Miles, J. H., Takahashi, T. N., Bagby, S., Sahota, P. K., Vaslow, D. F., Wang, C. H., Hillman, R. E., & Farmer, J. E. (2005). Essential versus complex autism: Definition of fundamental prognostic subtypes. *American Journal of Medical Genetics, 135,* 171–180.

Miles, J. H., Takahashi, T. N., Hong, J., Munden, N., Flournoy, N., Braddock, S. R., Martin, R. A., Bocian, M. E., Spence, M. A., Hillman, R. E., & Farmer, J. E. (2008). Development and validation of a measure of dysmorphology: Useful for autism subgroup classification. *American Journal of Medical Genetics, 146A,* 1101–1116.

Mirenda, P. (2001) Autism, augmentative communication and assistive technology: What do we really know? *Focus on Autism and Other Developmental Disabilities, 16*(3), 141–151.

Mirenda, P. (2003). Towards functional augmentative and alternative communication for students with autism: Manual signs, graphic symbols, and voice output communication aids. *Language, Speech and Hearing Services for Schools, 34,* 203–216.

Mouridsen, S. E., Rich, B., & Isager, T. (1999). The natural history of somatic morbidity in disintegrative psychosis and infantile autism: A validation study. *Brain and Development, 21*(7), 447–452.

Parmeggiani, A., Posar, A., Antolini, C., Scaduto, M. C., Santucci, M., & Giovanardi-Rossi, P. (2007). Epilepsy in patients with pervasive developmental disorder not otherwise specified. *Journal of Child Neurology, 22*(10), 1198–1203.

Pelco, L. E., Kissel, R. C., Parrish, J. M., & Miltenberger, R. G. (1987). Behavioral management of oral medication administration difficulties among children: A review of literature with case illustrations. *Journal of Developmental and Behavioral Pediatrics, 8*(2), 90–96.

Scahill, L., Chappell, P. B., Kim, Y. S., Schultz, R. T., Katsovich, L., Shepherd, E., Arnsten, A. F., Cohen, D. J., & Leckman, J. F. (2001). A placebo-controlled study of guanfacine in the treatment of children with tic disorders and attention deficit hyperactivity disorder. *American Journal of Psychiatry, 158*(7), 1067–1074.

Schopler, E., Reichler, R. J., & Renner, B. R. (1986). *The Childhood Autism Rating Scale (CARS) for Diagnostic Screening and Classification of Autism.* Irvington, NY: Irvington Publishers.

Souders, M. C., Freeman, K., DePaul, D., & Levy, S. E. (2002) Caring for children with autism who require challenging procedures, *Pediatric Nursing, 28*(6), 555–562.

Spence, S. J., & Schneider, M. T. (2009). The role of epilepsy and epileptiform EEGs in autism spectrum disorders. *Pediatric Review, 65,* 599–606.

Steffenburg, S., Steffenburg, U., & Gillberg, C. (2003). Autism spectrum disorders in children with active epilepsy and learning disability: Comorbidity, pre- and perinatal background, and seizure characteristics. *Developmental Medicine and Child Neurology, 45*(11), 724–730.

Trevathan, E. (2004). Seizures and epilepsy among children with language regression and autistic spectrum disorders. *Journal of Child Neurology, 19*, S49–57.

Tuchman, R., Alessandri, M., & Cuccaro, M. (2010). Autism spectrum disorders and epilepsy: Moving towards a comprehensive approach to treatment. *Brain Development, 32*(9), 719–730.

Tuchman, R. F., & Rapin, I. (1997). Regression in pervasive developmental disorders: Seizures and epileptiform electroencephalogram correlates. *Pediatrics, 99*(4), 560–566.

Tuchman, R. F., Rapin, I., & Shinnar, S. (1991). Autistic and dysphasic children II: Epilepsy. *Pediatrics, 88*(6), 1219–1225.

Volkmar, F. R., Cicchetti, D. V., Cohen, D. J., & Bregman, J. (1992). Brief report: developmental aspects of DSM-III-R criteria for autism. *Journal of Autism and Developmental Disorders, 22*(4), 657–662.

Volkmar, F. R., & Nelson, D. S. (1990). Seizure disorders in autism. *Journal of the American Academy of Child & Adolescent Psychiatry, 29*(1), 127–129.

Vorstman, J. A., Morcus, M. E., Duijff, S. N., Klaassen, P. W., Hieneman-de Boer, J. A., Beemer, F. A., Swaab, H., Kahn, R. S., & Van Engeland, H. (2006) The 22q11.2 deletion in children: High rate of autistic disorders and early onset psychotic symptoms. *Journal of American Academy of Child & Adolescent Psychiatry, 45*, 1104–1113.

Weinberg, P. M. (2006). Aortic arch anomalies. *Journal of Cardiovascular Magnetic Resonance, 8*(4), 633–643.

Zackai, E. H., McDonald-McGinn, D. M., Driscoll, D. A., Emanuel, B. S., Christensen, K. M., & Chien, P. (1996). Respiratory symptoms may be the first presenting sign of 22q11.2 deletion: A study of vascular rings. *In Proceedings of the Greenwood Genetic Center* (*vol. 15*, p. 137). Greenwood, SC: Greenwood Genetic Center.

Nursing Care of the Child With Autism Spectrum Disorder Scheduled for a Tonsillectomy

7

Brenda M. Holtzer

The purpose of this chapter is to provide nurses with evidence-based knowledge and guidelines for the pre- and postoperative nursing care for a child with autism spectrum disorder (ASD), using the exemplar case of a child hospitalized for complications after a tonsillectomy. This case is unique, in that most children with ASD are discharged home to the care of their parents immediately following recovery from surgery. The primary goal in caring for these children is to return them to their familiar environment and routines as soon as possible. There is limited research-based evidence for the care of hospitalized children with ASD having surgical procedures, although there are recent evidence-based guidelines for the care of children having tonsillectomies (Baugh et al., 2011; Seid, Sherman, & Seid, 1997; Sutters et al., 2004, 2007, 2010; Zeev, Mayes, Caldwell-Andrews, Karas, & McClain, 2006). The challenge nurses face in this situation is to incorporate the standards of practice for post-tonsillectomy care into the routine of care for a child with ASD. Most often, the situation requires an approach that is flexible but does not compromise the child's health.

BACKGROUND

The Centers for Disease Control and Prevention (CDC, 2009), estimated that 560,000 children across the United States have one of the three categories of ASD: classic autism disorder, Asperger's syndrome, or pervasive developmental disorder—not otherwise specified (a nonspecific disorder along the spectrum). The CDC (2010) stated that ASDs occur in all racial, ethnic, and socioeconomic groups, but are four times more likely to occur in boys than in girls. While more children than ever before are being diagnosed with an ASD, some of this increase is believed to be related to a broadened definition of ASD, along with improved screening and testing. Coplan (2010) listed events occurring in the past 25 years, starting with the 1975 enactment of Public Law 94-142, the Education for All Handicapped Children Act (p. 90). Since then, other federal legislation has mandated the development of early intervention programs for high-risk infants and preschool children; in 1992, mandatory reporting of autism by individual states became a federal requirement.

Revisions to the *Diagnostic and Statistical Manual of Mental Disorders* [American Psychiatric Association (APA), 2000]) have broadened the range of disability and criteria for inclusion into the ASD category (Coplan, 2010). In addition, the American Academy of Pediatrics, developed more specific standards of practice for screening, identification, and management of children with ASD, including two clinical reports and a toolkit for primary-care providers. The first report reviews identification procedures, the second report provides guidelines for management, and the toolkit includes all the screening tools. The AAP also called for screening of all children for ASD at their 18- and 24-month well-baby visits, so that intervention services are provided as soon as a developmental concern is noted.

As prevalence rates for ASD continue to rise, it is likely that nurses caring for children having tonsillectomies and other procedures in an acute-care setting will encounter more children with ASD. Refer to Chapters 1 through 5 for a more detailed discussion of the epidemiological, diagnostic, and screening considerations.

MANIFESTATIONS OF ASD

Pediatric nurses are highly likely to encounter children on the autism spectrum in many settings, including the hospital, and need the knowledge and skills required to provide safe and effective care to them. It is also imperative that nurses understand the wide variety of patient characteristics along the spectrum of autistic disorders. Children with ASD have impaired functioning in three domains: age-appropriate social interactions, language development, and communication patterns, and behaviors and/or interests (APA, 2000). Another clinically significant issue that is found in children with ASD is hypersensitivity to sensory stimuli, such as touch, lights, and sounds (Scarpinato et al., 2010). Admission to a busy hospital or outpatient clinic can exacerbate their maladaptive behaviors because of the auditory and visual stimulation.

Children on the autism spectrum of disorders vary in the severity of impairments they experience, as well as in the ways they display behaviors or characteristics. There is also variation in IQ. Some high-functioning individuals can be quite successful academically and in careers that fit their personalities and styles. Females with ASD are often the most cognitively impaired (CDC, 2010). Since their receptive and expressive communication patterns are different than those of typical children, children with ASD are especially challenging for a nurse to interact with appropriately without the family's presence and input.

Types of repetitive behaviors are well documented in the literature that describes case studies, approaches to assessment and diagnosis, and treatment. Clinicians may organize criteria to facilitate diagnosis. For example, Coplan (2010, p. 25) describes the types of repetitious behaviors that occur across the spectrum as falling into two broad categories that are motivated by either mental or physical drives. Mentally repetitious behaviors are

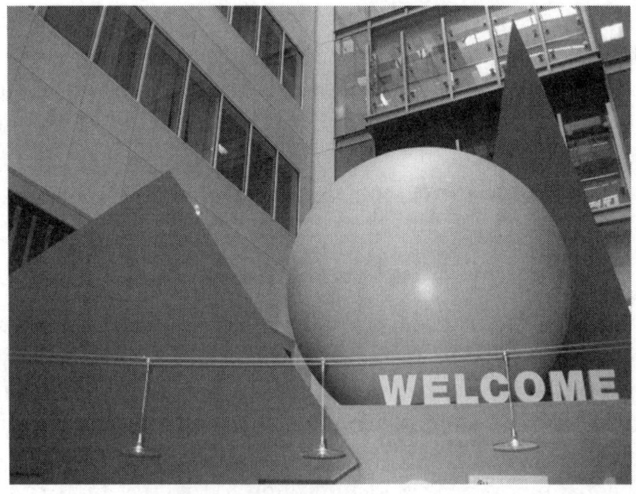

FIGURE 7.1 ■ Photograph courtesy of Andrea Segal and Brenda Holtzer.

usually motivated by a thought or idea. These include insistence on sameness of routine, difficulty making transitions, and stereotypical play. Furthermore, researchers have discovered that mentally repetitious behaviors are instrumental to learning for children with ASD. They are able to learn through repetition of play, stories, and visual experiences, eventually cataloging that information into categories that they understand and can apply to future experiences (Coplan, 2010, p. 26).

Physically repetitious behaviors do not appear to be driven by any thought and are unique behaviors for each child. These include hand-flapping, twiddling with fingers or an object, toe-walking, spinning, lap running and excessive rocking of self in chair or bed. (Coplan, 2010).

Physically repetitious behaviors are red flags for distress in children with ASD. The behaviors usually increase in response to changes in routine, environment, and patterns of daily living, all of which occur in an acute-care hospitalization. It is not unusual to see a parent or care assistant walking laps alongside the patients within our hospital unit or to see a child obsess with fingering objects, while avoiding human contact. These behaviors might be a form of stress control or self-stimulation, but usually decrease in frequency as the child grows older. They can also reappear in response to stressors later in life (Scarpinato et al., 2010).

Nurses learn about a child's specific routines, behaviors, and environmental triggers for agitated states by collaborating with the parents or the primary caregiver. The case of Shawn illustrates issues in the care of children with ASD in the acute-care perioperative setting. This case highlights the need for targeted nursing strategies and modifications in nursing approach to support child and family during a difficult health care experience.

CASE

Shawn is an 8-year-old boy scheduled for a tonsillectomy, due to a history of frequent sore throats, fevers, and positive throat cultures for group A beta-hemolytic *Streptococcus* over the past 3 years. He recently developed exudates on his tonsils, along with hypertrophy of the tonsils. His parents report a history of snoring and some sleep disturbances through the night, and he is often drowsy during the day. He had a sleep study 1 month prior to this visit and has documented sleep apnea with decreasing oxygen saturation to 88% to 90% by pulse oximetry. Shawn's symptoms meet the criteria for tonsillectomy, as described in recent clinical guidelines issued for tonsillectomy in children in the *Otolaryngology Head and Neck Surgery* journal (Baugh et al., 2011).

Shawn was born at 37 weeks of gestation. His Apgar scores were 7 at 5 minutes and 8 at 10 minutes after birth. He developed respiratory distress and required hospitalization in the high-risk nursery for 5 days after delivery. He needed oxygen therapy via nasal cannula for 3 days and antibiotics until his cultures were read as negative for any bacterial or viral infection. Shawn tolerated feedings through a nasogastric tube while tachypneic, and then began to breast-feed without any difficulty. He was discharged on day 5 of life. His parents report that his growth and development over the next 2 years was appropriate, but that he seemed to play with the same toys repeatedly, becoming upset with any changes in routines and activities. At the age of 2 years, his language consisted of two-word sentences, often repeating them and mimicking words he heard from others and from television shows.

(*Continued*)

CASE (Continued)

His parents report that he developed attachments to them and his older brother, but withdrew from interactions with his grandparents and aunts and uncles.

The intensity of mentally repetitious behaviors (resistance to changes in routines, difficulty in making transitions) increased, and Shawn began to demonstrate an increase in repetitive physical behaviors (rocking himself when sitting, fingering objects repeatedly, and covering his ears). These behaviors were noticeably worse with changes in routines or environments. When his parents reported their observations to their pediatrician, he referred them to a developmental pediatrician for an evaluation. Shawn was diagnosed with ASD, and enrolled in an early intervention program. Apart from the tonsillitis, Shawn has not had any other health problems nor has he been hospitalized since birth. His parents are concerned about how he will react to being prepared for surgery and shared their concerns with both the surgeon and the nurse practitioner from the anesthesia department during his preoperative visit and assessment.

EVIDENCE-BASED CARE

In order to provide the most effective nursing care to the child in this case, the standards of practice should be based on sound evidence. There is little documented research for the care children with ASD having traumatic procedures, and therefore there is little evidence-based guidance for hospital-based care of this specific population of children. There is evidence to support best practices in the care of children undergoing tonsillectomies, and more information than ever to promote understanding of individuals with ASD. When nurses understand the unique needs and characteristics of the child with ASD, they can provide safe and effective care, adapting the hospital policies and standards of care to the needs of the individual patient. Figure 7.2 is a photo of a pediatric unit's educational bulletin board, created by a nurse whose objective was to highlight the most common characteristics and special needs of autistic children for other nurses and hospital staff.

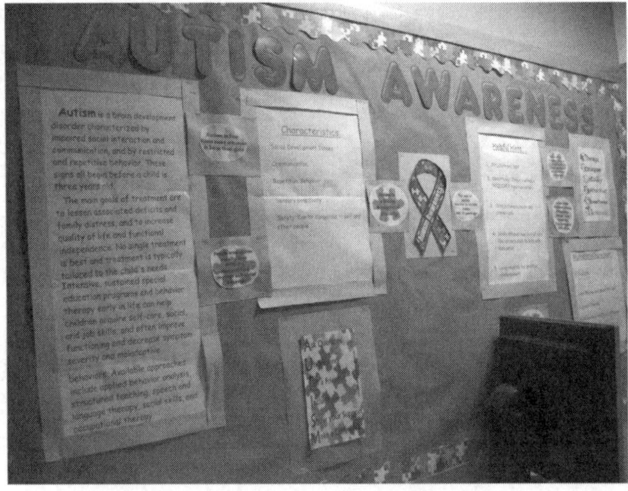

FIGURE 7.2 ■ Photograph courtesy of Andrea Segal and Brenda Holtzer.

Current Evidence to Guide Nursing Care

The postoperative care of children undergoing tonsillectomies and adenoidectomies includes vigilant nursing observations and interventions to prevent potential complications of dehydration, bleeding, and infection. Ineffective pain control contributes to each of those complications, simply because the child will not be able to swallow fluids without experiencing pain. Using the steps outlined for evidence-based practice (Newhouse, Dearholt, Poe, Pugh, & White, 2007; Titler et al., 2007), an extensive literature review was performed to determine the most current evidence and strategies for caring for children having a tonsillectomy. Search strategies, using CINAHL and OVID databases, were performed using the terms "tonsillectomy," "children," "pediatric," "pain assessment," and "autism." Since there was limited literature for children with ASD in the hospital setting, the literature searches were separated into three categories of evidence review, including essential pain relief measures for any child having a tonsillectomy. These included: tonsillectomy and pain relief in children without ASD; procedure-related pain and stress in children with ASD; and children with ASD and expression of pain.

In several studies, the authors described children's reports of pain severity and their emotional reactions to the pain (Sutters et al., 2004, 2007, 2010; Zeev et al., 2006). One study examined children's expectations of pain following a tonsillectomy, their perceptions of the efficacy of pain medications, and descriptions of nonpharmacological interventions that relieved pain (Sutters, et al., 2007). Table 7.1 summarizes these studies and findings.

Seid and colleagues (1997) discussed perioperative psychosocial interventions for children with ASD that were utilized in an otorhinolaryngology practice. The authors compared interventions and outcomes for two children requiring tonsillectomies. A team without prior knowledge of ASD-specific interventions saw the first child requiring a tonsillectomy; a second team received information and training about ASD-specific interventions and treated the second child. The second patient had an uncomplicated postoperative recovery, while the first child had more problems with pain and inadequate fluid intake. The authors believe the difference in outcomes occurred because the second team included the parents as consultants in every aspect of care (Seid et al., 1997). While their conclusion is not based on rigorous examination, the authors highlight the need for knowledge of the characteristics of ASD and the importance of a partnership with parents to enable clinicians to provide the most effective care to their patients.

Overall, there are limited data from controlled studies to support interventions aimed at hospitalized children with ASD. One study compared children with and without ASD (Ross Hazlett, Garret, Wilkerson, & Piven, 2005), to examine achievement of adequate sedation prior to an MRI. They found that children with ASD did not require more sedation than children without ASD and that children with ASD were responsive to behavioral interventions for calming prior to induction of anesthesia. Nordahl and colleagues (2008) studied 25 children with ASD who were having MRIs without sedation. The research team found that children who had a pretest visit to the environment needed less or no sedation. Other authors described interventions based on their best practice and experience with children with ASD in the hospital and clinic settings, detailed in Table 7.2.

In two studies, the authors analyzed pain assessment in children with ASD, comparing parental assessment to health care provider assessment. Nader and colleagues (2004) compared parental and trained observer ratings of pain expression after needle sticks in a group of children with ASD and a group of similar-age children without ASD. Parents rated pain as no more distressing than a bump from falling, while the trained observers differed, rating children with ASD as sensitive to pain. In the second study, Inglese (2008)

TABLE 7.1 ■ Tonsillectomy/Pain Relief Evidence Review: Children without ASD[a]

Article/journal	Author/date	Procedure	Results	Recommendations
A randomized clinical trial of the effectiveness of a scheduled oral analgesic dosing regimen for the management of postoperative pain in children following tonsillectomy *Pain*	Sutters et al., 2004	Random assignment to three treatment groups: one with PRN dosing of Tylenol with codeine; One with q 4 hr dosing; and one with q 4 hr dosing, along with nurse coaching.	Round-the-clock dosing does not cause opioid-related side effects, and is more effective in pain relief than PRN dosing. No difference between groups two (no RN coach) and three (RN coach)	Evidence that prescribed interval dosing is better than PRN dosing, in relieving pain.
Children's expectations of pain, perceptions of analgesic efficacy, and experiences with nonpharmacologic pain management strategies at home following tonsillectomy *Journal for Specialists in Pediatric Nursing*	Sutters et al., 2007	Qualitative Random assignment of patients having tonsillectomies to three different treatment groups Interviews of patients at home with parents on day 4 postoperative (This article focused on child responses.)	More children (65.4%) reported more pain than expected; 40% reported that taking medicine was difficult due to pain of swallowing.	Evidence shows that tonsillectomy is considered very painful by children, and they need careful preoperative education about their options for pain management.
A randomized clinical trial of the efficacy of scheduled dosing of acetaminophen and hydrocodone for the management of postoperative pain in children after tonsillectomy *Clinical Journal of Pain*	Sutters et al., 2010	Random, quasi-experimental Same procedures as in 2004, with different groups, and different opioid (hydrocodone and Tylenol)	Children receiving medication around the clock had better analgesic effect than those with PRN.	Reaffirms findings of research done in 2004, that around-the-clock dosing is better than PRN, with or without a nurse's coaching.
Preoperative anxiety, postoperative pain, and behavioral recovery in young children undergoing surgery *Pediatrics*	Zeev, Mayes, Caldwell-Andrews, Karas, & McClain, 2006	Controlled cohort study to assess the relationship of preoperative anxiety to increase in postoperative pain First of its kind in pediatrics There were 561 children recruited, all having elective tonsillectomy and adenoidectomy, exclusive of children with developmental, physical, or psychiatric problems. Utilized several assessment measures for anxiety, behavior, pain level, and child temperament; the group was split into two groups: those with greater preoperative anxiety and those without.	Results are similar to those found with adult populations. Individuals having higher levels of anxiety prior to surgery will have more difficulties with pain control, dietary intake, and sleeping.	In children without a diagnosis of ASD, there is an association of preoperative anxiety with the amount of postoperative pain and adjustment.

[a]PRN as needed; q every 4 hours; RN, registered nurse.

TABLE 7.2 ■ Procedure-related Pain/Stress in Children with ASD

Article/journal	Author/date	Procedure	Results	Recommendations
Perioperative psychosocial interventions for autistic children undergoing ENT surgery *International Journal of Otorhinolaryngology*	Seid, Sherman, & Seid, 1997	Nonexperimental comparison of two different approaches of care by surgeons, first without any training on ASD and second after training	As expected, the surgeons who had new knowledge adjusted their approach to the patient and their patient's induction and postoperative recovery was better than the first case.	Insufficient evidence or effectiveness due to methodology. However, does support the education and awareness of ASD that health care providers need to have, as well as inclusion of caretakers in provision of care.
Caring for children and adolescents with autism who require challenging procedures *Pediatric Nursing*	Souders, DePaul, Freeman, & Levy, 2002	Expert opinion and recommendations for alterations to environment of care and approaches by staff		Health care providers need to know what strategies help to gain a child's cooperation and compliance. Authors recommend specific behavioral strategies to employ when reviewing aspects of care in a hospital setting.
Moderate sedation for MRI in young children with autism *Pediatric Radiology*	Ross, Hazlett, Garret, Wilkerson, & Piven, 2005	Two-group comparison, children with ASD, and children without, receiving anesthesia	Children with ASD are not more difficult to sedate and do not require higher doses of sedatives.	If correct behavioral intervention strategies are utilized, children with ASD could be more compliant with procedures, and staff can be more flexible in approach.
Brief report: Methods for acquiring structural MRI data in very young children with autism without the use of sedation *Journal of Autism and Developmental Disorders*	Nordahl, Simon, Zierhut, Solomon, Rogers, & Amaral, 2008	Nonexperimental Reviewed care for 25 patients with ASD who made a visit to the MRI suite and registration area prior to the day of testing.	None of these children required sedation, just time spent for them to recognize the environment.	For children having elective procedures and studies, a previsit to familiarize them and the family is important for decreasing anxiety. This is a quality practice for both children with ASD and children without, but it does involve planning and investment of staff time.

surveyed parents of children with ASD. This researcher reported that parents felt they were the best judges of pain level for their children, as they had learned their children's expressions and responses. Survey respondents believed their children experienced pain, which often was manifested as nontypical behavior.

Summary of Evidence

There is scant evidence to support targeted nursing interventions for hospitalized children with a primary diagnosis of ASD. Most higher-quality studies related to the care of children undergoing tonsillectomies did not include children with ASD in their samples. Research involving children with ASD has been limited; more of the literature in this population describes best practices by health care providers and expert opinion. When preparing to care for children with ASD in the hospital setting, nurses often rely on parents and other family members to help adapt the environment. Other staff with expertise to support better care of children with ASD in the hospital setting include child life specialists, music and art therapists, and rehabilitation therapists.

BEST PRACTICES: NURSING CARE AND SURGICAL PROCEDURES

A surgical procedure of any type is challenging for a child. Pediatric nursing care always acknowledges the importance of parents and/or other primary caregivers as sources of comfort and support for children and as advocates and interpreters of their children's needs. When a child on the autism spectrum is the surgical patient, involvement of parents and others who know the child's patterns of behavior and unique needs is even more important.

Preoperative Assessment

The preoperative visit should be done in advance of the actual admission for surgery, in order to acquaint the child and family with the perioperative staff and routines. An advanced practice nurse (APN), such as a pediatric nurse practitioner or clinical nurse specialist, might be the initial hospital contact for the family. The APN is charged with the development of an individualized plan of care that acknowledges the child's needs, typical behavior and communication patterns, and other individual characteristics. The plan is communicated to, and followed by, all perioperative staff. Before examining the child, the APN should discuss with the parents the events that will occur and collaborate with them to determine the best approach to use with their child. When nurses are familiar with the typical problems experienced by children with ASD in the hospital, and with the unique characteristics of a particular child, they are able to collaborate more effectively with parents or other family members to develop the best and least traumatic plan of care for each child. Using the assessment questions in Table 7.4 as a guide, nurses can become knowledgeable about a child's behavior patterns and responses to the environment.

These questions can guide the nurse's preoperative assessment and engage the parents in a partnership with the health care staff in order to help their child through the operative experience. Since the domain (or core deficit) problems vary in severity among children with ASD, information from parents will contribute to the development of a truly individualized plan of care. The APN can determine the extent of parental involvement required for successful transition through perioperative and postoperative phases. Encouraging the

TABLE 7.3 ■ Children with ASD and Expression of Pain

Article/journal	Author/date	Procedure	Results	Recommendations
Expression of pain in children with autism *Clinical Journal of Pain*	Nader, Oberlander, Chambers, & Craig, 2004	Comparison of a group of children with ASD to a group without, receiving similar intravenous sticks, using two scales of pain assessment: reliable observers and parental report of child distress.	In the ASD group, parental reports of pain were negatively correlated to observer-documented facial response and behavioral response to pain of intravenous. In the other group, parental scores were more positively correlated to observed facial and behavioral responses.	Although the groups were not equal in number , both of them had similar reactions, according to observations of facial activity and of behavioral activity. Authors also noted that parents of autistic children had a hard time viewing the needle insertion as more painful or distressing than an everyday fall. However, the observations by trained recorders indicate that children with ASD are sensitive to pain. This study does point to differences in assessments made by parents versus care providers.
Pain perception and communication in children with autism spectrum disorder: New parental insights *Southern Online Journal of Nursing Research*	Inglese, 2008	Nonexperimental Three-question survey to 400 families to explore their perception of child's pain and pain expression.	Response rate was 22% ($n = 88$) 86% ($n = 76$) reported that their child reacts differently to pain than other children. 70% ($n = 62$) reported difficulty in determining child's pain level. These parents have learned to watch for certain behaviors or facial signals. Of these parents, 40 felt that providers could not assess their child's pain.	In contrast to the previous study, parents generally felt that once they learned the child's pain-related behaviors and responses, they (not health care providers) were the best judges of their children's pain.

TABLE 7.4 ■ Initial Assessment Questions Pertinent to the Hospitalized Child with ASD

Domain of potential problem	Assessment questions
Impaired social skills	• How does this child tolerate new faces? • How does this child react to other children his/her age? To adults? • Is this child sensitive to touch? Sensitive to noise? • What is this child's comfort with personal space? • What is the best way to approach this child (e.g., touch or stand back)?
Impairment in communication	• How does this child communicate? Verbally? Nonverbally? • Does he/she require the use of picture cards, writing, or drawing? • Is he/she uncomfortable with eye contact and prefer to • Communicate with you via alternative means? (For example, an adolescent patient might feel more comfortable communicating via text message than via the spoken word.) • Is he/she able to understand emotional cues? • How does this child report or show pain?
Restricted interests/ stereotyped behaviors	• Are there any items of fixation for this child? If yes, how does the family manage these? • What are some things that potentially agitate this child? Think especially of the current hospital environment. • What early warning signs might indicate that this child is becoming agitated? • When this child becomes agitated or overstimulated, what are the interventions that work best?
Inflexibility/ adherence to routine	• What is this child's schedule at home? How much can the hospital's routine mirror the child's home schedule? • How can you best prepare this child for any upcoming transitions (e.g., a room change or preparation for a test)? • What has the family or school done that helps with transitions?

Adapted from Scarpinato, Bradley, Kurbjun, Bateman, Holtzer, & Ely (2010).

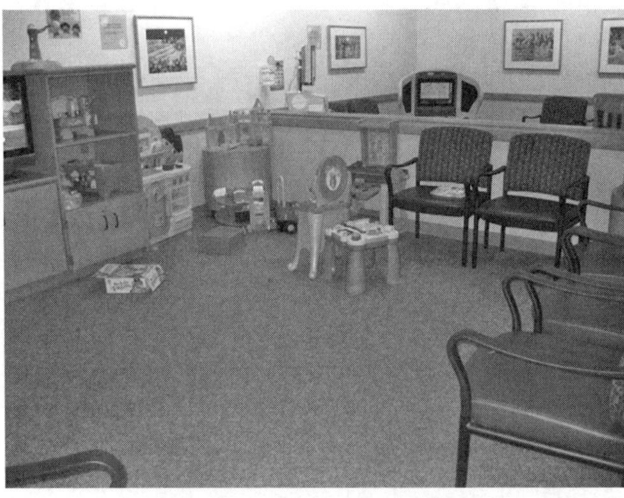

FIGURE 7.3 ■ Photograph courtesy of Andrea Segal and Brenda Holtzer.

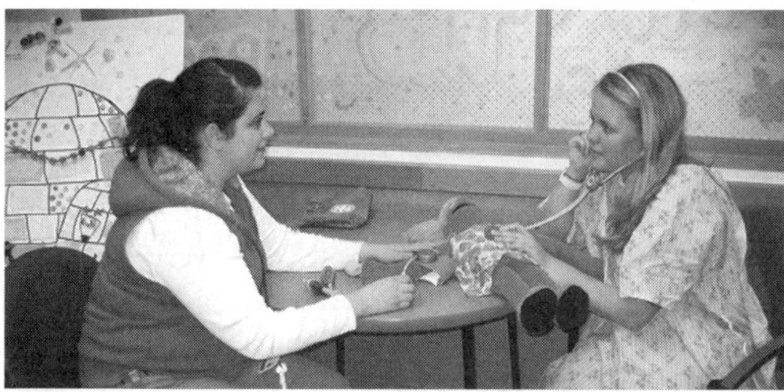

FIGURE 7.4 Preparation of a child for a procedure using medical play. Photograph courtesy of Andrea Segal and Brenda Holtzer.

child to see, touch, or explore some of the equipment that is likely to be encountered on the day of surgery can promote better coping.

The APN, or another nurse who is familiar to the child, should escort the family and child on a tour of the perioperative unit and other places the child is likely to encounter on the day of surgery. The registration process is best completed in a pleasantly decorated lounge, which can provide areas for family privacy and diversion activities for the child. The child can be shown the appealing items in this lounge and be offered the opportunity to touch and explore the toys (Figure 7.3).

A child life specialist (CLS) can intervene with more challenging children in the play area. Children might benefit from distraction or other forms of support. Medical play can be useful for many children. Medical play can allow a child to explore medical equipment, engage in pretend scenarios or imitation (if he or she has these skills), observe the CLS demonstrating play, and become familiar with some medical processes. In addition, by observing the way a child with ASD plays and/or explores the medical equipment, the APN or nurse can identify other behavior patterns and likes and dislikes (Figure 7.4).

The nurse also learns about the child's response to environmental changes and interaction with new people just by observing behaviors during the tour of the operative areas. The APN and CLS will often work together to identify key communication strategies and intervention approaches for the child. These keys or "pearls of knowledge" (see Exhibit 7.1) are documented in the chart and flagged so that all care providers have access to them.

EXHIBIT 7.1

Pearls of Knowledge

- Allow Shawn to keep his stuffed rabbit during preparation for surgery and postanesthesia.
- Involve parents in provision of care and allow them to stay at bedside pre- and postoperatively.
- Limit the numbers of care providers in his room at one time.
- Maintain consistency of care providers as is possible.

Perioperative Plan of Care

After observing the child's responses to environmental changes, new faces, and unfamiliar medical equipment, the APN is better equipped to select the surgical setting for the child's procedure. For example, use of a room in the back of the surgical suite, with low light and sound, might be indicated for a child who is highly sensitive to certain stimuli. Rooms used for preoperative preparation and postoperative recovery are filled with equipment, lights, and monitors that can overwhelm or overstimulate a child with ASD. The nurse and parents together decide how to structure the environment in order to decrease the incidence of strong emotional and behavioral reactions.

Nurses need to remember that children with ASD often become highly upset with disruptions of their routines. Child life staff in the operative suite areas can provide quiet music, videos, or play stations to distract or calm the child. Parents should be allowed to remain with their children to provide emotional support and interpret their behaviors to the staff if needed. Children will be hungry and might or might not understand the reasons for their "nothing by mouth" status. They might become upset that no food is permitted. Most will not tolerate waiting in the admission area or preoperative holding area for any length of time, and therefore need to be admitted as close to the surgical time as possible.

Anesthesia staff should prepare the child for the surgery as quickly as possible. To minimize the likelihood of distress or outbursts, the child can be allowed to keep his own clothes and shoes on until sedated. The anesthesiologist might decide to provide mask induction prior to starting any intravenous fluids and sedation. Monitoring might need to be delayed until the child is asleep. The actions in Exhibit 7.2 vary from the usual standards of practice. However, when the health care team is able to adapt their usual practices to meet the needs of a child with ASD, the child is likely to experience less distress and exhibit fewer maladaptive or disruptive behaviors.

When the procedure is completed, the operating room nurse accompanies the anesthesiologist and patient to the recovery room. Staff might need to discontinue intravenous fluids and minimize monitoring to avoid potential injury if the child is combative on awakening from anesthesia. Parental input about the child's likely responses during the recovery period, along with assessment of the child's physiological status, can guide these decisions. The smallest number of staff possible, along with parents, should be at the child's bedside as he or she is waking up. If possible, for consistency, the nurse who provided preoperative care and is familiar to the child should be assigned by the APN to care for the child in the recovery area. Pain medications are given as soon as the child is aroused and demonstrates any discomfort through facial expressions, behavior, and/or parent assessment of the child's pain.

EXHIBIT 7.2

Perioperative Plan of Care

- Have parents stay with patient pre-sedation.
- Place patient in a quiet room away from the central activity in the unit.
- Consider letting patient keep his clothes and shoes on until asleep, if he does not want to undress.
- Consider mask induction prior to the intravenous insertion.
- Decrease loud noises and dim lights to promote calming atmosphere.

Pain Assessment and Management

Assessment of pain every 4 hours is a standard of care for children recovering from surgery. Reassessment should occur after any medication intervention. Assessing pain in children with developmental delays and communication impairments is often challenging for nursing staff. Children unable to report their own pain, and especially those with cognitive impairment, are frequently undertreated for pain during hospitalizations (Malviya, Voepel-Lewis, Burke, Merkel, & Tait, 2006). Children with ASD have variations in the degree of impairment across the domains of language and communication, social interaction, and behaviors, which can result in variations in both perception of pain and expression of pain. When children have verbal skills but cannot interpret a facial expression–based pain scale or a numerical pain rating scale, the nurse should ask the parents to estimate the pain level. In one case, a verbal child who was unable to rate the pain with a number was able to state "a little" or "a lot" with the help of his parents. For nonverbal and cognitively impaired children with ASD, the r-FLACC scale can be used. The r-FLACC is a numerical rating scale based on observation of patient behavior, including postures, sounds, and activity levels of children (Malviya et al., 2006). Unresolved pain can increase sensitivity to other environmental factors in children with ASD. A carefully designed, individualized pain-management strategy, created in partnership with parents, can decrease risks for untreated pain in a child with ASD.

CASE–CONTINUED

Shawn's procedure was performed as planned. No complications occurred during the operative phase. He was transferred to the postanesthesia care unit, where he required oxygen by nasal cannula due to changes in blood oxygen saturation as measured by pulse oximetry. His parents had difficulty arousing him after the surgery. His intravenous infusion was maintained, and elbow restraints were applied to prevent him pulling out any medical devices. Due to concerns about his recovery, Shawn was transferred to the inpatient surgical nursing unit for overnight observation. On admission to the inpatient unit, he was sleepy but easily aroused. Both parents remained at his bedside. His nurse measured postoperative vital signs, assessed his status, ensured his comfort, and then met with his parents to complete the hospital admission documentation.

The nurse in the surgical area had limited experience in working with children with ASD, but was able to determine the best approaches to Shawn's care by consulting with his parents. She also pulled the information bullets that had been flagged by the APN on the child's electronic records. Shawn remained drowsy until the later part of the evening shift. Then he wanted to sit up in bed, and subsequently tried to remove the nasal cannula, intravenous line, and pulse oximetry probe. Since he was more alert, his oxygen status improved, and the nurse discontinued his oxygen. His parents thought that his gestures in the direction of a cup on the bedside stand meant he wanted a drink. He was permitted to drink clear liquids. He received pain medication based on his parents' assessment of his pain level. The rest of his night progressed well, and he managed to sleep for half of the night. Intravenous fluids were discontinued, and he was discharged home that morning.

Postoperative Care

In most instances, if a child with ASD undergoing a tonsillectomy is free of problems postoperatively, surgeons and parents prefer recuperation at home. So, hospitalizations for healthy children with ASD after tonsillectomies or similar procedures are rare. It is the exceptional case that creates the greatest challenges for nurses who are unfamiliar with children with ASD.

Care after Discharge

Children with ASD benefit from the return to the normal routine in their usual environments after discharge from the hospital. Recuperation is usually fast, and children are able to resume normal activities quickly. Returning to the hospital or clinic for a postoperative visit can be highly distressing. Parents can use the preparation strategies that were effective during the preoperative visit to minimize the stress associated with follow-up care.

SUMMARY

Hospitalization exposes children with ASD to multiple health care providers, medical equipment, and uncomfortable environments, as well as invasive and painful procedures that can cause distress, exacerbate behavioral difficulties, and increase the risk for complications or injuries. Communication deficits, compounded by anxieties and fears associated with the hospital environment, disruption of routines, and pain, add to the challenges that nurses need to meet as they take care of this population. Most nurses receive little preparation at the prelicensure or graduate level related to the care of children with special needs. In addition to providing direct care and modeling best practices for staff, APNs can support improved care of children with ASD through staff education. Integration of information about children with ASD into new employee-orientation programs, along with patient care rounds, formal and informal education sessions, and consultation can improve knowledge and facilitate skill development related to this population. The keys to success in caring for children with ASD involves recognition of the many types of disorders that occur in the ASD population, learning the individual characteristics of each patient encountered, and learning how to develop effective partnerships with the child's primary caregivers.

REFERENCES

American Psychiatric Association. (2000). *Diagnostic and statistical manual of mental disorders* (4th ed., text revision). Washington, DC: Author.

Baugh, R. F., Archer, S. M., Mitchell, R. B., Rosenfeld, R. M., Amin, R., Burns, J. J., . . . Patel, M. M. (2011). Clinical practice guideline: Tonsillectomy in children. *Otolaryngology Head and Neck Surgery.* doi: 10.1177/0194599810389949. Retrieved 1/14/11, http://www.entnet.org/HealthInformation/upload/CPG-TonsillectomyInChildren.pdf

Centers for Disease Control and Prevention. (2009). *Autism information center.* Retrieved from http://www.cdc.gov/ncbddd/autism/facts.html

Centers for Disease Control and Prevention. (2010). *Autism spectrum disorders facts.* Retrieved from http://www.cdc.gov/ncbddd/autism/facts.html

Coplan, J. (2010). *Making sense of autistic spectrum disorders: Create the brightest future for your child with the best treatment options.* New York: Bantam.

Inglese, M. D. (2008). Pain perception and communication in children with autism spectrum disorder: New parental insights [abstract]. *Southern Online Journal of Nursing Research, 8*(2). Retrieved from http://www.resourcenter.net/images/SNRS/Files/SOJNR_articles2/Vol08Num02I_K.html#inglese

Malviya, S., Voepel-Lewis, T., Burke, C., Merkel, S., & Tait, A. R. (2006). The revised FLACC observational pain tool: Improved reliability and validity for pain assessment in children with cognitive impairment. *Pediatric Anesthesia, 16,* 258–265.

Nader, R., Oberlander, T. F., Chambers, C. T., & Craig, K. D. (2004). Expression of pain in children with autism. *Clinical Journal of Pain, 20*(2), 88–97.

Newhouse, R., Dearholt, S., Poe, S., Pugh, L., & White, K. (2007). *Johns Hopkins nursing evidence-based practice: Model and guidelines.* Indianapolis, IN: Sigma Theta Tau International.

Nordahl, C. W., Simon, T. J., Zierhut, C., Solomon, M., Rogers, S. J., & Amaral, D. G. (2008). Brief report: Methods for acquiring structural MRI data in very young children with autism without the use of sedation. *Journal of Autism and Developmental Disorders, 38,* 1581–1590. doi: 1007/s10803-007-0514-x

Ross, A. K., Hazlett, H. C., Garret, N. T., Wilkerson, C., & Piven, B. (2005). Moderate sedation for MRI in young children with autism. *Pediatric Radiology, 35,* 867–871.

Scarpinato, N., Bradley, J., Kurbjun, K., Bateman, X., Holtzer, B., & Ely, B. (2010). Caring for a child with an autism spectrum disorder in the acute care setting. *Journal for Specialists in Pediatric Nursing, 15*(3), 244–254.

Seid, M., Sherman, M., & Seid, A. (1997). Perioperative psychosocial interventions for autistic children undergoing ENT surgery. *International Journal of Pediatric Otorhinolaryngology, 40,* 107–113.

Souders, M. C., DePaul, D., Freeman, K. G., & Levy, S. E. (2002). Caring for children and adolescents with autism who require challenging procedures. *Pediatric Nursing, 28*(6), 555–562.

Sutters, K. A., Miaskowski, C., Holdridge-Zeuner, D., Waite, S., Paul, S. M., Savedra, M. C., & Lanier, B. (2004). A randomized clinical trial of the effectiveness of a scheduled oral analgesic dosing regimen for the management of postoperative pain in children following tonsillectomy. *Pain, 110*(1-2), 49–55.

Sutters, K. A., Miaskowski, C., Holdridge-Zeuner, D., Waite, S., Paul, S. M., Savedra, M. C., Lanier, B., & Mahoney, K. (2010). A randomized clinical trial of scheduled dosing of acetaminophen and hydrocodone for the management of postoperative pain in children following tonsillectomy. *Clinical Journal of Pain, 26*(2), 95–103.

Sutters, K. A., Savedra, M. C., Miaskowski, C., Holdridge-Zeuner, D., Waite, S., Paul, S. M., & Lanier, B. (2007). Children's expectations of pain, perceptions of analgesic efficacy, and experiences with nonpharmacologic pain management strategies at home following tonsillectomy. *Journal for Specialists in Pediatric Nursing, 12*(3), 139–148.

Titler, M. (2007). Translating research into practice: Models for changing clinician behavior. *American Journal of Nursing, 17*(6), 26–33.

Zeev, N., Mayes, L. C., Caldwell-Andrews, A. A., Karas, D. E., & McClain, B. C. (2006). Preoperative anxiety, postoperative pain, and behavioral recovery in young children undergoing surgery. *Pediatrics, 118*(2), 651–658.

"Keep Calm and Carry On": The School Nurse and Students on the Autism Spectrum

8

Marian S. Byrnes and Marcia R. Gardner

Advances made in the diagnosis and treatment of children with special physical and emotional needs, together with federal and state mandates under the Individuals with Disabilities Education Act (IDEA) to provide each child with "the most appropriate" education to age 21, have resulted in ever-increasing numbers of special needs children enrolled in both private and public schools. The IDEA is an expansion of previous federal legislation relating to children with disabilities, and promotes the creation of the least restrictive educational environment possible for each child, the participation of parents, and the development of an individualized education plan (IEP) to meet the educational needs of students with disabilities (U.S. Department of Education, Office of Special Education Programs, n.d.). Autism is one of 13 disabling conditions defined by IDEA (Lewis & Bear, 2009). In the fall of 2007, 95% of students with disabilities ages 6 to 21 years were served in public schools; 1% were enrolled in private schools; and fewer than 1% were being educated in other settings (e.g., residential facilities) or were homeschooled. Approximately 90% of students with a diagnosis of autistic spectrum disorder (ASD) were enrolled in a "regular school" environment (National Center for Educational Statistics, 2011). These trends coincide with parental demands and expectations for inclusive education.

Data reported by the Autism and Developmental Disabilities Monitoring (ADDM) Network of the Centers for Disease Control (CDC, 2009) demonstrate that approximately 1 of every 110 children is diagnosed "on the spectrum," and these children come from every racial, ethnic, and socioeconomic group. According to the Autism Society of America (2006), recent diagnoses of ASD have increased 10% to 17% annually. Most researchers and clinicians agree that there are multiple reasons for this increase in numbers, including earlier screening and diagnosis and more inclusive diagnostic criteria.

Nurses in many settings, but particularly in school settings, *will* care for children on the autism spectrum. The prospect of reductions in federal, state, and local funding of educational programs, the recent economic downturn, as well as state and federal budget shortfalls, make it likely that students diagnosed with ASD will constitute an increasing percentage of students who will be enrolled in the nation's public educational system, rather than in private or specialized schools.

MULTIDISCIPLINARY SCHOOL-BASED TEAMS

A multiprofessional team, consisting of teachers, administrators, therapists, nurses, and others, in close partnership with parents and guardians, should collaborate to create the best possible educational approach for each student. The school setting is where families and students on the spectrum receive the highest level of ongoing formal and appropriate support services. School nurses have an integral role on the educational team, but also face ever-increasing challenges presented by the growing numbers of children with special needs. In order to provide appropriate and holistic care in the school setting, it is important that school nurses have a substantial knowledge base regarding manifestations of autism, associated health concerns, and treatment strategies specific to ASD, as well as an appreciation of the impact a child with autism can have on family dynamics.

This chapter describes the role of nurses caring for individuals with ASD in the school setting, and presents practice approaches and guidelines that can inform nursing care and assist school nurses, in collaboration with parents and the school community, to more effectively care for preteens and adolescents on the spectrum. Exemplified by the case of a young adolescent in middle school, this chapter focuses on manifestations associated with the more common forms of ASD: autistic disorder, Asperger's syndrome (AS), and pervasive developmental disorder–not otherwise specified (PDD-NOS; see Chapter 1).

AUTISM SPECTRUM DISORDERS IN THE SCHOOL HEALTH CONTEXT

The often-repeated adage that to know one child on the spectrum is to know one child on the spectrum reflects the experience of many who care for students diagnosed with an ASD. Like every individual, a student with ASD is unique, with unique patterns and personality traits. The diagnosis of ASD encompasses a very wide variety of complex clinical and behavioral presentations that are often especially challenging and frustrating for parents, educators, and health care providers.

Different Presentations in the School Environment

Clinicians and therapists often categorize individuals with autism according to cognitive abilities—high-functioning versus low-functioning autism (HFA, LFA)—although these categories are not universally accepted. The *Diagnostic and Statistical Manual of Mental Disorders, Fourth Edition, Text Revision* (*DSM-IV-TR*; American Psychiatric Association [APA], 2000) outlines the diagnostic criteria for each subtype of autism including: autistic disorder, AS, PDD-NOS, Rett syndrome, and childhood disintegrative disorder. Refer to Chapters 1 to 3 for a more detailed discussion of defining characteristics, core deficits, and types of ASD.

Diagnosis of the classic form of autism generally occurs earlier than other variants. This occurs because of the overt manifestations and, in general, follows from the identification of behavioral red flags by nurses, parents, teachers, or other caregivers (e.g., lack of social responsiveness, absence of shared attention, absence of face or eye contact, delayed or absent language development, atypical play, inflexible adherence to nonfunctional routines, repetitive motor mannerisms). Diagnosis is followed by formal evaluation by pediatric and developmental specialists (Trillingsgaard, Sorensen, Nemec, & Jorgensen, 2005).

Pervasive developmental disorder–not otherwise specified is typically diagnosed when children meet some, but not all, of the criteria for other autistic disorders; these children and those with AS usually fall into the high-functioning category. Rett syndrome and childhood disintegrative disorder are rare and are broadly characterized by apparently normal development of the infant and young child, followed by insidious loss of established communicative and developmental abilities. Recently, there has been controversy about whether to cluster AS with other forms of autism, and diagnostic definitions of AS are evolving (Woodbury-Smith & Volkmar, 2009). Nurses may encounter parents who resist having their child categorized with

PDD-NOS, fearing that they will not receive all possible services. In the school setting, individuals with AS continue to receive specialized services and need specialized school health intervention, based on their educational needs and not necessarily on the diagnosis (APA, 2000; Woodbury-Smith & Volkmar, 2009).

Children and adolescents diagnosed with AS often display near to above normal intelligence and capacity to learn, but can manifest wide discrepancies between functional abilities. Often, verbal expression abilities are strong, and the child's developmental history usually includes normal timing of language development but odd, pragmatic speech, and difficulties with peer and other social interactions (Woodbury-Smith & Volkmar, 2009). However, children with AS have significant difficulties recognizing and responding to social cues, such as the interpretation of others' body language and intonation; they also experience difficulty comprehending language subtleties, such as humor, idiom, and sarcasm. These hallmark symptoms of autism often leading to social awkwardness (Atwood, 2005). When the child reaches school age, social cues become increasingly important in navigating the social experiences of the school classroom, cafeteria, and recreational activities. The symptoms of ASD may worsen in students as they move up grades and face increasingly challenging social situations. These students may present to the nurse with physical or other complaints.

Difficulty processing stimuli, difficulty communicating information, sleep disorders, anxiety disorders, and depression are frequently observed comorbidities associated with AS (Woodbury-Smith & Volkmar, 2009). Co-occurring problems affect the student's ability to function in school. Farrugia and Hudson's (2006) review concluded that students with AS, aged 12 to 16 years, experienced significantly higher levels of anxiety than same-age adolescents in the general population. Negative thoughts and behavioral problems interfering with daily life were significantly more common in students with AS than in typical students. Nurses in school settings with preteens and adolescents must have a high index of suspicion for mood and anxiety disorders in their students with AS.

In summary, ASD can be viewed as a complex developmental disorder that is neurologically based, diagnosed by observation of behavioral patterns, and manifested by deficits in social interaction, reciprocity, and communication; common tendencies of the disorder include repetitive and stereotyped behaviors, sensory difficulties, and restricted interests (National Institute of Mental Health [NIMH], 2012). Autism spectrum disorder manifests along a range of subtle to overt behavioral indicators and along a range of cognitive and communication abilities (APA, 2000). Ellen Notbohm, in the book *Ten Things Your Student with Autism Wishes You Knew* (2004), compared communication between autistic and nonautistic students to that of the early PC and MAC computer programs. The author recommended that we think of the basic operating systems (hardwiring) of autistics and "neurotypicals" to be different and somewhat incompatible; this analogy can help nurses, parents, caregivers, teachers, and others to understand some of the communication difficulties and negative behaviors that students on the spectrum may display. The challenge for nurses is to assist parents, educators, and others who help these students to manage these difficulties. By doing this, we acknowledge and accept this basic and important neurological difference.

MANAGEMENT IN THE SCHOOL SETTING

Autism spectrum disorder is a lifelong condition. Management of the disorder's manifestations, therefore, must evolve in concert with the individual's growth, development, health status, and social and family circumstances. Management in the school setting must reflect this complex network of influences. Care for students on the autism spectrum involves a multimodal approach, with a focus on improvement of the quality of life for individuals with the condition in the context of the learning environment. Seigel, Ihle, Marco, and Hendren (2010) noted that "evidenced-based treatment for ASD begins with an understanding that the syndrome is heterogeneous in expression and that treatment plans must target ASD rather than the co-morbid disorders that may require integrated but separate treatment" (p. 38). Interventions should be individualized (personalized) with the goals of addressing the core features of ASD, which are social, communication, and behavioral deficits, as they intersect with the expectations of school personnel.

Early Intervention Follows Early Identification

To date, there is neither a cure nor a specifically determined biological or developmental etiology for autism, although there are many promising theories and extensive research. This fact has understandably led to a wide array of unproven and often controversial treatments. Discussing the future directions of ASD research, Seigel and colleagues (2010) noted that although progress is rapid, there are now many collaborative genetic studies and comparatively fewer studies about treatment. Current avenues of research illustrate the investigator's hypothesis that early identification and intervention will improve functional, and educational, outcomes. Elder and D'Allessandro (2009) pointed out that the treatment goals of psychopharmacological as well as behavioral therapies are to "alleviate the most troublesome behavioral symptoms that impair or distress the child and/or interfere with therapeutic efforts, such as intensive education and socialization" (p. 243).

Students with ASD experience a wide variety of educational strategies and integrated developmental therapies (i.e., occupational, physical, and speech therapies). Many benefit from small, structured classroom environments (Woodbury & Volkmar, 2009), with special education teachers and trained classroom paraprofessional aides. Inclusion education in classrooms with nonautistic students who model appropriate behaviors can help children and adolescents with autism, particularly high-functioning individuals such as those with AS, to develop age-appropriate skills (Woodbury & Volkmar, 2009). Any of these behavioral treatments should be selected based on the individual characteristics and needs of the student (Cade & Tidwell, 2001).

Resources for school nurses

In 2005, the National Autism Center (NAC, 2011) launched a project to comprehensively evaluate and analyze vast numbers of current ASD treatment modalities for children, adolescents, and young adults. A panel of nationally recognized researchers, scholars, and noted autism experts led this effort, and their findings were published in April 2011 in the National Standards Report (NAC, 2011). The purpose of this project was to provide parents, educators, service providers, and health care professionals, including nurses, with evidence-based, reliable guidelines for interventions targeting core autism characteristics. The National Standards Report is a useful resource for school nurses, and can be accessed at the National Autism Center website (NAC, 2011). Nurses might be invited to participate in educational research projects in which students are subjects. In these cases, nurses may refer to the NAC guidelines for information to critique the merit of research proposals before agreeing to be involved or to enroll students.

Evidence-based Intervention for Behavior Management

A well-recognized and evidence-based cornerstone in the management of the communicative, socialization, and behavioral challenges of those on the spectrum is applied behavioral analysis (ABA). "ABA is the process of applying interventions that are based on the principles of learning derived from experimental psychology research to systematically change behavior and to demonstrate that the interventions used are responsible for the observable improvement in behavior" (Myers & Johnson, 2007, p. 1164). Behavioral therapies utilize principles of classic operant conditioning to change, extinguish, or elicit behaviors, but do not attempt to determine their underlying meaning. Social skills training and/or elimination of problem behavioral issues, such as tantrums, can be achieved using these therapies. Educators have a long history of using versions of ABA in modifying student behaviors with positive reinforcement and positive punishment. This modality has its origins in behaviorist theories of learning (Skinner & Rogers, 1965).

ABA can be viewed as the updated form of behavior modification (Ciccarelli & White, 2010; NIMH, n.d.). Applied behavioral analysis is widely used in autism programming. For example, Stahmer, Collings, and Palinkas (2005) have reported that 72% of community-based early intervention programs in southern California incorporated some form of ABA as a primary intervention strategy for young children with autism.

When used by skilled practitioners, ABA combines many research-validated methods into a comprehensive and individualized approach for students with autism (Green, 2011). Applied behavioral analysis can make learning enjoyable, while engaging the learner in positive social interactions. Programs train parents in ABA methods so that learned communication skills and desired behaviors are transferred to other settings. Treatment goals are set and modified in small, incremental steps. Skills to be increased and reinforced (e.g., appropriate verbalization, eye contact) are rewarded, while maladaptive behaviors (e.g., stereotypical, self-injurious (SIB), aggressive, or disruptive behaviors) are not reinforced or rewarded, but are replaced by acceptable alternative behaviors.

Functional behavioral analysis

Effect treatment programs build on the child's interests, are highly structured, involve learning in small steps, and provide regular positive reinforcement for behavioral management (NIMH, 2012). Triggers and solutions for behavioral problems can be identified by detailed functional behavior analysis (FBA) performed by specially trained educators or psychologists, who then devise interventions. A nurse might also receive training in conducting FBA. Students on the spectrum may have individual behavior plans that target problematic behavioral issues and socialization goals through modeling, token rewards, and time-out reinforcement techniques. Functional behavior analysis plans are often developed in collaboration with the teacher, student, and parent, and are incorporated into the IEP. Dedicated, consistent, but flexible application of FBA principles to the student's behavioral and educational programs in all settings are important for progress.

Not all interventions used with students on the autism spectrum have a strong evidence base, nor do all educational providers have a full understanding of the concept of evidence-based intervention. Stahmer and colleagues (2005) also found that more than one-half of the community-based early intervention providers had an erroneous understanding of the research evidence for autism-related interventions and misclassified evidence-based and non-evidenced-based strategies. They also found that most utilized a variety of untested techniques in their programs. Considering the variety of intervention strategies, programs, and providers, the following guidelines might help parents to evaluate potential interventions, approaches, and programs for their child on the autistic spectrum. Nurses should encourage parents to consider:

- comparing the progress of other children in the program;
- how effectively children from the program integrate into regular school settings;
- whether all staff have had appropriate autism-specific training;
- if classrooms are organized and distraction-free;
- whether daily schedules and activities are predictable and routinized;
- the staff-to-child ratio and level of individual attention for each child;
- strategies used to measure children's progress;
- the level of individualization of tasks and reward systems;
- involvement of parents, including training of parents in the intervention strategies used with the child; and
- costs, time involved, and location of the program. (NIMH, n.d.; NIMH, 2012)

CASE

Tim is a 13-year-old student in the AM School. He was diagnosed with autism/PDD-NOS as a toddler, and now fits the criteria for AD. He is considered to be relatively high functioning. Tim lives at home with his parents, an older brother, who is an honors athlete at the high school, and a younger sister, who is in the fourth grade. His developmental milestones were somewhat delayed, and he had several years of early intervention in the form of speech, occupational, and physical therapy. His verbal communications are typically nonspontaneous; his responses to interaction are short phrases and single words with a monotonal, clipped quality. Tim avoids direct eye contact with others. His actions and verbalizations often seem disorganized. As an example, he speaks to himself nonsensically about favorite cartoon characters.

His motor skills are fairly good, and he enjoys running for short sprints and swimming. During recess, Tim often becomes engaged in gathering twigs and other debris from under trees. Tim sometimes displays robotic-like motions of his arms and hands, and has a restless, easily distracted energy. His IQ has been estimated to be in the low-normal range, with discrepancy between an average nonverbal and low-average verbal ability. He is participating in an inclusion program in his public middle school. His IEP calls for physical therapy twice per week, occupational therapy in individual and in group sessions twice per week, and twice-weekly lessons with a middle school reading specialist.

Tim generally appears to enjoy school. His classroom is highly structured and consists of six other developmentally delayed students, a special education teacher, and one assistant. His favorite home activity is watching SpongeBob videos on the computer, and computer gaming is a major positive reinforcement intervention strategy outlined in his behavioral plan. He habitually picks at his skin, particularly the cuticles, causing bleeding and occasional infection.

BEST PRACTICES: INDIVIDUALIZED EDUCATION AND HEALTH PLANS

Students with a diagnosis of ASD typically qualify for IEPs based on the IDEA. The IEP is updated at least once-yearly by all providers and educators involved with the child's school experience, in collaboration with parents. The plan typically outlines specific developmental goals and delineates the services that will be provided to meet these goals, such as physical, speech, and occupational therapies; use of a classroom aide; and direct nursing care when there are underlying medical issues that may require treatments (IDEA, 1990).

Role of the Nurse

The school nurse, as the health care professional on the team, will assist teachers, counselors, and others by providing and interpreting information about growth and development; coordinating health services; addressing health concerns, medications, and other treatments; educating staff; and advising the team on the integrated management of co-occurring health problems, including pharmacotherapy. The nurse should ensure that medically relevant information is included in the IEP.

Significant medical issues and personalized health interventions that may affect the educational process may also require an individualized health plan (IHP). The IHP is developed by the school nurse and is usually incorporated into the IEP. Integration of pertinent health-related data and information into the IEP and/or IHP optimizes the nursing role on the educational team and promotes a holistic view of the child's health and educational needs (Bellando & Lopez, 2009; Gardner, 2001). Refer to Table 8.1 for an example of an IHP for a *young* child with AS, developed by Gardner (2001). Bellando and Lopez (2009) provided a comprehensive six-point framework for this process to assist a team in addressing both health/safety needs and educational goals of students within the IEP/IHP. The framework is outlined in Table 8.2.

Nursing Roles in School Settings

A school nurse or school nurse practitioner is likely to be the health care professional who has the most contact daily with students with ASD. In addition to providing direct care, the nurse is an important liaison with parents, teachers, psychologists, primary-care providers, developmentalists, and medical or advanced practice nurse specialists. The liaison role includes coordinating information from multiple sources, monitoring and communicating health status, and making treatment recommendations and referrals.

A busy school nurse or school nurse practitioner is challenged throughout the day by a variety of issues ranging from the mundane to the true health emergency. The British adage "keep calm and carry on" reflects a style of staying organized and setting appropriate priorities when juggling the myriad of health issues that arise in the care of students with ASD. These can be especially challenging due to the wide range and degree of communicative, learning, and sensory integration difficulties that these students may exhibit.

The nurse's office is often seen as the place in which a friendly face, gentle touch, and expert care of injury are available. The health office can function as "safe harbor" in which students seek relief from a variety of physical and emotional stressors. School health nurses should recognize that students will display their individual personality styles, as well as the traits typifying the disorder. Each student should be treated as whole and unique; there is no "one size fits all" approach. Combining a deliberately centered and calm demeanor with a caring attitude is a recommended approach for the school nurse in meeting the

TABLE 8.1 Example of an IHP for a Young Child in the School Setting

Nursing diagnosis	Goals	Interventions
Impaired social interaction: R/T altered thought processes (atypical preoccupation with or perseveration on the presidents)	Student will: Show signs of pleasure when socializing Increase frequency of nonperseverative interactions by 50% by the end of the school year	Behavioral domain 1. Incorporate the behavior modification system used in Robbie's classroom: stickers for appropriate interactions noted while in health office (e.g., eye contact, appropriate affect, initiating interactions) 2. Give positive verbal feedback for social behaviors not involving the topics that preoccupy him. Pair Robbie with another child for visits to health office to increase socialization opportunities.
Risk for injury: R/T tantrums	Student will: Decrease overall tantrum frequency 25% in 3 months and 50% in 6 months Experience no tantrum-related injuries	Safety domain 1. Monitor Robbie's tantrum pattern of determine precipitating factors. 2. Ask classroom staff to prepare Robbie for transitions such as leaving the classroom to visit the nurse. 3. Clearly explain rules, expected behaviors, and consequences of behaviors. Use consistency in adhering to behavioral management plan. 4. Instruct classroom staff in appropriate response to tantrums: A. Do not placate. B. Maintain clam demeanor. C. Ensure safety. D. Ignore if possible until tantrum is over. E. Provide positive reinforcement for desired behavior. 5. Use health office as safe area for "cooling off" when classroom staff feel Robbie is beginning to lose control. 6. Provide structured, calm approach in health office. 7. Log frequency of tantrums. Ask parents to log frequency at home. 8. Refer to school psychologist if not improved.
Risk for loneliness	Student will: Demonstrate no signs of emotional distress	Behavioral domain: Coping 1. Consult with teachers about social behaviors exhibited. 2. Periodically observe Robbie in class and play situations for social integration. 3. Monitor for behavior changes consistent with depressive symptoms, loneliness, need for attention, or other issues. 4. Refer parents to state Division of Developmental Disabilities.

(*Continued*)

TABLE 8.1 ■ *Continued*

Nursing diagnosis	Goals	Interventions
		5. Support and coach parents in seeking friends and activities for Robbie. 6. Refer to psychologist if needed.
Altered communication: R/T inability to interpret language subtleties	Student will: Demonstrate comprehension of messages Express needs	Behavioral domain: Communication 1. Use concrete language with Robbie; avoid sarcasm or teasing. 2. Clearly explain rules and expected behaviors, and use consistent approach in applying these. 3. Point out nonverbal meanings of gestures, facial expression ("I see that you are smiling today. Are you feeling happy?"). 4. Check that Robbie comprehends what is said to him. 5. Reinforce appropriate reciprocal interactions.
Family coping: Potential for growth	Family members will: Seek assistance as needed Develop strategies for handling situations related to Robbie's disability Normalize family life to incorporate Robbie's special needs while continuing to meet their own needs	Family domain 1. Participate in parent-staff Individualized Educational Plan planning meetings. 2. Provide consistent feedback about Robbie's progress. 3. Use nonjudegmental listening to allow parents and sibling to express feelings. 4. Discuss situations that parents or other family members find difficult to handle, and teach strategies for coping. 5. Provide anticipatory guidance regarding sibling issues. 6. Ensure that all family members have adequate information about Asperger syndrome. 7. Coach parents in how to explain Robbie's condition to others. 8. Encourage parents to continue to meet their developmental, social, and emotional needs. 9. Refer parents to Asperger syndrome support group 10. Refer family, if needed, to therapist familiar with developmental disabilities issues.
Potential complication: Medication therapy adverse effects	Student will: Demonstrate decreased frequency of inattentive behaviors Be without signs of adverse effects of medications	Physiologic domain: Medication management 1. Determine evidence of decreased motor activity, decreased impulsivity, increased attention and focus, improved socializing. 2. Log frequency of target behaviors, and compare with baseline. 3. Provide parental feedback about behavior changes and therapeutic effects. 4. Evaluate family knowledge of adverse effects of medications. Teach, clarify, and reinforce.

(*Continued*)

TABLE 8.1 ■ *Continued*

Nursing diagnosis	Goals	Interventions
		5. Instruct classroom staff about adverse drug effects to be reported. 6. Consult with family about appetite changes; monitor eating patterns; suggest calorie-dense snacks if appetitue is diminished; monitor height and weight periodically; refer for weight loss or growth stagnation.
Knowledge deficit: Manifestations of the disorder, therapeutic and adverse effects	Parents, teachers, staff will: Demonstrate necessary knowledge of disorder and Robbie's treatment	Health system domain 1. Refer family and staff to autism and Asperger syndrome resources. 2. Develop list of providers who are knowledgeable about Asperger syndrome, use as referral source. 3. Assess family's understanding of disorder; teach, clarify, and reinforce. 4. Provide staff training.

Note: R/T = related to.

From Gardner, M. R. (2001). Understanding and caring for the child with Asperger Syndrome. *Journal of School Nursing, 17*(4), 178–184. Copyright © Sage Publications. Reprinted with permission of Sage Publications.

challenges presented by students on the spectrum. A calm and quiet approach and environment are crucial aspects of care tailored to needs of children with ASD.

Strategies to Facilitate Assessment of Students with ASD

Ideally, the health office is a nonchaotic, safe, low-stimulation environment in which students on the spectrum can expect familiar, predictable, and consistent responses to their needs. This type of environment can promote cooperation and minimize resistance to examination, evaluation, and treatment. A preliminary visit to the health office, before any care is needed, can help new students become familiar with the space and staff. A helpful way of getting to know students individually, and establishing familiarity and trust, is for the school nurse to participate occasionally in events outside of the health office, such as field day, off-campus excursions, family fun nights, and health and fitness activities. Some students will visit the health office when they need "down time," away from classroom demands; this intervention can be incorporated into the IHP.

Interacting with the student: Students with ASD generally are concrete thinkers who benefit from pictures and modeling, rather than words, to explain health-related procedures (Minchella & Preti, 2011). If a child is nonverbal, the child's usual communication modes should be used; these might include picture-exchange communication system (PECS) or other visual means (Souders, DePaul, Freeman, & Levy, 2002). When assessing children and adolescents, nurses should use simple, concrete, straightforward directions and avoid idioms, words with multiple meanings, and open-ended queries, such as "Tell me what is bothering you," or "How do you feel?" It is usually better to ask direct questions, such as "Does your ear

TABLE 8.2 Steps for Developing an Individual Health Plan

1. Define the nurse's role in the presenting problem	• What is the nursing role in this problem? • How cm nursing expertise facilitate medical care? • If this is not a nursing issue, who needs to be contacted to make sure the problem is addressed?
2. Characterization of the presenting problem	• What is the problem? • When is it happening? • Is there a pattern to the problem (frequency, duration, time)? • Are there people/events that make it better or worse? • What information should be gathered to be more informed?
3. How does the medical diagnosis contribute?	• Gather information about medical aspects of the presenting problem. • Talk to parents, community medical providers. • Begin to develop handouts and information you will need to educate, monitor, or devise a plan for the student's team about medical issues.
4. How do diagnosed developmental issues contribute?	• What developmental issues does the student have: cognitive, language, motor delays, and/or sensory issues? • How might they impact this situation? • What team members should be consulted to help get information to guide the IHP (occupational therapist, speech therapist)?
5. How are psychological/ behavioral issues contributing?	• What psychological diagnoses does the student have? • Is the student on medication (or these conditions? Which ones? Are they effective? • How do these diagnoses impact the current problem? • Are there environmental issues contributing to the problem? • What team members should be consulted to help get information to guide the IHP psychologist social worker)?
6. How to implement the IHP	• Have the plan in writing, free of medical jargon, and easy to understand. • Review the IHP with key team members/team meeting if possible. • Establish a time line to gather data, get back together to modify the plan, and discuss next treatment steps. • Establish guidelines as to what constitutes a medical emergency and when the student's doctor needs to be contacted. • If the student is involved in the plan, make sure you have consulted with therapists to make sure the plan is consistent with the student's needs and capabilities. • Make sure that all parties have signed the IHP/IEP (Individual Education Plan). • If student is involved in the plan, make sure he/she is aware of plan's implementation and his/her role.

Source: Reprinted from Bellando and Lopez (2009). The school nurse's role in treatment of the student with austim spectrum disorders. *Journal of School Nursing, 14*(3), 173–182. Reprinted with permission from Wiley Publishing, Wiley-Blackwell.

hurt?" Allow extra time for the student to process verbal cues, directions, and questions. Anticipate that responses might be slow in coming, and that unexpected experiences or sensations can result in vigorous behavioral responses. The student's teachers and parents are the best informants about the most effective communication and assessment strategies (Souders, DePaul, Freeman, & Levy, 2002), which should be documented as part of the IHP.

Sensory issues in the nurse's office: Many people with ASD are highly sensitive to tactile stimuli and react with distress, physical withdrawal, self-injury, or other maladaptive behaviors to touch or to other stimuli (Souders, DePaul, Freeman, & Levy, 2002). During a physical examination, the nurse should prepare the student for any touching; approach the student with a calm, quiet voice; use slow, deliberate motions; and provide focused, short explanations of each technique used. For example, before measuring the pulse, the nurse can tell the student, "I am going to touch your hand and wrist for a little while." Use the least invasive strategy possible. For example, an infrared scanning thermometer, rather than oral or axillary thermometer, might be easier to use and less anxiety-provoking with this population (Minchella & Preti, 2011).

Periodic health screenings, such as hearing screening, may present challenges. Practical strategies to facilitate accurate hearing screening with students on the autism spectrum and those with learning disabilities or with other special needs include the following:

1. Some special training prior to the test may be necessary. For example, the student may need to learn, "When you hear the beep, drop a block into the pan." Classroom aides or teachers can practice these skills with an individual prior to audiometry.
2. Prior to testing, allow the student to hear the audiometer tones without the use of earphones. These can be introduced later.
3. Present a loud practice tone first (e.g., 1000 Hz at 45 db) and gauge the child's response.
4. Follow the student's lead (e.g., he or she may not raise a hand, but may consistently reply "I hear it," "Beep," "Okay."). Observe nonverbal clues to hearing, such as consistent change in facial expression or shift in eye gaze or posture when the tone is played.
5. Allow for response delays. Students may have processing or initiation of response delays after each tone is introduced (e.g., every response is 3 seconds delayed).
6. Students who have been in specific auditory training programs do not wear headsets, even for hearing screening. Consultation or referral to a speech therapist may be necessary for their screening.

Cooperation during procedures should be positively reinforced with praise and encouragement. The nurse should also attempt to modify noncompliance. In some cases, the best strategy for noncompliance or negativity may be to offer the student having "a bad day" the choice to have the screening, or other procedure, performed at another time.

Clues to Health Problems

Behavior is a form of communication; signs of increasing stress and agitation or self-injury can reflect sensory issues, including pain (Oliver & Richards, 2010), illness, or other problems. Head-banging, striking walls, habitual picking and scratching and opening skin sores, and self-biting are examples of SIBs that can result in complications, such as bruising or infection, and need to be addressed as priorities. Difficulties with communication will also interfere with accurate identification of illness or assessment of causes of distress. Some students do not spontaneously seek out adults when ill, injured or in pain. If a trigger for behaviors (such as unexpected stimuli, hunger, schedule changes, or staff changes) is not apparent, the nurse should suspect illness, injury, or pain as contributing to the behavior.

Identification of signs and symptoms requires close attention to cues, and significant detective work. For example, an ingrown toenail may become seriously infected before it is identified, because the student may never have complained or called attention to the problem. The student might demonstrate only nonverbal clues, such as pacing, acting out, or withdrawal, and a thorough physical assessment might be needed to identify and treat the problem. The nurse should also keep in mind that individuals with ASD often perseverate on stressful thoughts or minor discomforts. For example, they might be unable to shift or refocus attention despite attempts at redirection. Such patterns can present additional challenges to accurate health assessment; ongoing redirection to the assessment question or health care task will be necessary.

CASE–EPISODES OF AGGRESSION

Tim's teachers and parents become concerned about his increasing episodes of aggressive, oppositional behaviors. These manifest as periods of agitation that occasionally erupt into tantrums. Tim can throw objects at others and flail against the floors and walls. Occasionally these incidents have escalated to the point of safety risks for his parent, and even teachers. His siblings are afraid of Tim's violent outbursts and go to their rooms when these behaviors occur at home. If these behaviors occur at school, Tim is escorted to the quiet room by trained members of a behavioral team until he calms and becomes cooperative. Triggers for the behaviors are the repeated, and unwanted, prompts to comply with his teacher's or parent's directives. Over time, classmates in the inclusion classes have become increasingly distant and have excluded Tim from activities.

Tim's psychiatrist has attempted to address his behavioral problems with ongoing medication adjustments. Currently prescribed medications are: aripiprazole (Abilify) daily at bedtime, guanfacine (Tenex) three times a day (crushed in applesauce), citalopram (Celexa) twice a day, and lorazepam (Ativan) as needed for agitation and aggressiveness. A functional behavioral plan (FBP) has also been formulated by Tim's teacher, occupational therapist, and school psychologist to be utilized at school and reinforced at home. This plan identifies triggers and outlines deescalation and reward strategies for compliance, improved performance, and acceptable behaviors.

As a member of the educational team, the school nurse is aware of the details of Tim's FBP and uses this behavior-management approach during encounters in the health office. The nurse creates a "routine" so that Tim is prompted to consistently come to the nurse's office after lunch to take his afternoon dose of guanfacine. He learns that coming to the health office at the appropriate time and displaying socially appropriate behaviors result in additional "points," in keeping with his FBP. During the medication time, Tim is carefully assessed for untoward effects of all of the medications he is taking, as well as for his general state of health. The nurse has good rapport with Tim's parents and teachers and shares information regarding changes in behaviors or physical condition or other health concerns. After parental consent is given, questions and concerns, as well as recommendations for treatment plan changes are discussed with other health care professionals, such as the student's primary-care provider and psychiatrist.

BEST PRACTICES

Medication Management

Management of medications is a major nursing responsibility in the school health setting. More than one-half of all individuals with ASD are treated with psychoactive medications that can have significant health risks (Canitano & Scandurra, 2011). Nurses must be familiar with medications commonly prescribed for children with ASD, along with multiple other drugs frequently used in the pediatric population for a variety of acute and chronic conditions. Considering the typical manifestations of children with ASD, particularly impairments in verbal expression, expert assessment and clinical skills along the lines described above are required to monitor children's therapeutic responses to their medications, to recognize side effects, and to ensure that accurate doses are prescribed and administered. Table 8.3 lists medications frequently used in this population of children along with their more common autism-specific indications. Also, see Table 8.1 for a detailed summary of medications used with individuals on the autism spectrum.

The nurse should discuss medication regimens with parents before the student attends school. Parents often share effective strategies for administering medications to their children and can provide information about their children's usual responses. The establishment of a consistent, individualized schedule and methods for daily medication administration at school is important. Some children with ASD are unable to swallow or are resistant to swallowing tablets. Medications can be administered in liquid form or crushed in applesauce or pudding if it is pharmacologically safe to do so. Rituals or routines associated with medication administration can support compliance. In small steps, with a large "dose" of patience and behavioral reinforcement, older children and adolescents can be taught to properly swallow pills. Older students should be encouraged to develop personal responsibility for their medications, such as coming to the health office on time and without prompting, and developing familiarity with the appearance and reason for each medication.

TABLE 8.3 ■ Medications Frequently Used to Manage School Children's ASD Manifestations[a]

Classification	Examples of drugs	Indications in ASD care
Atypical neuroleptics	Risperidone Olanzipine Aripriprizole	Aggression, self-injury, repetitive stereotypical behaviors, irritability
Selective serotonin reuptake inhibitors	Fluoxetine Escitalopram compulsion	Irritability, repetitive stereotypic, repetitive stereotypic behaviors
Stimulants	Methylphenidate Atomoxetine	Attention deficit hyperactivity disorder
Anticonvulsants	Topirimate Valproic acid	Seizure control, repetitive stereotypical behaviors
Agonists	Clonidine Guanfacine	Attention deficit hyperactivity disorder

[a]Many drugs are used in combination to maximize therapeutic effects.

Based on Aman, Farmer, Hollway, & Arnold (2008); Bellando & Lopez (2009); Canitano & Scandurra (2011); Farmer & Aman (2011); Rezaei et al. (2010); West, Brunssen, & Waldrop (2009).

Promoting Safety

Galinat, Barcalow, and Krivda (2005) emphasize the importance of environmental safety when caring for the ASD child in a school setting. They note that increased safety risks arise from several areas of autism-related vulnerability, including seizures, tantrums, self-stimulatory and SIBs, altered sensations to pain, pica, poor coordination, and impulsive behavior. Assessing classrooms, recreational areas, and time-out rooms for environmental dangers and removing them, educating staff, and monitoring children closely are practices that can help to reduce safety risks. Patterns and triggers for SIBs should be discussed with educational staff and parents, so that strategies can be immediately instituted to limit them. Behavioral staff should be trained and certified in proper procedures for restraining aggressive students.

The nurse should educate the school staff on how to recognize seizures and how to provide care and first aid and about other relevant health concerns (Bellando & Lopez, 2009). The school nurse may spearhead, develop, or participate in educational programs and committees in the school and/or community for school staff and parents. Pertinent topics for nurse-initiated programs could include health promotion, sexuality, comorbidities, pharmacotherapy, safety, prevention of bullying, or advances in autism research.

ADOLESCENCE AND ASD

Negotiating life's trials and tribulations throughout the period leading to adulthood is universally challenging. The physical changes of puberty combined with increased social, academic, and community expectations associated with the move from elementary to middle school can result in a bewildering mix of anxiety and excitement. Transitions of any type can be very difficult for children on the autism spectrum. The changes in daily routines and sensory overload associated with the middle school environment can be particularly challenging. One qualitative study that focused on transition issues reported that parents of children with ASD expressed the need for ongoing and meaningful communication among school staff, parents, and children (Stoner, Angell, House, & Bock, 2007). This is best served by a child-centered approach, respect for parents' knowledge of their children's transition challenges, and an "identify, observe, explore" approach to support smoother daily transitions, as well as major changes, such as entry into a new school (Stoner et al., 2007, p. 32). Transition to middle school, in particular, involves entering classes with larger student numbers, regular switching from one room to another, multiple teachers, lockers, and a less predictable environment than the elementary school setting. For adolescent students in inclusion classrooms, the increased emphasis on independence, organization, and self-care skills can be overwhelming and anxiety-provoking. Advance preparation, skills practice, and incremental exposure to new experiences and middle school expectations facilitates adjustment.

Health Instruction for the Student with ASD

The school nurse can expect to provide guidance and instruction to students about a wide variety of health concerns for this age group. Sensitive topics, such as puberty, sexuality, personal hygiene, body image, and masturbation can be presented creatively using storyboards, role-playing, and other visual methods. Health education can take place in groups or during individual sessions, depending on the cognitive and language abilities of the learners. Behavior such as masturbation and sexual overture can sometimes be problematic for lower-functioning people with autism. Socially inappropriate, offensive, or compulsive behaviors should be managed with consistent application of individualized behavioral plans and persistent redirection. Myles, Trautman, and Schelvan (2004) noted that although persons with socio-cognitive disabilities may have verbal skills:

> Their inability to develop social skills and interpret social nuances of those around them brings deep and lifelong challenges that impact their lives in a multitude of ways, including socially, emotionally, behaviorally.... personal safety and decision making can be at risk if people are not able to quickly and efficiently adapt to and read social cues and intuit the hidden rules that surround them at every turn. (p. 1)

Social Skills

Students who previously "fit in" with peer groups during elementary school may be slowly losing ground in middle school. Despite social and communication impairments, many high-functioning individuals, particularly those with AS, want to fit in, and attempt to find and maintain friendships (Woodbury & Volkmar, 2009). The behavioral traits of AS or autism can make this goal difficult to achieve, especially during the preteen and adolescent years, when "difference" is poorly tolerated by peers. Individuals with AS can seem eccentric or odd, have problems with reciprocal conversation, and, in general, do not understand the social culture and norms of their peers. Studies document negative attitudes of normal children toward peers with ASD, despite inclusion education approaches (Campbell, Ferguson, Herzinger, Jackson, & Marino, 2005; Morton & Campbell, 2008). Education about behaviors related to the condition has been associated with improved attitudes of school-aged children (Campbell, Ferguson, Herzinger, & Jackson, 2004). Morton and Campbell (2008) also found that older children had more positive attitudes toward peers with autism when information about the condition was provided by a health professional, rather than their parents. Education of classmates so that they understand their peers' health conditions is a strategy that school nurses often use. Although further research is needed, studies to date suggest that the school nurse might help facilitate integration of children with autism into the peer group through educational interventions in the classroom.

Children and adolescents with ASD are at risk for bullying; almost two-thirds of children and adolescents with AS have been targets of some form of bullying by peers (Carter, 2009). School nurses need to recognize risks, and to immediately intervene when physical and emotional signs of bullying behaviors are apparent. According to Carter (2009, p. 153), "mental health professionals need to consider victimization and shunning when performing evaluations on children who exhibit anxiety, depression, and school phobia." School nurses might be the first to treat students with injuries or responses that might indicate victimization, and should communicate these concerns to appropriate school authorities and parents.

Nurses can become partners with school staff to maintain a safe school environment by being alert to risks for bullying, and attending to high-risk areas, such as the lunchroom and schoolyard, by providing training to other professionals and taking active part in anti-bullying campaigns in the school and community (Carter, 2009). School staff can develop programs to recruit more mature, empathic, and responsible peers in the process of an anti-bullying campaign. Following education about both ASD and positive interaction and tolerance, these student leaders might help their classmates on the spectrum to form friendships, and can model acceptable social behaviors for their peers with and without autism (Freschi, 2011).

Electronic Media

Screen-based media, such as video games, television, and computers, are appealing to individuals on the autism spectrum, especially as related to preferences for visual input. Shane and Albert (2008) found that children with ASD were more likely to spend leisure time using electronic media than in other play activities. Many children and adolescents with autism are highly proficient in navigating the latest in high-tech electronics, but these activities do not require social awareness or reciprocal personal interaction (Mirenda, 2001; Moore, Cheng, McGrath, & Normann, 2005). However, these activities are also commonly used in social situations by "typical" preteens and adolescents; skills with electronic media might open the "gate" to social participation for some children with autism. Video gaming, television, and computer use can interfere with a healthy lifestyle by limiting physical activities, study time, sports participation, and even sleep. For higher-functioning individuals, Internet chat rooms and networking sites can become substitutes for real-life, face-to-face social interaction and relationship building. Naïve adolescents, such as individuals with AS, can misinterpret Internet solicitations for friendship and unknowingly place themselves in unsafe situations in which the potential for exploitation by predators is real. Internet websites that are provocative and illegal, such as child pornography sites, may be tempting to curious and incautious adolescents. Parents can benefit from education about potential risks and benefits associated with screen-based activities.

PREPARING FOR POST-HIGH SCHOOL LIFE

The school nurse can support a successful secondary transition to life after high school by preparing students to assume greater responsibilities for self-care and self-advocacy with regard to their health and well-being. Older adolescents who are capable should develop a basic awareness of any significant or chronic health conditions, learn about their medications, become responsible for taking them, and learn when and to whom they should disclose information. A student's IEP will outline specific goals for transition and may outline areas of vocational education, actual work experience, and mobility training (Johnson, n.d.; U.S. Dept. of Education, n.d.). The school nurse can assist the educational team and parents by developing a referral list of relevant community services, such as county mental health agencies, professional providers, support groups, in-home therapeutic and wraparound service and social organizations for adults with ASD. It may be difficult for families to find and access all of these services.

Shattuck and colleagues (Shattuck, Wagner, Narendorf, Sterlzing, & Hensley, 2011) reported that approximately 39% of young adults with ASD, 0 to 2 years post high school, received no mental health, medical evaluation/assessment, speech therapy, or case-management services. Discontinuation of services occurred more frequently in three populations: higher-functioning individuals, African Americans, and those from lower socioeconomic strata. Taylor and Seltzer (2011) reported that 25% of high-functioning young adults with autism who recently graduated from the public education system were not involved in any daily activities, compared with 8% of those with intellectual disabilities. Most individuals receiving formal services were lower functioning, with cognitive impairment; rates of employment and service use were low in both high- and low-functioning individuals. Findings such as these illustrate the significant gaps in services and community assistance for young adults with ASD post-high school.

Individual goals and preparation for adult life will require ongoing family support and access to important community and state-sponsored resources. The nurse should ensure that families are aware of and know how to contact their respective state departments of special education or offices serving people with developmental disabilities. Nurses should encourage parents to find services and programs designed for people with special needs. Every state has such a program. Services might differ across states and some Internet hunting may be necessary. The school nurse is an important partner with the young adult, parents, and the educational team in anticipating needs and accessing resources.

FAMILY SUPPORT

All professionals caring for those with ASD should recognize and acknowledge the enormous challenges families, particularly parents, face in caring for a child with a serious and lifelong developmental disability. Myers (2009) emphasized the need to consider and incorporate the entire family system into any treatment plan. Doyle and Iland (2003) described the importance of active, nonjudgmental listening to parents. The authors maintained that professionals can best serve families by encouraging open expression and keeping a realistic but hopeful attitude. They also suggested that most parents eventually recognize and discard unrealistic goals for their children with autism.

The significant stresses related to parenting children with autism have been well-documented. Caregiving for these children can affect spouse or partner relationships. High stress generated by the demands of caring for children with ASD might be associated with depression, decreased physical health, and other health problems (Anderson, 2009; Hartley et al., 2010; Kasari & Sigman, 1997; Meyers, 2007; Phetrasuwan & Miles, 2009; Seltzer et al., 2009; Seltzer, Krauss, Orsmond, & Vestal, 2001; Twoy, Connolly & Novak, 2007). School nurses should recognize the simple truth that students, other than those in residential facilities, spend most time at home, where parents do not have the luxury of "lunch breaks" or support from a team of colleagues. Consideration of parenting and family concerns and stresses should be integrated into the plan of care.

Sibling Issues

Families might be simultaneously dealing with the needs of more than one child on the spectrum; this is common. The recurrence risk for ASD in families with a diagnosed child has been reported to be in the range of 2% to 8% (Muhle, Trentacoste, & Rapin, 2004). Constantino and colleagues (Constantino, Zhang, Frazier, Abbacchi, & Law, 2010) reported that among families with a child with autism approximately 11% of siblings had ASD diagnoses, 20% of nondiagnosed siblings had a history of language delay, and one-half of those exhibited speech and language features consistent with autism. The financial burden for families with one or more children on the autism spectrum can also be considerable, since behavioral or other treatment options might not be covered by insurance, depending on state law. The intense responsibilities of caregiving for a child with autism can limit employment opportunities for the primary caregiver. It is easy to understand how affected families can become overwhelmed by caring and planning for special needs members.

The needs of siblings should also be considered when evaluating family stressors and dynamics. Elder and D'Allessandro (2009) noted that parents can experience guilt, because they perceived that their attention to the child with autism could rob their other children of attention and time and because they asked siblings to become caregiving helpers. Older children and adolescent siblings may resent the child with autism or feel embarrassed by the behaviors of their brother/sister and avoid inviting friends into the home. After studying siblings of young adults with autism and cognitive disabilities, Benderix and Sivberg (2007) reported that fear of violence, viewing challenging behaviors, and early assumption of responsibility were commonly expressed concerns. Family activities, routines, and focus might be skewed toward the needs and limitations of the child with a disability (Larson, 2006). Siblings of children with developmental disabilities have higher risks for depression and other psychiatric disorders (Orsmond & Seltzer, 2007) Elder and D'Allessandro (2009) suggested that parents acknowledge and accept siblings' feelings and encourage them to communicate their feelings openly and honestly. School nurses also encounter siblings of individuals with autism in their practices, and can be instrumental in assessing the needs of siblings, facilitating communication about issues of concern with teachers and parents, and ensuring appropriate referral and treatment.

Family strength, resiliency, and enduring sibling bonds are also important factors when planning for the future security of those family members with ASD. Concerned parents might count on siblings or other family members if their adult child with ASD requires lifelong guardianship and oversight to some degree. Mailick and colleagues (Mailick, Seltzer, Orsmond, & Esbensen, 2009) conducted one of the first studies to investigate relationships of adolescents and adults with their siblings with ASD. They reported associations between parental support for the sibling relationship and later involvement of the well sibling with the individual with autism, between behavioral symptoms and sibling involvement, and between gender and sibling involvement. These investigators referred to these findings to highlight the importance of providing support, anticipatory guidance, and resources related to sibling relationships to families and parents.

Community Support Services

Families benefit from access to effective support systems (Myers, 2009). Supports can include extended family, empathetic friends and neighbors, autism support and religious outreach groups, and respite programs, among others. Respite programs can be the source of much-needed energy renewal for families in danger of becoming burnt out from ongoing caregiving for disabled children. The school nurse can maintain referral lists for community services, including respite, recreational programs, and summer camps for the autistic population. The nurse can refer families to professionals, such as pediatricians, dentists, clinical psychologists, and social workers who can offer additional experience and expertise in treating children on the autism spectrum and their families. School nurses are in a good position to network families struggling with the issues of raising children with autism.

Complementary and Alternative Therapies

Parents of children with these lifelong and challenging conditions look for help in many arenas, both inside and outside traditional care. Parents often seek complementary and alternative medicine (CAM), in an effort to help manage difficult symptoms or even "cure" their children. Media reports, books or magazine articles, and particularly Internet websites reporting therapies or programs that ameliorate symptoms or "cure" autism are easy to find (Shute, 2010). Vitamin supplementation and dietary restriction have been reported to be some of the most frequently used alternative therapies (Senel, 2010). Current research findings suggest that a majority of children with ASD receive some form of CAM (Hanson et al., 2007; Myers & Johnson, 2007). Wong (2009) found that use of CAM by parents of children with autism, including frequency and type of therapy, varied with location and culture. While health care providers can be unaware of CAM interventions chosen by parents, a recent survey of a random sample of physicians in the United States found that more than one-half of the 539 respondents reported recommending at least one CAM therapy to families of children with autism. Most frequently recommended therapies included vitamins, melatonin, and probiotics; additionally, dietary management, such as elimination of gluten, casein, and sugar, was considered acceptable by a majority of respondents if parents had already chosen to use this strategy (Golnick & Ireland, 2009). The school nurse should be aware that students might be on restricted diets or might be receiving herbal supplements, atypical vitamin therapy, chelation therapy, or other alternative treatments that might affect health status or interact with prescribed medications (Bellando & Lopez, 2009).

Nurses and other health professionals should routinely include questions about complementary and alternative treatments in the health history and assessment. Alternative treatments might be attempted, despite weak or nonexistent scientific evidence to support efficacy or effectiveness (Levy & Hyman, 2008). However, evidence is a moving target as promising therapies undergo more rigorous testing (Hyman & Levy, 2005). School nurses can help parents evaluate interventions by following and interpreting the current research findings and directing them to authoritative sources of information (Abby, 2009; Bellando & Lopez, 2009). The National Standards Project, described earlier (NAC, 2011), is a relevant resource for both nurses and parents, particularly with respect to educational interventions. see Exhibit 8.1 for a list of general resources for parents and school nurses. Parents can be encouraged to

EXHIBIT 8.1

Assessment Aid: Resources for School Health Professionals and Families

- American Academy of Pediatrics (AAP) www.pediatrics.org
- Autism Alliance of Metro West—School Nurse Autism Packets www.autismalliance.org/nurses-packet.htm
- Autism Society of America www.autism-society.org (useful information about the IEP process)
- Autism Research Institute www.autism.com
- Autism Spectrum Quarterly (a wealth of informative articles for parents, and others caring for those on the spectrum)
- National Autism Center www.nationalautismcenter.org.
- National Standards Project www.nationalautismcenter.org/affiliates/reports.php
- National Institute of Mental Health (NIMH) www.nimh.nih.gov/health/publications/autism
- *Ten Things Your Student with Autism Wishes You Knew* by Ellen Notbohm (2004), published by Future Horizons. Practical suggestions for educators and other school staff.
- *Understanding Autism (for Dummies Series)* by Stephen M. Shore and Linda Rastelli (2006), published by Wiley, Inc. In-depth and practical information and resources for those caring for people with ASD over the lifespan.

share their concerns and use of various therapies with their children's health care providers, and to consider:

- Potential risks for harm from the treatment;
- The potential outcomes for child and family if treatment is not effective;
- Scientific evidence of effectiveness of the treatment;
- How the child will be assessed for treatment outcome;
- Integration of a treatment into the current plan of care. (NIMH, 2012; NIMH n.d.)

SUMMARY

"Keep calm and carry on" is a suitable philosophy for the school nurse in navigating a wide range of unique challenges when caring for children, preteens, and adolescents on the autism spectrum. The school health office can be a "safe harbor" for students with ASD. A nonjudgmental approach, balanced with expert knowledge, compassion, and sincere acceptance of each individual is essential. Caring for students with ASD often results in a mixture of success and challenge. The best school health outcomes are facilitated by knowledge of the core characteristics of autism and informed by an understanding of each child's strengths and challenges. Maintaining knowledge of evidence-based health management strategies, taking a creative approach, and acknowledging family issues, dynamics, and support needs are crucial assets for the school nurse working with students on the spectrum. Comprehensive and holistic care of the individual with autism in the school setting involves direct care, health education, referral to community support services and other health care providers, and education of parents, staff, and other family members on a wide array of autism-related issues. Above all else, nurses in school and other settings can experience a profound satisfaction in assisting young people on the courageous path of attaining personal, social, and educational achievement.

ACKNOWLEDGMENTS

The authors acknowledge and thank the speech and language therapists at the Vanguard School, Paoli, PA, for sharing recommendations for hearing screening.

REFERENCES

Abby, D. (2009). Helping families find the best evidence: CAM therapies for autism spectrum disorders and Asperger's disorder. *Journal for Specialists in Pediatric Nursing, 14*(3), 200–202.

Aman, M. G., Farmer, C. A., Hollway, J., & Arnold, L. E. (2008). Treatment of inattention, overactivity, and impulsiveness in autism spectrum disorders. *Child and Adolescent Psychiatric Clinics of North America, 17*(4), 713–738.

American Psychiatric Association. (2000). *Diagnostic and Statistical Manual of Mental Disorders* (4 ed., text revision). Washington, DC: Author.

Anderson, L. (2009). Mothers of children with special health care needs: Documenting the experience of their children's care in the school setting. *Journal of School Health Nursing, 25*(5), 342–351.

Atwood, T. (2005). *What is Asperger syndrome?* Retrieved from http://www.aspergersyndrome.org/Articles/What-is-Asperger-Syndrome-.aspx

Autism Society. (2006). *Facts and statistics.* Retrieved from http://www.autism-society.org/about-autism/facts-and-statistics.html

Bellando, J., & Lopez, M. (2009). The school nurse's role in treatment of the student with autism spectrum disorders. *Journal for Specialists in Pediatric Nursing, 14*(3), 173–182.

Benderix, Y., & Sivberg, B. (2007). Siblings' experiences of having a brother or sister with autism and mental retardation: A case study of 14 siblings from five families. *Journal of Pediatric Nursing, 22*(5), 410–418.

Cade, M., & Tidwell, S. (2001). Autism and the school nurse. *Journal of School Health, 71*(3), 96–100.

Campbell, J. M., Ferguson, J. E., Herzinger, C. V., Jackson, J. N., & Marino, C. A. (2004). Combined descriptive and explanatory information improves peers' perceptions of autism. *Research in Developmental Disabilities, 25*(4), 321–339.

Campbell, J. M., Ferguson, J. E., Herzinger, C. V., Jackson, J. N., & Marino, C. A. (2005). Peers' attitudes toward autism differ across sociometric groups: An exploratory investigation. *Journal of Developmental and Physical Disabilities, 17*, 281–298.

Canitano, R., & Scandurra, V. (2011). Psychopharmacology in autism: An update. *Progress in Neuro-Psychopharmacology & Biological Psychiatry, 35*, 18–28.

Carter, S. (2009). Bullying of students with Asperger syndrome. *Issues in Comprehensive Pediatric Nursing, 32*(3), 145–154.

Centers for Disease Control and Prevention. (2009). Prevalence of autism spectrum disorder-Autism and Developmental Disabilities Monitoring Network, United States, 2006. *Morbidity and Mortality Weekly Review, 58*(SS-10), 1–20.

Ciccarelli, S., & White, J. (2010). *Psychology: An exploration.* Upper Saddle River, NJ: Pearson.

Constantino, J., Zhang, Y., Frazier, T., Abbacchi, A., & Law, P. (2010). Sibling recurrence and the genetic epidemiology of autism. *American Journal of Psychiatry, 167*(11), 1349–1356.

Doyle, B., & Iland, E. (2003). *How educators and support professionals can help families.* Retrieved from http://marthalakecov.org/~building/spneeds/autism/doyle_families.htm

Elder, J., & D'Alessandro, T. (2009). Supporting families of children with autism spectrum disorder: Questions parents ask and what nurses need to know. *Pediatric Nursing, 35*(4), 240–253.

Farmer, C. A., & Aman, M. G. (2011). Aripiprazole for the treatment of irritability associated with autism. *Expert Opinion on Pharmacotherapy, 12*(4), 635–640.

Farrugia, S., & Hudson, J. (2006). Anxiety in adolescents with Asperger syndrome: Negative thoughts, behavioral problems, and life interference. *Focus on Autism and Other Developmental Disabilities, 21*(1), 25–35.

Freschi, D. (2011, January/February). Middle school transition: Curves in the road up ahead. *Autism Asperger's Digest*, 28–31.

Galinet, K., Barcalow, K., & Krivda, B. (2005). Caring for children with autism in the school setting. *Journal of School Nursing, 21*(4), 208–217.

Gardner, M. R. (2001). Understanding and caring for the child with Asperger syndrome. *Journal of School Nursing, 17*(4),178–184.

Golnick, A. E., & Ireland, M. (2009). Complementary alternative medicine for children with autism: A physician survey. *Journal of Autism and Developmental Disorders, 39*(7), 996–1005.

Green, G. (2011). *Applied behavior analysis for autism.* Retrieved from http://www.behavior.org/resource.php?id=300.

Hansen, E., Kalish, L. A., Bunce, E., Curtis, C., McDaniel, S., Ware, J., & Petry, J. (2007). Use of complementary and alternative medicine among children diagnosed with autism spectrum disorder. *Journal of Autism and Developmental Disorders, 37*(4), 628–636.

Hartley, S. L., Barker, E. T., Seltzer, M. M., Floyd, F., Greenberg, J., Orsmond, G., & Bolt, D. (2010). The relative risk and timing of divorce in families of children with an autism spectrum disorder. *Journal of Family Psychology, 24*(4), 449–457.

Hyman, S. L., & Levy, S. E. (2005). Introduction: Novel therapies in developmental disabilities—hope, reason, and evidence. *Mental Retardation and Developmental Disabilities Research Reviews, 11*(2), 107–109.

Johnson, D. R. (n.d.) *Key provisions on transition: IDEA 1997 compared to H. R. 1350 (IDEA 2004).* Retrieved from http://ncset.org/publications/related/ideatransition.asp

Kasari, C., & Sigman, M. (1997). Linking parental perceptions to interactions in young children with autism. *Journal of Autism and Developmental Disorders, 27*(1), 39–57.

Larson, E. (2006). Caregiving and autism: How does children's propensity for routinization influence participation in family activities? *ORJR: Occupation, Participation and Health, 26*(2), 69–79.

Levy, S. L., & Hyman, S. E. (2008). Complementary and alternative medicine treatments for children with autism spectrum disorders. *Child and Adolescent Psychiatric Clinics of North America, 17*(4), 803–820.

Lewis, K., & Bear, B. (2009). *Manual of school health: A handbook for school nurses, educators, and health professionals.* St. Louis, MO: Saunders-Elsevier.

Mailick, M., Seltzer M. M., Orsmond, G., & Esbensen, A. (2009). Siblings of individuals with an autism spectrum disorder: Sibling relationships and well being in adolescence and adulthood. *Autism, 13*(1), 59–80.

Minchella, L., & Preti, L. (2011). Autism spectrum disorder: Clinical considerations for the school nurse. *NASN School Nurse, 26*(3), 143–145.

Mirenda, P. (2001). Autism, augmentative communication, and assistive technology: What do we really know? *Focus on Autism and Other Developmental Disabilities, 16,* 141–151. doi:10.1177/108835760101600302

Moore, D., Cheng, Y., McGrath, P., & Norman, J. (2005). Powell Collaborative Virtual Environment Technology for people with autism. *Focus on Autism and Other Developmental Disabilities, 20,* 231–243. doi:10.1177/10883576050200040501

Morton, J. F., & Campbell, J. M. (2008). Information source affects peers' initial attitudes toward autism. *Research in Developmental Disabilities, 29,* 189–201.

Muhle, R., Trentacoste, S. V., & Rapin, I. (2004). The genetics of autism. *Pediatrics, 113,* e472–486. Retrieved from http://pediatrics.aappublications.org/content/113/5/e472.full.html

Myers, S. M. (2009). Management of autism spectrum disorders in primary care. *Pediatric Annals, 38*(1), 42–49.

Myers, S., & Johnson, C. (2007). Management of children with autism spectrum disorders. *Pediatrics, 120*(5), 1162–1180.

Myles, B., Trautman, M., & Schelvan, R. (2004). *The hidden curriculum: Practical solutions for understanding unstated social rules in social situations.* Shawnee Mission, KS: Autism Asperger Publishing.

National Autism Center. (2011). *National standards project.* Retrieved from http://www.nationalautismcenter.org/affiliates/reports.php

National Center for Education Statistics. (2011). *Fast facts.* Retrieved from http://nces.ed.gov/fastfacts/display.asp?id=59.

National Institute of Mental Health. (n.d.) *A parent's guide to autism spectrum disorder.* Retrieved from http://www.nimh.nih.gov/health/publications/a-parents-guide-to-autism-spectrum-disorder/parent-guide-to-autism.pdf

National Institute of Mental Health. (2012). *Autism spectrum disorders, Pervasive developmental disorders.* Retrieved from http://www.nimh.nih.gov/health/publications/autism/nimhautismspectrum.pdf

Notbohm, E. (2004). *Ten Things Your Student with Autism Wishes You Knew.* Arlington, Texas: Future Horizons.

Oliver, C., & Richards, C. (2010). Self-injurious behavior in people with intellectual disability. *Current Opinion in Psychiatry, 23*(5), 412–416.

Orsmond, G. I., & Seltzer, M. M. (2007). Siblings of individuals with autism spectrum disorders across the life course. *Mental Retardation and Developmental Disabilities Research Reviews, 13,* 313–320.

Phetrasuwan, S., & Miles, M. S. (2009). Parenting stress in mothers of children with autism spectrum disorders. *Journal for Specialists in Pediatric Nursing, 14*(3), 157–165.

Rezaei, V., Mohammadi, M., Ghanizadeh, A., Sahraian, A., Tabrizi, M., Rezazadeh, S., & Akhondzadeh, S. (2010). Double-blind, placebo-controlled trial of risperidone plus topiramate in children with autistic disorder. *Progress in Neuro-Psychopharmacology and Biological Psychiatry, 34*(7), 1269–1272.

Seigel, B., Ihle, E., Marco, E., & Hendren, R. (2010). Update on autism—Issues in treatment and comorbidity. *Psychiatric Times, 27*(10). Retrieved from http://www.psychiatrictimes.com/child-adolescent-psych/content/article/10168/1694995

Seltzer, M. M., Greenberg, J. S., Hong, J., Smith, L. E., Almeida, D. M., Coe, C., & Stawski, R. S. (2009). Maternal cortisol levels and behavior problems in adolescents and adults with ASD. *Journal of Developmental Disorders, 40*(4), 457–459.

Seltzer, M. M., Krauss, M. W., Orsmond, G. I., & Vestal, C. (2001). Families of adolescents and adults with autism: Uncharted territory. *International Review of Research on Mental Retardation, 23,* 267–294.

Senel, G. (2010). Parents views and experiences about complementary and alternative medicine treatments for their children with autistic spectrum disorder. *Journal of Autism and Developmental Disorders, 40*(4), 494–503.

Shane, H. C., & Albert, P. D. (2008). Electronic screen media for persons with autism spectrum disorders: Results of a survey. *Journal of Autism and Developmental Disorders, 38*(8), 1499–1508.

Shattuck, P., Wagner, M., Narendorf, S., Sterlzing, P., & Hensley, M. (2011). Post-high school service use among young adults with an autism spectrum disorder. *Archives of Pediatric and Adolescent Medicine, 165*(2), 141–146.

Shore, S., & Rastelli, L. G. (2006). *Understanding autism for dummies.* Hoboken, NJ: Wiley.

Shute, N. (2010). Desperate for an autism cure. *Scientific American, 303*(4), 80–85.

Skinner, B. F., & Rogers, C. R. (1965). Some issues concerning the control of human behavior: A symposium. *Science, 124,* 1057–1066.

Souders, S. C., DePaul, D., Freeman, K. G., & Levy, S. E. (2002). Caring for children and adolescents with autism who require challenging procedures. *Pediatric Nursing, 28*(6), 555–562.

Stahmer, A. C., Collings, N. M., & Palinkas, L. A. (2005). Early intervention practices for children with autism: Descriptions from community providers. *Focus on Autism and Other Developmental Disabilities*, *20*(2), 66–79.

Stoner, J. B., Angell, M. E., House, J. J., & Bock, S. J. (2007). Transitions: Perspectives from parents of young children with autism spectrum disorder. *Journal of Developmental and Physical Disability*, *19*(1), 23–39.

Taylor, J., & Seltzer, M. (2011). Employment and post-secondary educational activities for young adults with autism spectrum disorders during the transition to adulthood. *Journal of Autism and Developmental Disorders*, *41*(5), 566–574.

Trillingsgaard, A., Sorensen, E. U., Nemec, G., & Jorgensen, M. (2005). What distinguishes autism spectrum disorders from other developmental disabilities before the age of four years? *European Child and Adolescent Psychiatry*, *14*(2), 65–72.

Twoy, R., Connolly, P. M., & Novak, J. (2007). Coping strategies used by parents of children with autism. *Journal of the American Academy of Nurse Practitioners*, *19*, 251–260.

U.S. Department of Education. (n.d.). *Building the legacy: The Individuals with Disabilities Act 2004*. Retrieved from http://idea.ed.gov/explore/home

U.S. Department of Education, Office of Special Education Programs. (n.d.). *History: Twenty-five years of progress in educating children with disabilities through IDEA*. Retrieved from http://www2.ed.gov/policy/speced/leg/idea/history.html

West, L., Brunssen, S. H., & Waldrop, J. (2009). Review of the evidence for treatment of children with autism with selective serotonin reuptake inhibitors. *Journal for Specialists in Pediatric Nursing*, *14*(3), 183–191.

Wong, V. C. (2009). Use of complementary and alternative medicine (CAM) in autism spectrum disorder (ASD): Comparison of Chinese and western culture (Part A). *Journal of Autism and Developmental Disorders*, *39*(3), 454–463.

Woodbury-Smith, M. R., & Volkmar, F. R. (2009). Asperger syndrome. *European Child & Adolescent Psychiatry*, *18*(1), 2–11.

Adolescent Health and Development: The Unique Experience of the Adolescent With Asperger's Syndrome

9

Nina Scarpinato

COMPLEXITY OF PHYSICAL AND PSYCHOSOCIAL PROBLEMS

Adolescence is a difficult time of life. It can also be exciting and filled with new opportunities and experiences. Adolescence is a time of rapid physical development, specifically pubertal changes and emotional development, with heavy emphasis on peer relationships and intimacy. The approach to assessment of any adolescent must integrate the dynamic physical changes they are experiencing with the influence of academic challenges, peer relationships, sexuality, and mental health.

The following scenario provides a brief insight into a number of clinical issues relevant to the complex physical and psychosocial development of the adolescent male.

CASE

You are the nurse practitioner on an inpatient adolescent medical unit. You are conducting the initial assessment of a 14-year-old male, named Robert, who is sent to the hospital by his primary-care physician with bradycardia and dehydration. His heart rate is in the 40s while awake and drops to 28 while asleep. His mucous membranes are dry, his blood urea nitrogen and creatinine are elevated, and you notice the presence of lanugo on his skin. According to his mother, he has lost 20 lbs in the last 2 months. He reports a general sense of fatigue, lightheadedness, and nausea that has worsened in the last few weeks. His parents report the patient seems more depressed, is less interested in engaging in activities, and is having difficulty sleeping through the night. The patient is considered an "elite" track runner and he has restricted his diet to mostly fruits and vegetables and no more than 800 calories per day. His parents are also athletic and encouraged him to try out for the track team, as he has always had difficulty making friends, and they hoped his participation in sports would help improve his social skills. His school psychologist recently suggested to the family that the patient meets criteria for Asperger's syndrome (AS).

Planning Care

When prioritizing care, the first goal is medical stabilization and a diagnostic workup to rule out an organic cause for the weight loss and the reported change in sleep and activity level. Some of the more common medical comorbidities associated with autistic spectrum disorders (ASD) reported by clinicians are seizures, sleep disturbances, gastrointestinal (GI) disorders, and psychiatric disorders (Bellando & Lopez 2009; Leyfer et al., 2006; Manning-Courtney et al., 2003; Myers, Johnson, & the Council on Children with Disabilities, 2007). This chapter, first addresses evaluation of the patient's weight loss given the severity of his malnutrition and then discusses some of the unique challenges faced by the adolescent with an ASD. A nurse may use a screening tool such as the high-functioning Autism Spectrum Screening Questionnaire to quickly assess the types of behavioral issues faced by a person with AS.

The diagnostic workup begins with ordering a series of laboratory tests, including:

- Complete blood count
- Comprehensive metabolic panel
- Phosphorous
- Magnesium
- Albumin and pre-albumin
- Alkaline phosphatase
- Estimated sedimentation rate
- Thyroid panel
- Urinalysis

Additional laboratory tests may be considered by the nurse, based on laboratory results or findings on physical assessment. Other important tests include an electrocardiogram, potential imaging studies, such as an MRI, and consulting GI specialists to consider scopes or specialty laboratory tests. Along with the GI specialist, other specialists to consult include nutrition, cardiology, and psychiatry to obtain their evaluations of potential causes of weight loss and consequences of malnutrition. Given the severity of this adolescent's nighttime heart rate, telemetry is warranted. Interventions include stabilization with IV fluids, depending on the severity of his laboratory results and his ability or willingness to take fluids by mouth, and the development of a slow and careful nutrition plan.

GI DISORDERS WITH ASD

The phenomenon of GI disturbances is of particular interest regarding the ASD population. Gastrointestinal complaints are common among the general pediatric population, with constipation, for example, occurring at a rate of 0.7% to 29.6% (van den Berg, Benninga, & Di Lorenzo, 2006). Patients with an ASD may be more at risk for GI and eating-related issues, due to the intensity of their focus on selected items of interest (food being a potential source) and their insistence on sameness of routine and sensory issues (Ibrahim, Voigt, Katusic, Weaver, & Barbaresi, 2009). For example, a person with ASD may restrict his or her diet to include only soft textured foods and may avoid any foods that are found to provide an unpleasant taste or sensation. Other food-related behaviors associated with ASDs include overeating, rumination, food refusal, or pica. These restricted or altered diets may produce nutritional deficits, causing GI symptoms such as diarrhea or constipation. Results of studies looking at association between organic GI disorders and food sensitivities or allergies (e.g., celiac disease) in the ASD population have been mixed in their final conclusions (Horvath et al., 1999; Jyonouchi, Sun, & Itokazu, 2002; Pavone, Fiumara, Bottaro, Mazzone, & Coleman, 1997).

There are even fewer studies in which investigators looked at the diagnosis of anorexia and ASD. "Some have postulated that autism and anorexia nervosa form part of a spectrum of severe developmental disorders of empathy which also include obsessive-compulsive and personality disorders and Tourette's syndrome" (Gravestock, 2003, p. 75). Diagnosis and classification of eating disorder behaviors require careful assessment of the patient's physiological state and thought processes regarding food, eating practices, and body image. The *Diagnostic and Statistical Manual of Mental Disorders, Fourth Edition, Text Revision* (*DSM-IV-TR*; American Psychological Association [APA], 2000) criteria for diagnosis of anorexia nervosa (AN) include:

- Refusal to maintain body weight at or above normal parameters for height/weight
- Intense fear of gaining weight or becoming fat
- Disturbance in body image
- Amenorrhea for at least three consecutive cycles

These criteria set forth some important assessment points when attempting to distinguish between differential diagnoses for weight loss or altered food intake. First, is the patient's refusal to gain or maintain a healthy weight, as opposed to inability or lack of interest? Second, is the patient's intense fear of gaining weight or distorted perception of "becoming fat"? Again, this is not a fear of feeling sick or avoidance of taste or texture.

Coombs and colleagues (2011) published a report of the relationship between eating disorders and autistic symptomatology. There is a positive correlation. Selective eating patterns of behavior are quite common among children and adolescents with AS and can be conceptualized as part of the ritualism of the disorder. Problems with food and mealtime behaviors in individuals with ASD have a multifactorial etiology. Clinicians should not overlook the diagnosis of AN in an adolescent male who is underweight and has abnormal eating patterns. The presence of altered eating practices must be carefully evaluated in patients with AS. Do they stem from a primary diagnosis of anorexia, whereby the motivation behind restrictive eating is to lose weight and avoid "getting fat"? Or is the patient's restrictive eating pattern an accommodation to their desire to avoid certain tastes, texture, and/or smells that they find displeasing?

While AN and AS are two separate clinical disorders, they do share a few cognitive and behavioral traits. Personality traits, such as obsessive–compulsiveness, perfectionism, an insistence on sameness, and social impairment can be seen in patients with both diagnoses (Coombs et al., 2011; Zucker et al., 2007). A number of studies have also found that diagnosis with AS or high-functioning autism (HFA) has been made at later ages, even into adolescence, in contrast with diagnoses of more globally impacting symptoms of autism (Howlin & Asgharian, 1999; Wing, 1997). This is similar to the pattern of diagnosis of AN, which is often diagnosed in adolescence, although symptoms of anxiety or depression may be present in childhood. Table 9.1 lists some of the shared or similar characteristics of ASD and AN. This table provides some of the more common or generalizable traits of each condition, but by no means captures the spectrum of illness experienced by each individual.

TABLE 9.1 ■ Similar Characteristics of Autism Spectrum Disorder (ASD) and Anorexia Nervosa (AN)

	AS	AN
Character traits	Insistence on sameness Strive for order and routine Obsessive–compulsive thinking	Cognitive rigidity Perfectionism Obsessive focus on food, weight, calories
Behavioral traits	Repetition Fixation on items of particular interest	Strict adherence to routine and behaviors surrounding food, weight, calories, and exercise Potential for ritualized behaviors present during meals (e.g., cutting food into small pieces, moving food systematically around plate)
Social traits	Avoidance of social interaction or lack of desire to participate in social interactions or odd, socially awkward interaction Social anxiety	Social withdrawal Social anxiety

CASE–CONTINUED

Robert reports that he began restricting his diet because his peers on the track team were also "cutting out fats and meats." His peers would comment on how lean he looked and that "they really liked my abs." He reports that talking about food and calories enabled him to join in conversations with his peers, something he is not often able to do, as he usually does not know what to say. He states that school often makes him feel stressed and that running gives him the opportunity to "be part of a team, but still be by myself." He earns straight As in school and describes himself as a "perfectionist." He worries that gaining weight will result in a loss of his competitive edge and that his peers will no longer see him as athletic.

DEVELOPMENTAL TASKS OF ADOLESCENCE

Without question, adolescence is a time of intense social and emotional development. It is the developmental task of the adolescent to learn and develop new relationships with peers, including romantic relationships, to begin to achieve emotional independence from his or her parents, and to develop a healthy sense of self and identity within his or her social and familial environment. These tasks, along with the physical changes of puberty, are challenging enough for adolescents without ASD, let alone those adolescents who struggle to understand the nuances of social experience. What makes the adolescent with AS or HFA more vulnerable to social isolation than perhaps their more affected peers on the spectrum is that adolescents with AS or HFA are aware of their social deficits and actually *desire* social interaction (Bauminger & Kasari, 2000; Myles & Simpson, 2002). What they often lack, however, is the skill to interact effectively. Myles and Simpson's (2002) article on the characteristics of AS notes that "Children and youth with AS do not acquire greater social awareness and skill merely as a function of age. Rather, individuals diagnosed with AS may find themselves more and more in conflict with prevailing social norms as they move through adolescence and young adulthood when social growth is the norm" (Myles & Simpson, 2002, p. 133).

Adolescents with AS may be perceived by their peers as cognitively inflexible, rigid, lacking emotional connection or self-centered, possessing poor physical boundaries, and only capable of rudimentary methods of interaction (Myles & Simpson, 2002). They might use odd words or blurt out responses that seem out of context. Adolescents with AS have to work at interpreting the subtle meanings of communication among peer groups, including interpreting verbal and nonverbal cues, and understanding facial expression of emotion. Koning and Magill (2001) pointed out that individuals with AS might be able to recognize and understand facial expressions of their peers when interacting individually, but struggle to translate that meaning to a larger group setting and context. The restricted range of interests, often seen in adolescents with AS, also limits their ability to find a group of peers with whom they can share a particular interest or activity. For the young man described in this case, track became a shared interest with his peers and one for which he has received positive attention and praise. That kind of reinforcement is essential to his sense of self-worth and confidence in his ability to socialize; however, the extremes to which he had gone to excel and feel included have now had serious repercussions on his health.

A theory frequently cited by investigators, which seeks to explain the root of the social deficits that young people with AS experience, is called the Theory of Mind (Solomon, Goodlin-Jones, & Anders, 2004; Cashin, Sci & Barker 2009; Stichter et al., 2010). In the Theory of Mind, the originators hypothesized that an effective social interaction requires that an individual be able to identify a peer's thoughts and beliefs as different from their own and then make inferences about what that peer is thinking or feeling and decide on an appropriate social behavior or action in response (Frith & Frith, 2003; Hill & Frith, 2003; Stichter et al., 2010). For the child or adolescent with AS, this can be a daunting task. They must incorporate facial expression recognition with understanding of context and meaning and then provide a socially appropriate response. Many treatment approaches use this theory to help develop targeted interventions to improve the social skills of children and adolescents with AS. A combination of cognitive-behavioral approaches, social skills training, and facial recognition have been shown to be effective in improving the social skills of young people with AS (Solomon, Goodlin-Jones, & Anders, 2004; Stichter et al., 2010).

While there is much that is different about children and adolescents with AS when compared with their typically developing peers, there is also much that is the same. A study by Bauminger, Solomon, and Rogers (2010) examined friendship quality in a sample of 164 children from the United States and Israel. Forty-four children with HFA and 38 age-matched typically developing children and 82 friends (as identified by the children enrolled in the study) were administered a series of scales measuring attachment and mother–child relationships, friendship quality, and one measurement on theory of mind skill. The researchers hypothesized that for both typically developing children and those with HFA, security of attachment to caregivers and theory of mind skills would contribute to friendship quality. The investigators found similar friendship predictors and developmental patterns in both the typically developing and HFA group as well as the security of attachment to their caregivers. For children in the ASD group, the quality of friendships were positively affected, by higher verbal skills, and the ability to develop intimacy in friendships was correlated highly to a child's security of attachment to his or her caregiver; even more so than among the typically developing children. The researchers pointed out that children with ASD, like their typically developing peers, generalize their models of attachment in friendship after their relationships with caregivers. Again, this highlights the importance of a close, supportive family system in helping children with ASD develop healthy social relationships with peers.

In thinking about the case, track or running is an activity that has allowed Robert to connect with his parents and transfer that skill to his peers. It has set the stage for him to have a sense of belonging in his family and among his age group. This fact cannot be underappreciated, as the need for him to stop participating until he is healthy enough to rejoin means he is losing a sense of connection on the most important levels of his life.

With all of the social challenges faced by children and adolescents with ASD, one might wonder if they are more likely to experience loneliness than their typically developing peers. Several researchers have looked at the experience of loneliness among children and adolescents with HFA or a diagnosed ASD. Many found that children and adolescents with HFA or an ASD reported a sense of loneliness more often than their typically developing peers (Bauminger & Kasari, 2000; Bauminger, Shulman, & Agam, 2003; Lasgaard, Nielsen, Eriksen, & Goosens, 2010). Bauminger and Kasari (2000) found in their sample of 22 high-functioning children and 19 typically developing peers, that children with HFA reported feeling lonelier more often than their typically developing peers and rated the quality of their friendships as poorer (quality was defined as companionship, security, and help). More recently, Lasgaard and colleagues (2010) found in a sample of 39 adolescent boys with ASD that 21% reported feeling lonely often or always. Protective factors against feelings of loneliness were: perceived support by parents, caregivers, and a close friend. Looking more closely at the results of this study, the authors pointed out that more than one-half of the adolescent boys with ASD reported having difficulty making friends, but not everyone reported feeling lonely, reinforcing that adolescents with ASD can and do make friendships that are satisfactory to them.

Aggression and Bullying

Experiencing bullying can have serious physical and emotional consequences for children and adolescents. Current prevalence rates estimate that the experience of having bullied others or having been bullied at school at least once in the last 2 months were 20.8% physically, 53.6% verbally, 51.4% socially, and 13.6% electronically. These statistics were reported by Wang and colleagues on a representative sample of children in grades 6 to 10 ($N = 7182$; Wang, Iannotti, & Nansel, 2009). Multiple studies have data to show that children with special needs, physical deformities, psychiatric conditions, and even obesity are at higher risk of being victims of bullying (Twyman et al., 2010). Among children with ASD or AS, the risk of being the victim of bullying is high. Children or adolescents with social/communicative disorders are at increased risk, because of their difficulties with making friendships or understanding social cues or their engaging in odd, stereotyped behaviors that might make them a vulnerable target of peers (Bauminger & Kasari, 2000; Hill & Frith, 2003; van Roekel, Scholte, & Didden, 2010). Recently, researchers explored whether adolescents with AS could accurately perceive bullying behaviors by peers and found that adolescents with AS had accurate perceptions of bullying behaviors; however, the more often they were bullied or engaged in bullying, the more likely they were to misperceive bullying (van Roekel et al., 2010).

Wang and colleagues (2009) studied the prevalence of adolescent bullying. They reported that adolescents with more friends were more likely to be bullies. Apparently, having more friends reduces the likelihood of becoming the victim of physical, verbal, or relational bullying. This puts adolescents with ASD or AS at an additional disadvantage, given that they are less likely to have a large network of friends to protect them from bullying behaviors. In 2000, a study by Little surveyed the mothers of 411 children with AS (ages 4 through 17) via a questionnaire on their perception of the frequency of their children experiencing peer victimization or shunning (Little, 2002). Little reported that 94% of the mothers responding felt their child had been victimized by peers in the last year. Additionally, 33% of the sample respondents reported that their child had not been invited to a friends' birthday party in the last year, 31% were almost always picked last for teams, and 11% of the children sat alone at lunchtime every day (Little, 2002). She also found that the risk of becoming a victim of shunning or bullying increased in junior high and high school, ostensibly when social skills are becoming more complex (Little, 2002). Other authors have found the rates of bullying among adolescents with ASD to be lower than those found in Little's study and also note that the level of victimization was lower among adolescents with AS in special education schools than in general education settings (van Roekel et al., 2010).

While children and adolescents with an ASD or AS are at risk of being the victims of bullying, they are also at risk of being the perpetrators. There are a number of elements that may be factored into an explanation for bullying behaviors. Children and adolescents who have been the victims of bullying are more likely themselves to engage in bullying. Additionally, there is a higher prevalence of diagnosis of ASD or AS in boys than in girls, and boys are more likely to bully than girls (Montes & Halterman, 2006, 2007; Twyman, Saylor, Taylor & Comeaux, 2010).

Those most at risk of bullying others seem to be children or adolescents diagnosed with comorbid attention deficit hyperactivity disorder (ADHD) or aggressive behaviors. Utilizing data from the National Survey of Children's Health, Montes and Halterman (2007) found that among their sample of 322 children with autism, roughly one-half had a comorbid diagnosis of ADHD; of those children with ADHD and autism, 71% had or have behavior or conduct problems and 60.3% had anxiety or depressive problems. Children with autism and comorbid ADHD were four times more likely to bully than their peers in the general population (Montes & Halterman, 2007). Given that children with autism but no ADHD were not at greater risk of engaging in bullying than the general population, the moderating factor appears to be the impulsive and hyperactive behaviors of ADHD.

Intimacy

Among the greater challenges for adolescents, both typically developing and on spectrum, is learning the nuances of romantic relationships and sexuality. Adolescents with ASD again have some unique challenges to conquer as they try to understand the physical changes in their bodies and conceptualize intimacy and a relationship with another. These individuals are generally concrete thinkers who struggle to grasp subtleties in their and others feelings, words, and actions. Many parents of children with ASD rank explaining sexual feelings and practices and protecting their child/adolescent from harm or exploitation among the biggest of their concerns. Just like their typically developing peers, children and adolescents with ASD must be taught about privacy, sexual feelings, when masturbation is appropriate versus inappropriate, safe sex practices, and so on. These are all complex and critically important concepts that must be explained to a young person who is already struggling to understand social rules and relationships.

In a 2010 intervention study, Nichols and Blakely-Smith reported that in their sample of 21 parents of children with ASD, all of the parents expressed concern that their children would be bullied, teased, or possibly sexually exploited (Nichols & Blakely-Smith, 2010). They also worried that their children, without intending harm and understanding the meaning of their actions, might touch another person inappropriately. As the authors pointed out, touching of oneself in public or inappropriate exposure of private parts is often understood in younger children as part of social learning and development. In an older child or adolescent, these behaviors take on a deviant or offensive context that can have legal consequences (Nichols & Blakely-Smith, 2010). Sex education is critical to preventing these kinds of behaviors. Some authors have proposed the use of social stories to help teach about issues related to sexuality and/or providing sex education utilizing a training method that is visual, concrete, and repetitive, such as anatomically correct dolls or body charts (Sperry & Mesibov, 2005; Tissot, 2009; Tarnai & Wolfe, 2008). Important content related to sexual health behaviors starts with personal hygiene practices, identifying private and public parts of the body, rules for sexual touching, and identifying abusive behaviors.

It is vital to teach concepts of sexuality, and that sexuality is not to be used as a means to compensate for social skills deficits (Tissot, 2009, p. 32). Other important questions to assist the adolescent to answer are: What does it mean to feel attracted to a peer? What do I do with these feelings? What is a date and how do I act on it? How do I handle rejection by a peer or love interest?

Although sparse, data in the literature on sexuality and children/adolescents with ASD show young people with ASD as having sexual feelings and desiring intimate relationships. They possess less knowledge than their typically developing peers on how to successfully and safely accomplish this important developmental goal. Stokes and Kaur (2010) conducted a comparison study of sexuality and sexual behaviors in typically developing children and children diagnosed with AS or HFA, ranging in age from 10 to 15 year of age. In their study, they reported that at 15 years of age, adolescents with HFA displayed sexualized behavior similar to that of a 10-year-old, typically developing child. Overall, the authors found that adolescents with HFA displayed poorer and more inappropriate sexual behaviors, as well as less privacy awareness, and possessed less sexual education (Stokes & Kaur, 2010).

While the young man in the case did not present with issues or concerns related to sexuality, his admission still presented an opportunity to explore or identify any sexual health concerns he may have had but felt unable to ask. Given the above information that adolescents with HFA possess less sexual health education than their peers, nursing professionals need to ask pointed and specific questions about what the adolescent with ASD understands about his/her body, its functioning, and safe sexual health practices. In this population, it is particularly ill-advised to assume that the adolescent has "gotten the education" in school or from parents. Information might have been given, but how it was interpreted or understood might be vastly different than intended. By confidently and calmly inquiring about adolescents' thoughts on sexuality and their bodies, the nurse normalizes the experience for a patient and helps send a message of acceptance.

MANAGEMENT OF AS CHARACTERISTICS IN THE CLINICAL SETTING

CASE–CONTINUED

The nursing staff who care for Robert notice that at mealtimes the patient insists on a certain number of salt and pepper packets and will request separate plates on which to place his food. He insists on eating his favorite "fat-free chocolate pudding" at every meal and will become tearful if none is available. He times his meals on his cell phone and text messages his parents constantly to "make sure they're okay." He successfully completes his meals but

(*Continued*)

CASE–CONTINUED (Continued)

will ruminate on the "loss of my abs." Nursing staff defers on commenting on his physical appearance in order to not reinforce his perseveration and gently remind him that his body is healing and that healing is taking place throughout his body.

Most clinicians reading the above scenario would suspect this adolescent is suffering from obsessive–compulsive disorder (OCD) and/or another anxiety disorder or eating disorder. However, when diagnosing a child/adolescent with an ASD with a comorbid psychiatric disorder, clinicians must be careful to identify symptoms that are not better attributed to the ASD itself. For example, is this patient's insistence on sameness with the salt and pepper packets a long-standing preoccupation or does it meet criteria for true obsessive ideation? Assessment questions might include:

- When did you first notice that the patient began to focus on salt and pepper packets?
- What happens if the "right" number of salt and pepper packets are not available?
- Are there any other fixations on numbers of items pertaining to food or otherwise?
- Was there any history of similar focus?

For children and adolescents with ASD, symptoms of psychiatric disturbances include depressive and anxiety symptoms, and these must be carefully evaluated via a thorough history to understand whether a given symptom is long-standing or is it changing over time in intensity, frequency, or duration? In evaluating for depression, for example, a flattening of affect or social isolation may be a standing aspect of that child's experience of ASD and not classically anhedonic as a symptom of depression. Anhedonia is a psychological condition characterized by inability to experience pleasure in acts that normally produce such joy. Because of the considerable overlap of symptoms in ASD and other psychiatric disorders, the evaluation of comorbid psychiatric illness in a child with ASD is a complex process that involves careful assessment, history gathering, and treatment planning. As one author clearly explains, "The symptom must also be part of the cluster of mental state phenomena that define the comorbid disorder syndrome and the syndrome must be significantly impairing. An isolated symptom is not considered a disorder (Leyfer et al., 2006, p. 858).

There is an increasing body of evidence to support the proposition that psychiatric comorbidities in children and adolescents with ASD are the norm, not the exception. Prevalence rates range from 40% to 74% in clinically referred samples (Ghaziuddin, 2002; Hess, Matson, & Dixon, 2010; Leyfer et al., 2006, Mattila et al., 2010). Many of these investigators also point out that compared with their typically developing peers, children with ASD endorse a higher number of psychiatric symptoms and meet criteria for more than one comorbid psychiatric disorder (Hess et al., 2010; Leyfer et al., 2006). Commonly co-occurring disorders include mood disorders (e.g., depression), ADHD, and anxiety disorders (social phobia and OCD). Given the complexities of the case described, a consultation with psychiatry is warranted to help tease out the differential diagnoses.

Depression and Mood Disorders

Among individuals with AS, prevalence rates of depression have been as high as 41% (Toth & King, 2008). Some have theorized that because children and adolescents with AS or HFA have a better degree of insight into their social impairments, they may be more at risk of developing a co-occurring depression; however, researchers point out that there is no simple, direct relationship between awareness of disability and the development of emotional symptoms (Green, Gilchrist, Burton, & Cox, 2000). Other investigators have found a lower prevalence of depression in their study sample of children and adolescents with AS/HFA, but a higher degree of impairment (Mattila et al., 2010). Complicating the assessment of depression in individuals with ASD is the core feature of the disorder itself: expression and understanding of emotion. These children and adolescents are less likely to verbally report changes in mood. Clinicians and caregivers must closely monitor the patient for signs of depressed or changing mood, such as changes in sleep, appetite, or deterioration in personal hygiene. The patient in the case shows signs of depression. His sleep suffered and his interest in activities diminished. His parents' assessment of his overall mood provided objective data to consider a comorbid depression.

As with typically developing peers, the expression of depression in children and adolescents with an ASD may not always be one of "classic" report of sad mood and tearfulness. In fact, new onset or worsening of aggressive or self-injurious behavior was frequently seen in children and adolescents with an ASD (Stewart, Barnard, Pearson, Hasan, & O'Brien, 2006).

The presence of aggressive behavior is a symptom and one that can be associated with several psychiatric disorders. In 2008, Ming and colleagues found in their study of 160 children with a diagnosis of an ASD (ages 2 through 18) that 26% (42) had symptoms of a mood disorder and 32% (51) displayed self-injurious/aggressive behavior (Ming, Brimacombe, Chaaban, Zimmerman-Bier, & Wagner, 2008). Interestingly, this team also pointed out differences between subjects diagnosed with autism, pervasive developmental disorder – not otherwise specified (PDD-NOS), and AS. They found that children with a diagnosis of PDD-NOS or autism were more likely to have a comorbid medical disorder, whereas subjects with AS were more likely to have a psychiatric comorbidity (Ming et al., 2008).

As mentioned above, prevalence rates for comorbid ADHD in children and adolescents with ASD can range from 38% to 52% (Leyfer et al., 2006, Mattila et al., 2010; Montes & Halterman, 2007). The symptoms of hyperactivity and impulsivity are common among individuals with AS and HFA and present a diagnostic quandary for many clinicians, as the *DSM-IV-TR* states that ADHD cannot be diagnosed during the course of a pervasive developmental disorder (APA, 2000). However, many clinicians feel that the degree of impairment presented by the hyperactive, impulsive, and inattentive symptoms warrants the diagnosis and appropriate treatment (Ghaziuddin, 2002). Mattila and colleagues (2010) studied a community- and clinic-based sample of 67 children and adolescents with AS or HFA (ages 9 through 16). The most common psychiatric comorbidities were behavioral disorders, including ADHD and oppositional defiant disorder, anxiety disorders, and tic disorders (Mattila et al., 2010).

Obsessions and Compulsions

While the core symptoms of ASD can complicate an already complex diagnostic scenario, perhaps no traditional psychiatric disorder is as closely related to the core symptoms of ASD as OCD. The *DSM-IV-TR* includes a core feature of ASD to be: "an encompassing preoccupation with one or more stereotyped and restricted patterns of interest that is abnormal either in intensity or focus" (APA, 2000, p. 75). A core feature of OCD is "recurrent and persistent thoughts, impulses or images that are experienced . . . as intrusive and inappropriate and that cause marked anxiety or distress" (APA, 2000, p. 462). Two very distinct descriptions on paper can be more difficult to distinguish in the clinical setting. A few elements of assessment are important to consider when working with a child or adolescent with an ASD and OCD or OCD-like symptoms. Does the obsession or fixation cause distress? Children or adolescents with an ASD often enjoy talking about or engaging in their topic of interest, whereas someone suffering with OCD is distressed by the recurrent thought and wishes to extinguish its presence (Ghaziuddin, 2002). Are compulsions present and are they used to alleviate anxiety or are they simply repetitive in nature? Some questions that might help investigate this behavior include: What happens if the child/adolescent is unable to perform his/her ritual? Does he/she become tearful and distressed or can he/she be redirected? How often is the child seen engaging in the repetitive behavior? Does the child verbalize how engaging in this compulsion makes him/her feel? Better? Worse? Is there a certain number of times in which the behavior must be engaged?

One study of 109 children with autism (ages 5 through 17 years) contained data that 37% of their sample met *DSM-IV-TR* criteria for OCD and that nearly 50% of them had compulsions that involved needing others to do things a certain way (Leyfer et al., 2006). An example was requiring the parent to perform certain daily routines or greeting and separating rituals and having to ask parents the same question repeatedly (Leyfer et al., 2006). Leyfer and colleagues (2006) found specific phobias to be the most common *DSM-IV-TR* lifetime diagnosis in their sample, with 32% reporting fear of needles or crowds. Ten percent of the children had a fear of loud noises, a phobia not often seen in typically developing children, and the more common childhood phobias of flying, standing in lines, or bridges were seen less often in the children with autism (Leyfer et al., 2006).

A number of investigators have reported that children with AS or HFA are at higher risk for anxiety disorders than their typically developing peers (Kuusikko et al., 2008; Mattila et al., 2010). Interestingly, the nature of their anxieties and fears appears to be specific and focused on one area versus a generalized sense of anxiety or even a separation anxiety disorder. Social anxiety disorder is difficult to distinguish in the ASD population. A core feature of ASD includes a desire for social isolation and impaired social skills. One recent study contained a report on whether children and adolescents with AS or HFA experienced symptoms of social anxiety. The authors came to a few notable conclusions. One is that children and adolescents with AS/HFA might experience and report more social anxiety symptoms than their typically developing peers (Kuusiko et al., 2008). Another is that social anxiety *increased* for children and adolescents with AS or HFA as they got older, while it *decreased* for their typically developing peers (Kuusiko et al., 2008).

Self-Destructive Behaviors

Thinking cumulatively about the social and psychological struggles faced by adolescents with AS or HFA, one immediately becomes concerned about an increased risk of suicide. There is little current research available looking specifically at suicide in adolescents with ASD; however, the general literature on adolescent suicide provides clinicians with important risk factors for suicide. Suicide is still the third leading cause of death among youth ages 15 to 24 (American Association of Suicidology, 2010). Risk factors include history of suicide attempts, diagnosis of a mental health disorder, substance abuse, and familial stress. There is a substantial body of literature on peer victimization and suicidality. Investigators generally conclude that victims of bullying by peers display more depressive symptoms and exhibit more suicidal ideation than do nonvictims (Klomek, Marrocco, Kleinman, Schonfeld, & Gould, 2008). The potential combined risk of increased exposure to peer victimization, the impulsivity of ADHD, and the prevalence of mood and anxiety disorders in this population pose substantial concern. A small study conducted in Japan was designed to examine 12 adolescents diagnosed with PDD who were admitted to the hospital after a suicide attempt. The investigators found predisposing factors common to the adolescents who repeated suicide attempts; these factors were failed attempts at developing relationships and feelings of social isolation (Mikami et al., 2009). Speculatively, the concrete thinking and rigidity associated with ASD might also make it more difficult for these adolescents to "bounce back" from failed relationships or find hope that the future will bring positive change. Even without prevalence statistics to support the potential for increased risk for suicide among this population, clinicians and families *must* closely monitor for behaviors or statements that indicate suicidal ideation. Given the significant comorbidities of anxiety, depression, and perceived loss in the case example, it is important to assess Robert's coping abilities and risk of harm to himself as a consequence of being unable to participate in sports. It is also important to have a frank discussion with his family about the risk for suicide and develop a safety plan. Potential questions include:

- [Patient name], I know not being able to participate in track until your body is healthy enough is a very big disappointment for you. How will you cope with those feelings?
- [Patient name], I know this hospitalization and the days leading up to it have been really stressful. Have you found yourself having any thoughts of wanting to hurt yourself or wishing you were dead?"
- [Patient name], I worry about your safety. Are you able to talk with me or with your parents if you have any thoughts of wanting to hurt yourself?

BEST PRACTICES

There is a body of literature on ASD and the social, emotional, and cognitive abilities of these children and adolescents that offers guide to nurses who care for this population. The true expert, and primary source of information on any individual with ASD, is that person and his or her family. Best nursing practice for this patient population begins with a partnership with the patient and the family. Family input is critical. Our responsibility as nursing caregivers is to take the information provided by families, develop individually based treatment plans, and in turn, educate the family on lessons gathered from the evidenced based literature. The nursing process of assessment, diagnosis, treatment planning, implementation, and evaluation continues to provide a framework for us to consider the developmental and mental health needs of the adolescent with AS or HFA. In addition to the expected questions posed during a nursing evaluation, some additional considerations reflective of understanding of ASD are described in Table 9.2.

Consider some of the potential causes for weight loss in this patient. The algorithm in Figure 9.1 can be used by the nurse to identify potential sources of a chief complaint of "weight loss" and its subsequent physiological effects. Weight loss can be due entirely to a physiological condition such as viral illness, the effects of a medication or treatment, or GI/malabsorptive diseases, or it can be the symptom of a psychiatric illness. It can result

TABLE 9.2 ■ Assessment and Treatment Planning Considerations for the Patient with an ASD

Assessment	Diagnosis	Treatment plan
What has the patient's experience with ASD been so far? What realms of the disorder has he/she been most affected by (i.e., more social deficits or communicative deficits, etc.)?	Is the presenting problem reflective of a core symptom of ASD or perhaps a comorbidity, such as OCD or ADHD?	What is the most appropriate treatment intervention for the presenting problem and the patient's developmental/social needs? Modalities such as social skills groups, play or art therapy, or cognitive or behavioral therapy?
Does ASD impact the patient's ability to provide information on his/her health (e.g., expression of pain, alternate forms of communication)?	If a comorbid psychiatric disorder is present, are there any pharmacological interventions warranted for treatment of that psychiatric disorder?	How does this patient best learn new information? Visually? Orally? Role playing?
Are there any immediate safety risks to the patient or others?	Is the patient's current cognitive and developmental function at expected age level or delayed? Advanced?	Develop a safety plan with the patient and family Anticipate and reevaluate for safety concerns

from a combination of both. When evaluating for a psychiatric illness as the source of weight loss, it is critical to understand the patient's thought process.

- Is the patient bothered by his/her weight loss? How does he/she feel about his/her body?
- Did the patient intentionally restrict food or excessively exercise to lose weight (e.g., as in AN)?
- Did the patient "just not feel like eating," "have no energy to eat," or feel "nothing sounds good" (e.g., as in a depressive episode)?
- Is the patient scared to eat, because "I might throw up" or "It hurts"? (e.g., anxiety in a patient recovering from a bad gastritis)
- Is the patient scared to eat, because "Someone's been poisoning my food," "I can only eat foods I've seen prepared, because it might be contaminated" (e.g., a patient with paranoia or severe OCD)?
- Does the patient restrict his/her diet to avoid certain textures, tastes, or smells he/she finds displeasing (as in a patient with an ASD)?

The above questions are part of the assessment process and are not diagnostic of any of the illnesses cited as examples, unless supported by other symptoms or evidence to meet criteria for diagnosis of psychiatric illness. However, effectiveness of a treatment plan depends on the nurse understanding the root of the weight loss and determining what interventions (pharmacological, psychotherapies, medical tests and treatments, and so on) will treat the underlying disease and not just the symptom of "weight loss."

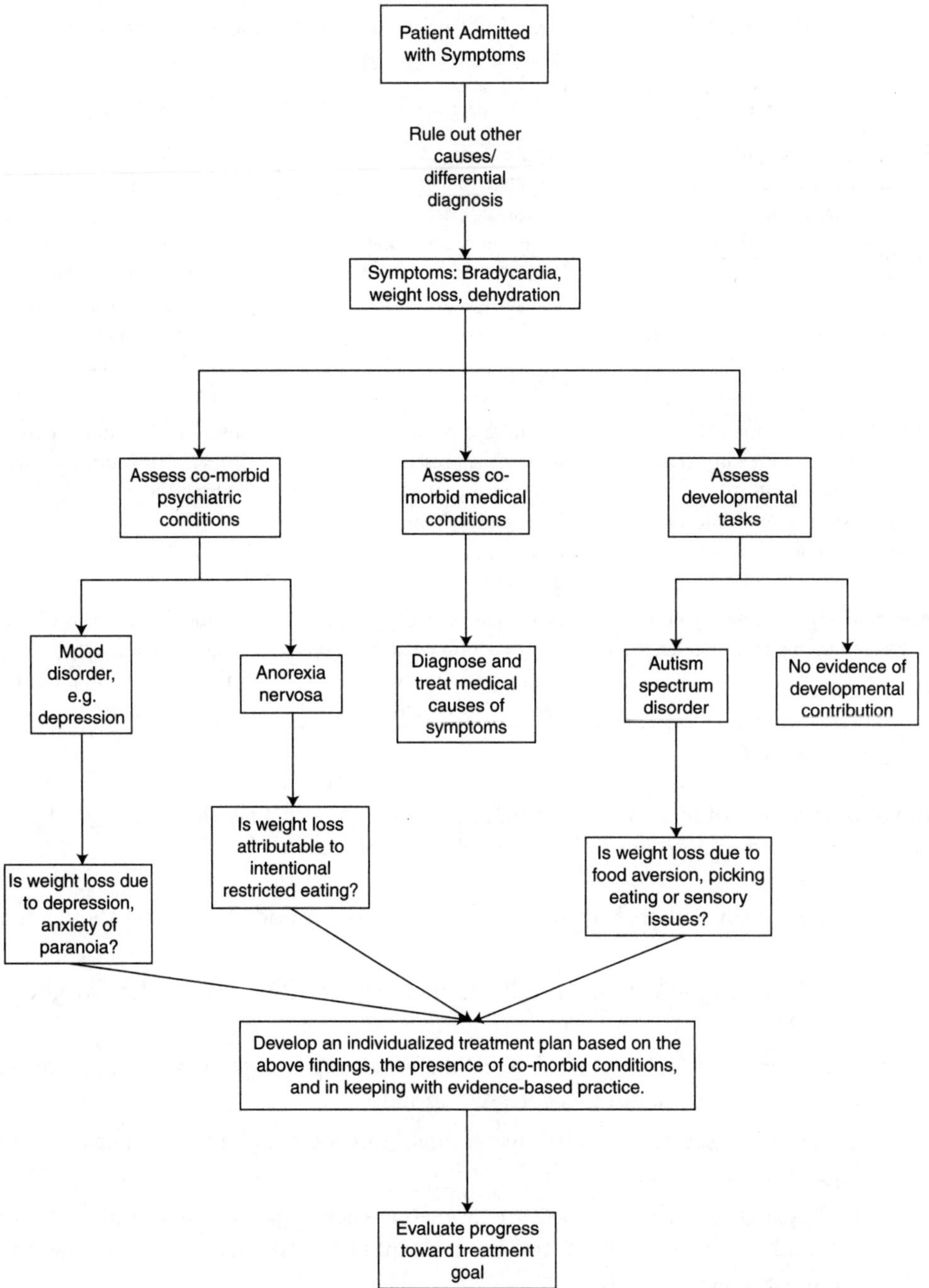

FIGURE 9.1 ■ Algorithm for evaluating symptoms in a patient with ASD.

SUMMARY

Every child, regardless of diagnosis, possesses skills or strengths. Helping that child and family to find and use these strengths is useful in reinforcing a positive self-image and the experience of success in the child, and is fundamental to treatment planning. Nurses have the opportunity to partner with adolescents with ASD and take their unique experience of the world and teach them skills in a way tailored just to them that promotes a course of safe and healthy development and successful transition to adulthood.

REFERENCES

American Association of Suicidology. (2010). *2007 Data rates, numbers, and rankings of each state.* Retrieved from http://www.suicidology.org/web/guest/stats-and-tools/statistics

American Psychiatric Association. (2000). *Diagnostic and statistical manual of mental disorders* (4 ed., text revision). Washington, DC: Author.

Bauminger, N., & Kasari, C. (2000). Loneliness and friendship in high functioning children with autism. *Child Development, 71*(2), 117–156.

Bauminger, N., Shulman, C., & Agan, G. (2003). Peer interaction and loneliness in high-functioning children with autism. *Journal of Autism and Developmental Disabilities, 33*(5), 489–507.

Bauminger, N., Solomon, M., & Rogers, S. (2010). Predicting friendship quality in autism spectrum disorders and typical development. *Journal of Autism and Developmental Disabilities, 40*(6), 751–761.

Bellando, J., & Lopez, M. (2009). The school nurses' role in treatment of the student with autism spectrum disorders. *Journal for Specialists in Pediatric Nursing, 43*(3),173–182.

Cashin, A., Sci, D. A., & Barker, P. (2009). The triad of impairment in autism revisited. *Journal of Child & Adolescent Psychiatric Nursing, 22*(4), 189–193.

Coombs, E., Brosnan, M., Bryant-Waugh, R., & Skevington, S. M. (2011). An investigation into the relationship between eating disorder psychopathology and autistic symptomatology in a non-clinical sample. *British Journal of Clinical Psychology, 50*(3), 326–338.

Frith, U., & Frith, C. (2003). Development and neurophysiology of mentalizing. *Philosophical Transactions of the Royal Society of London, 358*(1431), 459–473.

Ghaziuddin, M. (2002). Asperger syndrome: Associated psychiatric and medical conditions. *Focus on Autism and Other Developmental Disabilities, 17*(3), 138–144.

Gravestock, S. (2003). Diagnosis and classification of eating disorders in adults with intellectual disability: The diagnostic criteria for psychiatric disorders for use with adults with learning disabilities/mental retardation (DC-LD) approach. *Journal of Intellectual Disability Research, 47*(1), 72–83.

Green, J., Gilchrist, A., Burton, D., & Cox, A. (2000). Social and psychiatric functioning in adolescents with Asperger syndrome compared with conduct disorder. *Journal of Autism and Developmental Disorders, 30*(4), 279–293.

Hess, J., Matson, J., & Dixon, D. (2010). Psychiatric symptom endorsement in children and adolescents diagnosed with autism spectrum disorders: A comparison to typically developing children and adolescents. *Journal of Developmental and Physical Disabilities, 22*(5), 485–496.

Hill, E., & Frith, U. (2003). Understanding autism: Insights from the mind and brain. *Philosophical Transactions of the Royal Society of London, 358*, 281–289.

Horvath, K., Papadimitriou, J. C., Rabsztyn, A., Drachenberg, C., & Tildon, J. T. (1999). Gastrointestinal abnormalities in children with autistic disorders. *Journal of Pediatrics, 135*(5), 565–563.

Howlin, P., & Asgharian, A. (1999). The diagnosis of autism and Asperger's syndrome: Findings from a survey of 770 families. *Developmental Medicine and Child Neurology, 41*, 834–839.

Ibrahim, S., Voigt, R., Katusic, S., Weaver, A., & Barbaresi, W. (2009). Incidence of gastrointestinal symptoms in children with autism: A population based study. *Pediatrics, 124*(2), 680–686.

Jyonouchi, H., Sun, S., & Itokazu, N. (2002). Innate immunity associated with inflammatory responses and cytokine production against common dietary proteins in patients with autism spectrum disorder. *Neuropsychobiology, 46*(2), 76–84.

Klomek, A., Marrocco, F., Kleinman, M., Schonfeld, I., & Gould, M. (2008). Peer victimization, depression, and suicidality in adolescents. *Suicide and Life-Threatening Behavior, 38*(2), 166–180.

Koning, C., & Magill-Evans, J. (2001). Social and language skills in adolescent boys with Asperger's syndrome. *Autism, 5*(1), 23–36.

Kuusikko, S., Pollock-Wurman, R., Jussila, K., Carter, A., Mattila, M., Ebeling, H., Pauls, D., & Moilanen, I. (2008). Social anxiety in high-functioning children and adolescents with autism and Asperger's syndrome. *Journal of Autism and Developmental Disabilities, 38*, 1697–1709.

Lasgaard, M., Nielsen, A., Eriksen, M., & Goosens, L. (2010). Loneliness and social support in adolescent boys with autism spectrum disorders. *Journal of Autism and Developmental Disorders, 40*, 218–226.

Leyfer, O., Folstein, S., Bacalman, S., Davis, N., Dinh, E., Morgan, J., Tager-Flusberg, H., & Lainhart, J. (2006). Comorbid psychiatric disorders in children with autism: Interview development and rates of disorders. *Journal of Autism and Developmental Disorders, 36*, 849–861.

Little, L. (2002). Middle-class mothers' perceptions of peer and sibling victimization among children with Asperger's syndrome and nonverbal learning disabilities. *Issues in Comprehensive Pediatric Nursing, 25*(1), 43–57.

Manning-Courtney, P., Brown, J., Molloy, C. A., Reinhold, J., Murray, D., Sorensen-Burnworth,, & ... Kent, B. (2003). Diagnosis and treatment of autism spectrum disorders. *Current Problems in Pediatric Adolescent Health Care, 33*(9), 283–304.

Mattila, M., Hurtig, T., Haapsamo, H., Jussila, K., Kuusikko-Gauffin, S., ... Moilanen, I. (2010). Comorbid psychiatric disorders associated with Asperger syndrome/high functioning autism: A community and clinic based study. *Journal of Autism and Developmental Disabilities, 40*(9), 1080–1093.

Mikami, K., Inomata, S., Hayakawa, N., Ohnishi, Y., Enseki, Y., Ohya, A., ... Matsumoto, H. (2009). Frequency and clinical features of pervasive developmental disorder in adolescent suicide attempts. *General Hospital Psychiatry, 31*(2), 163–166.

Ming, X., Brimacombe, M., Chaaban, J., Zimmerman-Bier, B., & Wagner, G. (2008). Autism spectrum disorders: Concurrent clinical disorders. *Journal of Child Neurology, 23*(1), 6–13.

Montes, G., & Halterman, J. S. (2006). Characteristics of school-age children with autism in the United States. *Dev Behav Pediat, 27*, 379–385.

Montes, G., & Halterman, J. (2007). Bullying among children with autism and the influence of comorbidity with ADHD: A population based study. *Ambulatory Pediatrics, 7*(3), 253–257.

Myers, S. M., Johnson, C. P., the Council on Children with Disabilities. (2007). Management of children with autism spectrum disorders. *Pediatrics, 120*(5), 1162–1192.

Myles, B., & Simpson, R. (2002). Asperger's syndrome. An overview of characteristics. *Focus on Autism and Other Developmental Disabilities, 17*(3), 132–137.

Nichols, S., & Blakeley-Smith, A. (2010). "I'm not sure we're ready for this...": Working with families toward facilitating healthy sexuality for individuals with autism spectrum disorders. *Social Work in Mental Health, 1*, 72–91.

Pavone, L., Fiumara, A., Bottaro, G., Mazzone, D., & Coleman, M. (1997). Autism and celiac disease: Failure to validate the hypothesis that a link might exist. *Biological Psychiatry, 42*(1), 72–75.

Solomon, M., Goodlin-Jones, B., & Anders, T. (2004). A social adjustment enhancement intervention for high functioning autism, Asperger's syndrome, and pervasive developmental disorder NOS. *Journal of Autism & Developmental Disorders, 34*(6), 649–668.

Sperry, L. A., & Mesibov, G. B. (2005). Perceptions of social challenges of adults with autism spectrum disorder. *Autism, 9*(4), 362–376.

Stewart, M., Barnard, L., Pearson, J., Hasan, R., & O'Brien, G. (2006). Presentation of depression in autism and Asperger syndrome. *Autism, 10*(1), 103–116.

Stichter, J., Herzog, M., Visovsky, K., Schmidt, C., Randolph, J., Schultz, T., & Gage, N. (2010). Social competence intervention for youth with Asperger syndrome and high-functioning autism: An initial investigation. *Journal of Autism and Developmental Disabilities, 40*(9), 1067–1079.

Stokes, M., & Kaur, A. (2005). High-functioning autism and sexuality. A parental perspective. *Autism, 9*(3), 266–289.

Tarnai, B., & Wolfe, P. (2008). Social stories for sexuality education for persons with autism/pervasive developmental disorder. *Sexuality & Disability, 26*(1), 29–36.

Tissot, C. (2009). Establishing a sexual identity: Case studies of learners with autism and learning difficulties. *Autism, 13*(6), 551–566.

Toth, K., & King, B. (2008). Asperger's syndrome: Diagnosis and treatment. *American Journal of Psychiatry, 165*(8), 958–963.

Twyman, K., Saylor, C., Saia, D., Macias, M., Taylor, L., & Spratt, E. (2010). Bullying and ostracism experiences in children with special health care needs. *Journal of Developmental and Behavioral Pediatrics, 31*(1), 1–8.

Twyman, K., Saylor, C., Taylor, L. A., & Comeaux, C. (2010). Comparing children and adolescents engaged in cyberbullying to matched peers. *Cyberpsychology, Behavior and Social Networking, 13*(2), 195–199.

van den Berg, M. M., Benninga, M. A., & Di Lorenzo, C. (2006) Epidemiology of childhood constipation: A systematic review. *American Journal of Gastroenterology, 101*, 2401–2409.

van Roekel, E., Scholte, R., & Didden, R. (2010). Bullying among adolescents with autism spectrum disorders: Prevalence and perception. *Journal of Autism and Developmental Disorders, 40*(1), 63–73.

Wang, J., Iannotti, R., & Nansel, T. (2009). School bullying among US adolescents in the United States: Physical, verbal, relational, and cyber. *Journal of Adolescent Health, 45*(4), 368–375.

Wing, L. (1997). The autistic spectrum. *Lancet, 350*, 1761–1767.

Zucker, N. L., Losh, M., Bulik, C., LaBar, K., Piven, J., & Pelphrey, K. (2007). Anorexia nervosa and autism spectrum disorders: Guided investigation of social cognitive endophenotypes. *Psychological Bulletin, 133*(6), 976–1006.

II Discussion Questions

CHAPTER 4

1. What are the barriers to seeking and accessing care in minority ethnic/cultural groups in which there is risk for autism or other developmental disabilities?
2. What can nurses do to encourage utilization of existing resources for families?
3. Considering the case of Ms. Martinez, how should her partner be included in the decision-making process related to prenatal care, genetic testing, and other prenatal and postnatal services?
4. Create a plan to help Ms. Martinez prepare her child for the birth of a new sibling.

CHAPTER 5

1. How does culture influence developmental expectations of parents? What is the influence of culture on screening and early identification of autism spectrum disorder (ASD)? How do "American" cultural expectations influence primary-care practices related to anticipatory guidance, developmental surveillance, and screening for ASD?
2. It can be emotionally difficult for parents to hear that a child of theirs is at risk for, or diagnosed with, an ASD. How should clinicians address positive screening results with parents? How should the diagnosis of an ASD be presented to parents? What strategies should be used to individualize the approach to "giving the news" to parents and other family members?
3. Siblings of children with ASD are at higher risk for an ASD diagnosis themselves. Discuss the surveillance and screening approach to ASD for these siblings.
4. A family includes three children aged 2 months, 3 years, and 6 years. The 3- and 6-year-olds have been diagnosed with autistic disorder already. Develop a family support plan of care for this vulnerable family unit.
5. Many chapters in this text discuss the importance of community services. What services for individuals with ASD, and their families, are available in your own community? What is missing? How would you advocate to eliminate service gaps in your community?
6. What are the major red flags for ASD?
7. Differentiate screening and diagnostic instruments used for identification of children with an ASD.

CHAPTER 6

1. What is the nurse's role in the acute care of the child with complex ASD?
2. What settings support the most effective management of children with complex autism?
3. How can nurses assume leadership roles on a multidisciplinary team to develop and plan the long-term care of a child such as Joey? What are the unique contributions that nurses are able to make on the multidisciplinary team? Which team members are essential?
4. What support do families need to effectively care for children like Joey? What is the evidence for the effectiveness of such support?
5. In light of the evidence about families of children with ASD, and the evidence about disclosure of genetic testing results in general, discuss the impact of genetic findings for Joey's siblings and other relatives.

CHAPTER 7

1. A 7-year-old male is admitted to the neurology unit for a 72-hour video monitoring for seizures. He also has been diagnosed with Asperger's syndrome (AS). The procedure requires taping and securing of several leads and wires to the patient's scalp, and he must remain inside the room. His parents report that he has excellent verbal skills, but has difficulty listening and interpreting other people's conversations. He copes better with short instructions and conversations.
   (a) What information does the admitting nurse need in order to develop a plan of care that insures quality and successful outcomes of care?
   (b) What activities, hospital support staff, and conversation cues could the nurse consider in helping this patient cope with the hospitalization?
2. The nurse is preparing a 17-year-old with ASD for an endoscopy in the gastrointestinal (GI) suite, but has not been able to obtain a history from the parents or a set of vital signs before the procedure. This particular patient has challenging physical behaviors and will hit others at times. The father had to hold the teenager to avoid any escape from the room. The nurse has an incomplete database to send to the GI suite. What actions are indicated? What are liability issues are to be considered? What should the procedures team do to prevent future problems like this one?

CHAPTER 8

1. How should the nurse in the school setting address a family's use of unproven alternative therapies for their preteen with autism? Which alternative therapies have the strongest evidence to support their effectiveness? Should health care professionals recommend complementary and alternative medicine to families with children with autism?

2. Students with AS are at risk for depression and other psychiatric conditions. Describe the evidence-based plan of care to assess for and intervene with an adolescent with AS, as related to these conditions. What factors contribute to depression and other conditions? What strategies facilitate the most accurate assessment for depression and anxiety in adolescent students with autism?
3. Many parents, especially those with autistic children, are reluctant or unwilling to have them routinely immunized as infants. This situation remains true, despite recent studies disproving causation of autism by vaccines. Should the school nurse offer recommendations or even discuss this important issue with the parents? If so, how?
4. Discuss risks for bullying in children with ASD. Do you remember any bullying in school of yourself or peers because of perceived "differences" and "odd" behavior? Will the widespread recognition of autism as a set of neurologically based disorders alter people's perceptions and interactions with those affected?
5. Propose practical nursing strategies for the administration of medications to children who have severe food selectivity or who cannot or will not swallow pills.
6. Discuss the meaning and forms of "resilience" in families.
7. Describe ways life may be more difficult and more rewarding for the person with ASD and their family.
8. How does culture influence the family experience when a young child is diagnosed with an autism spectrum disorder?
9. When parents suspect that their child may have an ASD, what steps should the nurse take first?
10. What strategies can be used to support parents' decision making about immunizations in this child and siblings?
11. In rereading the case scenario in Chapter 8, would you diagnose this patient with co-occuring psychiatric conditions? If so, which? and why?

CHAPTER 9

1. How would ask you an adolescent with an ASD if they have been sexually active? What follow-up questions might you ask regarding their understanding of what constitutes sexually activity?
2. An adolescent with AS tells you that they want to ask a peer to prom. How might you help them prepare to ask a peer on a date?
3. What are some of the warning signs that might indicate to you a patient is at risk for suicide?
4. A parent of an adolescent with AS asks you what they can do to protect their child from being the victim of bullying. What are some protective factors and interventions you might suggest the parents and the school can take?
5. Reread the case scenario in Chapter 9. Would you diagnose this patient with any psychiatric comorbidities? If so, which? and why?

CHAPTER 10

1. What are some of the warning signs that indicate a patient with ASD is at risk for suicide?
2. Prepare a care plan to facilitate an adolescent's transition out of high school into the community.
3. You are developing a plan of care for an adolescent who has never held a job before and has little knowledge of budgeting. How would you use principles of pivotal response training and natural environment training to help him learn how to manage his money?

ADDITIONAL CASES FOR PRACTICE

YouTube Video Clips: Communication

Echolalia and Autism

Summary:

A young boy named Gavin with echolalia and his mother working on a reading lesson.

Length of clip: 2:27 min.

Link: http://www.youtube.com/watch?v=B0A9BU-pcc8 &feature=related

Discussion Questions

1. Describe the phenomena of echolalia and list the different instances of echolalia that you observed in this video.
2. What makes you believe that Gavin understands, or does not understand, the task that he was being asked to perform? Describe the indicators of his understanding or lack of understanding that you saw in the video.
3. Place echolalia in the context of learning a health-promoting behavior, such as learning the name and dosage of one's asthma medication. How would you know that your patient has learned the skill/information?
4. Discuss the mother's teaching technique. What seemed to work well? Would you do anything differently? Prepare an instructional session for the mother for a home visit.

Using Visuals to Teach Autistic Students

Summary:

This video describes simple communication tools and techniques that can be used to assist children on the autism spectrum.

Length of clip: 2:59 min.

Link: http://www.youtube.com/watch?v=RO6dc7QSQb4 &feature=related

Discussion Questions

1. List the different types of communication aids that are available. Elaborate on how these communication aids might be transferred or applicable to your clinical practice area.

2. Discuss the concept of using reward structures to encourage desirable behavior. Do you think rewards are an appropriate motivational strategy for autistic children? Why or why not?
3. Discuss the use of computers as a vehicle for communication with children with ASD.
4. How might computers be integrated with the clinical care of children with ASD?
5. What are the advantages and disadvantages of this technology in the development of communication skills?

Possible Asperger's Syndrome: Three-year-old Girl

Summary:

A mother asks a 3-year-old girl to repeat her and introduce herself to the camera.

Length of clip: 0:28 min.

Link: http://www.youtube.com/watch?v=TuUSS73zBn4 &NR=1

Discussion Questions

1. Describe the language development of this child. How does it differ from other children her age?
2. Do you think this is an example of echolalia. Why or why not?
3. Interpret the meaning of her vocalization.
4. Develop an appropriate approach to further evaluate this child's language ability during a brief encounter prior to her annual physical exam.

Autistic Child Negotiates Verbally with Mom

Summary:

A mother trying to convince her 7-year-old daughter to play in a soccer tournament, while the daughter expresses her disinterest both verbally and nonverbally.

Length of clip: 3:00 min.

Link: http://www.youtube.com/watch?v=v5xKlVVzK5o &feature=related

Discussion Questions

1. Describe the elements of verbal and nonverbal communication that you observed in this video.
2. Describe how you would conduct a functional analysis of this encounter.
3. Evaluate the techniques the mother is using to gain cooperation. Describe the child's response.
4. Resistance may develop during a clinical encounter. What solutions would you suggest for motivating this child?
5. Describe the challenges that make verbal communication more difficult with the child in this video clip, as compared with other children of the same age.

YouTube Video Clips: Socialization

Excuse me, SHE'S AUTISTIC: Lunchtime

Summary:

A young girl with autism eats lunch with her mother's direction.

Length of clip 5:42 min.

Link: http://www.youtube.com/watch?v=W3bf1-E1-98

Discussion Questions

1. What is the approximate age of the child? What developmental expectations do you have for a child this age?
2. What is the child doing to engage her environment?
3. Analyze the events of this lunchtime. Do you think this is typical of a lunchtime for children of this age?
4. What are your thoughts on the role of the parent in terms of teaching social conventions and manners to a child who is on the autism spectrum? Is this important? Why or why not?
5. Analyze the mother's communication style. List the aspects you think are effective and contrast them with what you think are ineffective.
6. Propose an intervention plan to improve the next lunchtime experience.

Kid with Asperger's Syndrome

Summary:

A brief interaction between two middle-school-age friends, a boy and a girl, both on the autism spectrum. Part of a BBC documentary on autism.

Length of clip 1:21 min.

Link: http://www.youtube.com/watch?v=V0DBHxS5Zv0 &feature=related

Discussion Questions

1. Discuss the challenges these two children might face in forming friendships with one another and with other children their age.
2. Identify the instances of sarcasm in this clip and the children's responses to them.
3. What does the literature say about children's (this age) ability to understand sarcasm/humor? Is this different for children with ASD?
4. How might sarcasm present itself in the health care environment? Give an example.
5. Propose a way to create a therapeutic environment in a shared hospital room for the children in this video clip. Would your plan be different if one of the children were neurotypical?
6. How would you manage "flirting" between same-sex patients in a shared hospital room?

Special Siblings—SpecialSiblings.org—Autistic Children

Summary:

A promotional clip for a documentary about children growing up with a sibling who has autism.

Length of clip: 1:05 min.

Link: http://www.youtube.com/watch?v=4vThd_vFrwY &feature=related

Discussion Questions

1. Discuss family dynamics in regard to having a family member with autism. What effects might this have on the other children in the family?
2. What suggestions do you have for family activities that would be appropriate to include the boy with autism in the video? What activities would you suggest for the young girl and her sister?
3. Describe how you would engage the help of a sibling if his/her brother/sister with autism is scheduled for a surgical procedure?

My Autistic Brother

Summary:

A 10-year-old boy makes a short video about his teenage brother who has autism.

Length of clip: 2:07 min.

Link: http://www.youtube.com/watch?v=hCbIGeOk0Ls& feature=related

Discussion Questions

1. In the video, Anthony's mother discusses her vision for Anthony as an adult. Make a list of the options you know of that are available for teens like Anthony after they graduate from high school.
2. If you were to design an assisted-living program for Anthony what would be the key features?
3. Elaborate on your observations about the way that Anthony behaves in the video clips. Contrast his behavior in the first few clips with his behavior in the latter clips.

YouTube Video Clips: Repetitive Movements and Restricted Interests

A Three-year-old Knows the Presidents

Summary:

A 3-year-old autistic savant identifies all the presidents using flash cards.

Length of clip: 2:13 min.

Link: http://www.youtube.com/watch?v=Su5MDM0nGxA& feature=related

Discussion Questions

1. Discuss what you know about autistic savants. At what age do these talents usually appear?

2. What do you notice about Drake's attention span? What nonverbal signals does he give?
3. Propose strategies to capitalize on his strengths and mitigate his difficulties and limitations.
4. List the potential difficulties that Drake might have socializing with other children of his age. How do you think this might change as Drake grows up?
5. If Drake arrives at the pediatrician's office with a seasonal allergy and asthma, how might you use his special skills to improve the quality and outcome of the visit?

Repetitive Behaviors at a Department Store

Summary:

A 7-year-old boy in the aisle of a department store.

Length of clip: 1:32 min.

Link: http://www.youtube.com/watch?v=GRR9BXFLjoU& feature=related

Discussion Questions

1. Break down the child's overall action into specific behaviors. What actions are exactly repetitive? Which are similar but different? Do you identify a pattern?
2. In the description of the video, the mother reports that this behavior had been going on for 15 minutes before she started filming. Discuss the parent's role in setting limits on repetitive behaviors.
3. Describe the challenges that Mikey will face during a clinical encounter.
4. What strategies would you propose to "unstick" the child? Which of these would work best in your practice area?

Matthew "Stimming" on Sword

Summary:

Video depicting a young boy handling a plastic light sword.

Length of clip: 1:20 min.

Link: http://www.youtube.com/watch?v=Kwxo9KFCpSg& feature=related

Discussion Questions

1. What is meant by the term "stimming"?
2. Describe the sequence of behaviors observed in this video. Hypothesize the purpose of the behaviors.
3. Based on this video clip, prioritize your list of concerns for Matthew in the home environment. Propose an intervention for the parents.
4. Matthew's mother asks you why he does this. What do you tell her?

Charlie Pretending

Summary:

A toddler is playing by himself in his kitchen, pretending he is on a train.

Length of clip: 3:28 min.

Link: http://www.youtube.com/watch?v=FxqMNhwnf3Y

Discussion Questions

1. What is unusual or atypical in this video? Summarize the repetitive behaviors that you noted in this video clip.
2. How do you distinguish nonfunctional from functional play?
3. Evaluate the aspects of this child's behavior that might be converted to strengths or seen as assets, rather than as deficits.
4. What criteria would you use to assess a child of this age to make a diagnosis of AS?

Zach's Autistic Stimming

Summary:

A teenager sits in front of the computer listening to music.

Length of clip: 1:25 min.

Link: http://www.youtube.com/watch?v = ASZhpnz0de0

Discussion Questions

1. List the ways that Zach's behavior in this video clip exemplify the behavior of a typical teenager. Which aspects of his behavior are "atypical"? Can you identify a possible purpose for any of these behaviors?
2. The video notes that Zach stops when he notices he is being videotaped. List and explain the factors that might influence a person to self-regulate behavior.
3. The mother comments that "hopefully we can eliminate 'string time' altogether when we go out." What are your thoughts on this? Do you think it is possible, how might this be achieved, and is it necessary for Zach?
4. If Zach were admitted for a short hospital, stay how would you manage this behavior?

III

Introduction: Adulthood and Midlife

Ellen Giarelli

This section highlights the role of nurses in providing health promotion and disease prevention services for people with autism spectrum disorder (ASD) as they transition out of pediatric care and into adult services and community living. Adults with ASD require cardiovascular monitoring and preventive care, such as cancer screening (i.e., colonoscopy, mammography), self-management of diabetes, pre- and postnatal care, and so on. To effectively engage in primary, secondary, and tertiary prevention, one must acquire a very specific set of skills that can be taught through skills training. Preparation for health self-management begins long before the age of 21.

ADAPTIVE SKILLS TRAINING

Without skills training, some people with ASD might acquire patterns of behavior that are difficult to overcome and become barriers to health management, future employment, and successful civic involvement. Outcome data show that approximately 40% of children who enter intensive behavioral intervention programs by the age of 60 months will make successful transitions (Krantz & McClannahan, 1999; Kregel & Wehman, 1997). These data have led to the formation of adult life-skills programs that engage life-skills coaches (McClannahan, MacDuff, & Krantz, 2002; Chadwick et al., 2005). There is still the need to incorporate health messages into transitioning services, because up to one-half of people with ASD have additional medical and psychiatric conditions diagnosed at the same time as the ASD, including seizure and genetic disorders, such as tuberous sclerosis, Fragile X syndrome, and schizophrenia (see Table S3.1).

Among adults, adaptive skills are those daily activities required to support personal and social self-sufficiency (Doll, 1953). These skills are a primary determinant of overall functioning and adjustment (Goldberg, Dill, Shin, & Nhan, 2009; Lifshitz, Merrick, & Morad, 2008). Lack of these skills is especially conspicuous among adults with ASD living in the community. As a result, deficits in this area are a primary impediment to independent living (Soenen, Van Berckelaer-Onnes, & Scholte, 2009). These skills include a wide range of tasks, from basic dressing skills to competitive employment (Dawson, Matson, & Cherry, 1998). Without effective intervention, difficulties appear early and tend to persist throughout t\he individual's life (Chadwick, Cuddy, Kusel, & Taylor, 2005; Rojahn, Matson, Naglieri, & Mayville, 2004). Nurses caring for adults with ASD in any service setting should assess their adaptive skills as part of an overall treatment plan.

TABLE S3.1 ■ Skill Sets for Participation in Adult Health Care Activities

Behavioral skill	Value to patient		
	Primary prevention	Secondary prevention	Tertiary prevention
Accepting of guidance without being disruptive			
Waiting for progressively longer periods before getting "rewards"			
Delivering one's own rewards			
Requesting assistance			
Using social conventions (e.g., saying "please" and "thank you")			
Putting hands in pocket to control finger stereotypy and repetitive behaviors			
Selecting and sequencing one's own activities			
Following photographic and written schedules			
Personal hygiene			

Goal planning, followed by skills development for adults, might include: preparing for school examinations; teaching medication management; practicing contacting medical/accident insurance providers; training on the use of prosthetic or assistive technology; training on the use of contraceptives, and the steps involved in family planning and child care.

DELAYED OR MISSING DIAGNOSIS

Assessing adults with possible ASD and evaluating the medical needs of adults already diagnosed are areas attracting increasing awareness and concern. Some older adults might never have received a definitive diagnosis, but have experienced the psychosocial consequences of core features and report failed marriages, persistent social isolation, a history of employment difficulties, and delayed or misdiagnosed medical conditions. This unusual situation is more common among older adults. These individuals might still be assessed and receive a diagnosis, and this might be highly useful to clinicians, who can then design plans of care that provide medical treatments augmented with provision for the special needs of people with ASD. Nurses might employ a newly validated instrument called the Ritvo Autism Asperger Diagnostic Scale–Revised (RAADS-R) to assist in the diagnosis of ASD in adults (Ritvo et al., 2011). This instrument was designed to address a major gap in screening services for adults with ASD. The authors noted that the increased prevalence of the disorder and the fact that adults are being referred or are self-referring for services make their instrument a useful clinical tool, especially for those who are high functioning and age 18 years and older. The instrument was developed based on criteria from *Diagnostic and Statistical Manual of Mental Disorders, Fourth Edition, Text Revision* (*DSM-IV-TR*; American Psychiatric Association [APA], 2000) diagnostic criteria and compatible with the proposed DSM-V criteria (APA, 2010). The RAADS-R is a highly specific (100%) and sensitive (97%) instrument. A score of 65 or higher is consistent with a diagnosis of ASD. The questions are administered in a clinical setting and the items are designed for individuals with average IQ and above (Ritvo et al., 2011; see Exhibit S3.1). The RAADS-R is reprinted with permission from the author.

EXHIBIT S3.1

RAADS-R©

Ritvo Autism-Asperger's Diagnostic Scale – Revised

All information on this scale is strictly confidential

* 1. Your name ____________________

* 2. Your address ____________________

____

* 3. Your phone number (____) ____________

* 4. Today's date ____________________

* 5. Your age in years ____________________

Your gender: * 6. Male ☐ * 7. Female ☐

Marital status: * 8. Single ☐ * 9. Married ☐ * 10. Divorced ☐

* 11. Not married but in a significant relationship ☐

Do you have children? * 12. Yes ☐ * 13. No ☐

* 14 If yes, list their sexes, ages and any psychiatric or neurological disabilities they may have including autism and Asperger's Disorder:

a. ____________________

b. ____________________

c. ____________________

d. ____________________

e. ____________________

Do you have or have you ever had a driver's license? Yes ☐ No ☐

* 17. The highest grade passed or degree earned in school ____________________

* 18. Was this in regular class? ☐

* 19. Or special education? ☐

* 20. Have you ever been diagnosed or labelled as having Autistic Disorder, Asperger's Disorder, High Functioning Autism, Pervasive Developmental Disorder, Dyslexia, Mental Retardation, Learning Disability or another psychiatric or neurological disorder?
If so, please name the diagnosis or label, when it was given and by whom (name the doctor, clinic or a school). Please use other paper if necessary.

Diagnosis: ____________________

Name of doctor, clinic or other: ____________________

Date of diagnosis: ____________________

When did you begin speaking?

* 21. I began at the usual time (around my second birthday at 24 months of age) ☐

* 22. I began speaking late (at or later than age 2½ or 30 months) ☐

* 23. I have no information as to when I began speaking or early language problems. ☐

It will take you about an hour to answer all the questions.

Please stop if you become tired and start again when you are rested. It is important to read each question completely and think of the answer carefully before checking only one of the four columns headed with these words:

1. **This is true or describes me now and when I was young.**
2. **This is true or describes me only now (refers to skills acquired, applies to negatively worded questions).**
3. **This was true only when I was young (16 years or younger).**
4. **This was never true and never described me.**

Please answer the questions according to what is true for you and only what you feel is true and correct, not what you think others expect you to say or taught you to say.

Please continue on the next page.

(*Continued*)

EXHIBIT S3.1 (Continued)

Some life experiences and personality characteristics that may apply to you	Check only one column: True now and when I was young	True only now	True only when I was younger than 16	Never true
1* I am a sympathetic person.	☐	☐	☐	☐
2. I often use words and phrases from movies and television in conversations.	☐	☐	☐	☐
3. I am often surprised when others tell me I have been rude.	☐	☐	☐	☐
4. Sometimes I talk too loudly or too softly, and I am not aware of it.	☐	☐	☐	☐
5. I often don't know how to act in social situations.	☐	☐	☐	☐
6* I can "put myself in other people's shoes."	☐	☐	☐	☐
7. I have a hard time figuring out what some phrases mean, like "you are the apple of my eye."	☐	☐	☐	☐
8. I only like to talk to people who share my special interests.	☐	☐	☐	☐
9. I focus on details rather than the overall idea.	☐	☐	☐	☐
10. I always notice how food feels in my mouth. This is more important to me than how it tastes.	☐	☐	☐	☐
11* I miss my best friends or family when we are apart for a long time.	☐	☐	☐	☐
12. Sometimes I offend others by saying what I am thinking, even if I don't mean to.	☐	☐	☐	☐
13. I only like to think and talk about a few things that interest me.	☐	☐	☐	☐
14. I'd rather go out to eat in a restaurant by myself than with someone I know.	☐	☐	☐	☐
15. I cannot imagine what it would be like to be someone else.	☐	☐	☐	☐
16. I have been told that I am clumsy or uncoordinated.	☐	☐	☐	☐

Please continue on the next page

(*Continued*)

EXHIBIT S3.1 (Continued)

Some life experiences and personality characteristics that may apply to you	Check only one column: True now and when I was young	True only now	True only when I was younger than 16	Never true
17. Others consider me odd or different.	☐	☐	☐	☐
18* I understand when friends need to be comforted.	☐	☐	☐	☐
19. I am very sensitive to the way my clothes feel when I touch them. How they feel is more important to me than how they look.	☐	☐	☐	☐
20. I like to copy the way certain people speak and act. It helps me appear more normal.	☐	☐	☐	☐
21. It can be very intimidating for me to talk to more than one person at the same time.	☐	☐	☐	☐
22. I have to "act normal" to please other people and make them like me.	☐	☐	☐	☐
23* Meeting new people is usually easy for me.	☐	☐	☐	☐
24. I get highly confused when someone interrupts me when I am talking about something I am very interested in.	☐	☐	☐	☐
25. It is difficult for me to understand how other people are feeling when we are talking.	☐	☐	☐	☐
26* I like having a conversation with several people, for instance around a dinner table, at school or at work.	☐	☐	☐	☐
27. I take things too literally, so I often miss what people are trying to say.	☐	☐	☐	☐
28. It is very difficult for me to understand when someone is embarrassed or jealous.	☐	☐	☐	☐
29. Some ordinary textures that do not bother others feel very offensive when they touch my skin.	☐	☐	☐	☐
30. I get extremely upset when the way I like to do things is suddenly changed.	☐	☐	☐	☐
31. I have never wanted or needed to have what other people call an "intimate relationship."	☐	☐	☐	☐
32. It is difficult for me to start and stop a conversation. I need to keep going until I am finished.	☐	☐	☐	☐

Please continue on the next page

(*Continued*)

EXHIBIT S3.1 (Continued)

Some life experiences and personality characteristics that may apply to you	Check only one column			
	True now and when I was young	True only now	True only when I was younger than 16	Never true
33* I speak with a normal rhythm.	☐	☐	☐	☐
34. The same sound, color or texture can suddenly change from very sensitive to very dull.	☐	☐	☐	☐
35. The phrase "I've got you under my skin" makes me very uncomfortable.	☐	☐	☐	☐
36. Sometimes the sound of a word or a high-pitched noise can be painful to my ears.	☐	☐	☐	☐
37* I am an understanding type of person.	☐	☐	☐	☐
38. I do not connect with characters in movies and cannot feel what they feel.	☐	☐	☐	☐
39. I cannot tell when someone is flirting with me.	☐	☐	☐	☐
40. I can see in my mind in exact detail things that I am interested in.	☐	☐	☐	☐
41. I keep lists of things that interest me, even when they have no practical use (for example sports statistics, train schedules, calendar dates, historical facts and dates).	☐	☐	☐	☐
42. When I feel overwhelmed by my senses, I have to isolate myself to shut them down.	☐	☐	☐	☐
43* I like to talk things over with my friends.	☐	☐	☐	☐
44. I cannot tell if someone is interested or bored with what I am saying.	☐	☐	☐	☐
45. It can be very hard to read someone's face, hand and body movements when they are talking.	☐	☐	☐	☐
46. The same thing (like clothes or temperatures) can feel very different to me at different times.	☐	☐	☐	☐
47* I feel very comfortable with dating or being in social situations with others.	☐	☐	☐	☐
48* I try to be as helpful as I can when other people tell me their personal problems.	☐	☐	☐	☐

Please continue on the next page

(*Continued*)

EXHIBIT S3.1 (Continued)

Some life experiences and personality characteristics that may apply to you	Check only one column: True now and when I was young	True only now	True only when I was younger than 16	Never true
49. I have been told that I have an unusual voice (for example flat, monotone, childish, or high-pitched).	☐	☐	☐	☐
50. Sometimes a thought or a subject gets stuck in my mind and I have to talk about it even if no one is interested.	☐	☐	☐	☐
51. I do certain things with my hands over and over again (like flapping, twirling sticks or strings, waving things by my eyes).	☐	☐	☐	☐
52. I have never been interested in what most of the people I know consider interesting.	☐	☐	☐	☐
53* I am considered a compassionate type of person.	☐	☐	☐	☐
54. I get along with other people by following a set of specific rules that help me look normal.	☐	☐	☐	☐
55. It is very difficult for me to work and function in groups.	☐	☐	☐	☐
56. When I am talking to someone, it is hard to change the subject. If the other person does so, I can get very upset and confused.	☐	☐	☐	☐
57. Sometimes I have to cover my ears to block out painful noises (like vacuum cleaners or people talking too much or too loudly).	☐	☐	☐	☐
58* I can chat and make small talk with people.	☐	☐	☐	☐
59. Sometimes things that should feel painful are not (for instance when I hurt myself or burn my hand on a stove).	☐	☐	☐	☐
60. When talking to someone, I have a hard time telling when it is my turn to talk or to listen.	☐	☐	☐	☐
61. I am considered a loner by those who know me best.	☐	☐	☐	☐
62* I usually speak in a normal tone.	☐	☐	☐	☐
63. I like things to be exactly the same day after day and even small changes in my routines upset me.	☐	☐	☐	☐
64. How to make friends and socialize is a mystery to me.	☐	☐	☐	☐

Please continue on the next page

(*Continued*)

EXHIBIT S3.1 (Continued)

Some life experiences and personality characteristics that may apply to you	True now and when I was young	True only now	True only when I was younger than 16	Never true
	Check only one column			
65. It calms me to spin around or to rock in a chair when I am feeling stressed.	☐	☐	☐	☐
66. The phrase, "He wears his heart on his sleeve," does not make sense to me.	☐	☐	☐	☐
67. If I am in a place where there are many smells, textures to feel, noises or bright lights, I feel anxious or frightened.	☐	☐	☐	☐
68* I can tell when someone says one thing but means something else.	☐	☐	☐	☐
69. I like to be by myself as much as I can.	☐	☐	☐	☐
70. I keep my thoughts stacked in my memory like they are on filing cards, and I pick out the ones I need by looking through the stack and finding the right one (or another unique way).	☐	☐	☐	☐
71. The same sound sometimes seems very loud or very soft, even though I know it has not changed.	☐	☐	☐	☐
72* I enjoy spending time eating and talking with my family and friends.	☐	☐	☐	☐
73. I can't tolerate things I dislike (like smells, textures, sounds or colors).	☐	☐	☐	☐
74. I don't like to be hugged or held.	☐	☐	☐	☐
75. When I go somewhere, I have to follow a familiar route or I can get very confused and upset.	☐	☐	☐	☐
76. It is difficult to figure out what other people expect of me.	☐	☐	☐	☐
77* I like to have close friends.	☐	☐	☐	☐
78. People tell me that I give too much detail.	☐	☐	☐	☐
79. I am often told that I ask embarrassing questions.	☐	☐	☐	☐
80. I tend to point out other people's mistakes.	☐	☐	☐	☐

Thank you for your cooperation!

(*Continued*)

EXHIBIT S3.1 (Continued)

RITVO AUTISM ASPERGER'S DIAGNOSTIC SCALE – REVISED

Instructions for Scoring the Scale

The scale contains two types of questions; (a) 64 "positively worded questions" describing specific symptoms of autism and Asperger's Disorder, and (b) 16 " negatively worded questions" to elicit "normally expected responses. The longer a symptom has been present the more serious it is considered to be, and the higher the score it will receive. To assess longevity and severity, each question can be answered: "True Now and when I was young"–" True Only Now," – "True Only When I Was Young," or –"Never True." The "negatively worded questions" are identified an asterisk by their number and are scored in reverse order. Column reflects acquired social and language skills. The "only true now." The scores for each answer are:

TABLE 1 ■ Scores for the Four Possible Answers

Answer checked by the subject	True now and when I was young	Only true now	True only when I was young	Never true
Positively Worded N = 64 Example: "I take things too literally so I often miss what people are trying to say". (No asterisk after question number).	3	2	1	0
Negatively Worded N = 16 Example: "I * "I am a sympathetic person". (Asterisk after question number).	0	1	2	3

EXECUTIVE FUNCTION

Executive functioning (EF) is defined as a cognitive construct that contributes to maintaining an appropriate problem-solving set to guide future behaviors (Norman & Shallice, 2000). Executive functioning affects abilities such as planning, organization, self-monitoring, attention shifting, and flexibility in thinking. People with EF deficits might have difficulty listening to directions or following instructions and acting on them at the same time (Holland & Low, 2010). They might have problems planning and organizing tasks and goals or knowing how to systematically accomplish a task. They have difficulty problem solving and might use the same approach to solving a problem, regardless of the specific situation (Elliot, 2003; Holland & Low, 2010). Nurses might observe that people with EF deficits have significant difficulty being independent at home, at work, and in the community (Pisula, 2010). Impairment in EF has been associated with behavior difficulties that include distractibility, impulsivity, inability to delay gratification, repetitive behavior, inflexibility, self-monitoring, and problems in self- regulation and mutual regulation (Christ, Kanne, & Reiersen, 2010).

Moreover, there is strong evidence to suggest that individuals with autism show atypicalities in multiple cognitive domains, including EF, central coherence, and theory of mind. Theory of mind is the ability to attribute mental states—beliefs, intents, desires, pretending, knowledge, and so on—to oneself and others and to understand that others have beliefs, desires, and intentions that are different from one's own (Teufel, Fletcher, & Davis, 2010). Pellicano (2010) found that early domain-general skills play a critical role in shaping the developmental trajectory of children's theory of mind.

The mental decisions (executive function) and control processes governing adaptive behavior are cumbersome for people with autism (Monette, Bigras, & Guay, 2011; Reck & Hund, 2011). This confusion can cause the individual on the spectrum greater frustration and cause or extend meltdown behavior and inappropriate behavior responses. Ozonoff's (1998) research associated deficits in EF with the behavior of focusing on selective and often irrelevant details, which causes the individual with ASD to lose the meaning of an event, interaction, or picture. This neurological deficit might be observed and labeled as willful noncompliance and will be especially difficult to accurately assess across cultures (Lan, Legare, Ponitz, Li, & Morrison, 2011).

CLINICAL RELEVANCE OF EF FOR NURSING CARE

Patient-centered health care places emphasis on informed decision making by patients after they receive sufficient and accurate information on risks, benefits, and uncertainties associated with treatment. This creates a significant problem for health professionals who care patients whose area of functional disability is receptive communication. Risks and benefits might be couched in concrete terms, but uncertainties are more abstract and might be difficult or impossible to convey in a way that would meet expectations for informed decision making. The core elements of the information needed by men to assist in their decision making regarding prostate cancer screening are listed in Chapter 13.

Nurses cannot assume that adults with autism have had routine preventive health care. They might not get regular immunizations, blood pressure checks, or vision and hearing screenings. The adult with ASD might have received deficient preventive care if other health concerns took precedence, such as seizure disorders or aggression. Health history data might be difficult to obtain and as fragmented as previous medical care. For the older adult, parents might be deceased or have relinquished guardianship. The legal guardian might be the only source of health history information, and the adult with limited communication skills might not be able to provide missing information. Accurate health information might be essential to provide best and responsible care. The ideal situation would be access to a portfolio of information collected over the years and transported with the patient. The portfolio would include records of physicians' names and contact information, preferences, core and associated features of the ASD, communication skills and deficits, cognitive ability, immunizations, surgeries, medications and dosages, metabolic and hematological tests, and relevant family histories.

Nurses should remember that the brain continues to mature and develop connections well into adulthood, and a person's EF abilities are shaped both by physical changes in the brain and by life experiences in the classroom and in the world at large. Early attention to developing efficient skills in this area can be very helpful. As a rule, direct instruction, frequent reassurance, and explicit feedback are recommended (National Center for Learning Disabilities, 2008).

Section III expands on nursing care of individuals by considering the unique issues faced by adults with ASD who have functional deficits in socialization, adaptive skills, and executive function. In Chapter 10, the authors discuss the nurse's role in facilitating developmental task achievement for adolescents and young adults as they find the path to independence. They discuss decision-making, sex education, and relationship counseling with older adolescents and young adults with ASD. In Chapter 11, the authors present a case of a pregnant woman with Asperger's syndrome and a seizure disorder preparing for labor, delivery, and parenting. This chapter points out myths about people with ASD and develops the idea that such individuals can lead relatively typical lives and can successfully thrive with specialized attention after difficult physical and emotional events. This chapter addresses the challenges of labor and delivery and the need to prepare instruction in concrete terms and conduct frequent home visits. Chapter 12 develops the roles of the emergency nurse when receiving and treating a patient with ASD, including rapid intake or admission and assessment of the potential for aggression and emotional meltdowns and the need for a safe, quiet, and low-stress/unintrusive environment. Lastly, the authors of Chapter 13 describe the nursing care from screening and diagnosis to recovery for a man with autism diagnosed with prostate cancer. This chapter begins with a discussion of disparities in cancer incidence among people with disabilities and explores the idea that people with ASD are less likely to receive cancer screening, less likely to benefit from primary prevention, and less likely to maximize their benefit from secondary prevention once diagnosed with cancer. The chapter explores the circumstances needed promote wellness, prevent cancer, and mitigate morbidity through early intervention.

REFERENCES

American Psychiatric Association. (2000). *Diagnostic and statistical manual of mental disorders* (4 ed.), Washington, DC: Author.

American Psychiatric Association. (2010). *Diagnostic and statistical manual of mental disorders* (5 ed.), Washington, DC: Author. Retrieved July 20, 2011 from http://www.dsm5.org/pages/default.aspx

Bruner, J. S. (1981). Intention in the structure of action and interaction. In L. P. Lipsitt, & C. K. Rovee-Collier (Eds.), *Advances in infancy research* (*Vol. 1*, pp. 41–56). Norwood, NJ: Ablex.

Chadwick, O., Cuddy, M., Kusel, Y., & Taylor, E. (2005). Handicaps and the development of skills between childhood and early adolescence in young people with severe intellectual disabilities. *Journal of Intellectual Disability Research, 49*, 877–888.

Christ, S. E., Kanne, S. M., & Reiersen, A. M. (2010). Executive function in individuals with sub-threshold autism traits. *Neuropsychology, 24*(5), 590–598.

Dawson, J. E., Matson, J. L., & Cherry, K. E. (1998). An analysis of maladaptive behaviors in persons with autism, PDD-NOS, and mental retardation. *Research in Developmental Disabilities, 19*, 439–448.

Doll, E. A. (1953). Vineland social maturity scale. *American Journal of Orthopsychiatry, 5*, 80–188.

Elliot, R. (2003). Executive function and their disorders. *British Medical Bulletin, 65*(suppl. 1), 49–59.

Goldberg, M. R., Dill, C. A., Shin, J. Y., & Nhan, N. V. (2009). Reliability and validity of the Vietnamese Vineland Adaptive Behavior Scales with preschool-age children. *Research in Developmental Disabilities, 30*, 592–602.

Hobson, R. P. (1995). *Autism and the development of mind*. Hillsdale, NJ: Lawrence Erlbaum.

Holland, L., & Low, J. (2010). Do children with autism use inner speech and visuospatial resources for the service of executive control? Evidence from suppression in dual tasks. *British Journal of Developmental Psychology, 28*(part 2), 369–391.

Krantz, P. J., & McClannahan, L. E. (1999). Strategies for integration: Building repertoires that support transition to public schools. In P. M. Ghezzi, W. L. Williams, & J. E. Carr (Eds.), *Autism: Behavior-analytic perspectives* (pp. 221–231). Reno, NV: Context Press.

Kregel, J., & Wehman, P. (1997). Supported employment: A decade of employment outcomes for individuals with significant disabilities. In W. E. Kiernan, & R. L. Schalock (Eds.), *Integrated employment: Current status and future directions* (pp. 31–47). Washington, DC: American Association of Mental Retardation.

Lan, X., Legare, C. H., Ponitz, C. C., Li, S., & Morrison, F. J. (2011). Investigating the links between the subcomponents of executive function and academic achievement: A cross-cultural analysis of Chinese and American preschoolers. *Journal of Experimental Child Psychology, 108*(3), 677–692.

Lifshitz, H., Merrick, J., & Morad, M. (2008). Health status and ADL functioning of older persons with intellectual disability: Community residence versus residential care centers. *Research in Developmental Disabilities, 29*, 301–315.

McClannahan, L. E., MacDuff, G. S., & Krantz, P. J. (2002). Behavior analysis and intervention for adults with autism. *Behavior Modification, 26*(1), 9–26.

Monette, S., Bigras, M., & Guay, M. C. (2011). The role of the executive functions in school achievement at the end of grade 1. *Journal of Experimental Child Psychology, 109*(2), 158–173.

National Center for Learning Disabilities. (2008). *Executive function fact sheet.* Retrieved from http://www.ldonline.org/article/24880/

Norman, D. A., & Shallice, T. (2000). Attention to action: Willed and automatic control of behaviour. In M. S. Gazzaniga (Ed.), *Cognitive neuroscience: A reader.* Oxford, UK: Blackwell.

Ozonoff, S. (1998). Assessment and remediation of executive dysfunction in autism and Asperger syndrome. In E. Shopler, G. B. Mesibov, & L. J. Kunce (Eds.), *Asperger syndrome or high functioning autism?* (pp. 263–290). New York: Plenum.

Pellicano, E. (2010). Individual differences in executive function and central coherence predict developmental changes in theory of mind in autism. *Developmental Psychology, 46*(2), 530–544.

Pisula, E. (2010).The autistic mind in the light of neuropsychological studies. *Acta Neurobiologiae Experimentalis, 70*(2), 119–130.

Reck, S. G., & Hund, A. M. (2011). Sustained attention and age predict inhibitory control during early childhood. *Journal of Experimental Child Psychology, 108*(3), 504–512.

Ritvo, R. A., Ritvo, E. R, Guthrie, D., Ritvo, M. J., Hufnagel, D. H., McMahon, W., ... Eloff, A. (2011). The Ritvo Autism Asperger Diagnostic Scale-Revised (RAADS-R): A scale to assist the diagnosis of autism spectrum disorder in adults: An international validation study. *Journal of Autism & Developmental Disorders, 41*, 1076–1089.

Rojahn, J., Matson, J. L., Naglieri, J. A., & Mayville, E. (2004). Relationships between psychiatric conditions and behavior problems among adults with mental retardation. *American Journal on Mental Retardation, 109*, 21–33.

Soenen, S., Van Berckelaer-Onnes, I., & Scholte, E. (2009). Patterns of intellectual, adaptive and behavioral functioning in individuals with mild mental retardation. *Research in Developmental Disabilities, 30*, 433–444.

Teufel, C., Fletcher, P. C., & Davis, G. (2010). Seeing other minds: Attributed mental states influence perception. *Trends in Cognitive Sciences, 14*(8), 376–382.

Transition to Community: Adolescence, Employment, and Companionship

10

Lauren Blann, Lori Ioriatti, Adrienne P. Robertiello, and Louise Walpin

The transition from an insulated, somewhat protected, environment of home and secondary school to adult life presents challenges for most people. This time encompasses shifts in self-awareness, sexual interest, work, and independence that have significant emotional and psychological effects. For those with an autism spectrum disorder (ASD), additional difficulties present themselves. Many adolescents on the spectrum have less-developed social skills compared to their nondisabled peers. They may not understand the hormonal and sexual changes they are experiencing. These individuals, who had previously relied on parental and administrative leadership, must now engage in self-determination and self-advocacy. In addition, they must now pursue support for their ongoing development of emotional, relationship, career, and life skills.

Transition is defined as the adolescent's movement out of high school and into independent living, employment, or higher education (Giarelli & Ruttenberg, unpublished manuscript). Transitioning is influenced by the adolescent's developmental needs and neurobehavioral problems; contextual factors, such as family support; school-based training; and the receptivity and flexibility of employers. The following case study illustrates the complex nature of the process of transitioning for adolescents with ASD and demonstrates the significant role a nurse may play in this important and essential developmental mandate.

CASE–DARYL'S STORY

It is September, and Daryl, a 17-year-old male with an ASD, is feeling increasingly anxious. Transitioning back to school after summer has always been difficult for him, but this year has been the worst. He is entering his senior year in high school and is considering his vocational options.

Daryl's cognitive level is generally functional in daily living scenarios. His attention and memory skills are sound. His thinking skills are marked by difficulties in analyzing situations, selecting appropriate strategies from multiple approaches, processing multistep instructions, and long-term planning. Daryl has an average attention span, but has a tendency to obsess on thoughts and situations. His general language skills are sound, but he is challenged with understanding abstract or symbolic conversation. He has good listening skills but needs some assistance in processing, organizing, and expressing information. Daryl's problem-solving skills require guidance, but he is able to implement skills previously learned.

(*Continued*)

CASE–DARYL'S STORY (Continued)

Daryl could not stop thinking about earlier experiences and fears that he would never succeed. As a sophomore, Daryl attempted part-time employment at a local fast-food restaurant. The noise of machinery and customer chatter was too much for him. He wanted to cover his ears and run. What did the manager mean when he said, "A busy mind is a healthy mind." Literal thinking made it difficult for Daryl to understand what the manager meant. Daryl wondered how could he make his mind busy while trying to work with his hands. Escape seemed the only solution, so, when he was asked to throw out the trash, he left for home.

Soon after, he asked a female classmate out on a date. She laughed at him and refused. Daryl became increasingly anxious and depressed. He was hospitalized due to suicidal ideation. He wondered if he would he ever be able to be successfully employed, attend college, or have an intimate relationship.

Daryl had an appointment to see Kim, an advanced practice nurse (APN), who was his psychiatric provider and therapist. During the session, Daryl described his ruminating thoughts: panic and fear of failure, as well as difficulty sleeping. His parents reported he had been increasingly irritable at home. While he denied thoughts of suicide, he reported hopelessness and negative thoughts about himself, the world, and the future. In addition to increasing his antidepressants, the APN talked with him about his strengths and challenges.

Daryl conveyed that he had always been in inclusive classes with in-class support. He excelled in math and science, but struggled with reading. He had difficulty with following multistep directions and completing long-term projects, but did well when the instructions were broken down into component parts, and short-term deadlines were set. Daryl emphasized that he learned best by watching and doing—not by listening or reading. He disliked loud noises and fluorescent lighting. Daryl loved animals. He had his own dog and had been taking care of his neighbors' pets when the neighbors were on vacation. He remarked that he felt calm when touching the soft fur of a cat or dog. Daryl proudly told the APN that he knew a great deal about the needs of various breeds of dogs and cats.

Throughout his life, Daryl was often bullied by others. He has had only a couple of good friends, who valued his loyalty and honesty. However, he understands that sometimes he makes inappropriate comments or stands too close to others. Daryl lacks some other social skills, as he has the tendency to miss cues when others are getting bored and can dominate conversations.

On further inquiry, the APN learned that Daryl's individualized education plan (IEP) included only general plans for transition out of high school. She contacted the case manager to suggest that Daryl be linked with the Division of Vocational Rehabilitation (DVR). The APN explained that the DVR could provide mentors or job coaches to support Daryl in appropriate vocational placement. She also suggested that school personnel assist Daryl in contacting local veterinarians, animal shelters, and rescue organizations to explore opportunities for volunteer or paid employment that could lead to a career. Perhaps he could help groom or walk the animals or provide clerical assistance in the operation of the shelter. The APN informed Daryl about the Americans with Disabilities Act and required accommodations.

They closed the session by talking about the need to think about employment options that would make use of Daryl's strengths, while limiting noise, multiple demands, and long-range planning. The APN made an appointment to see Daryl in one month.

In this interaction, the APN used the time to understand Daryl's interests, challenges, and goals. The APN also presented Daryl with some appropriate resources and topics of consideration to nurture continued discussion at their next session.

CASE–DARYL'S NEXT SESSION WITH THE APN

At the next session, Daryl reported the prospect of volunteering at a local animal rescue organization. His job duties would include feeding and grooming animals, as well as providing some clerical assistance in the operation of the shelter. He said that this position could lead to paid work and that his school would provide a job coach for him. This particular coach was new to the field and did not have much experience working with individuals on the spectrum.

Daryl was excited about working with the animals. However, the thought of dealing with supervisors as part of his clerical duties frightened him. He was unsure of how to introduce himself; what would happen if they asked him to do something he did not understand; what would happen if he became overwhelmed and could not perform a particular task; and what would happen if he refused and walked away.

Toward the end of the session, Daryl mentioned that he was thinking about attending a local community college. He also revealed his concern about whether or not he would ever date or have a long-term relationship. The APN assured him that they would discuss these topics at their next session in 2 weeks.

Connecting with the Job Coach

With Daryl's permission, the APN contacted the job coach during their treatment session. They talked about Daryl's learning style and ways that the job coach could model appropriate behavior and conversation. They agreed to work to build upon skills that Daryl had previously mastered and then observe his attempts at generalizing these skills. The APN encouraged Daryl to identify reinforcers that would motivate him to attempt new tasks, to focus on mastering new skills, and to participate in nonpreferred activities. At this time, Daryl was able to convey more detailed, personal difficulties and aspirations. The APN was able to ascertain Daryl's preferred method of learning. She also guided Daryl to reflect upon areas of motivation and inspiration so as to apply these to functional life skills. The APN continued to assess Daryl's challenges and identify his personal and functional needs and desires.

CASE–DARYL RETURNS FOR ADDITIONAL COUNSELING

At the next appointment, the APN asked Daryl about his knowledge and comfort level regarding the college application process. While he knew how to get an application, he told her that he was afraid of failing, because he had previously needed academic support in school. The APN assured Daryl that the college had offices for disability services and student assistance. She also emphasized that it was his choice to identify himself as a student with special needs. If he did, he would be entitled to accommodations similar to those he had had throughout elementary, middle, and high school. The APN pointed out

(Continued)

CASE–DARYL RETURNS FOR ADDITIONAL COUNSELING (Continued)

that he would now have to be active in terms of getting this assistance. In order to register, he would need to bring proof of his diagnosis, such as his IEP, to the college.

The APN suggested that Daryl visit the college to familiarize himself with the campus and to speak with a staff member in the disability services office before deciding to apply. They discussed the possibility of part-time registration, beginning with one course in an area of high interest. The APN assured Daryl that she had not forgotten about his concerns with dating and relationships. She wanted to be sure they had enough time to devote to the topic, so she suggested he make a list of questions that they could focus on to address those issues.

The APN began working with Daryl on planning goal-related strategies. She identified options and helped Daryl understand opportunities and alternatives. Based on Daryl's goals, the APN set forth an appropriate action plan and thoroughly explained his responsibilities and the significance of his actions.

CASE–NOT GOING AS PLANNED

At the next session, Daryl would not look at the APN. Instead, he paced and flicked his fingers at his side repetitively. When the APN mentioned that he looked upset, Daryl said he could not stop thinking about the time a girl had laughed at him in high school, and he was sure no one would ever want to marry him. Upon further questioning, the APN learned that he had never spoken to the girl before he had asked her to go on a date. She told Daryl that there are social rules for dating and just as he had learned the social rules for making friends when he was younger, he could learn these rules too.

She asked him whether he was interested in dating females, males, or both. Daryl responded that he thought he was interested in dating only females, but did not know how he would know for sure, since he had never dated anyone. The APN asked Daryl whether he ever pictured himself living with someone or kissing, touching, or having sexual relations. After Daryl affirmed he had, the APN asked whether he thought about males and/or females at those times. His reply was "only females." The APN explained to Daryl that these thoughts give us information about our sexual preference. She told him that his expressions suggested his interest in dating females.

In this session, the APN assessed Daryl's concerns with dating. She guided the discussion to help Daryl identify his personal interests and preferences. She also assured him that they could work together on skills to build his confidence in dating.

CASE–MORE DISCUSSIONS OF SEXUALITY

Over the next couple of sessions, the APN assessed Daryl's knowledge of body parts, sexual intercourse, reproduction and masturbation, and the distinction between appropriate public and private behaviors. While he had an adequate knowledge of facts, he had little

(*Continued*)

CASE–MORE DISCUSSIONS OF SEXUALITY (Continued)

understanding of putting these facts into practice for dating or developing relationships. Since Daryl was a visual learner, the APN gave him some videos and instruction sheets with pictures to provide clear, detailed steps regarding the process of getting to know someone and asking them out on a date. She also provided specific verbal and written information about laws (for instance age of consent) and sexual health and safety (sexually transmitted infections, condoms, Internet dating, etc.). They talked in detail about the fact that the word "no" means "no."

The APN believed it was necessary to make sure that Daryl understood these dating skills, but was concerned that he might be confused if she engaged in these role-playing exercises with him. As she did not want to damage their therapeutic relationship, with Daryl's permission, the APN asked a male colleague, Sam, to join them. Daryl consented that Sam could provide additional counseling and answer questions—helping Daryl work through solutions of various social situations. Based on his learning style, these types of role-playing exercises helped Daryl anticipate and respond to common relationship issues.

As the APN and Daryl continued their sessions, she reinforced relaxation strategies that he found helpful, including deep breathing and yoga. In order to develop a positive self-regard, they practiced ways to challenge Daryl's negative beliefs, such as "I always fail" with facts and positive affirmations in their place. The APN continued to educate Daryl about the effects physical health has upon mental health. At the request of the APN, Daryl maintained a 7-day diet and an exercise log, which they reviewed for healthy changes.

Through their ongoing sessions, Daryl became more comfortable expressing his concerns and his need for guidance. After assessing his needs, goals, and learning style, the APN was able to analyze the basis and characteristics of Daryl's struggles. With this information in place, the APN planned strategies to guide and educate Daryl in a method that would optimize the effectiveness of therapeutic interventions. She continued to guide and support his development to promote functional, independent, and meaningful adolescent transitions.

APPROACH TO CLINICAL MANAGEMENT

Children diagnosed with ASD often receive therapeutic interventions to assist with communication skills, social interactions, and behavior modification as part of their academic curricula. As these children reach adolescence, additional factors and challenges arise. During this time, there are increased demands and desires for independent, functional living skills, multifaceted social interactions, purposeful career planning, and the development of meaningful, mature relationships. During this transition period, adolescents with ASD benefit most from interventions designed to guide and support their successful passage from a structured, school-based system to self-determining, self-advocating adult life.

Legal Mandates

In 1975, the passage of the Education for All Handicapped Children Act (1975) mandated special education services for all children with disabilities within the public education system. Over time, parents and professionals realized that this act was inadequate to improve postschool outcomes for children with disabilities. In 1990, amendments were made to the EAHCA that provided for transition services to adulthood and employment. The new law became the Individuals with Disabilities Education Act (IDEA, 1990). Multiple modifications have been implemented to fine-tune educational services.

Under IDEA (1990), each student's IEP must include annual directives about the need for transition services commencing as early as age 14 and usually by age 16 years. The IDEA is set forth to prepare a child with a disability for further education, employment, and independent living. The stipulations contain language that mandates that IEP transition goals are to be based on the person's interests, needs, abilities, aspirations, and personal choices. This act was created to turn the focus on lifelong outcomes, team collaboration, and interagency coordination. Transition services are to be implemented by the student, along with the parents and with help from the educational team. Team members may include educators, job coaches, therapists, service providers, and community members. The emphasis of the transition planner should be the student's goals related to postsecondary education, employment, and/or independent living.

When advocates prepare adolescents for future employment, it is essential to shift the focus of programming from academics to more functional life skills and vocational tasks. Federal mandates require the IEPs of learners age 14 and older to include a statement of transition needs, although state codes may require a transition statement at a younger age. Therefore, their educational goals need to focus on preparing them for employment and adult life.

Under the IDEA (1990), all school-aged students have a right to a free and appropriate education. However, once a student graduates from high school, legal rights change, as the person falls under the protection of the Americans with Disabilities Act (1990, 2008). The ADA differs from the IDEA in that it grants no specific rights, except that a person cannot be excluded from participation based solely on his disability. Reasonable accommodations are provided for students, but only to the extent that they do not alter a college program or academic standards. As part of ADA requirements, colleges and universities must ensure that their programs are accessible to all qualified students. Students can request and receive auxiliary aids and services as well as educational modifications that would encourage equal participation. Unlike the IDEA, in a college environment, a student must self-identify as disabled, submit valid documentation of disability, and make the request for accommodation(s) (Dell, 2004). The student or family must self-advocate and request accommodations from professors and employers. Colleges and work sites are often better equipped to accommodate people with physical or learning disabilities than with the behavioral issues associated with ASD (Pacer Center, 2011). Because of these issues, it is essential that the transition process and planning for postsecondary education occur early in the student's high school career and involve all relevant team members (Geller & Greenberg, 2010).

Employment Statistics for ASD

Current employment rates for individuals with ASD are discouraging. According to the U.S. Department of Labor March 2011 disability employment statistics (U.S. Department of Labor, 2011), the employment rate for people with disabilities in the labor force was 21%. The employment rate for persons with no disability in the labor force was 69.7% (U.S. Department of Labor, 2011). The unemployment rate for those with disabilities was 15.6%, compared with 8.9% for persons with no disability (U.S. Department of Labor, 2011). Some authors indicate unemployment rates over 75% (Cimera & Cowan, 2009; U.S. Department of Labor, 2011). In the United States, adults with ASD continue to be underemployed, possibly due to inadequate or inappropriate transition planning, and to some extent, limited interest in supporting adult learners, particularly those with cognitive or behavioral challenges (Bateman, 2005; Coulter, 2001; Grandin, 1996; Nuehring & Sitlington, 2003).

As recently as 2011, Taylor and Seltzer (2011) reported that adolescents with ASD, but without intellectual disability, were three times more likely to have no daytime activities and low rates (56%) of employment in the community. Similar patterns have been observed over the last 15 years. Ballaban-Gil, Rapin, Tuchman, and Shinnar (1996) reported that among a sample of 45 adults with ASD, 27% had some sort of work, but were generally poorly paid. About one-half of these were competitively employed, while the other one-half were in supported or sheltered workshops, and the remaining had no employment. Forty-five percent of a sample of young adults with ASD had never been employed, and only one was able to financially support himself (Eaves & Ho, 2008). Behavioral profiles for young adults with ASD may worsen after exiting high school, due to lack of stimulation (Taylor & Seltzer, 2010); follow-up services and greater independence have been associated with few behavioral problems (Howlin, Goode, Hutton, & Rutter, 2004).

Preparing for Transition

When an adolescent prepares for the transition from high school to higher education and/or employment, it is essential that there are sufficient and appropriate resources in place to support the functioning and independence. Well-trained agency personnel can foster independence by providing both living and vocational supports. Deficits in social interaction and communication, as well as the propensity to engage in restrictive and repetitive behaviors, may serve to increase the challenges.

Receiving and Responding Styles

People with ASD have difficulty interpreting social cues and interacting with peers. Their interactions are egocentric, rather than reciprocal. This difference can becomes conspicuous in the workplace or any other social setting that demands sophisticated interpersonal skill sets (Hendricks, 2010). In addition, the adolescent with ASD may have impairments with executive functioning, which can affect organizational skills and attention (Lawrence, Alleckson, & Bjorklund, 2010), making transitioning from adolescence to adulthood especially difficult as expectations increase.

Generally, adolescents with ASD learn routines quickly, but they often lack an understanding of the purpose. It is difficult for them to tolerate changes in routine due to an inability to solve problems and formulate new or alternative solutions to fit changing situations. At times, these difficulties result in severe anxiety and behavioral problems. As an individual transitions from the familiar world of living at home and attending high school to the unpredictable adult life of college and/or the workplace, he or she will face new situations and changes in his or her routines (Schall & McDonough, 2010a). These situations have the potential to result in significant negative behaviors (Schall & McDonough, 2010b).

Dysfunctional Responses

For people with ASD, a negative behavior may be triggered by multiple antecedents. For instance, a person may engage in head-banging or biting in an attempt to indicate pain, hunger, anxiety, or frustration (Cermak & Ben-Sasson, 2007). He or she may have difficulty understanding or communicating feelings appropriately by using words, which may result in physical manifestations of feelings. People with ASD often depend on those around them to understand those expressions and make changes in the environment based on their behavior. If the nurse misses these early warning signals, behaviors may escalate to a severe level. Effective supports are based on accurate interpretations of behavior to provide the individual with tools necessary to adapt to environmental changes (Janzen, 2003). Even those individuals with highly developed language skills or special intellectual talents may regress to dysfunctional behavior when faced with a problem they cannot easily resolve.

An environment with bright lights, loud sounds, or intense smells can cause a person with ASD to demonstrate problematic behaviors (Janzen, 2003). This occurs because people with ASD often lack the ability to ignore, modulate, or organize sensory information (Janzen, 2003).

Principles for Successful Transitioning

There are nine principles used to guide a successful transition: 1) self-determination and student choice; 2) level and intensity of support; 3) family and student attitudes; 4) person-centered planning; 5) secondary curriculum reform; 6) inclusion; 7) career development; 8) longitudinal curricula; and 9) business connections and alliances (Miller-Kuhaneck, 2001). These principles are described below. See Figure 10.1 for an illustration of the relationship among the nine principles.

Self-Determination and Student Choice

The principle of self-determination is defined as taking steps as the primary agent in one's life and making quality-of-life decisions that are free from undue external influence or interference (Wehmeyer, 1992). In higher education, the principle of self-determination is used to direct students to take an active role in goal setting and for professionals to recognize this

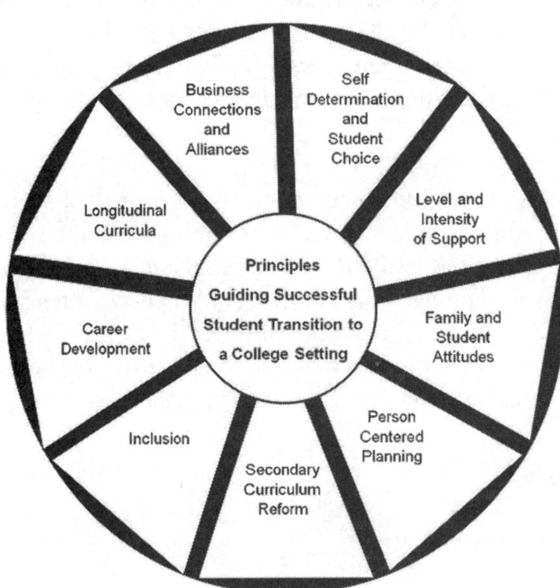

FIGURE 10.1 ■ The figure illustrates a conceptualization of the association among the nine principles.

effort, listen to students, and validate their goals by supporting them in their endeavors. As referenced in the case study, the APN first developed a comfort level with Daryl in order to allow him to openly express his needs, interests, and goals. Based on this information, she was able to determine and acquire the support that would be most beneficial for Daryl.

Level and Intensity of Support

Skills and resources needed to make a successful transition vary greatly from one person to another. Some students require only generic support that would be available to all individuals, regardless of the presence of a disability (McDonough & Revell, 2010). Other students require temporary supports, such as vocational training. Individuals with more severe disabilities may need intensive and continuous support as they transition. An example of this is supported employment in integrated work settings, in which individuals have equal opportunities to work with supports in a cohesive and competitive work setting with nondisabled peers.

Determining need for support: There are structured tools available that help determine the level and intensity of support needed to participate as a part of the community. One such tool is the American Association on Intellectual and Developmental Disabilities (AAIDD, 2011) Supports Intensity Scale (SIS). The SIS is used to measure a person's support needs with respect to work-related and social activities. The SIS can help users identify the types and intensity of the supports an individual requires. The SIS was designed to be part of person-centered planning processes that help all individuals identify their unique preferences, skills, and life goals. The supports approach helps advocates to recognize that individuals' needs change over time and that supports must change as well. They must be developed and delivered in age-appropriate settings with the understanding that, regardless of intellectual abilities or limitations, people should have the opportunity to engage in activities and life experiences just like any other person (AAIIDD, 2011).

The SIS has three sections. The first section measures the support needs related to a person's life activity domains, which include home living, employment, community life, health and safety, lifelong learning, and social activities. The second section—the supplemental protection and advocacy scale—provides data to assist in the development of personalized support plans. The last section identifies exceptional medical and behavioral supports needs (North Carolina Division of Mental Health, Developmental Disabilities and Substance Abuse Services, 2011).

In the case study, the APN assessed Daryl's learning style and recognized his need for direct instructions and short-term deadlines in both school and work environments. The APN acknowledged Daryl's potential stressors, such as fluorescent lighting, noises, and proximity of people. She also assessed for social and behavioral challenges. Concurrently, she was able to help Daryl hone in on his motivators and interests. Evaluating all of these factors collectively on an ongoing basis enabled the APN to provide least restrictive and optimally relevant supports, thus enabling Daryl to work on adaptations and skill development.

Family and Student Attitudes

Families play an integral role in the development of the transition plan. Parents are most familiar with their children and are often their strongest advocates. Many of the goals and services that were written as part of the transition plan will be carried out after the student leaves secondary education. As the student matures, he or she will gradually take on self-advocacy.

During the transition, family members can help young people meet their goals by listening openly to their concerns and interests, while encouraging them to embrace opportunities for independent thinking and increased independence. The family can set aside samples of assignments and projects that represent the individual's strengths. Families might also provide their young adult child with increasingly complex information about his or her disability to increase self-awareness. Parents can work with their children to identify accommodations that have been successful in the past in order to ascertain similar supports in the future. In addition, parents should help their children understand how and when to reveal appropriate disability-related information to others (Pacer Center, 2011).

Person-centered Planning

The principle of person-centered planning is best described as the development of individualized strategies based on a person's needs and aspirations. Instead of focusing on physical capacity, service entitlement, and need, this type of approach emphasizes choice and control. Person-centered planning is used by those who are concerned with the quality and preferences of a person's life, not just the need for services (Helen Sanderson Association, n.d.).

This principle informs an approach to transitioning that involves supporting the student and his or her family members and service providers in achieving the student's goals. Nurses are well prepared to take a person-centered approach to therapeutic relationships with the adolescent who is transitioning. They are able to assist in the facilitation of the health care transition process from pediatric to adult medical providers. Nurses have clinical proficiency and understanding related to disability concerns, the influence of coexisting health problems, and the associated needs for supports and services.

In practicing person-centered planning, nurses can provide guidance and support to all members of the family through the transition process and familiarize them with the community services and resources available, including, assistive technology, vocational educators, employment specialists, social workers, recreation providers, housing agencies, and transportation services. Support personnel can nurture appropriate methods to support friendship development and prevent social isolation for adolescents with ASD. They should also discuss health care concerns that may affect work-related tasks and should help determine the most appropriate accommodations or assistance. Person-centered strategies should contain planning based on the student's vision of life postgraduation.

For Daryl, short-term goal setting and action planning were beneficial. The APN conscientiously explained Daryl's responsibilities and possible outcomes of his actions in the plan options. Using her expertise and knowledge of resources, the nurse offered and described options from which Daryl could decide. On a continual basis, the APN guided Daryl by exposing him to an increasing quantity and array of community exchanges, assisting him in developing self-sufficiency in routine and significant matters, encouraging situations where he could engage in meaningful and functional activities, identifying opportunities for social networking, and facilitating relationships.

Secondary Curriculum Reform

The principle of secondary curriculum reform emphasizes the need for students to participate actively in community experience before exiting school. Advocates should foster a close relationship between the secondary education institution and the workplace environments. This is essential for supporting students with disabilities as they transition to adulthood.

Functional life and job-related skills, such as learning how to budget, shop, and use public transportation are critical in school curricula (Miller-Kuhaneck, 2001). There are academic programs that are designed with structured internships in restaurants, banks, and other businesses. For instance, a student that is placed in a work environment may perform routine tasks while learning task prioritization, categorization, and communication skills (Humphrey & Lewis, 2008).

Some college environments are arranged to include peer mentors as a means to practice social interactions. A number of colleges have disability counselors who have developed programs that enable the practice of chosen professions, providing opportunities for interning in specific fields on college grounds. Academic institutions have coordinated interagency collaborations to support job sampling, training, and placement. Work–study positions develop various skills that translate readily to real-world jobs.

The APN explained to Daryl what he could gain from mentors or job coaches. She made recommendations for educational representatives to support partnerships with neighboring businesses to investigate opportunities for experiential learning.

Inclusion

Inclusion is a vital principle for the comprehensive education of individuals with ASD. This principle is applied to guide the creation of opportunities for students to interact and participate in daily life alongside their peers who are neurotypical. An inclusive environment can be set up to foster a student's ability to work on social skills, language development, and relationships, which are crucial to successful participation in the community (Haring, 1992). In an inclusive educational environment, Daryl experienced increased exposure to and participation in pragmatic social interactions. As a result, he developed appropriate social skills and cultivated various types of social relationships.

In 2004, the U.S. Legislature reauthorized IDEA in order to better include parents in the process. Among other changes, the reauthorization mandated that parents be included in decisions of their child's eligibility, placement, and services (IDEA, 2004). According to the IDEA (2004), students must be educated in the least restrictive environment and included in a classroom with typically developing children to the fullest extent possible. To support these mandates, school district administrators are placing children of various abilities and disabilities in inclusive general education environments with appropriate, more advantageous supports. This approach is applied to support the assertion that both general education and special education students can thrive in inclusive and cooperative environments, both in school and in larger social systems.

Families with children who have ASD often experience feelings of separation from many typical societal activities. With the reauthorization of IDEA, parents are now empowered to express their desire to integrate their children within diverse, plentiful learning environments typical of general education. On a larger scope, these expressions have demonstrated the importance of reframing public perception of the meanings of "ability" and "disability" toward "differently-abled."

Career Development and Employment

Career development is a principle that includes consideration for an individual's choice of his or her life work and goal setting for employment. Organizations such as the Missouri Planning Council for Developmental Disabilities (2010) supports a commitment to full community participation for persons with disabilities. Such programs help job seekers in planning for, and achieving, community-based employment with competitive wages, and benefits. Tools and resources are available to assist individuals and service providers to help individuals with ASD and other developmental disabilities with prevocational, employment, and career-planning processes (Missouri Planning Council for Developmental Disabilities, 2010). One example is the Missouri Planning Council for Developmental Disabilities (2010) handbook, *A Guide for Career Discovery*, which walks the reader through the career-planning process.

Adjusting to a work environment is one of the most difficult tasks that an individual with ASD faces in his or her life. Ideally, employment should be gainful, as society places considerable value on productive work. However, it may begin as unpaid work that allows the young adult to practice skills, develop personal strengths, and contribute to the community. This may not provide a salary at first, but it provides other cultural and "social capital," such as social cohesion and personal investment in the community that has a different value (Bowles & Gintis, 2002).

There is a critical need to review the ways in which learners are prepared for adult life beyond the classroom, in the community, and on the job. It is important to consider all learners to be "employment-ready," to view first jobs as learning experiences, to promote creativity in job development, to provide coworker training, and to develop active ties with the local business community.

Daryl's work history in a local fast food restaurant was affected by environmental and social challenges. From these experiences and the identification of his interests and goals, Daryl was able to receive support and direction to investigate prospective appropriate employment opportunities. Ongoing, recurring, and evolving assessments and supports help identify and make valuable use of his personal strengths, as well as recognize and manage his challenges, in order to set a path for a meaningful and purposeful career path.

Longitudinal Curricula

Educators design longitudinal curricula to assure that there is career education across the student's academic life. As part of early childhood development, children begin developing work-related interests and proficiencies. Within their educational experience, children with ASD should be involved in functional and interactive work experiences to help identify and cultivate vocation awareness, desire, and related skills. With the identification and emergence of new competencies and interests, teachers can make associations with functional, work-related applications. As part of the process, other personal qualities can be encouraged and developed, such as cooperation, responsibility, self-reliance, and self-motivation. Repetitive and generalized application of proficiencies over the course of a child's academic life sets the course for more focused interests and refined skills at the time of adolescent transitioning.

An activity such as taking out the garbage develops responsibility, motivation, execution of routines, performance of repetitive tasks, and increased independence. The simplest of skills can be used to support career development and self-sufficiency (Lundine & Smith, 2009).

Business Connections and Alliances

It is essential that community agencies have personnel to support students with ASD. Nurses can foster supportive business connections and alliances can be as simple as providing staff to work with individuals on writing a resumé, job exploration, and job readiness. Such personnel can set up environments to support relationship building, social skill development, communication strategies, and experiential learning, as well as prevocational skills such as following directions, task completion, problem solving, and attention to safety.

Collaboration among leaders in educational institutions and local businesses will lead to opportunities for students to take on internships and paid work. According to Miller-Kuhaneck (2001), students with ASD are most likely to be employed after leaving school if they held paid jobs during high school.

In the case study, the APN provided a reference to the DVR, an organization that could provide Daryl with mentors or job coaches. Other connections included veterinarians, animal shelters, and rescue organizations. The school administrator could have formed partnerships with these organizations to create enriching experiences for adolescents.

INTIMACY AND SEXUALITY

Sexuality is a complex aspect of our personality and "self." Our sexuality is defined by sexual thoughts, desires and longings, erotic fantasies, and experiences. In many ways, sexuality is the force that empowers us to express and display strong, emotional feelings for another person and is a natural stimulus for the procreation of our species. The thing that attracts one person to another may not always be sexual—it could be sense of humor, personality, "likeability," compatibility, or intelligence. Sex or sexuality may only be a secondary consideration (Hellemans, Colson, Verbraeken, Vermeiren, & Deboutte, 2007; Stokes & Kaur, 2005; Tissot, 2009).

Many individuals with ASD face challenges similar to those of their neurotypical peers with regard to intimacy and sexuality. Social awareness increases during adolescence, and there is an overall desire to fit in and experience companionship with others. For individuals with ASD, this can be especially difficult, due to impulsivity, lack of insight on socially appropriate behavior, lack of empathy and an inability to apprehend others' perspectives, and difficulty understanding the consequences of behavior. While some adults with ASD choose not to pursue intimate relationships, those who do often remain ill prepared and have no one, outside their family, with whom they can discuss difficulties with (National Autistic Society, 2011).

Nurses can work with an adolescent to facilitate the development of relationships and to promote proper sexual health care. A nurse should maintain a rapport conducive to open discussion of topics of sexuality, relationships, and dating. Counseling with various options and strategies should be made based on the individual's cognitive, attitudinal, communication, and behavioral levels. Key relationship concepts include self-esteem and types and rules of relationships (respect and reciprocity) and gradually process to sexual intimacy. Related social skills themes include grooming and hygiene, body language, privacy, appropriate and inappropriate touching, listening, expression and understanding of feelings, cooperation, intimidation, and conflict resolution (Rao, Beidel, & Murray, 2007).

Sex Education

Attwood (2009) notes that the source of information on relationships for adolescents with Asperger's syndrome, for example, can be pornography for males and television "soap operas" for females. The person with Asperger's syndrome might assume that the actions in pornographic material provide a script of what to say or do on a date, but this misunderstanding might lead to a charge of sexual harassment or, rarely, a criminal charge for sexual offense (Attwood, 2009). The content of sex education for individuals with ASD is the same as for neurotypical adolescents and young adults. The best venue is a small group or one-to-one interaction with an instructor or trusted adult who is knowledgeable about the thinking and behavior of people with ASD. These might include teachers, counselors, or health care professionals with whom the individual has established rapport. It is important to include another individual to monitor the discussion for signs of potential abuse or misinterpretation of intent. Planning for sex education should include both the parent as well as the individual whenever possible and should be individualized according to the individual's learning style and social competence (Janzen, 2003).

Sex education for older adolescents may include content on sexual versus other kinds of attraction, sexual feelings, and masturbation. When and where appropriate, include sexual preference, love versus sex, depth and growth of relationships. Educate regarding safe sexual practices, including pregnancy, sexually transmitted diseases, and laws regarding consensual sex. Individuals with autism may not understand the social inappropriateness of masturbation. For them, masturbation may be an unreserved public expression of comfort, stress-relief, or diversion. The act may also be a method of entertaining predictable, animated responses from others (Human Sexuality Education and the Student with ASD, 2005). Diagrams labeling appropriate and inappropriate times, locations, and people can aid in guiding behavior.

As Daryl is a visual and active learner, responding least to listening and written text, effective teaching tools for Daryl include anatomically correct dolls, videos, body charts, interactive games, role-playing, social stories, and the like.

Sexual Behaviors

Adolescents with ASD may engage in behaviors such as public undressing, unrestricted fondling of genitalia, nonconsensual touching of others, or inappropriate sexual conversation or gestures. Other important educational targets include role-playing potentially unsafe situations and establishing clear cues to stop unacceptable activities. It is important to work with the individual on recognition and expression of sexual feelings and self-regulation of related behaviors (Mandell, Walrath, Manteuffel, Sgro, & Pinto-Martin, 2005; Spencer et al., 2005).

Nurses may teach private and personal care behaviors in the context of personal routines and use visual aids whenever possible. In addition, staff should avoid behavior that might be misinterpreted when observed by an individual with ASD. For instance, hugging and flirting with a person with ASD can arouse sexual feelings, and if the learner does not understand the context of the interaction, he or she has the potential to read the behavior differently than it was originally intended.

Risk for Abuse

People with ASD have the potential to be exploited by others due to their literal interpretation of words and actions, cognitive challenges, difficulty communicating their own thoughts and feelings, and general trusting and naïve nature (Janzen, 2003). Individuals with ASD who need assistance with self-care may be at additional risk for exploitation due to the ambiguity of body boundaries (Hellemans et al., 2007).

From early childhood, many individuals with an ASD have been taught compliance. This attribute, as well as common challenges with the interpretation of social cues and/or intellectual disabilities, contributes to vulnerability to abuse and victimization (Howlin & Clement, 1995). This same vulnerability may lead to the individual being a perpetrator of abuse. As individuals with ASD often lack understanding of appropriate social behaviors, they may not understand the meaning or consequences of their actions. Understanding and attitude toward sex and the capacity of consent should be assessed, as well as comprehension of abusive sexual behaviors. During counseling, one may reinforce the difference between acceptable and unacceptable sexual behaviors, establish strategies to prevent dangerous or unsolicited sexual activity, and aid in the discrimination between reasonable and unreasonable requests. Organizations like the Network of Victim Assistance (NOVA, 2008) have outreach experts who provide supports, counseling, and education programs for people with disabilities. This is one such organization from which a student may get specialized help when he or she has been the victim of a crime.

COMORBIDITIES THAT AFFECT TRANSITIONING

The most common comorbid psychiatric conditions in adolescents and young adults with ASD are anxiety, depression, and attention deficit hyperactivity disorder (ADHD; Klin & Volkmar, 2003). Anxiety may stem from having to deal with fast-paced social situations, which they are ill equipped to handle. Anxiety may worsen during adolescence, as young people face an increasingly complex social milieu and often become more aware of their differences and interpersonal difficulties. Large-scale epidemiological studies have not been conducted on the prevalence of co-occurring anxiety disorders in ASD, however, the studies reviewed here indicate that between 11% and 84% of children with ASD experience some degree of impairing anxiety (White et al., 2009).

Depression may be the result of multiple social failures. According to Ghaziuddin, Ghaziuddin, and Grede (2002), there is evidence that depression is the most common comorbid psychiatric disorder with individuals with ASD, and a person's depressive state depends upon their level of intelligence, age, gender, associated medical conditions, genetic factors, and life events.

ADHD and ASD are neurodevelopmental disorders with distinct diagnostic symptoms. ADHD is a result of difficulty with organization, executive functioning, and impulse control. Anxiety and poor stress management are common concerns in clinical samples of children with ASD. Those with combined symptoms of ASD and ADHD may exhibit more intense challenges in controlling behavior, focusing, and general functioning. For a detailed description of the comorbidities manifested in children with ASD, see Levy and colleagues (2010).

BEST PRACTICES: NURSING PLAN OF CARE

The social impairments in individuals with ASD involve deficits in speech, linguistic conventions and interpersonal interaction, social pragmatics, and poor speech prosody. Autism spectrum disorder consists of deficits in social reciprocity skills, regardless of cognitive or language ability. As a child grows into adolescence and young adulthood, social interactions becomes a more vital part of that individual's life. With increased awareness of his or her social differences, there may be a rise in anxiety, and this may lead to withdrawal, oppositional behaviors, increased need for routines or rituals, self-stimming behaviors, mood problems, and/or academic or occupational underachievement (Howlin & Goode, 1998; Myles, Bock, & Simpson, 2001; Schopler & Mesibov, 1983; Tantam, 2003). Individuals with ASD often report a desire for more peer social interaction and the desire to attend college and obtain employment in which they can gain independence. In turn, they also report more loneliness than their typically developing peers and a decrease in self-esteem (Bauminger & Kasari, 2000).

By utilizing the nursing process, nurses can develop a best practices care plan for adolescents with ASD to assist them in achieving their social, academic, and occupational potential. The nursing process includes assessment, diagnosis, planning, intervention, and evaluation (Souders, Levy, DePaul, & Freeman, 2002).

Assessment

During the assessment phase, the nurse takes a holistic approach to collecting information about the adolescent's health history and psychosocial and physical condition. Specific assessment tools are used when appropriate (Souders et al. 2002). For the purpose of this Chapter, we will discuss assessment tools that may be useful for the adolescent diagnosed with ASD.

Autistic Diagnostic Interview-Revised

The Autistic Diagnostic Interview-Revised (ADI-R; Lord, Rutter, & Le Couteur, 1994) is a structured interview that covers the individual's full developmental history and includes current behavior as well as past behaviors. It is administered by a licensed professional trained in using the ADI-R. Nurses can receive training in the clinical use of this tool. Currently, the interview consists of 93 questions spanning the main behavioral areas: communication, social development play, repetitive and restricted behavior, and general behavior.

The section of the ADI-R most useful for the transitioning adolescent encompasses current behaviors and how they are perceived differently by the adolescent and the caregiver. If there is a qualitative difference between these perceptions, this can be used by the nurse to predict the way employers or others in the community will experience the adolescent's behaviors. The assessment, administered to a caregiver familiar with the person with ASD, also contains questions about behaviors such as self-injury, aggression, and overactivity that help in developing treatment plans.

Autistic Diagnostic Observation Schedule

The Autistic Diagnostic Observation Schedule (ADOS; Lord, Rutter, DiLavore, & Risi, 2001) consists of interactive assessment modules tailored for individuals ranging in age from toddler to adult, with various activities providing observation of social and communication behaviors. For adolescents and adults, the ADOS Module IV can provide specific information about social behaviors and communication skills, such as reciprocal conversations and understanding of nonverbal gestures. This tool can also help the nurse to determine the person's interest in others' thoughts and emotions and his or her understanding and perceptions of relationships.

Stress Survey Schedule for Persons with Autism and Other Developmental Disabilities

The Stress Survey Schedule for Persons with Autism and Other Developmental Disabilities (Groden, Diller, Bausman, Velicer, Norman, & Cautela, 2001) was designed as a tool to measure stress in people with ASD. The tool is used to identify factors that impact stress levels for an individual on the autism spectrum. Through procedural analysis, various sources and dimensions of stress can be identified. These include anticipation/uncertainty, changes and threats, unpleasant and pleasant events, sensory/personal contact, food-related activity, social/environmental interactions, and ritual-related stress (Goodwin, Groden, Velicer, & Diller, 2007).

The Adolescent/Adult Sensory Profile

The Adolescent/Adult Sensory Profile (Brown & Dunn, 2002) is a tool that can be used to identify sensory-processing patterns and effects on functional performance. From this questionnaire, the nurse can cull information about the impact of common sensory experiences on behavior in different settings. The results can aid the nurse in raising awareness and developing supportive strategies (Brown & Dunn, 2002). People with ASD are often seen by others as acting in ways to receive additional sensory input or "sensory seeking." These behaviors may include rocking back and forth, spinning, head-banging, jumping, hand-flapping, or biting. These atypical behaviors often have a chilling effect on social interactions, leading to isolation (Miller-Kuhaneck, 2001). Problems with sensory processing and integration can interfere with ability to tolerate stress, handle change, maintain social relationships, and participate in society (Lawrence et al., 2010).

Child Behavior Checklist

The Child Behavior Checklist (CBCL) is a standardized checklist of behavioral problems that allows parents to evaluate their child's behavioral problems and social skills (Achenbach, 1991). The CBCL has extensive normative data, is widely used in national and international research, and has good psychometric properties. There is a Youth Self Report (YSR) version for older adolescents and adults. Total behavior problems, broad-band behavior problems (e.g., internalizing behavior problems, externalizing behavior problems), and more narrow-band behavior problems (e.g., attention problems, anxious/depressed moods, aggressive problems, delinquent problems) are assessed.

Other Tools

The Pervasive Developmental Disorder Behavior Inventory: The PDDBI (Cohen & Sudhalter, 2005) contains rating forms that are completed by parents, caregivers, and teachers. It provides a broader view of the person's behavior. These diagnostic tools provide the nurse with an understanding of the person's strengths and challenges, and problems that may affect the adolescent's transitioning and functionality as an adult. With this information, the nurse is equipped to initiate a qualified plan of care with appropriate interventions. In addition, a sensory evaluation is an important part of the process. There are a few simple steps to assessing sensory problems with the aim of recommending occupational therapy (see Exhibit 10.1).

Interventions

Individuals diagnosed with ASD have a strong need for uniformity in various aspects of home, social, academic, and occupational experiences. Slight changes in the course of a day can cause significant anxiety. Pragmatics of language, understanding sarcasm, and interpreting body language are often deficient in individuals with ASD. As nurses develop care plans, they should consider external stimuli and variables in the environment, such as talking, music,

EXHIBIT 10.1

Elements of Adolescent Occupational Therapy Sensory Evaluations

Conduct Interviews

Communicate with individual, educators, employers, parents, caretakers, and other appropriate individuals to identify and assess the individual's responses to environmental stimulation (likes, dislikes, challenges).

Create an Occupational Profile

Gather information from individual, educators, employers, parents, caretakers, and other appropriate individuals about individual's needs, challenges, skills, and concerns.

Observation

Observe how the individual responds in applicable environments. Extract information about the individual's responses to various sensory stimuli, and ascertain sensory-processing deficits that impact functioning and participation in routine activities.

lights, and noise from machines. The nursing care plan can serve as a guide through these experiences, providing strategies to maintain feelings of calm and preventing feelings of overwhelming anxiety that may lead to socially unacceptable behaviors. Providing tools for problem solving and techniques for self-calming are essential components in a nursing plan of care (Souders, Levy, DePaul, & Freeman, 2002).

Individualized Behavior Management

Students with ASD face various challenges during the transition process. Service providers must recognize these difficulties and tailor programs and services to their needs. Moreno and O'Neal (1999) identified several important principles in teaching and coaching individuals with ASD. These include support around organizational skills, appreciation of uneven skill development, need for literal and clear communication, social awareness, and the need for consistency among providers (Moreno & Neal, 1999).

Individualized behavior management practices are included as part of the transition plan. These should use positive, age-appropriate language (Miller-Kuhaneck, 2001). Selected approaches to behavioral management are described below. All are appropriate for the transitioning adolescent (Ikeda, 2002).

Applied Behavior Analysis

Applied behavior analysis (ABA) is a form of behavior modification used to reinforce positive behaviors; to build skills to improve social interaction, communication, and activities for daily living; and to reduce problem behaviors in learners with ASD of all ages. In this process, behaviors are broken into incremental steps and repeated opportunities to learn and practice skills in a variety of settings with positive reinforcement are offered. The nurse can use specific types of instruction, prompting, and reinforcement and can customize the steps according to the strengths and needs of the individual. Performance is measured continuously by direct observation, and intervention is modified as needed to advance and enable independent functioning in a variety of environments (Cohen, Amerine-Dickens, & Smith, 2006; Cooper, Heron, & Heward, 2007; Martin & Pear, 2011).

Naturalistic Approaches to Behavioral Management

Individuals with an ASD have difficulty transferring skills learned in one situation to another context. Naturalistic teaching strategies can be used by a nurse in a variety of naturally occurring environments or situations. In this approach one presumes that behaviors are more likely to be generalized to other situations when teaching sessions are gradually less structured, driven by the student's interests, take place in a variety of locations, and use a variety of stimuli. Furthermore, behaviors are more likely to be generalized when the reinforcements or consequences occur naturally and are not directed by the teacher (Dawson & Osterling, 1997; Mahoney & Perales, 2003).

In Daryl's case, the APN recognized his fondness for animals and experience walking the neighbor's dog. She also assessed his fears and concerns which included interacting with authority figures, struggling with social situations, and having low self-esteem. To work on these issues, she contacted a job coach and case manager and recommended making a connection with local veterinarians, animal shelters, and rescue organizations. In natural settings where Daryl had some comfort level, he would begin grooming and walking the animals. Job coaches and mentors can prompt, encourage, and expand positive social interactions in this environment until Daryl becomes more confident in generalizing and using these skills independently.

Pivotal Response Training: Pivotal response training (PRT) is one naturalistic approach. The goals of PRT are to teach a child to be responsive to multiple learning opportunities in a natural setting by providing multiple cues for responses. Pivotal response training is part of a comprehensive behavioral program and is used to teach motivation and responsiveness to multiple environmental cues that are commonly recognized as problems for people diagnosed with ASD (Harris, Handleman, & Jennett, 2005). The hope is that the student will generalize his or her response to the critical and relevant features of stimuli in novel situations (Koegel et al., 1999). Responsiveness to environmental cues is necessary to enable a student to attend to both visual and auditory stimulation. This, in turn, is necessary to enhance learning. When using PRT, the nurse should teach self-management and self-initiation (Souders, Levy, DePaul, Freeman, 2003).

Pivotal response training can be used in a one-to-one teaching setting or in the adolescent's natural environment. A cue is presented by the teacher, the adolescent produces a behavioral response, and a consequence is given for the behavior. This method is equally useful in a natural environment setting, and it decreases the prompting dependence that often develops in children with ASD (Miller-Kuhaneck, 2001).

Natural Environment Training: Sundberg and Partington (1998) developed the method of natural environment training (NET). In this method, the instructor assesses the current motivation and works to create an increase in the learner's spontaneity (Sundberg & Partington, 1998). The ability to make requests is the initial skill targeted by the nurse (Sundberg &

Partington, 1998). The instructor counts the learner's spontaneous requests with the aim of increasing frequency. The instructor serves as an agent of reinforcement, which builds rapport. Gradually, the instructor combines requests with instructional context and incrementally adds small delays in the receipt of desired items. The interaction includes the instructor's demands with the learner's requests, which builds rapport. Both NET and PRT interventions are based on the principles of ABA. The nurse emphasizes the use of internal motivation, teaching in natural contexts, and focusing on the student's interests to guide language instruction.

Sensory Integration

Sensory integration (SI) is a term used to describe the neurological function that involves organizing sensory information for use (Ayers, 1979). Sensory integration is used by the nurse to help the individual to process and integrate sensations experienced in the environment. Spitzer (1999) describes SI as a dynamic process of interactions that impact behavior and abilities based on the individual's ability to process internal and external stimuli. A sensory threshold refers to the level of strength that a stimulus must reach in order to be detected. Sensory-processing disorder (SPD) is a condition that exists when sensory signals are not organized into appropriate responses. A person with SPD finds it difficult to process and act upon information received through the senses. This may be observed by others as motor clumsiness, behavioral problems, anxiety, depression, or school failure (Sensory Processing Disorder Foundation, 2011).

Daryl responded best through visual observation and direct hands-on activity. He struggled in areas involving listening and reading. While he found certain noises and lighting problematic, the sensation from brushing the fur of animals was calming. These sensory factors affected Daryl's functioning and participation in activities.

People with ASD have to cope with constantly changing stimuli in a work or college environment such as changes in temperature, noise, and lighting. Another important sensory factor to consider is a person's proprioception, or internal sensory processing that provides information about the body's position in space. Appropriate proprioception is essential for the brain and body to communicate effectively and adapt to changing environments (Minshew, Sung, Jones, & Furman, 2004; Molloy, Dietrich, & Bhattacharya, 2003; Vernazza-Martin et al., 2005).

If an individual is overwhelmed by sensory stimulation and is not able to process these stimuli, negative behaviors may manifest and may result in increased anxiety, disruptive behavior, and aggression (Barnhill, 2007). An occupational therapy evaluation is useful in assessing an individual's sensory processing in order to generate methods of adaptive responses to environmental challenges.

Peer Mentors

An important goal for any adolescent as he or she is transitioning out of high school and into adulthood is to fit in and belong to a social group (Giarelli & Ruttenberg, unpublished manuscript). The adolescent with ASD struggles to form satisfying social relationships (Miller-Kuhaneck, 2001; Giarelli & Ruttenberg, unpublished manuscript). People with ASD tend to have false perceptions that affect social interactions and relationships (Locke, Ishijima, Kasari, & London, 2010). For example, individuals with ASD may understand words and language only in the most literal sense, have trouble seeing others' perspectives in situations, and believe that everything spoken is the absolute truth (Miller-Kuhaneck, 2001).

EXHIBIT 10.2

Resources and Supports for Nursing Interventions for Transitioning

Attainment Company, Inc. (2007). *Everybody's working: Learn how to become a successful employee.* Verona, WI: Author.

Autism Society (2007). *Autism information for child abuse counselors.* Retrieved from http://www.leanonus.org/images/CHILD_ABUSE_COUNSELORS.pdf

Autism Society of Canada (2005). *Human sexuality education and the student with ASD, Appendix E.* Retrieved from http://www.autismsocietycanada.ca/DocsAndMedia/KeyReports/MB_Supp_Schls_appendixe.pdf

Baker, J. (2006). *Preparing for life: The complete guide for transitioning to adulthood for those with autism and Asperger's syndrome.* Arlington, TX: Future Horizons.

Baker, J. (2003). *Social skills training for children and adolescents with Asperger syndrome and social-communications problems.* Shawnee Mission, KS: Autism Asperger Publishing.

Bruey, C., & Urban, M. (2009). *The autism transition guide: Planning the journey from school to adult life.* Bethesda, MD: Woodbine House.

Cowardin, N., & Stanfield, J. (1989). *Life facts 1: Sexuality, and Life facts 2: Sexual abuse prevention.* Santa Monica, CA: James Stanfield Publishing.

Dalrymple, N., Gray, S., & Ruble, L. (1991). *Sex education: Issues for the person with autism. Part of "functional programming for people with autism: A Series:"* Bloomington, IN: Indiana Resource Center for Autism, Indiana University.

Do2learn (2011). *Job tips.* Retrieved from http://www.do2learn.com/JobTIPS//index.html

Dunn Buron, K. (2007). *A 5 is against the law! Social boundaries: Straight up!* Overland Park, KS: Autism Asperger Publishing.

Faherty, C. (2000). What does it mean to me? *A workbook explaining self-awareness and life lessons to the child or youth with high functioning autism or Asperger's.* Arlington, TX: Future Horizons.

Fenwick, E., & Walker, R. (2004). *How sex works: A clear, comprehensive guide for teenagers to emotional, physical and sexual maturity.* London, UK: Dorling Kindersley.

Foxx, R. M. (1983). Stacking the deck: Teaching social skills to retarded adults with a modified table game. *Journal of Applied Behavior Analysis, 16*, 157–170.

Gerhardt, P. F., & Holmes, D. L. (2005). Employment: Options and issues for adolescents and adults with Autism. In F. Volkmar, R. Paul, A. Klin, & D. Cohen (Eds.), *Handbook of autism and pervasive developmental disorders* (pp. 1087–1101). New York: Wiley.

Gerhardt, P. F. (2007). Effective transition planning for learners with ASD. *Exceptional Parent, 37*(4), 26–27.

Getzel, E. E., & deFur, S. (1997). Transition planning for students with significant disabilities: Implications for student-centered planning. *Focus on Autism and Other Developmental Disabilities, 12*, 39–48.

(*Continued*)

EXHIBIT 10.2 (Continued)

Goldstein, A., & McGinnis, E. (1997). *Skill-streaming the adolescent: New strategies and perspectives for teaching prosocial skills.* Champaign, IL: Research Press.

Gray, S., Ruble, L., & Dalrymple, N. (1996). *Autism & sexuality: A guide for instruction.* Indianapolis, IN: Autism Society of Indiana.

Henault, I. (2005). *Asperger's syndrome and sexuality from adolescence through adulthood.* Philadelphia, PA: Jessica Kingsley.

Hendricks, D., Smith, M., & Wehman, P. (2009). Teaching youth for success: From classroom to community. In P. Wehman, M. Datlow Smith, & C. Schall, *Autism and the transition to adulthood: Success beyond the classroom* (pp. 109–136). Baltimore, MD: Paul H. Brookes.

Hingsburger, D., & Harber, M. (1998). *The ethics of touch: Establishing and maintaining appropriate boundaries in service to people with developmental disabilities.* DVD and manual, Ontario, Canada: Diverse City Publications.

Hingsburger, D., & Jobes, J. (2008). *The whole truth: An abuse prevention programme for people with intellectual disabilities.* Ontario, Canada: Diverse City Publications.

Hingsburger, D. (1995). *Hand-made love: A guide for teaching about male masturbation through understanding and video.* Ontario, Canada: Diverse City Press.

Hingsburger, D. (1995). *Just say know: Understanding and reducing the risk of sexual victimization of people with developmental disabilities.* Ontario, Canada: Diverse City Press.

Hingsburger, D. (1995). *Under Cover Dick: Teaching men with disabilities about condom use through understanding and video.* Ontario, Canada: Diverse City Press.

Hoke, S. (1995). *My body is mine, my feelings are mine.* Plainview, NY: Childswork/Childsplay.

Jackson, L. (2002). *Freaks, geeks and Asperger syndrome.* Philadelphia, PA: Jessica Kingsley.

Karakoussis, C., Calkins, C., & Eggeling, K. (1998). *Sexuality: Preparing your child with special needs—how to develop a plan for sex education and sexual abuse prevention.* Retrieved from http://www.moddrc.org/user_storage/File/SexualityPreparingYourChildwithSpecialNeeds.pdf

Keel, J. H., Mesibov, G. B., & Woods, A. V. (1997). TEACCH-supported employment program. *Journal of Autism and Developmental Disorders, 27,* 3–9.

Korpi, M. (2007). *Guiding your teenager with special needs through the transition from school to adult life: Tools for parents.* Philadelphia, PA: Jessica Kingsley.

Mahler, K. (2009). *Hygiene and related behaviors for children and adolescents with autism spectrum and related disorders: A fun curriculum with a focus on social understanding.* Overland Park, KS: Autism Asperger Publishing.

Maurer, L. (1999). *Talking sex! Practical approaches and strategies for working with people who have developmental disabilities when the topic is sex.* Ithaca, NY: Planned Parenthood of Tompkins County.

(*Continued*)

EXHIBIT 10.2 (Continued)

McIlwee Myers, J. (2010). *How to teach life skills to kids with autism or Asperger's.* Arlington, TX: Future Horizons.

Meyer, R. (2002). *Social skills and work: Advice for advanced level job seekers.* Retrieved from http://www.rogernmeyer.com/employment_social_skills_and_work.html

Meyer, R., & Attwood, T. (2001). *Asperger syndrome employment workbook: An employment workbook for adults with Asperger syndrome.* Philadelphia, PA: Jessica Kingsley.

Missouri Planning Council for Developmental Disabilities. (2011). *A Guide for career discovery.* Retrieved from http://www.mpcdd.com/pageDownload.php?docID= 3354

Müller, E., Schuler, A., Burton, B., & Yates, G. (2003). Meeting the vocational support needs of individuals with Asperger syndrome and other autism spectrum disabilities. *Journal of Vocational Rehabilitation, 18*, 163–175.

Newport, J. & Newport, M. (2002). *Autism-Asperger's & sexuality: Puberty and beyond.* Arlington, TX: Future Horizons.

Nietupski, J.A., & Hamre-Nietupski, S. (2000). A systematic process for carving supported employment positions for people with severe disabilities. *Journal of Developmental and Physical Disabilities, 12*(2), 103–119.

Organization for Autism Research. (2006). *Life's journey through autism, a guide for transition to adulthood.* Retrieved from www.researchautism.org/resources/reading/documents/transitionguide.pdf

Planned Parenthood of Northern New England (2010). *Developmental disabilities and sexuality curriculum sexuality education for adults with developmental disabilities.* Retrieved from http://www.plannedparenthood.org/ppnne/development-disabilites-sexuality-31307.htm

Rioux, M. (1997). *Out of harm's way: A safety kit for people with disabilities who feel unsafe and want to do something about it.* Ontario, Canada: Roeher Institute.

Schall, C., Cortijo-Doval, E., Targett, P. S., & Wehman, P. (2006). *Applications for youth with autism spectrum disorders.* In P. Wehman (Ed.), *Life beyond the classroom: Transition strategies for young people with disabilities* (pp. 535–575). Baltimore, MD: Paul H. Brookes.

Segar, M. (1997). *Coping: A survival guide for people with Asperger syndrome.* Nottingham, UK: The Early Years Diagnostic Centre.

Shalock, R. L., & Jensen, C. M. (1986). Assessing the goodness-of-fit between persons and their environment. *Journal of the Association for Persons with Severe Handicaps, 11*, 103–109.

Siperstein, M., & Rickards, E. (2003). *Promoting social success: A curriculum for children with special needs.* Baltimore, MD: Paul H. Brookes.

Smith Myles, B., Trautman, M., & Schlevan, R. (2004). *The hidden curriculum: Practical solutions for understanding unstated rules in social situations.* Overland Park, KS: Autism Asperger Publishing.

Smith, M.D., Belcher, R.G., & Juhrs, P.D. (1995). *A guide to successful employment for individuals with Autism.* Baltimore, MD: Paul H. Brookes.

(*Continued*)

EXHIBIT 10.2 (Continued)

Specialisterne (2004). *From unique skills to unique results.* Retrieved from http://specialisterne.dk/english/index.html

Stanford, A. (2003). *Asperger syndrome and long-term relationships.* Philadelphia, PA: Jessica Kingsley.

Coalition for Positive Sexuality (2011). Retrieved from http://www.positive.org/Home/index.html

National Autistic Society (2003). *Good practice guidelines for services—adults with Asperger syndrome.* Retrieved from http://www.sacramentoasis.com/docs/8-22-03/taking_responsibility.pdf

National Autistic Society (2011). *Social skills for adolescents and adults.* Retrieved from http://www.autism.org.uk/living-with-autism/communicating-and-interacting/social-skills/social-skills-for-adolescents-and-adults.aspx

Ticoll, M. (1992). *No more victims: Manual for counselors and social workers.* Ontario, Canada: Roeher Institute.

Unger, D., & Luecking, R. (1998). Work in progress: Including students with disabilities in school-to-work initiatives. *Focus on Autism and Other Developmental Disabilities, 13*(2), 94–100.

Unger, D., Parent, W., Gibson, K., Johnston, K., & Kregel, J. (1998). An analysis of the activities of employment specialists in a natural support approach to supported employment. *Focus on Autism and Other Developmental Disabilities, 13*(1), 27–38.

Visual Aids for Learning (2009). *The complete adolescent pack.* Retrieved from http://www.visualaidsforlearning.com/adolescent-pack-learning.htm

Wehman, P., Datlow Smith, M., & Schall, C. (2008). *Autism & the transition to adulthood: Success beyond the classroom.* Baltimore, MD: Paul H. Brookes.

Wrobel, M. (2003). *Taking care of myself: A healthy hygiene, puberty and personal curriculum for young people with autism.* Arlington, TX: Future Horizons.

Young Adult Institute (YAI) Network. *Relationships and Sexuality.* Retrieved from http://www.yai.org/resources/r-c/topic-relationships-and-sexuality.html

Young Adult Institute (YAI) Network (2010). *Relationship series.* Retrieved from http://www.youtube.com/watch?v=QXNi5YRpJ_A

Zaks, Z. (2006). *Life and love: Positive strategies for autistic adults.* Shawnee Mission, KS: Autism Asperger Publishing.

In the case study, Daryl obsessed about fears of failure. During a short-lived employment experience, he was unable to comprehend the meaning of, "A busy mind is a healthy mind," as he understood literal expressions verbatim. He deliberated over possibilities of misinterpretations, being overwhelmed, and ineptitude. Daryl was preoccupied with a high school relationship encounter, which he felt impaired the success of any future personal relationships. He had limited comprehension of social rules or interpersonal skills. This lack of understanding and mounting frustration contributed to his feelings of failure.

Video modeling, role-playing, social skills groups, social comic strips, and peer mentors are examples of some effective tools that could be used to improve Daryl's social skills set. See Exhibit 10.2 for a comprehensive list of resources available to nurses as they assist adolescents in managing their behavioral problems.

People with ASD are often viewed as different because of their limited and restricted interests and unusual behaviors. Because of this, they are at high risk for being targeted by bullies and victimized (Shtayerman, 2007). Adolescents with ASD might become increasingly isolated and depressed due to social failure. Young people with ASD may therefore gravitate toward superficial relationships, such as through social networking sites on the Internet, in which they do not need to have close physical proximity or reciprocal communication with another person. While this not necessarily unhealthy, it may replace other social experiences. A peer mentor can be particularly valuable for adolescents during this difficult time to serve as a role model, a confidant, and a guide for social skill development (Lawrence et al., 2010). Peer mentors are paired with people with ASD to assist with challenges, provide supports, offer encouragement, and cultivate relationships. They can provide social, personal, academic, and/or work-related guidance and support.

Social Skills Training

Social skills training for individuals with ASD may be helpful to increase social awareness, competence, and overall independence. Therapeutic intervention for social skill development in adolescents employs the techniques of modeling and role-playing. Adolescents gain competence and confidence in handling mature social interactions and conflicts and can gain the skills necessary to self-regulate behaviors and emotions (Goldstein & McGinnis, 1997; Scattone et al., 2002). Adolescents can benefit from social skill development, such as planned classroom interactions, peer relationship and friendship development, practice sessions for understanding and managing emotions and related behaviors, conflict resolution, stress and anger management, and problem solving.

Because each person exhibits unique strengths and deficits, these exercises should be tailored to an individual's needs. Most naturally occurring day-to-day interactions are not ideal opportunities to learn these social skills. Structured groups that specifically work on social skills are often more useful (Miller-Kuhaneck, 2001; Mackay, Knott, & Dunlop, 2007). Social skill groups can be designed to match the needs of children at all levels of ability. The groups are ideal for children with autism or Asperger's syndrome, as these children are frequently included in school or community settings, yet lack the natural ability to interact with others socially. Peer groups are especially effective (Middleton, Zollinger, & Keene, 1986). Goals may be set for each group with an emphasis on solving interpersonal problems or developing friendships. These groups may be most successful when they occur outside of a traditional clinic setting and in a more natural environment in the community (Janzen, 2003; Solomon, Goodlin-Jones, & Anders, 2004).

A first step in developing social objectives and articulating the methods for measuring and evaluating progress toward those goals is to continually ask the question, "How will we measure a satisfactory outcome?" For example, for the objective of improved conversational reciprocity, the focus should be on identifying "How will we know when his/her reciprocal conversation skills have improved?" Precise behaviors related to this outcome can then be observed and measured in naturally occurring and contrived situations. For example, outcomes associated with this objective for a particular learner may be: (a) an increased number of conversational exchanges; (b) an increased number of questions directed to the conversational partner; and (c) an increase in the demonstration of eye contact linked with verbal statements (Kraijer, 2000).

Social support groups, facilitated by a nurse, can bridge skill development when a person with ASD is no longer in school and therefore has fewer opportunities for practice. Such groups can be held in community settings and should start and end with a familiar routine. Social support groups are beneficial to individuals with ASD, as they provide an environment in which others understand their unique issues and in which they can have fun and learning new coping skills (Janzen, 2003).

Personal hygiene: Teaching self-care skills to adolescents is important, because these abilities will increase adolescent success in getting ready for work, as well as influence how employers and coworkers will perceive them. In fact, maintaining a neat appearance and following a dress code are requirements for most jobs. Skills training can include written or pictorial schedules that prompt the person to go to the restroom and check their appearance.

Fears, obsessions, and/or resistance to elements of personal hygiene are common in people with ASD. In addition, there is often a lack of awareness or understanding of the necessity of hygienic practices, the differentiation between public and private hygiene, appropriate use of personal care items, as well as the relationship of hygiene in social interactions. Consideration of sensitivity to soaps, deodorants, toothpastes, shampoos, and other products may be a factor. For the adolescent with ASD, understanding hormonal changes and related personal care is an additional challenge. In this regard, teaching personal and oral cleanliness and care is associated with daily routines.

Stress Management

A person experiences stress as a natural response to circumstances and conditions presented in life. Psychologists and educators have researched the function and relevance of various types of stress at different points of developmental ages (Baron, Groden, Groden, & Lipsitt, 2006). Researchers have determined that people with ASD encounter increased stress levels in comparison with those who are typically developing or have other disabilities (Hess, 2009). Due to the prevalence of anxiety in this population, Hess (2009) recommends that those serving these individuals have resources with which to measure the extent and the nature of their anxiety.

For a young adult with autism, the college environment can trigger heightened stress levels in many of these categories. When developing the plan of care, the nurse should discuss how the individual's ASD characteristics interface with the new environment in order to develop appropriate strategies to prepare, reduce, and respond to stressful situations. Yoga, deep breathing, and meditation are some techniques used for self-calming (Doman & Lockhart, 2003). Other interventions are social stories, video modeling, and materials that can familiarize the person with situations to reduce fears and anxieties. Nurses can help counsel on recognizing the need for calming techniques and can help with identifying appropriate locations and applications of these techniques. Lytle and Todd (2009) advise that understanding the stress response in the typical individual and the irregularities of the response in individuals with ASD can help the nurse better comprehend why stress-reduction strategies are important in planning learning environments for these students.

Sensory Stimulation

Sound stimulation has been used in conjunction with therapeutic, neurodevelopmental, academic, and behavioral programs in an effort to improve listening by facilitating the integration and organization in sensory and motor systems (Baranek, 2002). Some practitioners use sound stimulation in attempts to increase the rate of acquiring skills and desired outcomes. Desensitization to sound may be a way to create a more comfortable environment and eliminate the need to protect oneself from undesirable or uncomfortable sounds (Doman & Lockhart, 2003).

Sensory stimulation is not limited to sound. Individuals may be agitated or calmed by touch. Certain fabrics, textures, seams in clothing, or tags can be a source of significant distress for certain individuals. The nurse may suggest seamless socks, tagless clothing, or a change in fabric or texture, all of which may provide more comfort and potentially reduce sensory agitation. Desensitizing is a behavior modification technique that can be used by the nurse to help individuals become tolerant of different textures, such as sand, dirt, or grass (Ayers, 1979). Strategies are taught to help the young adult learn to wear certain fabrics in work environments and more tolerable fabrics in other settings. Modifications or alternatives to uniform requirements may need to be discussed with an employer. See Table 10.1. for a sample of a nursing care plan for Daryl.

TABLE 10.1 ■ Nursing Plan of Care for Daryl

Areas of concerns	Details	Interventions
Anxiety	Concern of future failure based on past events/ruminating thoughts of failure, as well as hopelessness and negative thoughts	• Teach behavior modification techniques for decreasing anxiety (e.g., yoga, deep breathing). • Provide positive reinforcement of successes, redirect repetitive discussion.
	Mood/affect in the home setting, becoming irritable	• Teach Daryl and his family to replace irritable behavior with an acceptable technique to release stress. • Acknowledge the changes occurring as Daryl matures to adulthood. • Utilize ABA techniques to encourage positive behaviors, replacing ineffective coping skills.
Managing change	Change from high school to college	• Utilize educational counseling for life coaching and support in the college setting. • Teach Daryl and his family how to find colleges that offer educational assistance for special needs students. • Reinforce positive educational experiences Daryl has had in the past. • Remind Daryl and his family to execute the process in small steps. Provide positive reinforcement as each step is accomplished.
	Obtain and retain a job where he will increase his	Helping Daryl find a job working with animals at the veterinary office was a good idea.

(*Continued*)

TABLE 10.1 ■ Continued

Areas of concerns	Details	Interventions
	independence and be successful (enjoys working with animals, easily agitated by loud noise and fluorescent lights)	Interventions may include: • Teach Daryl to adapt to loud noises and lights using ABA techniques and to express his concerns through coaching. Daryl can learn how to explain his strengths and weaknesses to his boss. • Help Daryl work with his boss to develop a collaborative work environment conducive to Daryl's special needs and job requirements.
	Unexpected changes	Daryl may encounter unexpected changes • Utilize ABA techniques to teach adaptive skills. • Support Daryl's use of calming techniques, such as deep breathing, when anxiety arises from unexpected occurrences. For instance, he can calm himself with a piece of soft cloth by taking a few minutes to rub the fabric in order to decrease his anxiety. • Help Daryl arrange to have a coach or counselor he can access as needed.
Social skills	Friends/relationships	• Use role modeling and reinforcement techniques to help Daryl understand issues of personal hygiene, personal space, and conversational speech. • Utilize a group approach to teach and reinforce social skills. • Have ongoing discussions regarding various relationship situations, emphasizing how a relationship develops in small, simple steps. • Raise awareness of appropriate human touch. Help Daryl express his comfort level regarding touch. Teach socially acceptable behaviors. • Maintain ongoing discussions and use videos to ensure Daryl's clear understanding of legal implications of verbal and physical sexual activity.

SUMMARY

This chapter has focused on the issues faced by adolescents diagnosed with ASD in their transition to adulthood. As Daryl's case study shows, these young adults face challenges associated with social skill and communication deficits, anxiety, and sensory issues. These factors can have an impact on the individual's abilities to function with less structure in a more complex, mature environment. In order to appropriately intervene, nurses must be aware of the legal mandates, principles, and resources that are available to support individuals with ASD and their families as they cope with the challenges of transitioning. The IDEA mandates transition planning in preparation for post-high school experiences. Validated tools are available to evaluate the individual's functioning.

Teaching and mentoring techniques should be conducted in naturalistic environments, keeping in mind the principles of ABA. As depicted in the case study, the transition plan should be developed by the nurse based on the individual's challenges and strengths and should focus on the need for advocacy and planning. While career planning is essential, the nurse must also be aware of the need to help the individual develop social skills and increase knowledge in order to meet their intimacy, sexuality, and personal care needs. A team approach to developing an individualized, person-centered plan of care that incorporates the guiding principles for successful transition will help to facilitate success and support a meaningful and functional adult life for the individual with ASD.

REFERENCES

Achenbach, T. M. (1991). *Integrative guide to the 1991 CBCL/4-18, YSR, and TRF profiles.* Burlington, VT: Department of Psychology, University of Vermont.

American Association on Intellectual and Developmental Disabilities. (2011). Supports Intensity Scale. Retrieved from http://www.aaidd.org/content_918.cfm?navID=96

Americans with Disabilities Act (ADA). (1990). Retrieved from http://www.ada.gov/archive/adastat91.htm

Attwood, T. (2009, March 16). Romantic lives of young adults with Asperger's. *Opposing Views.* Retrieved from http://www.opposingviews.com/i/romantic-lives-of-young-adults-with-asperger-s

Ayers, A. (1979). *Sensory integration and the child.* Los Angeles, CA: Western Psychology Services.

Ballaban-Gil, K., Rapin, L., Tuchman, T., & Shinnar, S. (1996). Longitudinal examination of the behavioral, language, and social changes in a population of adolescent and young adults with autistic disorder. *Pediatric Neurology, 15,* 217–223.

Baranek, G. T. (2002). Efficacy of sensory and motor interventions for children with autism. *Journal of Autism and Developmental Disorders, 32,* 397–422.

Barnhill, J. (2007). Outcomes in adults with Asperger's syndrome. *Focus on Autism and Other Developmental Disabilities, 2,* 116–136.

Baron, M. G., Groden, J., Groden, G., & Lipsitt, L. P. (2006). *Stress and coping in autism.* New York: Oxford University Press.

Bateman, B. D. (2005). Legal requirements for transition components of the IEP. Retrieved from http://www.wrightslaw.com/info/trans.legal.batement.htm

Bauminger, N., & Kasari, C. (2000). Loneliness and friendship in high functioning children with autism. *Child Development, 71,* 447–456.

Bowles, S., & Gintis, S. (2002). Social capital and community governance. *The Economic Journal, 112,* 419–436.

Brown, C., & Dunn, W. (2002). *Adolescent/Adult Sensory Profile manual.* San Antonio, TX: Psychological Corporation.

Cermak, S. A., & Ben-Sasson, A. (2007). Sensory processing disorders in children with autism nature, assessment, and intervention. In R. L. Gabriels, & D. E. Hill (Eds.), *Growing up with Autism; Working with school-age children and adolescents* (pp. 95–123). New York: Guilford Press.

Cimera, R. E., & Cowan, R. J. (2009). The costs of services and employment outcomes achieved by adults with autism in the US. *Autism, 13*(3), 285–302.

Cohen, H., Amerine-Dickens, M., & Smith, T. (2006). Early intensive behavioral treatment: Replication of the UCLA model in a community setting. *Journal of Developmental and Behavioral Pediatrics, 27*(suppl), S145–S155.

Cohen, I. L., & Sudhalter, V. (2005). *The PDD Behavior Inventory.* Lutz, FL: Psychological Assessment Resources.

Cooper, J. O., Heron, T. E., & Heward, W. L. (2007). *Applied behavioral analysis* (2 ed.). Upper Saddle River, NJ: Pearson.

Coulter, D. (2001). *Asperger syndrome: Transition to college and work.* Retrieved from http://www.coultervideo.com.

Dawson, G., & Osterling, J. (1997). Early intervention in autism: Effectiveness and common elements of current approaches. In M. J. Guralnick (Ed.), *The effectiveness of early intervention: Second generation research* (pp. 307–326). Baltimore, MD: Paul H. Brookes.

Dell, A. G. (2004). Transition: There are no IEP's in college. *TECH-NJ, 15*(1). Retrieved from http://www.tcnj.edu/~technj/2004/transition.htm

Doman, A., & Lockhart, D. L. (2003). Using the Listening Program in the treatment of autism. *Autism Asperger's Digest (May–June).* Retrieved from http://www.thelisteningprogram.com/PDF/Case_Studies/7_Article_Using_TLP_Autism_2.pdf

Eaves, L. C., & Ho, H. H. (2008). Young adult outcomes of autism spectrum disorders. *Journal of Autism and Developmental Disorders, 38*, 739–747.

Education of All Handicapped Children Act (1975). *Public Law 94-142*. Retrieved from http://www.scn.org/~bk269/94-142.html

Geller, L., & Greenberg, M. (2010). Managing the transition process from high school to college and beyond: Challenges for individuals, families, and society. *Social Work in Mental Health, 8*, 92–116.

Gerhardt, P. F. (2006/2007). Effective transition planning for learners with ASD approaching adulthood. *Impact, 19*(3). Retrieved from http://ici.umn.edu/products/impact/193/over11.html

Ghaziuddin, M., Ghaziuddin, N., & Grede, J. (2002). Depression in persons with autism: Implications for research and clinical care. *Journal of Autism and Developmental Disorders, 32*(4), 299–306.

Giarelli, E., & Ruttenberg, J. (unpublished manuscript). "Staying afloat in a sea-change": Transition to community by adolescents with Asperger's syndrome.

Goodwin, M., Groden, J., Velicer, W., & Diller, A. (2007). Brief report: Validating the stress survey schedule for persons with autism and other developmental disabilities. *Focus on Autism and Other Developmental Disabilities, 22*, 183–189.

Goldstein, A., & McGinnis, E. (1997). Skill-streaming the adolescent: New strategies and perspectives for teaching prosocial skills. Champaign, IL: Research Press.

Grandin, T. (1996). *Making the transition from the world of school into the world of work.* Center for the Study of Autism. Retrieved from http://www.autism.org/temple/transition.html

Groden, J., Diller, A., Bausman, M., Velicer, W., Norman, G., & Cautela, J. (2001). The development of a stress survey schedule for persons with autism and other developmental disabilities. *Journal of Autism and Developmental Disorders, 31*(2), 207–217.

Haring, T. G. (1992). Social relationships. In L. H. Meyer, C. A. Peck, & L. Brown (Eds.), *Critical issues in lives of people with severe disabilities* (pp. 195–218). Baltimore, MD: Paul H. Brookes.

Harris, S. L., Handleman, J. S., & Jennett, H. K. (2005). Models of educational intervention for students with autism: Home, center, and school-based programming. In F. R. Volkmar, R. Paul, A. Klin, & D. J. Cohen (Eds.), *Handbook of autism and pervasive developmental disorders* (vol. 2, 3 ed., pp. 1043–1054). Hoboken, NJ: Wiley.

Hendricks, D. (2010). Employment and adults with autism spectrum disorders: Challenges and strategies for success. *Journal of Vocational Rehabilitation, 32*(2), 125–134.

Helen Sanderson Associates (n.d.). *What is person centered planning?* Retrieved from http://www.helensandersonassociates.co.uk/media/14189/what%20is%20person%20centred%20planning.pdf

Hellemans, H., Colson, K., Verbraeken, C., Vermeiren, R., & Deboutte, D. (2007). Sexual behavior in high-functioning male adolescents and young adults with autism spectrum disorder. *Journal of Autism and Developmental Disorders, 37*(2), 260–269. Retrieved from http://ovidsp.ovid.com/ovidweb.cgi?T=JS&PAGE=reference&D=medl&NEWS=N&AN=16868848.

Hess, K. (2009). Stress for individuals with Autism Spectrum Disorders: Effects of age, gender, and intelligence quotient. *Educational Psychology and Special Education Dissertations. Paper 58.* Retrieved from http://digitalarchive.gsu.edu/epse_diss/58

Howlin, P., & Goode, S. (1998). Outcome in adult life for people with autism and Asperger's syndrome. In F. R. Volkmar (Ed.), *Autism and pervasive developmental disorders* (pp. 209–241). New York: Cambridge University Press.

Howlin, P., & Clement, J. (1995). Is it possible to assess the impact of abuse on children with pervasive developmental disorders? *Journal of Autism & Developmental Disorders, 25*(4), 337–354.

Howlin, P., Goode, S., Hutton, J., & Rutter, M. (2004). Adult outcome for children with autism. *Journal of Child Psychology and Psychiatry, 45*, 212–229.

Human sexuality education and the student with ASD (2005). In Manitoba Education, Citizenship and Youth (Eds.), *Supporting inclusive schools: A handbook for developing and implementing programming for students with autism spectrum disorder* (pp. 107–112). Winnipeg, Manitoba: Crown in Right of Manitoba. Retrieved from http://www.autismsocietycanada.ca/DocsAndMedia/KeyReports/MB_Supp_Schls_appendix.pdf

Humphrey, N., & Lewis, S. (2008). "Make me normal": The views and experiences of pupils on the autistic spectrum in mainstream secondary schools. *Autism, 12*(1), 23–46.

Ikeda, M. J. (2002). Best practices for supporting students with autism. In A. Thomas, & J. Grimes (Eds.), *Best practices in school psychology* (IV, vol. I, pp. 1501–1512). Bethesda, MD: The National Association of School Psychologists.

Janzen, J. (2003). *Understanding the nature of autism* (2 ed.). San Antonio, TX: Therapy Skill Builders.

Klin, A., & Volkmar, F. (2003). Asperger syndrome: Diagnosis and external validity. *Child and Adolescent Psychiatric Clinics of North America, 12*, 1–13.

Koegel, L. K., Koegel, R. L., Shoshan, Y., & McNerney, E. (1999). Pivotal response intervention, II: Preliminary long-term outcomes data. *Journal of the Association of Personality and Severe Handicaps, 24,* 186–198.

Kraijer, D. (2000). Review of adaptive behavior studies in mentally retarded persons with autism/pervasive developmental disorder. *Journal of Autism and Developmental Disorders, 30*(1), 39–47.

Lawrence, D., Alleckson, D., & Bjorklund, P. (2010). Beyond the roadblocks: transitioning to adulthood with Asperger's disorder. *Archives of Psychiatric Nursing, 24,* 227–238.

Levy, S. E., Giarelli, E., Lee, L.-C., Schieve, L. A., Kirby, R., Cunniff, C., … Rice, C. (2010). Autism spectrum disorder and co-occurring developmental, psychiatric, and medical conditions among children in multiple populations of the United States. *Journal of Developmental & Behavioral Pediatrics, 31*(4), 267–275.

Locke, J., Ishijima, E. H., Kasari, K., & London, N. (2010). Loneliness, friendship quality and the social networks of adolescents with high-functioning autism in an inclusive school setting. *Journal of Research in Special Educational Needs, 10*(2), 74–81.

Lord, C., Rutter, M., & Le Couteur, A. (1994). Autism Diagnostic Interview-Revised: a revised version of a diagnostic interview for caregivers of individuals with possible pervasive developmental disorders. *Journal of Autism and Developmental disorders.*

Lord, C., Rutter, M., DiLavore, P. C., & Risi, S. (2001). *Autism Diagnostic Observation Schedule.* Los Angeles, CA: Western Psychological Services.

Lundine, V., & Smith, C. (2009). Transitioning from high school to work—Preparing students with autism for adulthood. *ACT-Autism Community Training.* Retrieved from http://www.youtube.com/watch?v=D0P93zn5OZ8

Lytle, R., & Todd, T. (2009). Stress and the student with Autism Spectrum Disorders: Strategies for stress reduction and enhanced learning. *Teaching Exceptional Children, 41*(4), 36–42.

Mackay, T., Knott, F., & Dunlop, A. W. (2007). Developing social interaction and understanding in individuals with autism spectrum disorder: A groupwork intervention. *Journal of Intellectual & Developmental Disabilities, 32,* 279–290.

Mahoney, G., & Perales, F. (2003). Using relationship-focused intervention to enhance the social-emotional functioning of young children with autism spectrum disorders. *Topics in Early Child Special Education, 23,* 77–89.

Mandell, D. S., Walrath, C. M., Manteuffel, B., Sgro, G., & Pinto-Martin, J. A. (2005). The prevalence and correlates of abuse among children with autism served in comprehensive community-based mental health settings. *Child Abuse & Neglect, 29*(12), 1359–1372.

Martin, G., & Pear, J. (2011). *Behavior modification: What it is and how to do it* (9 ed.). Upper Saddle River, NJ: Pearson.

McDonough, J. T., & Revell, G. (2010). Accessing employment supports in the adult system for transitioning youth with autism spectrum disorders. *Journal of Vocational Rehabilitation, 32*(2), 89–100.

Middleton, H., Zollinger, J., & Keene, R. (1986). Popular peers as change agents for the socially neglected child in the classroom. *Journal of School Psychology, 24,* 343–350.

Miller-Kuhaneck, H. (2001). *Autism: A comprehensive occupational therapy approach.* Bethesda, MD: American Occupational Therapy Association.

Minshew, N. J., Sung, K., Jones, B. L., & Furman, J. M. (2004). Underdevelopment of the postural control system in autism. *Neurology, 63*(11), 2056–2061.

Missouri Planning Council for Developmental Disabilities (2010). *A guide for career discovery.* Retrieved from http://www.mpcdd.com/pageDownload.php?docID=3354

Molloy, C. A., Dietrich, K. N., & Bhattacharya, A. (2003). Postural stability in children with autism spectrum disorder. *Journal of Autism and Developmental Disorders, 33*(6), 643–652.

Moreno, C., & O'Neal, C. (1999). *Tips for teaching high functioning people with autism.* Crown Point, IN: MAAP Services.

Myles, B. S., Bock, S. J., & Simpson, R. L. (2001). *Asperger syndrome diagnostic scale.* Austin, TX: Pro-Ed.

National Autistic Society. (2002). *Good practice guidelines for services—Adults with Asperger syndrome.* Retrieved from http://www.sacramentoasis.com/docs/8-22-03/taking_responsibility.pdf

National Autistic Society. (2011). *Social skills for adolescents and adults.* Retrieved from http://www.autism.org.uk/socialskills

Network of Victim Assistance. (2008). *At risk groups—People with disabilities.* Retrieved from http://www.nova-bucks.org/atriskgroups.html

North Carolina Division of Mental Health, Developmental Disabilities and Substance Abuse Services (2011). *Support Planning Process Supports Intensity Scale.* Retrieved from http://www.ncdhhs.gov/mhddsas/sis/index.htm

Nuehring, M. L., & Sitlington, P. L. (2003). Transition as a vehicle: Moving from high school to an adult vocational service provider. *Journal of Disability Policy Studies, 14*(1), 23–25.

Pacer Center (2011). *Help your young adult learn about accessing accommodations after high school.* Retrieved from http://www.pacer.org/parent/php/php-c165.pdf

Rao, P., Beidel, D., & Murray, M. (2007). Social skills interventions for children with Asperger's syndrome or high-functioning autism: A review and recommendations. *Journal of Autism and Developmental Disorders, 38*, 353–361.

Scattone, D., Wilczynski, S. M., Edwards, R. P., & Rabian, B. (2002). Decreasing disruptive behaviors of children with autism using social stories. *Journal of Autism and Developmental Disorders, 32*, 535–543.

Schall, C. M., & McDonough, J. T. (2010a). Autism spectrum disorders: Transition and employment. *Journal of Vocational Rehabilitation, 32*(2), 79–80.

Schall, C. M., & McDonough, J. T. (2010b). Autism spectrum disorders in adolescence and early adulthood: Characteristics and issues. *Journal of Vocational Rehabilitation, 32*(2), 81–88.

Schopler, E., & Mesibov, G. (1983). *Autism in adolescents and adults.* New York, NY: Plenum.

Sensory Processing Disorder Foundation. (2011). *About SPD.* Retrieved from http://www.spdfoundation.net/about-sensory-processing-disorder.html

Shtayerman, O. (2007). Peer victimization in adolescents and young adults diagnosed with Asperger's syndrome: A link to depressive symptomatology, anxiety symptomatology and suicidal ideation. *Issues in Comprehensive Pediatric Nursing, 30*(3), 87–103.

Solomon, M., Goodlin-Jones, B., & Anders, F. (2004). A social adjustment enhancement intervention for high functioning autism, Asperger's syndrome, and pervasive developmental disorder-NOS. *Journal of Autism and Developmental Disorders, 34*, 649–668.

Souders, M., Levy, S., DePaul, D., & Freeman, K. (2002). Caring for children and adolescents with autism who require challenging procedures. *Pediatric Nursing, 28*(6), 555–562.

Spencer, N., Devereux, E., Wallace, A., Sundrum, R., Shenoy, M., Bacchus, C., & Logan, S. (2005). Disabling conditions and registration for child abuse and neglect: A population-based study. *Pediatrics, 116*(3), 609–613.

Spitzer, S. (1999). Dynamic systems theory: Relevance to the theory of sensory integration and the study of occupation. *Sensory Integration Special Interest Section Quarterly, 22*(6), 1–4.

Stokes, M. A., & Kaur, A. (2005). High-functioning autism and sexuality: A parental perspective. *Autism, 9*(3), 266–289.

Sundberg, M. L., & Partington, J. W. (1998). *Teaching language to children with autism or other developmental disabilities.* Pleasant Hill, CA: Behavior Analysts.

Tantam, D. (2003). The challenge of adolescents and adults with Asperger's syndromes. *Child and Adolescent Psychiatric Clinics of North America, 12*(1), 143–163.

Taylor, E., & Seltzer, M. M. (2010). Changes in the autism behavioral phenotype during the transition to adulthood. *Journal of Autism and Developmental Disorders, 40*(12), 1431–1446.

Taylor, J. L., & Seltzer, M. M. (2011). Employment and postsecondary educational activities for young adults with autism spectrum disorder during the transition to adulthood. *Journal of Autism and Developmental Disorders, 41*, 566–574.

Tissot, C. (2009). Establishing a sexual identity: Case studies of learners with autism and learning difficulties. *Autism, 13*(6), 551–566.

U.S. congress. Individuals with Disabilities Education Act, 1990 (IDEA). Retrieved from http://www.idea.ed.gov/. Accessed March 3, 2012.

U.S. Department of Justice (2008). *Americans with Disabilities Amendments Act of 2008* (P.L. 110–325). Retrieved from http://www.ada.gov/pubs/ada.htm

U.S. Department of Labor, Office of Disability Employment Policy (2011). *Disability employment statistics released.* Retrieved from http://www.dol.gov/odep/

Vernazza-Martin, S., Martin, N., Vernazza, A., Lepellec-Muller, A., Rufo, M., Massion, J., & Assaiante, C. (2005). Goal directed locomotion and balance control in autistic children. *Journal of Autism and Developmental Disorders, 35*(1), 91–102.

Wehmeyer, M. L. (1992). Self-determination and the education of students with mental retardation. *Education and Training in Mental Retardation and Developmental Disabilities, 27*, 302–314.

White, S., Oswald, D., Ollendick, T., & Scahill, L. (2009). Anxiety in children and adolescents with autism spectrum disorders. *Clinical Psychology Review, 29*(3), 216–229.

Caring for Women With Asperger's Syndrome During the Childbearing Cycle

11

Joan Rosen Bloch, Karen J. Lecks, and Patricia Dunphy Suplee

While the published literature on autistic spectrum disorders (ASD) has substantially increased over the last two decades, and more individuals have been formally diagnosed with Asperger's syndrome (AS), insufficient evidence-based guidelines exist to guide those caring for women with AS during their reproductive years, especially during pregnancy and childbirth. Prior to the 1990s, few females were given diagnoses of AS, but that changed in the 1990s (Hollander, Kolevzon, & Coyle, 2011). Girls who were diagnosed then are now reaching their adult years. Increasingly, obstetrical health care providers will be caring for women who present to prenatal care with a confirmed diagnosis of AS. It is possible that in the past, health care providers cared for women who were previously undiagnosed or misdiagnosed, and the formal diagnosis of AS was not integrated into their plan of care. Today, that is different. In addition, many individuals diagnosed with AS have a variety of medical and behavioral therapeutic plans that have important implications for their health and well-being during childbearing.

The objective of this chapter is to provide guidance to nurses, based on the existing evidence, on how to better understand the diagnosis of AS and the related nursing care needs for women with AS during the childbearing period. In reviewing the literature for this chapter, the absence of research to guide health care professionals as they care for women with AS during their reproductive years was compelling. Thus, the authors researched, synthesized, and integrated evidence-based literature related to AS to inform and guide the nursing care of women with AS during pregnancy and postpartum and further into the mothering period. Information gathered from reaching out to mothers with AS themselves also informed this chapter. We reached out in order to promote a better understanding of their childbearing experiences and to seek recommendations about the ways that clinicians can better provide nursing care during their pregnancy and childbirth experience.[1]

Advanced practice nurses (APNs) managing care during pregnancy, childbirth, and postpartum need to understand key components of the disorder, its treatment, and the potential comorbidities that could impact physiological and psychosocial maternal infant health outcomes. A collaborative approach among the woman's perinatal health and behavioral health team members is needed.

[1]The Institutional Review Board of Drexel University granted permission to use these data to inform this chapter. The identifiers were removed, and anonymity of data was protected at all times.

CASE

M.K. is a 27-year-old Gravida-1, Para- 0 (G1P0) who presents for her first prenatal care visit at 7 weeks gestation and identifies herself as an "Aspie." She explains that she was diagnosed with AS when she was in kindergarten and has a history of being on an array of medications (Ritalin, Prozac, chlorpromazine, dextroamphetamine, and valproate) since the age of 8 years. As a child, she was told she had Tourette syndrome, due to several tics (involuntary movements such as hand-flapping and finger-flicking, no verbal tics). Her tics were well managed on chlorpromazine; however, at the age of 24, under medical supervision, she stopped her medication for the Tourette syndrome. Despite stopping this medication, neither she nor her family report the return of these symptoms. With regard to her other medications, she consulted with a perinatalogist, as advised by her neurologist and psychiatrist, for preconception advice. She was advised to go to the Organization of Teratology Information Specialists (OTIS) website to get the most comprehensive information about the teratology of all her medication. After careful review of the scientific information, and multiple discussions with her perinatologist and neurologist, she decided to stop her medications and is closely monitored for neurological and psychiatric symptoms related to her AS.

M.K. married her high school boyfriend 3 years ago, after dating for 7 years. She is a PhD student in physics at a prestigious university. Her husband has a good job as a computer programmer. They live in a small town-house community close to both of their families.

The advanced practice nurse (APN) is quite impressed with all the detailed information that M.K. presents at the first prenatal visit. Unfamiliar with caring for women who present with AS during pregnancy, and not sure why medications more commonly used to treat depression, anxiety, seizures, and psychosis had been prescribed, she asks M.K. for more information. Using the typical approach to establish a nonjudgmental, trusting nurse–patient relationship, she asks open-ended questions in a nonthreatening way. Development of a trust-based clinician–patient relationship is an important goal during all first prenatal visits, and especially for vulnerable populations who might be marginalized because of the stigma of being on psychiatric medication.

As the visit continues, M.K.'s responses become more terse. The APN feels she cannot "connect" with her. M.K. is avoiding eye contact. In response to questions about medications taken, she provides detailed information and appears to understand the mode of actions, why the medications helped her when they did, and why she needed to be switched to another medication. After obtaining her 22-year medication history, the APN is exhausted and uncomfortable, and senses that M.K. does not like her as a health care provider. She comes to this conclusion based on nonverbal clues during the interaction (loud tone of voice, lack of eye contact, and her stiff-appearing stature). In preparing to assess vital signs, the nurse touches her to wrap the blood pressure cuff around her arm and M.K. jumps away.

The APN begins to wonder if there are better approaches to care, specific nursing measures to take, or approaches to avoid. What additional knowledge is needed to best meet this woman's needs and help facilitate optimal health for her and her baby? After the visit, the APN and colleagues go to the computer to learn more about caring for a woman with AS during pregnancy and childbirth. A literature search on CINAHL and PubMed yields nothing. However, they are able to learn about AS itself. They obtain permission from M.K. to consult with her other providers.

REVIEW OF ASPERGER'S SYNDROME

Asperger's syndrome is a neurodevelopmental disorder affecting key aspects of social awareness and interaction, language usage, and sensory integration (Kleinhans et al., 2009; Miller & Ozonoff, 2011; Simone, 2010). People with this disorder are often regarded as having a high-functioning form of autism and, in general, often have difficulty with social interactions and repetitive behaviors and might appear clumsy. People with AS usually have little to no delay in cognitive development, often have above-average intelligence, and excel in a variety of fields, including computer technology, the arts, and science. Independent living skills, including activities of daily living, are often not problematic for individuals with AS, but interpersonal skills are often compromised (Pijnacker, Hagoort, Buitelaar, Tenisse, & Geurts, 2009; Spek, Schatorje, Scholte, & van Berckelaer-Onnes, 2009). Due to their difficulty reading social cues, people with AS often respond awkwardly in normal social situations, are rigid about their routines or rituals, and might appear insensitive to the emotions of people around them (Jellema et al., 2009; National Institute of Neurologic Disorders and Strokes, 2005). A major difference between people with AS and those with autism is that most people with AS want intimate relationships with others, as opposed to people with autism, who tend not to have the same need for personal relationships (Aston, 2003).

The prevalence of AS is greater among males compared to females (Manning, Baron-Cohen, Wheelwright, & Sanders, 2001) with a male-to female ratio range of 4:1 (Mattila et al., 2007). The majority of the research on AS has been conducted on males. However, there are documented gender differences that generally indicate that females with AS seem to have more empathy and might have less severe communication deficits (Nichols, Moravick, & Tenenbaum, 2009). Many girls are able to imitate social actions and mannerisms and develop social scripts based on their observations of peers or from television. As author Willey (1999) writes in her book *Pretending To Be Normal*, they might "pretend to be normal," yet often still appear socially awkward and unnatural. Unfortunately, females with AS can experience lifelong struggles in understanding and interpreting interactions in the world, which are full of double meanings, nonverbal communication, and social demands (Aston, 2003).

To understand potential nursing care needs of women with AS during the childbearing cycle requires appreciation of the growing culture of AS, a knowledge base of common comorbidities associated with AS, and existing and new pharmacological and therapeutic approaches employed to help individuals with this syndrome. The interactions among these factors and the physiological, psychosocial transitions due to pregnancy and childbirth require serious attention.

Understanding the Culture of the Aspie or "Aspergirl"

The growing online community base and power of social media to connect individuals at a distance provided an avenue for evolution of a culture of AS (Miller & Ozonoff, 2011). This is exemplified by M.K.'s self-identification as an "Aspie" when she presents for her first prenatal visit. Individuals with AS often refer to themselves as Aspies as a way to distinguish themselves from those who do not have an ASD (known as neurotypicals, often abbreviated as NT; Willey, 1999). "Aspergirl" is another recently coined term for females with AS (Simone, 2010). These terms are viewed as empowering, rather than derogatory, when used by individuals with AS to describe themselves.

While a woman might refer to herself as an Aspie, it would be inappropriate, perhaps even disrespectful, for the nurse to reference the patient with this label. However, the nurse should keep in mind that if a woman describes herself as such, it is an important message to the nurse that the woman self-identifies in a perhaps empowering way with herself as part of the larger community of others with AS. This could also indicate a proclivity to use the Internet as an important means of obtaining information.

In the last decade, the explosion of information available through the Internet and the synergies between autism advocacy groups (Jordan, 2010) and the academic research centers have made a plethora of information available to the public and the provider. Simple Internet searches using "Asperger's syndrome," "Aspie," and "Aspergirl" yield thousands of websites. Likewise, using the term "pregnancy" to search the Internet yields equally large numbers of results. Childbearing has been referred to as a cycle that includes: preconceptual, prenatal, intrapartum, postpartum, and continued mothering throughout the child's life cycle. Considering the social and communication deficits challenging those who have AS, using a computer is a preferred method of learning for many individuals, particularly when compared to one-on-one teaching during office visits or even formal group childbirth and parenting classes. However, it is important to recognize that much misinformation is available through the Internet. It is imperative to provide reliable websites for patients to reference information. Exhibit 11.1 provides a few reliable websites that can be used by women. It is advisable for all health care practices to screen Internet websites and choose those they would like their clients to visit.

EXHIBIT 11.1

Childbearing-Related Websites Sponsored by Reputable Professional Organizations

March of Dimes
http://www.marchofdimes.com/pregnancy/pregnancy.html
This link is designed for those who have questions about pregnancy. Pre-conceptual to postpartum issues are addressed, with the overall aim of promoting optimal birth outcomes. It is a thorough, excellent site that is interactive with excellent informative videos.

American College of Nurse-Midwives Consumer section:
http://www.midwife.org/Consumer-Information
www.mymidwife.org is a link to help women take an active role in making the right choices for themselves and their families. It explains about midwifery, women's health and choices.
www.gotmom.org is a link to a site created by the American College of Nurse-Midwives to provide breast-feeding information and resources for mothers and families.

Organization of Teratology Information Specialists (OTIS)
http://www.otispregnancy.org/
OTIS provides accurate evidence-based, clinical information to patients and health care professionals about exposures during pregnancy and lactation.

US National Library of Medicine – LactMed
http://toxnet.nlm.nih.gov/cgi-bin/sis/htmlgen?LACT
LactMed is a peer-reviewed database of drugs that provides information to health care providers and breast-feeding women or those considering breast-feeding regarding: drug levels, possible effects to the neonate, and possible drug alternatives.

It is also important for health care providers to remember that ASD is a spectrum disorder, and every patient with a diagnosis of AS will not be the same or have the same needs. Although there are common traits, their individual needs and preferences might vary considerably, so make no assumptions. There is great deal of individual variation in presentation, degree of language and interpersonal/social skills, sensory processing, and comorbidities associated with AS. Individualized, nonjudgmental nursing care is of utmost importance.

Diagnosis of AS among Females

Diagnosis of AS might not occur during the early childhood years, especially for girls (Miller & Ozonoff, 2011; Simone, 2010). The traits associated with AS that appear early on (e.g., verbal expression, memory, intelligence) might not be as unusual for little girls compared to little boys, who are expected to be much more active (Giarelli et al., 2010). However, for girls, the social deficits and difficulties in making friends that become painfully apparent usually command the attention of parents or teachers later in childhood or even as late as adulthood (Miller & Ozonoff, 2011; Simone, 2010). It is challenging to differentiate the diagnosis from comorbidities that coexist.

Diagnosing females with AS is difficult because, at the present time, there is no consensus-based diagnostic instrument for AS, such as the gold standard tool Autism Diagnostic Observation Scale (ADOS), which is used for diagnosing autistic disorder. Due to this limitation, Miller and Ozonoff (2011) warn those reviewing the scientific literature that there is a wide variance on the criteria used to diagnose AS, so caution is needed when comparing findings from published AS research. Clinicians should clarify how the diagnosis was made and by whom (see also Section I and Chapters 5 and 6). It is also important to keep in mind that as more information becomes available about AS via social media, some individuals who suspect they possess AS-like features/characteristics might self-diagnose without ever receiving a formal evaluation and/or professional diagnoses.

There are general social deficits associated with the AS diagnosis. However, women appearing for pregnancy-related care can vary in terms of their psychoeducational and/or pharmacological treatment histories. One woman might have been diagnosed since early childhood, while another woman might have recently learned of her formal AS diagnosis after an extensive family workup when one of her children was diagnosed with autism.

It is important to acknowledge that not all women identify with their AS diagnosis, and some work very hard to appear normal (Willey, 1999). This can be problematic, because the desire to act normal and conceal anxiety about social interactions might interfere with the actual interaction during a health care encounter. For example, the woman might have learned social cues, like nodding one's head when someone is speaking to her. A clinician might interpret head nodding as a sign of understanding, when in reality it might be used by the woman with AS to conceal sensory overload or shutting down. The nurse needs to be acutely aware of these possibilities when interacting with women with AS.

PREGNANCY: A TIME OF TRANSITION

Pregnancy is a time of transition for all women (Meleis, 2010). The growing fetus causes tremendous physiological changes that can influence a mother's physical and mental perceptions of well-being, even if there are no medical problems or complications (Gabbe, Niebyl, & Simpson, 2007). If there are medical or psychological problems, dealing with their related manifestations creates additional challenges. Additionally, psychosocial transitions related to multiple roles occur during this time (Meleis, 2010). For example, the daughter–mother role evolves, as the daughter becomes a mother; the lover–partner role evolves, as parenting becomes a priority—with an enormous amount of responsibility for caring for the newborn. A professional woman needs to incorporate the role of mother, along with the other roles she manages, in the work environment. For women who have an ASD, transitions present enormous challenges.

Nurses must be especially sensitive to the influence of the transitions of pregnancy on the experiences and coping abilities of women with AS; it is possible that such transitions can lead to crisis in these women. Tailoring perinatal nursing care to all women is important (Suplee, Dawley, & Bloch, 2007); however, it is especially important to consider the unique concerns and needs in this population of women. Nurses need to carefully rethink some of the routine nursing interventions used during the provision of perinatal nursing care. Avoiding sensory overload is important. For example, maternal child health nurses traditionally consider teaching an important part of their responsibility. Attending childbirth preparation and infant care classes are assumed to be vital responsibilities of expectant parents. Traditional methods of health teaching might need to be modified for AS women during the childbearing cycle. Alternative methods might include providing suggestions for books, websites, and videos with reliable educational information regarding pregnancy, childbirth, lactation, breast-feeding, and early parenting.

Women with AS are typically aware of societal and gender expectations regarding motherhood and parenting. In attempt to "be normal," they might be more inclined to research and study the information in great depth continuously throughout the childbearing cycle.

Routine prenatal care entails monthly visits until 28 weeks gestation, then biweekly until 36 weeks, followed by weekly visits until delivery. High-risk pregnancies require more visits (Bloch, Dawley, & Suplee, 2009). Women with AS might not be considered by all obstetric clinicians to fit into a high-risk pregnancy category. However, effects of drugs prescribed for AS-related issues, comorbidities they might have or develop, and communication and social considerations increase the need for surveillance and interdisciplinary management of care.

Physiological changes in pregnancy affect just about every system in the human body; there are multiple hormonal and metabolic changes as well. The impact of these physiological changes on the neurobiological factors associated with AS has not been explored. For the purpose of review, Table 11.1 lists key physiological changes in pregnancy. The magnitude of the effects of pregnancy-related changes on women with AS is certainly a fascinating area for further study.

CASE–CONTINUED

It is Monday morning, and the waiting room is full, with a set of 10-month-old triplets screaming loudly in the waiting room. M.K. appears unannounced at the office to find out the results of her screening test for Down syndrome and neural tube defects (QUAD screen), which was performed at the laboratory last week. She is now 17 weeks pregnant. Pacing the room, tapping her foot, she demands her results. She is repeating this demand over and over and appears quite agitated, as if a temper tantrum is about to occur.

The APN is confused about why M.K. has appeared without an appointment and is so insistent about hearing the results of her tests. She brings M.K. into her office and closes the door to block out the loud noises from the crowded waiting room. The APN asks M.K. about her concerns and why she came to the office without calling or making an

(*Continued*)

CASE–CONTINUED (Continued)

appointment. M.K. explains in a monotone voice that the lab technician told her to get the results in a week from her prenatal care provider. She read online that it is important to get the results quickly in case further testing, like an amniocentesis, is needed, because time is of the essence. The APN now appreciates M.K.'s concerns. She provides details about the method used to inform patients of their results when abnormal. After a 10-minute explanation, M.K. stands up within 1 foot of the APN and repeats loudly, "I want my results now." The APN realizes that M.K. probably did not process anything she just said. Unfortunately, the QUAD results are not back from the lab yet.

To try to minimize M.K.'s anxiety, the APN informs the patient that she will call her each morning by 9 a.m. to let her know if the results are back. Although this is not common practice, appreciating the characteristics associated with AS, the nurse tailors the approach specifically to meet M.K.'s need. M.K. might not be able to function for the rest of the day if she does not know, first thing in the morning, if the results are back. Additionally, the APN is able to adjust the office environment when M.K. comes for care. Carefully scheduled, she is given extended appointment times when the number of people and amount of noise in the waiting room are minimal.

TABLE 11.1 ■ Overview of Common Physiological Changes in Pregnancy[a]

Organ System	Physiological Change
Integumentary	Darkened skin pigment of areola and genital skin—hyperpigmentation Formation of linea nigra, striae gravidarum, or melasma
Musculoskeletal	Joint laxity due to increased progesterone and relaxin Lordosis due to compensation for the shift in the growing abdomen
Gastrointestinal	Gums soften, might swell or bleed easily Heartburn related to decreased lower esophageal sphincter tone Reflux related to decreased tone and mobility of stomach Constipation and flatulence related to decreased tone and mobility of intestines Gall stone formation due to decreased tone of gallbladder
Carbohydrate metabolism	Mild fasting hypoglycemia and postprandial hyperglycemia Hyperinsulinemia and Insulin resistance
Hemotologic	Hemoglobin and hematocrit decreased Platelets decrease Activated coagulation cascade
Cardiovascular changes	Increase in blood volume and cardiac output Peripheral vasodilatation and decreased systemic vascular resistance Increase in heart rate Slight drop in blood pressure in second trimester
Respiratory	Increased awareness of breathing and/or dyspnea due to increased progesterone and estrogen and elevation of diaphragm due to growing uterus
Renal system	Glomerular filtration rate increases Bladder capacity changes
Endocrine	Pituitary and thyroid enlarge slightly Prolactin increases

[a]*Note*: Table is not inclusive of all physiological changes that occur with pregnancy. Information compiled from Cohen (2011); Gabbe et al. (2007); Ricci and Kyle (2008).

Despite possibilities of leading productive work lives and seemingly normal personal lives, women with AS often have distinctive impairments—core deficits—that interfere with multiple dimensions of life. Knowledge of these helps the nurse understand awkward, perhaps even frustrating, interactions that might even leave the nurse feeling inept. Common nursing cues, such as open-ended questions or facial expressions used to encourage deeper exploration of feelings about pregnancy might not result in the expected outcome from the woman with AS, since she might not be able to interpret them correctly.

Theory of Mind

Theory of mind (TOM), posited by Simon Baron-Cohen, a leading ASD expert, provides tremendous insight into the autistic mind. Theory of mind refers to the ability to attribute mental states and thoughts to others (Baron-Cohen, 2011). It describes an individual's ability to be able to see the perspective of another individual. People with autism tend to view the world in very narrow, concrete terms. They see the world as black and white and do not have the ability to put themselves in another person's shoes (Aston, 2003). Individuals with ASD are delayed in the development of TOM, leaving them with "mindblindness" (Zalla, Sav, Stopin, Ahade, & Leboyer, 2009). Because they are often unable to interpret other people's behaviors, they often feel quite confused and frightened by others. This lack of perspective is more severe in those diagnosed with autism than with AS, yet in both disorders it can cause serious difficulties in developing and maintaining relationships with partners, family members, work colleagues, and others in the individual's social network. Theory of mind can help nurses understand patients with AS and helps explain the social and communication impairments (Pijnacker et al., 2009; Spek et al., 2009) and resulting lack of empathy that can be manifested (Blackshaw, Kinderman, Hare, & Hare, 2001).

More recently, Baron-Cohen expanded his theory to include the empathizing–systemizing (E-S) theory, explaining that TOM is only the cognitive component of empathy. Empathizing–systemizing theory explains that empathy is considered to be below average, while the psychological skill involved in systemizing is above average. Systemizing is a term used to describe the drive to analyze or construct systems, noting regularities and paying close attention to rules. This theory additionally helps explain social-communication difficulties, such as having narrow interests, repetitive behaviors, and resistance to change with a need for sameness (Baron-Cohen, 2011). Framing nursing care in the E-S theory directs practical AS-friendly interventions that appreciate the distinct learning style that is different from neurotypical individuals. Such care profiles strengths as well as weaknesses, so teaching can be tailored to harness learning strengths and avoid pitfalls.

Best Practices: Nursing Approach to Social-Communication Impairments

Social impairments, specifically core deficiencies in reciprocal social behavior, are incompletely understood, but are a fundamental component of impairment in autism. Deficits in conversation, social communication, and interpreting social cues are major impediments to social functioning (Gold, Faust, & Goldstein, 2010; Jellema et al., 2009; Samson & Hegenloh, 2010). It is important to keep in mind that the person with AS uses more concrete (versus abstract) cognitive processes. Interpreting social cues is, at most times, an automatic process for neurotypical individuals. The person with AS often struggles to interpret the meaning of others' verbal and social cues, which leads to anxiety and frustration (Jellema et al., 2009). While some people with AS have keen senses of humor, producing excellent puns, riddles, or sarcasm, they might not understand the punch line of a joke when it is told in person, because understanding the humor often depends on interpreting social cues, such as facial expression (Gold et al., 2010; Samson & Hegenloh, 2010). When caring for women with AS, avoid social innuendos. Language should be literal and to the point.

Minimizing Social Environment Stressors During Prenatal Care

A key component in management of AS is to minimize the extent to which social environments are overwhelming, confusing, or overtly hostile. A useful strategy, if possible, would be to minimize the likelihood of new social encounters. During prenatal care, schedule appointments when the office is not so crowded. Of special concern is the waiting room environment. Is it possible to schedule an appointment 15 minutes before normal hours, so there is no one in the waiting room while the AS patient waits for her appointment? Continuity of care should be a priority with the prenatal care provider. If at all possible, the same practitioner should be the provider of care during the prenatal, intrapartum, and postpartum periods. Perhaps a midwifery model of care or doula support would serve the woman better in terms of continuity of care. However, these models of care typically involve extensive social interaction and communication, particularly during teaching and coaching sessions; this might not be what the woman needs. Having a chatty nurse, midwife, or doula who uses extensive nonverbal communication modalities, typically effective with neurotypical women, might not serve the woman with AS very well.

During prenatal teaching, nurses should avoid using metaphors when preparing women for childbirth and the changes that occur in pregnancy. Research conducted by Gold and her associates (2010), demonstrated that AS persons had difficulty comprehending novel, as well as conventional, metaphors. It would be helpful for the APN to provide a brief, concise, written summary of information or topics discussed at each visit for the pregnant woman's future reference. This intervention can help to mitigate auditory-processing issues. Another suggestion that might help to reduce anxiety is to encourage the woman to keep a journal between visits, which can be reviewed with her at each prenatal visit. The APN managing care should avoid directing the woman to group childbirth classes and to the increasingly popular group models of prenatal care, such as centering pregnancy (Baldwin, 2006; Reid 2007). These models of care focus on creating social capital among participants, with the assumption that the participants are interested in new social relationships. Such an environment could potentially trigger anxiety in a woman with AS.

Best Practices: Nursing Approach to Sensory-Processing Issues

Individuals with AS can have sensory-processing difficulties that reflect unusual sensory response patterns: hypersensitivity, hyposensitivity, and/or sensory overload causing a "shutdown" (Aylott, 2010; Pfeiffer, Kinnealey, Reed, & Herzberg, 2005; Willey, 1999). Such sensory modulation dysfunction can result from sound, vision, touch, smell, proprioception and vestibular responses. The triggers for sensory overload for women with AS are almost everywhere. How this will change during pregnancy is unknown in general and specifically for each individual woman.

Women enter many entirely new environments, including unfamiliar health offices, the birthing center/hospital, and the pediatric office during the perinatal period. Physiological changes of pregnancy often result in altered sensitivities. Simone (2010) conducted extensive interviews with Aspergirls and received long lists from women identifying a multitude of triggers. Importantly, she notes that in addition to recognizing common triggers, the nurse needs an understanding of the intensity of the disturbance—the associated anxiety that is so painful, the distress of feeling so "out of control." Simone's vivid descriptions help us develop insight into the intense pain resulting from these hypersensitivities: the hyperawareness of the sounds most do not hear and things most do not notice. The following vignette about florescent lights and grocery stores illustrates these challenges; the health care environment, especially the hospital labor and delivery environment might be even more disturbing for people with AS.

> We all know that Autistics and Aspies have an aversion to fluorescent lights because they flicker and hum at a rate we can detect even when others can't. But there are many other visual processing difficulties, such as from too many objects or people in motion. The objects in a grocery store aren't in motion but we are, causing a maelstrom of images in our minds that make us dizzy like we're riding a scrambler at the county fair. Grocery stores are hell on earth for autistic children and grownup Aspergirls . . . and yes, they can still cause us to have temper tantrums. (Simone, 2010, pp. 37–38)

Managing Sensory Overload

The health care team needs to be particularly sensitive to potentials for sensory overload and to adjust the actions and environment to minimize overload. A tailored program of care can be developed with input from the patient and her family, in order to avoid her particular triggers when possible. Providing a written or online questionnaire for the mother might be most productive; with this strategy, she can provide guidance to those caring for her without the anxieties that might be exacerbated during in-person conversations.

Engaging the Family in the Process

A pregnant woman with AS might be more likely to depend on her family members as a bridge between the health care providers and herself—usually her family understands her communication style and needs (Aylott, 2010). The patient's partner, family member, or friend should be an integral part of the communication team. A person who knows and understands the patient's needs can accompany her to all prenatal visits and serve as a second "pair of ears" to help bridge the communication and auditory-processing gaps. Clinicians should summarize and repeat all instructions at the end of each visit. Providing visual information is helpful. For practical coping techniques, it might be helpful to refer the family to the list of strategies that Willey identifies (1999, pp. 124–133). For example, for auditory sensitivity, bring earplugs to prenatal visits or to the hospital; to avoid smells that might be too disturbing, pack nose plugs; use sunglasses to avoid fluorescent lighting. There are many other excellent strategies in Willey's classic reference for those living with AS.

CASE–CONTINUED

At 32 weeks of pregnancy, M.K. tells the APN that she is extremely irritable and depressed, withdrawing even from talking and interacting with her husband. Determined not to take her former medication (selective serotonin reuptake inhibitors) during the pregnancy, she started complementary alternative therapies for these symptoms. She reports that she has not

(*Continued*)

CASE (Continued)

slept for about a week. She is fearful that she will suffer from postpartum psychosis after she delivers. M.K. states that she is happy about having a baby, thinks she will be a good mother, and her baby will love her, despite her AS. She is researching everything she must "know" to be a good mother. She says she will hug her baby often, even if it does not come naturally. She continues meeting weekly with her psychotherapist, who has experience treating individuals with AS. She has not seen her psychiatrist for six months.

The APN is aware that the onset of serious psychiatric disorders usually occurs during the second and third decade of life. M.K.'s sleep disruption can be a result of stress and anxiety, or even of the common discomforts of pregnancy. However, of most concern is to differentiate her inability to sleep as a symptom of mania, a symptom of bipolar disorder. A critical question to further assess this is to ask M.K. if she is tired. In response to this question, M.K. reports that she is exhausted and reports that the physiological pregnancy changes make her uncomfortable. Additionally, her sheets at night irritate her, as she hears all the movements she makes in an attempt to get comfortable. The patient does not report any heightened awareness to other symptoms nor excessive changes in behavior during the day. The APN assesses that her sleeplessness is probably not a symptom of mania, because she is aware that patients that are manic usually do not report being tired, despite the fact that they have not slept for several days. Therefore, she provides guidance to help improve M.K.'s sleep quality, such as purchasing sheets that address her hypersensitivity issues, a body pillow for more comfortable positioning, a white noise machine for auditory sensitivity, along with a follow-up visit in a week to reassess the situation. She refers M.K. to her psychiatrist for an immediate visit as well.

COMORBID CONDITIONS AND PREGNANCY

A variety of comorbidities accompany AS, and there is a growing body of evidence that suggests children with ASD develop psychiatric diagnoses during adulthood. Common comorbid psychiatric syndromes associated with AS are anxiety, mood disorders (including depression), and obsessive–compulsive disorder (Hurtig et al., 2009; Tager-Flusberg & Dominick, 2011). It is not clear if these are truly comorbidities, an extension of the individual's AS, or separate coexisting conditions. However, for clinical purposes, these common syndromes are important to assess for, so appropriate psychosocial and psychopharmacological treatments can be provided (Tager-Flusberg & Dominick, 2011).

In the case described above, M.K. planned her pregnancy and decided to stop her medications before conceiving. However, some patients might be on their psychotropic medication throughout the pregnancy. Considering that almost one-half of all pregnancies are unplanned (Centers for Disease Control and Prevention, 2010), some women might be on medications without knowing they are pregnant. Nursing care must include attention to the need for mothers to find the most reliable information about use of their medications during pregnancy. With this information, they can actively participate in decision making about continuation or discontinuation of drug therapy. The APN managing care must be astute in differentiating common physiological discomforts and symptoms related to pregnancy from somatic manifestations of psychological distress related to AS and its comorbidities. These pregnancy-related physical symptoms include: headaches, muscle tension, dyspepsia, abdominal pain, and sleep disturbance, as exemplified in the case above (Gabbe et al., 2007; Myles, 2003; Souders et al., 2009).

Mood Disorders

Depression is the most common mood disorder in ASD, and even more prevalent among those diagnosed with AS (Tager-Flusberg & Dominick, 2011). Poor sleep quality associated with autism (Souders et al., 2009) and with pregnancy and the postpartum period can certainly exacerbate depression (Posmontier, 2008). Nurses unaccustomed to caring for those on the autism spectrum, need to be aware that it might be challenging to distinguish depressive symptoms from typical AS behavior, such as the preference to be alone.

Depression is more prevalent in individuals with ASD who have higher IQ scores. It often develops in adolescence, escalating in young adulthood, as the person becomes aware of social differences. This seems to be particularly true for females (Simone, 2010; Tager-Flusberg & Dominick, 2011). There is no current literature that examines incidence of depression in pregnant females with AS. It is also important to recognize that any pregnant woman is at risk for depression if she perceives that she has a poor relationship with her partner (Bloch et al., 2010). It might also be helpful to refer the woman and partner to couples therapy with a therapist experienced with working with individuals with AS; if accessible, such support can promote optimal family health during the transition from pregnancy to parenthood.

Anxiety

Reported rates of anxiety subtypes among those with AS vary across studies (Tager-Flusberg & Dominick, 2011). Anxiety symptoms observed in high-functioning adults with AS interfere with quality of life (Myles, 2003; Hurtig et al., 2009). Females with AS report having awareness of their own social confusion and report experiencing anxiety while trying to interpret social cues and attempting to mimic neurotypical behavior to meet perceived societal expectations in social situations (Attwood, 2007). Management of anxiety involves a variety of behavioral and pharmacological therapeutic approaches (Myles, 2003).

Obsessive–Compulsive Disorder

The relationship between OCD and autism, in general, is unclear. Perseverative thoughts and repetitive behaviors associated with OCD are also features associated with autism, making it difficult at times to distinguish between the two. It has been suggested that there might be a genetic association between ASD and OCD, because children with ASD are more likely to have a parent that has been diagnosed with OCD (Tager-Flusberg & Dominick, 2011). The clinical relevance is that if OCD behaviors interfere with an individual's quality of life, medical therapy might be indicated. Especially during the postpartum period, rigid adherence to infant feeding schedules, diaper changes, standards of cleanliness, and similar concerns might be very important to the mother, and should be respected, as long as none of the practices are harmful to the infant's well-being.

Tics and Tourette Syndrome

The existence of tics in people with ASDs, including AS, is well recognized (Ringman & Jankovic, 2000). Tics are defined as brief, involuntary, and intermittent movements (motor tics) or sounds (phonic or vocal tics) that tend to occur abruptly. Tourette syndrome (TS) is diagnosed, after an extensive medical workup, if there are multiple tics that include one or more vocal tics persisting for more than a year (Ringman & Jankovic, 2000; Robertson, 2011). The mean age of onset is 5 to 7 years. Tics are frequently most severe between ages 10 to 12 years, and can improve with age (Robertson, 2011). Tourette syndrome is a complex neurobiological disorder that can coexist with other neurobehavioral conditions, such as OCD and/or depression (Robertson, 2011). The etiopathogenesis of the spectrum of phenotypes of TS is multifactorial, and can be linked to the interaction of genetic susceptibility, epigenetic factors, environmental factors, and neurobiological factors active in the brain.

In many instances, symptoms of TS are concerning enough to warrant medical management, often with clonidine and/or neuroleptic medications. Ascertaining medication safety during pregnancy and lactation of the drugs used to treat symptoms of TS is of foremost importance. Medical management of TS in pregnant women with AS should be in tandem with a neurologist or psychiatrist and perinatologist. Surveillance of the subtleties of interaction between TS and the physiological changes of pregnancy requires collaborative expertise. Caution with dosage is needed; medication doses of neuroleptics are small for those with AS and TS in comparison with their use for schizophrenia or mania (Robertson, 2011). Table 11.2 summarizes the safety profile of some of the most commonly used drugs for comorbidities described above.

Eating Disorders

Although there is little research examining eating disorders in individuals with ASDs, food selectivity, a refusal to eat all but a select group of foods, has been reported to occur more frequently in individuals with ASD (Kalyva, 2009; Schreck &Williams, 2006). As reported in a published interview (Campbell, 2007) with Janet Treasure, an eating disorder researcher, more than one in five individuals with anorexia nervosa met the criteria for having an ASD. Similarly, Attwood (2007) reported that between 18% and 23% of teenage girls who suffer from anorexia nervosa also meet some or all of the diagnostic criteria for AS. A review of 32 studies conducted in various countries reported that individuals with anorexia nervosa are more likely to have an ASD, as well as an anxiety disorder, compared with those in the general population (Berkman, Lohr, & Bulik, 2007). Individuals with AS and ASD who have sensory hypersensitivity might restrict themselves to narrow dietary choices due to an inability to tolerate specific textures, tastes, and smells of many foods and might even experience nausea when attempting to ingest certain foods. They might also require unusual food preparation or meal routines (Copley, 2009). Avoidance of many foods can lead to extremely low body mass index and/or malnutrition, although obesity is also possible if only high-calorie foods are tolerated. These issues have important nursing implications when assessing and caring for women with ASDs who present for prenatal care.

As part of routine care, the nurse should inquire about dietary restrictions, as well as meal routines at the initial prenatal visit and monitor for appropriate weight gain during pregnancy. If the patient reports having a history of having an eating disorder, it is important to inquire if the patient is in the active phase of the disorder and what, if any, treatment she is receiving. If the woman reports a history of treatment with a psychotherapist and/or dietitian, the nurse should recommend that the patient contact them for counseling during pregnancy and postpartum, and include them as part of the multidisciplinary care team. Nurses should provide written educational materials about good nutrition in pregnancy and postpartum. It is important to discuss risks to the patient herself, the fetus, and the baby associated with disordered eating, including poor nutrition, dehydration, cardiac

TABLE 11.2 ■ Common Medications Used to Treat Comorbidities Associated with AS[a]

Classification	Medication (Generic/ Trade name)	Uses	FDA category[b,c]	Risks to fetus/newborns	Risks for breast-feeding
Anticonvulsants	Topiramate (Topamax)	Anticonvulsant	D	Animal studies: crosses the placenta in animals; might cause limb and vertebral malformations. Human studies: increased development of cleft lip and/or cleft palate.[d]	Passes into breast milk.
	Valproic acid (Depakote)	Anticonvulsant, Antimanic	D	Might cause neural tube defects (especially if used in first trimester); might also cause increase in atrial septal defects, cleft palates, hypospadias, polydactyly, and craniosynostosis Children might score lower on cognitive tests[e]	Passes into breast milk. No unquestionable adverse reactions to this drug during breast-feeding have been reported.
	Carbamazepine (Tegretol)	Anticonvulsant, mood stabilizer	D	Might cause increased risk of neural tube defects, facial abnormalities, cardiac defects, and growth restriction.	Passes into breast milk, AAP[b] and WHO[b] note compatibility with breast-feeding.
Antidepressants (SSRIs)[b]	Bupropion (Wellbutrin)	Depression	C	Same as general public.	Passes into breast milk, one report of infant seizures.
	Citalopram (Celexa)	Depression, generalized anxiety disorder	D	Might cause neonatal PPHN,[b,f] septal and valve defects, congenital lung defects, cranial defects, clubfoot, gastroschisis, and other abdominal wall defects. Neonatal abstinence syndrome has also been reported.	Passes into breast milk. A few cases of drowsiness or fussiness in the neonate have been reported, but no adverse effects on development have been found in infants during the first year of life.
	Sertraline (Zoloft)	Depression, anxiety disorder, OCD	D	Has been associated with PPHN[b] when taken during the last half of pregnancy.[f] Newborn: might see jitteriness, increased muscle tone, irritability, altered sleep patterns, tremors, difficulty eating, and some problems with breathing.	Passes into breast milk. Recommended drug for breast-feeding use

Antipsychotics	Chlorpromazine (Thorazine)	Bipolar and anxiety disorders	C	When taken in the third trimester, there is an increase in withdrawal symptoms in newborns, including: agitation, tremors, sleepiness, and difficulty in feeding. In some newborns, the symptoms subside within hours or days; others might require longer hospital stays	Unknown
Mood stabilizers	Lithium (Lithobid)	Bipolar disorder, depressive disorder, impulsivity	D	Mother: possible development of a goiter Fetus: cardiac defects Newborn: Reversible thyroid and kidney toxicity	Passes into breast milk. Might adversely affect the infant.
	Carbamazepine (Tegretol)	Bipolar disorder, seizure control	D	Increased risk of facial deformities, cleft lip, and neural tube and heart defects.	Passes into breast milk, AAP[b] and WHO[b] note compatibility with breast-feeding
Stimulants	Methylphenidate (Concerta, Ritalin)	Attention deficit hyperactivity disorder	C	No human studies available; possible cardiac defects in animals when given high doses.	Limited data exist, low levels have appeared in breast milk.
	Dexmethylphenidate (Focalin)	Attention deficit hyperactivity disorder	C	No human studies available.	Limited evidence shows low levels in breast milk.

[a]Note: This table summarizes commonly used medications. Not an exhaustive list of medications that can be used to treat comorbidities associated with AS. References for table: OTIS & LactMed; Jentink et al., 2010; drugs.com.

[b]AAP, American Academy of Pediatrics; FDA, Food and Drug Administration; PPHN, persistent pulmonary hypertension of the newborn; SSRIs, selective serotonin reuptake inhibitors; WHO, World Health Organization.

[c]FDA Category C: Either studies in animals have revealed adverse effects on the fetus and there are no adequate or well-controlled studies in women OR no studies have been conducted on animals and there are no well-controlled or adequate studies in pregnant women. (Retrieved from http://perinatology.com)

FDA Category D: Observational or adequate well-controlled studies have demonstrated fetal risk, but the benefits from use in pregnant women might be acceptable if they outweigh the risk. (Retrieved from http://perinatology.com)

[d]FDA Drug Safety Communication – 2011. Retrieved from http://www.fda.gov/NewsEvents/Newsroom/PressAnnouncements/ucm245594.htm

[e]FDA Drug Safety Communication – 2011. Retrieved from http://www.fda.gov/Safety/MedWatch/SafetyInformation/SafetyAlertsforHumanMedicalProducts/ucm261610.htm

[f]FDA Drug Safety Communication – 2006. Retrieved from http://www.fda.gov/Drugs/DrugSafety/PostmarketDrugSafetyInformationforPatientsandProviders/DrugSafetyInformationforHeathcareProfessionals/ucm084267.htm

irregularities, gestational diabetes, severe depression during pregnancy, premature birth, labor complications, difficulties nursing, and postpartum depression (National Eating Disorders Association, 2005).

The APN should also discuss the benefits of breast-feeding and encourage women to consider this option. It is important to stress that there is evidence that long-term breast-feeding fosters a positive maternal–child bond, aids in postpartum weight loss, and provides the mother with an opportunity to reestablish healthy eating habits for her infant (Carwell & Spatz, 2011).

BEST PRACTICES: NURSING APPROACH TO INTRAPARTUM CARE

Admission to the hospital or birth center during labor can be very overwhelming for any woman. Staff often rush to obtain initial signatures on consent forms with complex written language. Women with AS might be confused by the request to sign a consent for care form for a baby who has not yet been born. These consents can be explained to the mother during prenatal visits so that she is not surprised by requests to sign them during admission to the labor suite. Moving among different departments or physical spaces, such as from emergency department to exam room to labor room, can be stressful for a woman with AS. One solution would be to make arrangements for the woman to be admitted directly to her labor room. Specific strategies that are effective with each woman should be documented in the prenatal chart and communicated in writing (with the prenatal chart or by other means) to staff in the labor and delivery setting by about 36 weeks gestation (i.e., in advance of the woman's admission for delivery). After admission, the nurse should become familiar with the expectations and preferences the woman has for her labor and delivery experience. The nurse should review the expected sequence of events.

Health care providers tend to instruct women to be flexible during their labors and deliveries, and typically inform them that unplanned events can, and often do, occur. Situations resulting in care that is different from what was expected (e.g., change in pain control mode, change in method of delivery) are likely to be difficult for a woman with AS to cope with. During the labor process, women in general are challenged to relinquish control over their bodies; a woman with AS can find this to be very upsetting. Aston (2003) stated "control is as essential to adults with AS as air is to breathe" (p. 49). With this quote in mind, consider the following scenario: Repetitive late decelerations, possibly indicating poor placental perfusion, are seen on the fetal heart rate monitor during labor. The nurse will reposition the patient, administer oxygen via face mask, check her cervical dilation status, and notify the provider all within seconds to a few minutes. These interventions might drastically increase the anxiety level of a woman with AS. They occur very quickly and expose the patient to significant amounts of unanticipated tactile stimulation. Other interventions that are frequently used in the labor setting, such as assisting with position changes and massaging might be perceived as unpleasant or even noxious stimuli. Numerical pain rating scales (see Exhibit 13.3) can help the woman with AS communicate her level of discomfort or labor-related pain. There is little evidence specific to AS and pregnancy to guide practice in this area of perinatal management.

The rationales for procedures and interventions should be explained in concrete terms before they are implemented. The nurse should remember that too much information or too much auditory stimulation can cause the woman with AS to shut down. It is important to assess the woman for cues that overload is occurring. If the woman requires a cesarean section, careful and deliberate explanations need to be provided. Often, surgical delivery is emergent/unplanned and staff are rushing. The nurse should make every effort to minimize noise, provide concrete explanations about the expected sequence of events, and explain why the health care team needs to move quickly. If possible, describe the delivery/surgery setting to prepare her for the lights, temperature, sounds, and sensations. The nurse should also assess the woman for rising anxiety, and the need for positive reinforcement that she is doing well. If possible, the more familiar labor nurse should remain with the patient in the delivery room, while another nurse circulates during the procedure.

A woman should be encouraged to become familiar with the setting in which the delivery will take place, whether birthing center, hospital, or other environment. She and her partner and/or a family member should be encouraged to visit and take notes to help anticipate what to put in her labor and delivery "toolbox" of comfort items, to eliminate or mitigate the effects of triggers for sensory overload. These can include blanket, sheets, and pillows that feel good against the skin; headphones, earmuffs or ear plugs to block noise; music for relaxation; and a nightgown or bedclothes that feel comfortable. In addition, a squishy toy or hand manipulative might provide comfort during periods of sensory overload (Simone, 2010). Ideally, a labor floor or birthing unit will have a sensory-friendly birthing room styled and equipped to meet the needs of women with AS or others with similar sensory challenges.

Pregnant women with AS might also "stim" (behavior done to self-soothe) when they have experienced sensory overload; such behaviors can include rocking, swaying, humming, hand-flapping, or finger-flicking (Simone, 2010). If self-stimulatory behaviors are seen, reassessment of the nursing approach and environment is indicated. Figure 11.1 summarizes a best-practices set of nursing interventions for control of the environment during labor and delivery.

Immediately after the delivery, once again explain what the woman can expect (i.e., vital sign assessment, fundal height and vaginal bleeding assessment, monitoring of intake and output—especially first void, when she might be transferred to another room, where the baby will be transported to, if necessary). Remember that the patient might have been intensely overstimulated by the delivery and might be anxious or withdrawn/shutdown. Minimizing noise and interactions is prudent. Nurses should also be aware of olfactory hypersensitivity and the likelihood that the scent of the amniotic fluid, urine or feces, blood, perspiration, and/or even bad breath can become a disruptive stimulus. Provide for personal hygiene and dispose of anything that has been soiled from delivery. Personal cleanliness might be a priority for a woman with AS. Avoid assuming that her lack of desire to hold the baby immediately postbirth is an indication of a problem; she might need time to regroup and gain control prior to exposure to the additional stimuli.

The labor and delivery process can be extremely overwhelming to all women; responses to the experience might be heightened in women with AS. Nurses should be cognizant of the potential for posttraumatic stress disorder (PTSD), which has been reported after childbirth and has a prevalence rate of 1.5% to 6% in the general population (Beck, 2006). Little is known about the prevalence of PTSD in women with AS after childbirth. Research is needed in this area.

BEST PRACTICES: NURSING APPROACH TO POSTPARTUM CARE

The crisis associated with the transitioning to the role of a parent has been documented in the literature (Meleis, 2010). Mothering is never easy, and adapting to the mothering role with a newborn is a huge adjustment. From a theoretical perspective, framed by the TOM insights, we might wonder if a new mother with AS is able to read and respond to her newborn's cues

Labor

- Assign room far away from nurse's station
- Place a sign on door to decrease visitors & staff
- Decrease number of providers
- Do not use fluorescent lights, use lamps & overhead lights for delivery
- If using a fetal heart rate monitor, keep muted
- Use manual BP cuff if possible (automatic BP cuff may startle patient each time it inflates causing undo stress and elevated BP)
- Respond to alarms on I.V. pumps & monitors quickly
- Inform woman prior to any touching
- Offer every opportunity for patient to control the room environment (i.e. blinds open or closed, where chairs are placed, where personal belongings are placed, etc.)
- If woman agrees to massaging to assist with pain control, use a firm touch

Delivery

- If at all possible have the woman deliver in the same room she labored in
- Minimize the number of personnel in the room
- Ask the woman if she would like to hold the infant immediately after birth; if so place an extra blanket on the woman's chest while she is pushing
- Keep lighting directed on perineum, decrease use of fluorescent lights as much as possible
- If counting for the woman while she bears down is necessary, speak softly
- Once the baby is born– keep the level of noise in the room at a minimum
- If breastfeeding, may want to wait until woman is out of stirrups (if used) and has been cleaned & covered to minimize the amount of different stimuli happening to her body
- If breast feeding, assist with latching on & discussing all new sounds the newborn may make
- Clean the room as quickly as possible & remove all soiled materials
- Make every attempt to restore a sense of order & control for the woman

FIGURE 11.1 Control of the physical and interactional environment during labor and delivery.

and meet the newborn's needs. After all, the newborn does not communicate with words, but instead gives ambiguous cues to discomfort or distress. Typical mothers learn to read and interpret these cues, mediated by time and experience.

Will she attach to her newborn? How well can she nurture? Can she rehearse and study the details on how to care for a newborn such that she is an expert caregiver? Perhaps her strengths in systematization will guide the mother to be a meticulous caregiver, studying all the right things to do—as if the newborn is her project. Certainly there are particular risk factors for physical and psychiatric disorders, such as postpartum depression/psychosis. Thoughts the provider should consider include: "Can she adapt to all the changes?" and "Will she experience sensory overload and shut down—perhaps endangering the newborn by neglect?"

There is no evidence to prove the mother will not be able to fulfill her maternal role. Absence of empathy and attachment are considerations for children with ASD. Yet they are not well-studied in adults. While it is well established that most people with ASDs do poorly on TOM tasks, social competency does improve over time in a proportion of adults. For higher-functioning people with ASD, social competency is a delayed but not fully absent developmental process. Some evidence suggests that people with autism form attachments, but in idiosyncratic ways; they might not express their attachment behaviors nor engage in relationships in ways that are typical or normal (Taylor, Target, & Charman, 2008). The influence of oxytocin, a neuropeptide that is increased throughout pregnancy and the postpartum period (Feldman, Weller, Zaboory-Sharon, & Levine, 2007). Attachment capacities in women with AS during the childbearing cycle is also unexplored.

From mothers themselves who have AS, the authors learned that most were diagnosed after their children were diagnosed with an ASD. Simone also found this phenomenon to be prevalent in her research for her book *Aspergirls* (Simone, 2010). Thus, there probably are many mothers with AS who are not identified; there is little mothering research in this population. It is not possible to draw conclusions about the relationship between AS and mothering; there are many unanswered questions. However, Aston (2003) has summarized key points about AS and parenting in her book, *Aspergers in Love: Couple Relationships and Family Affairs*, one of which is that "having Asperger syndrome does not make a person a bad parent" (p. 105).

BEST PRACTICES: NURSING APPROACH TO THE FIRST YEAR OF PARENTHOOD

Assessment of maternal functioning during the first postpartum year is critical for maternal and infant well-being. Accurate assessment, especially of mothers who have psychosocial risk factors that potentially interfere with the ability to competently care for their infants is critical. Reliable and valid instruments that assess maternal status and function can help to identify women at high risk for ineffective maternal caregiving, and facilitate appropriate intervention. An example is the Barkin Index of Maternal Functioning (BIMF; Barkin et al., 2010). The BIMF was developed by researchers studying mental illness during childbearing years. They needed a tool that could assess the mother's ability to meet both her self-care needs and the dependent-care needs of her infant from birth through the first year of life. Building upon previous maternal functional status research conducted several decades ago by prominent nurse researchers (Fawcett & Tulman, 1988), Barkin, a biostatistician and epidemiologist, created the BIMF to accurately assess maternal functioning. It is currently used in multiple research projects, including clinical trials of efficacy of drug treatment and light therapy in expectant and new mothers (J. Barkin, personal communication, January 19, 2011). Content validity was achieved using an expert panel and focus groups. Internal reliability in a cohort of 109 women was reported as Cronbach's alpha of 0.87 (Barkin et al., 2010). For clinical use, one should look at the items individually to assess maternal functioning; areas tailored to help the new mother can be of use (Barkin et al., 2010).

BIMF has great promise as a clinical tool to assess maternal functioning. With permission, we have reproduced a copy of this written tool so it can be used for clinical purposes (Exhibit 11.2). A method for use might be to allow the mother with AS to read and complete it herself. Both mother and clinician can review the responses and assess maternal functioning and need for intervention.

ADDITIONAL PREGNANCY-RELATED ISSUES

Safe Medication Management of AS Symptoms during Pregnancy and Lactation

There is no specific drug treatment for AS per se, but medications are used to treat the disturbing symptoms women with AS experience. Multidisciplinary approaches often include psychotropic medications, along with social skills training, behavioral therapy, and educational interventions (Thompson, Thompson, & Reid, 2010). A critical component of

EXHIBIT 11.2

Barkin Index of Maternal Functioning[1,2,3]

	Strongly disagree	Disagree	Somewhat Disagree	Neutral	Somewhat Agree	Agree	Strongly Agree
1. I am a good mother.							
2. I feel relaxed.							
3. I am comfortable with the way I've chosen to feed my baby (either bottle or breast, or both).							
4. My baby and I understand each other.							
5. I am able to relax and enjoy time with my baby.							
6. There are people in my life that I can trust to care for my baby when I need a break.							
7. I am comfortable allowing a trusted friend or relative to care for my baby (can include baby's father or partner).							
8. I am getting adult interaction.							
9. I am getting enough encouragement from other people.							
10. I trust my own feelings (instincts) when it comes to taking care of my baby.							
11. I take a little time each week to do something for myself.							
12. I am taking good care of my baby's physical needs (feedings, changing diapers, doctor appointments).							
13. I am taking care of my physical needs (eating, showering, etc.)							
14. I make good decisions about my baby's health and well-being.							
15. My baby and I are getting into a routine.							
16. I worry about how other people judge me (as a mother).							
17. I am able to take care of my baby and my other responsibilities.							
18. Anxiety or worry often interferes with mothering ability.							
19. *As time goes on*, I am getting better at taking care of my baby.							
20. I am *satisfied* with the job I am doing as a new mother.							

[1]The copyright for this tool is owned by the University of Pittsburgh. Changes in the BIMF are not allowed. Permission to Dr. Bloch to replicate the BIMF for use in this book was granted directly by Dr. Barkin, without charge, due to the educational purpose of this book. For questions about the development of the BIMF, contact Jennifer L. Barkin, PhD; e-mail barkinj@gmail.com. For commercial use of the BIMF, contact the Office of Technology Management at the University of Pittsburgh at 412–648–2206.

[2]This table is replicated from Barkin et al. (2010). Development of the Barkin Index of Maternal Functioning. Journal of Women's Health, *19*(12): 2239–2246.

[3]Scoring: Add all 20 items (after the reverse scoring of items 16 and 18). The range of score is from 0 to 120. The higher the score is interpreted as a greater the level of maternal functioning.

obstetrical care for the woman with AS is to make sure medications are safe for her and her developing fetus during the pregnancy, and into the postpartum period if she is breastfeeding. The influence of the biology of pregnancy, birth, and postpartum on medication needs, dosage requirements, and effect profiles, as well as the influence of these drugs on the developing fetus and growing child have not yet been fully examined.

The most commonly prescribed psychotropic medications are antidepressants, stimulants, and antipsychotics. Anticonvulsants and antiparkinson medications are also often used, even without history of seizures or epilepsy (Esbensen, Greenberg, Seltzer, & Aman, 2009). There is a plethora of published research reports about a variety of these drugs used during pregnancy, and ongoing trials whose findings are not yet in print. Simply reading research reports on a drug or drugs is insufficient to correctly understand the risks to the mother and fetus, because most of the studies are observational epidemiological studies, not randomized control trials. Therefore, much caution is needed to reach absolute conclusions. For the most current and reliable up-to-date information in the public domain, the OTIS website and the LactMed website are suggested, along with a thorough discussion between provider and patient. Also, women need to consider the time frame for discontinuing the use of a drug prior to becoming pregnant to make sure it is cleared from their system. They also need to weigh whether taking the drug is more beneficial than detrimental, or if taking the drug is more detrimental to fetal development than to the benefit of the mother. To make good decisions in collaboration with their health care providers, women with AS need to know:

- if their medications cross the placenta;
- if there are adverse effects on fetal development;
- whether there are increased risks for infertility, spontaneous abortions, or prematurity with continued administration;
- if the drug crosses into breast milk and the likely effect on the infant.

For a list of common medications used to treat comorbidities associated with AS, see Table 11.2.

A New Area of Science: The Role of Oxytocin in Human Social Behavior

In recent years, there has been a growing interest in examining the role of the hormone oxytocin in human social behavior. Earlier animal studies with sheep, rats, and prairie moles, provided considerable evidence that oxytocin plays an important role in facilitating bonding with offspring, as well as with partners (Bartz & Young, 2011). Overall, it is clear from basic neuroscience studies that oxytocin has an important role in regulating affiliative behaviors, social-information processing, and social attachment (Ross & Young, 2009). Increasing oxytocin levels has improved social behavior and cognition in animals.

Perinatal Risk Factors for Autism

An important component of preconceptual and prenatal care is avoidance of exposures that could harm the embryo and growing fetus. Although the focus of much research is on the genetic associations with autism (Turunen et al., 2008), it is quite plausible that environmental exposures during intrauterine life might elevate the risk for an infant to have an ASD. Prematurity, infectious agents, and drugs during pregnancy are associated with neurodevelopmental disorders in children (Gillberg & Cederlun, 2005), but causation has not been established. It is likely that mothers with AS will be concerned about potential genetic and environmental exposure risks and might seek the nurse's guidance. Maternal age has been studied most frequently; research findings definitely suggest that increased maternal age (>35 years of age) and advanced paternal age (>40 years of age) increase the risk of autism (Grether et al., 2009; Reichenberg, Gross, Kolevzon, & Susser, 2011). Advanced maternal and paternal age has been found to be associated with a variety of physical and psychiatric disorders. Proposed causation includes spontaneous genomic alterations, epigenetic dysfunction triggered by advanced parental age, or even accumulated exposure to environmental toxins over the lifespan, possibly resulting in genomic or epigenetic alterations in germ cells. (Reichenberg, Gross, Kolevzon, & Susser, 2011).

Markers for newborns at risk for subsequent neurodevelopmental disorders include history of preterm birth, low birth weight, or being small for gestational age due to intrauterine growth restriction (Institute of Medicine, 2007). Only recently have these adverse perinatal outcomes become the subject of scientific examination. However, researchers must account for confounders, such as genetic susceptibility for both autism and obstetrical suboptimality (Reichenberg et al., 2011). More research is under way to shed more light on these very important questions pertaining to the etiology of autism. For example, the longitudinal National Children's Study will examine a broad range of environmental and other exposures during pregnancy and will follow 100,000 children to 21 years of age (National Research Council and Institute of Medicine, 2008).

BEST PRACTICES: TRANSLATING THE EVIDENCE

Overall, and specifically for each woman with AS, clinicians must ask, "Will pregnancy and childbirth improve, exacerbate, or have no effect on AS symptoms and issues?" As of this writing, there is not enough evidence to predict how women with AS fare during this time of their lives. Figure 11.2 illustrates the possible effects of pregnancy and childbirth in a woman with AS. Exacerbation can be due to any or all of the changes that occur. Yet, it is possible that a woman with AS will have a smooth pregnancy and postpartum course as a function of high-quality interdisciplinary care, complemented by her own strengths and a highly supportive network, including her partner, family, clinicians, and/or friends. Integrating current state of the science evidence about women with AS with evidence-based, tailored care for the childbearing cycle (Suplee et al., 2007), we have formulated summary guidelines to consider when a woman with AS is pregnant (Figure 11.3).

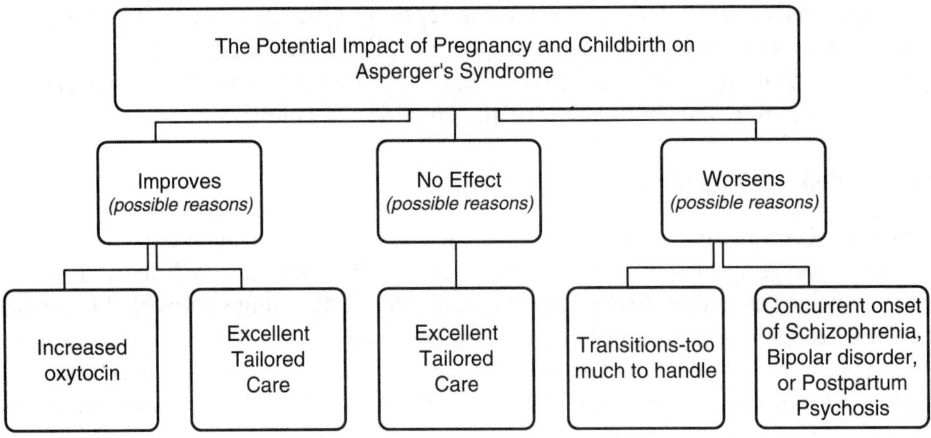

FIGURE 11.2 ■ Best practices: Assess the impact of pregnancy and childbirth on AS.

Prenatal Care & Childbirth Preparation

- Establish preferred method of communication
- Keep health teaching instructional, supplement with written & visual information
- Instruct patient to keep a journal & to bring it with her to all visits
- Be thorough! Explain all procedures
- Provide concrete answers to all questions
- Address all sensory issues & coping strategies
- Avoid innuendos & jokes
- Group childbirth classes probably not good idea—provide accurate websites for reference
- Encourage partner/friend to attend all visits
- Encourage using behaviorial therapist for help with new experiences during pregnancy & childbirth transitions

↓

Pharmacologic Management

- Asperger's symptoms may change with pregnancy & warrant changes in medical management
- Hormonal changes of pregnancy may exacerbate depression in neurotypic women—is it the same for Aspergirls—assess at each visit
- Monitor medication safety for pregnancy & lactation
- Oxytocin production may eliminate need for medical management of pre-pregnancy AS symptoms
- If choice made to discontinue medications for comorbidities during pregnancy—monitor woman carefully & more frequently
- May need to assess for pain management during labor more frequently

↓

Sensitivities

- Touch—find out preferences—have patient bring own sheets, pillow, gown, gloves. Discuss "touching" during visits (BP, physical assessment, cervical exams, position changes. etc.)
- Light—often too bright in healthcare settings—encourage use of sunglasses, lamps in offices & DR
- Loud Noises—limit as much as possible—adjust appoinment schedule, room preference, posting of signs
- Too many people-decrease number of providers, staff caring for patient as much as possible
- Smell—prepare mother for new smells (hospital, rupture of membranes, lochia, breast milk, infant)
- Taste—food selections vary in healthcare settings—may want to bring food from home

↓

Postpartum Functioning

- Understudied area—May be high risk for severe postpartum depression
- Home visiting encouraged
- Assess bio-psycho-social health of mother & her ability to care for new infant
- Reassess relationships b/w patient and partner, family, friends
- Administer Barkin Maternal-Functioning Scale
- Encourage Breastfeeding—additonal benefits may incur from increased oxytocin levels during lactation
- Be in communication with pediatric health care provider

FIGURE 11.3 ■ Nursing care guidelines for the pregnant woman with AS.

SUMMARY

Transitioning to motherhood is a challenge for all new mothers. Support and encouragement is needed, and even more so for women with AS. Modifications of the clinical environment, and of the interpersonal, interactional, and educational approaches for prenatal, intrapartum, and postpartum nursing care are likely to help women with AS stay in control, tolerate interventions, and feel empowered in treatment and health care management decision making. Nurses must be careful to avoid making assumptions about pregnancy and motherhood for women with AS—that a woman with AS will not tolerate labor and delivery, will not comply with treatment, or will not be a good mother because she has AS. There is not yet research-based evidence to support or disprove these assumptions. The following quote by Liane Holliday Willey (1999), noted author and mother diagnosed with AS, describes her early parenting experience: "there were never mornings when I did not wake up and tell myself I was doing my best to give my babies the best parts of me. I realized early on, way before I heard the words Asperger's Syndrome, that I reacted to the world in unusual ways, but I never told myself this would mean I could not become a loving and good mother. I was not put together like other moms, but I was still my daughters' mom and I was determined they would have the kind of care they needed from me" (p. 77).

Perhaps many women with AS will be determined to follow rules to be responsible, competent mothers *because* of some of the traits associated with AS. We are not dismissing the potentially detrimental influences of the deficits associated with AS and the related treatment modalities (especially medications), on pregnant women and their fetuses, infants, and children. However, with close monitoring, appropriate intervention, a partnership with the woman, and a collaborative, multidisciplinary perspective, potential problems can be prevented or identified early, so that optimal family well-being is promoted.

All pregnant women and new mothers benefit from nonjudgmental, unbiased, compassionate, evidence-based nursing care that is tailored to their individual needs during these times of intense transition. We need a better understanding of the intersection between the neurobiology of AS and the physiological changes of pregnancy, along with a better understanding of the needs of pregnant women with AS in order to develop appropriate and effective intervention strategies.

ACKNOWLEDGMENT

The authors would like to thank all of the women and mothers with AS who offered their time to be interviewed about their experiences in pregnancy, childbirth, and early parenting. The input and insight they provided was invaluable and helped us frame care and nursing interventions tailored to better help meet their needs during this time of their lives. We would also like to acknowledge the following authors who graciously provided guidance during the interview process: Maxine Aston, Michael John Carley, Isabelle Henault, Shana Nichols, and Rudy Simone. Finally, we would like to thank the staff and members of the Women's Autism Network.

REFERENCES

Aston, M. (2003). *Aspergers in love.* Philadelphia, PA: Jessica Kingsley.

Attwood, T. (2007). *The complete guide to Asperger's syndrome.* Philadelphia, PA: Jessica Kingsley.

Aylott, J. (2010). Improving access to health and social care for people with autism. *Nursing Standard, 24*(27), 47–56.

Baldwin, K. A. (2006). Comparison of selected outcomes of Centering Pregnancy versus traditional prenatal care. *Journal of Midwifery & Women's Health, 51*(4), 266–272.

Barkin, J. L., Wisner, K.L., Bromberger, J. T., Beach, S. R., Terry, M. A., & Wisiewski, S. R. (2010). Development of the Barkin Index of Maternal Functioning. *Journal of Women's Health, 19*(12), 2239–2246.

Baron-Cohen, S. (2011). The autistic mind: Empathizing-systematizing theory. In E. Hollander, A. Kolevzon, & J. T. Coyle (Eds.), *Textbook of Autism Spectrum Disorders* (pp. 39–48). Washington, DC: American Psychiatric Publishing.

Bartz, J. A., & Young, L. J. (2011). Oxytocin, social cognition and autism. In E. Hollander, A. Kolevzon, & J. T. Coyle (Eds.), *Textbook of Autism Spectrum Disorders* (pp. 265–276). Washington, DC: American Psychiatric Publishing.

Beck, C. T. (2006). The anniversary of birth trauma: Failure to rescue. *Nursing Research, 55*(6), 381–390.

Berkman, N., Lohr, K., & Bulik, C. (2007). Outcomes of eating disorders: A systematic review of the literature. *International Journal of Eating Disorders, 40*(4), 293–309.

Blackshaw, A. J., Kinderman, P., Hare, D. J., & Hare, C. (2001). Theory of mind, causal attribution and paranoia in Asperger syndrome. *Autism, 5*(2), 147–163.

Bloch, J. R., Dawley, K., & Suplee, P. D. (2009). Application of the Kessner and Kotelchuck Prenatal Care Adequacy Indices in a preterm birth population. *Public Health Nursing 26*(5), 449–459.

Bloch, J. R., Webb, D., Mathew, L., Dennis, E., Bennett, I., & Culhane, J. (2010). Beyond marital status: The quality of the mother-father relationship and its influence on reproductive health behaviors and outcomes among unmarried low income pregnant women. *Maternal and Child Health Journal, 14*(5), 726–734.

Campbell, K. (2007, August 17). Is anorexia the female Asperger's? *The Sunday Times.* Retrieved from http://www.timesonline.co.uk/tol/life_and_style/health/features/article2272080.ece

Carwell, M. L., & Spatz, D. L. (2011). Eating disorders and breastfeeding. *Maternal Child Nursing, 36*(2), 112–117.

Centers for Disease Control and Prevention. (2010). U.S. medical eligibility criteria for contraceptive use. *Morbidity and Mortality Weekly Report, 59*(RR-4), 1–86.

Cohen, A. (2011, July). *Physiologic Changes of Pregnancy.* Fundamentals Course presented at the Department of Obstetrics and Gynecology, Albert Einstein Medical Center, Philadelphia, PA.

Copley, J. (2009). Asperger's syndrome and anorexia: The link between eating disorders and autism spectrum disorders. Retreived from http://www.suite101.com/content/aspergers-syndrome-and-anorexia-a110610

Esbensen, A. J., Greenberg, J. S., Seltzer, M. M., & Aman, M. G. (2009). A longitudinal investigation of psychotropic and nonpsychotropic medication use among adolescnets and adults with autism spectrum disorders. *Journal of Autism & Developmental Disorders, 39*(9), 1339–1349.

Fawcett, J., & Tulman, L. (1988). Development of the inventory of functional status after childbirth. *Journal of Nurse-Midwifery, 33*(6), 252–260.

Feldman, R., Weller, A., Zagoory-Sharon, O., & Levine, A. (2007). Evidence for a neuroendocrinological foundation of human affiliation: plasma oxytocin levels across pregnancy and the postpartum period predict mother-infant bonding. *Psychological Science, 18*(11), 965–970.

Gabbe, S. G., Niebyl, J. R., & Simpson, J. L. (Eds.). (2007). *Obstetrics: Normal and problem pregnancies.* Philadelphia, PA: Elsevier.

Giarelli, E., Wiggins, L. D., Rice, C. E., Levy, S. E., Kirby, R. S., Pinto-Martin, J., & Mandell, D. (2010). Sex differences in the evaluation and diagnosis of autism spectrum disorders among children. *Disabilities Health Journal, 3*(2), 107–116.

Gillberg, C., & Cederlun, M. (2005). Asperger syndrome: Familial and pre- and perinatal factors. *Journal of Autism & Developmental Disorders, 35*(2), 159–166.

Gold, R., Faust, M., & Goldstein, A. (2010). Semantic integration during metaphor comprehension in Asperger syndrome. *Brain & Language, 113*(3), 124–134.

Grether, J. K., Anderson, M. C., Croen, L. A., Smith, D., & Windham, G. C. (2009). Risk of autism and increasing matrnal and paternal age in a large north American population. *American Journal of Epidemiology 170*, 1118–1126.

Hollander, E., Kolevzon, A., & Coyle, J. T. (Eds.). (2011). *Textbook of autism spectrum disorders.* Washington, DC: American Psychiatric Publishing.

Hurtig, T., Kuusikko, S., Mattila, M. L., Haapsomomo, H., Ebeling, H., Jussila, K., Pauls, O., & Moilanen, I. (2009). Multi-informant reports of psychiatric symptoms among high-functioning adolescents with Asperger syndrome or autism. *Autism, 13*(6), 583–598.

Institute of Medicine. (2007). *Preterm birth: Causes, consequences, and prevention.* Washington, DC: National Academies Press.

Jellema, T., Lorteije, J., van Rijn, S., van t'Wout, M., de Haan, E., ven England, H., & Kemner, C. (2009). Involuntary interpretation of social cues is compromised in autism spectrum disorders. *Autism Research, 2*(4), 192–204.

Jordan, C. J. (2010). Evolution of autism support and understanding via the world wide web. *Intellectual & Developmental Disabilities, 48*(3), 220–227.

Kalyva, E. (2009). Comparison of eating attitudes between adolescent girls with and without Asperger syndrome: Daughters' and mothers' reports. *Journal of Autism & Developmental Disorders, 39*(39), 480–486.

Kleinhans, N. M., Richards, T., Weaver, K. E., Liang, O., Dawson, G., & Ayward, E. (2009). Brief report: Biochemical correlates of clinical impairment in high functioning autism and Asperger's disorder. *Journal of Autism and Developmental Disorders, 39*(7), 1079–1086.

Manning, J., Baron-Cohen, S., Wheelwright, S., & Sanders, G. (2001). The 2nd to 4th digit ratio and autism. *Developmental Medicine & Child Neurology, 43*(3), 160–164.

Mattila, M. L., Kielinen, M., Jussila, K., Linna, S. L., Bloigu, R., Ebeling, H., & Moilanen, I. (2007). An epidemiological and diagnostic study of Asperger syndrome according to four sets of diagnostic criteria. *Journal of the American Academy of Child & Adolescent Psychiatry, 46*(5), 636–646.

Meleis, A. I. (Ed.). (2010). *Transitions theory.* New York: Springer Publishing.

Miller, J. S., & Ozonoff, S. (2011). Asperger's syndrome. In E. Hollander, A. Kolevzon, & J. T. Coyle (Eds.), *Textbook of autism spectrum disorders* (pp. 77–87). Washington, DC: American Psychiatric Publishing.

Myles, B. S. (2003). Behavioral forms of stress management for individuals with Asperger syndrome. *Child & Adolescent Psychiatric Clinics of North America. 12*(1), 123–141.

National Eating Disorders Association. (2005). *Eating disorders and pregnancy: Some facts about the risk.* Retreived from http://www.nationaleatingdisorders.org/nedaDir/files/documents/handouts/Pregnant.pdf

National Institute of Neurologic Disorders and Strokes. (2005). Asperger syndrome information page. Retreived from http://www.ninds.nih.gov/disorders/asperger/asperger.htm

National Research Council and Institute of Medicine. (2008). *The National Children's Study Research Plan: A review.* Washington, DC: National Academies Press.

Nichols, S., Moravick, G. M., & Tenenbaum, S. P. (2009). *Girls growing up on the autism spectrum.* Philadelphia, PA: Jessica Kingsley.

Pfeiffer, B., Kinnealey, M., Reed, C., & Herzberg, G. (2005). Sensory modulation and affective disorders in children and adolescents with Asperger's disorder. *American Journal of Occupational Therapy, 59*(3), 335–345.

Pijnacker, J., Hagoort, P., Buitelaar, J., Tenisse, J. P., & Geurts, B. (2009). Pragmatic inferences in high-functioning adults with autism and Asperger syndrome. *Journal of Autism and Developmental Disorders, 39*(4), 607–618.

Posmontier, B. (2008). Sleep quality in women with and without postpartum depression. *Journal of Obstetric, Gynecologic, & Neonatal Nursing, 37*(6), 722–735.

Reichenberg, A., Gross, R., Kolevzon, A., & Susser, E. S. (2011). Parental and perinatal risk factors for autism. In E. Hollander, A. Kolevzon, & J. T. Coyle (Eds.), *Textbook of autism spectrum disorders.* Washington, DC: American Psychiatric Publishing.

Reid, J. (2007). Centering Pregnancy: A model for group prenatal care. *Nursing for Women's Health, 11*(4), 382–388.

Ricci, S., & Kyle, T. (2008). *Maternity and pediatric nursing.* Philadelphia, PA: Lippincott, Williams and Wilkins.

Ringman, J. M., & Jankovic, J. (2000). Occurrence of tics in Asperger's syndrome and autistic disorder. *Journal of Child Neurology, 15*(6), 394–400.

Robertson, M. M. (2011). Gilles de la Tourette syndrome: The complexities of phenotype and treatment. *British Journal of Hospital Medicine, 72*(2), 100–107.

Ross, H. E., & Young, L. J. (2009). Oxytocin and the neural mechanisms regulating social cognition and affiliative behavior. *Frontiers in Neuroendocrinology, 30*(4), 534–547.

Samson, A., & Hegenloh, H. (2010). Stimulus characteristics affect humor processing in individuals with Asperger syndrome. *Journal of Autism and Developmental Disorders, 40*(4), 438–447.

Schreck, K. A., & Williams, K. E. (2006). Food preferences and factors influencing food selectivity for children with autism spectrum disorders. *Research in Developmental Disabilities, 27*(4), 353–363.

Simone, R. (2010). *Aspergirls.* Philadelphia, PA: Jessica Kingsley.

Souders, M., Mason, T. B., Valladares, O., Bucan, M., Levy, S. E., Mandell, D. S., Weaver, T. E., & Pinto-Martin, J. (2009). Sleep behaviors and sleep quality in children with autism spectrum disorders. *Sleep, 32*(12), 1566–1578.

Spek, A., Schatorje, T., Scholte, E., & van Berckelaer-Onnes, I. (2009). Verbal fluency in adults with high functioning autism or Asperger syndrome. *Neuropsychologia, 47*(3), 652–656.

Suplee, P. D., Dawley, K., & Bloch, J. R. (2007). Tailoring peripartum nursing care for women of advanced maternal age. *Journal of Obstetrical, Gynecologic, and Neonatal Nursing, 36*(6), 616–623.

Tager-Flusberg, H., & Dominick, K. (2011). Comorbid disorders. In E. Hollander, A Kolevzon, & J. T. Coyle (Eds.), *Textbook of autism spectrum disorders* (pp. 209–217). Washington, DC: American Psychiatric Publishing.

Taylor, E. L., Target, M., & Charman, T. (2008). Attachment in adults with high-functioning autism. *Attachment & Human Development, 10*(2), 143–163.

Thompson, L., Thompson, M., & Reid, A. (2010). Neurofeedback outcomes in clients with Asperger's syndrome. *Applied Psychophysiology & Biofeedback, 35*(1), 63–81.

Turunen, J., Rehnstrom, K., Kilpinen, H., Kuokkanen, M., Kempas, E., & Ylisaukko-Oja, T. (2008). Mitochondrial aspartat/glutamate carrier SLC25A12 gene is associated with autism. *Autism Research, 1*(3), 189–192.

Willey, L. H. (1999). *Pretending to be normal.* Philadelphia, PA: Jessica Kingsley.

Zalla, T., Sav, A. M., Stopin, A., Ahade, S., & Leboyer, M. (2009). Faux pas detection and intentional action in Asperger Syndrome. A replication on a French Sample. *Journal of Autism & Developmental Disorders, 39*(2), 373–382.

12 Emergency Nursing Care of Patients With Autism Spectrum Disorder

Kathleen Patrizzi and Ellen Giarelli

The nurse in the emergency department plays an important role in the receiving, treatment, and management of the patient on the autism spectrum who presents for emergency care. As the number of children diagnosed with ASD increases (Centers for Disease Control and Prevention, 2009) and the population ages, adult emergency departments (EDs) are likely to encounter an increased number of patients with autism spectrum disorder (ASD).

McDermott, Zhou, & Mann (2008) examined the differences in the frequency and type of injury for children with autism and pervasive developmental disorder (PDD) compared with typically developing peers when both groups are insured by Medicaid. The relative rate (RR) of emergency/hospital treatment of injury for children with autism or PDD compared with controls was 1.20 (95% confidence interval [CI], 1.04 to 1.39) after controlling for age and gender. Children with autism or PDD had a higher rate for head, face, and neck injuries (RR = 1.47, 95% CI, 1.13 to 1.90) and a lower rate for sprains and strains (RR = 0.54, 95% CI, 0.32 to 0.91). Treatment for poisoning was 7.6 times as frequent, and self-inflicted injury was also 7.6 times as frequent for children with autism or PDD than for controls. In addition, individuals with developmental disabilities are four to 10 times more likely to be victims of crime (Sobsey, Wells, Lucardie, & Mansell, 1995) and may be taught "compliance" from a very young age, making them easy targets for abuse. Crime victimization of individuals with autism may result in injuries that require an emergency medical response and care. When addressing physical and sexual assaults, professionals face additional challenges in trying to preserve evidence while providing appropriate medical treatments.

Sometimes the ED staff will have advance notice that a patient has ASD; however, it is more likely that the patient will arrive without this information. Outside resources with more knowledge and experience about caring for autistic patients may not be available when the patient arrives, especially during night and weekend hours. Therefore, knowledgeable nurses have a critical role in recognizing which patients have ASD and must include this information when planning care to meet their specials needs during the visit. Nurses are on the front line for modifying the physical environment in the ED to ensure a safe and therapeutic encounter.

In this chapter, we develop the role of the emergency nurse in assessing and treating the patient with ASD, including rapid assessment and treatment and management of potential aggression and emotional "meltdowns."

THE EMERGENCY DEPARTMENT EXPERIENCE

Upon arrival to the ED, a patient is typically greeted by a triage nurse who performs a quick assessment of the patient to determine the severity of the chief complaint. Following this initial assessment, the patient will go through several more steps until a decision can be made to admit the patient to the hospital, discharge the patient home, or transfer the patient to an outside facility. During this process, a patient encounters several different staff members and can be involved in a variety of tests and procedures. People experience EDs in different ways. Many of these processes take place concurrently, and it may seem to the patient that an intolerable number of activities are happening at once. On the other hand, a patient can also sit idle for long periods of time while waiting for procedures to be prescribed and performed. This is the unpredictable nature of triage.

During triage, the patient is evaluated by a nurse and asked several questions about his or her presenting complaint, past medical history, and current medications. Following the initial intake, a patient is registered by a staff member who collects insurance information and a copayment. After this, the patient may wait in a public area until called into the ED to be seen, or if triage warrants, he or she may be moved to a treatment room immediately. On placement in the examination room, the patient is seen first by a nurse and then a physician.

If admitted to a teaching hospital, a patient may also be approached by nursing students, medical students, and/or medical residents, who may repeat questions and ask additional questions. Throughout one's stay, and depending on one's needs, a patient may encounter other members of the health care team, including social workers, case managers, physical therapists, radiology technicians, respiratory therapists, and phlebotomists, among others. This process is disorienting. Any one of these steps may cause significant distress for patients with ASD who have problems with socialization, cognition, and communication (Blake, 2010; Parish, Moss, & Richman, 2008; Vessey, 1988).

Patients may have several tests completed while they are in the ED, including having phlebotomy, portable radiology, transport to the radiology department for scanning, electrocardiography, or other diagnostic testing A typical visit to the ED may include wound suturing, intravenous (IV) placement, or dislocation reduction. The majority of patients in the ED also receive some type of medication, either topically, orally, or intravenously. After the initial evaluation and testing, the team makes a decision about the type of care the patient requires, whether he or she can be discharged home to follow up with his or her own provider, admitted to the hospital, or transferred to another facility (Nelson & Amplo, 2009). Consider all the ways the patient with ASD might become distressed.

The process of emergency care is complicated and can be overwhelming for any patient. In addition, the crowded, busy environment of the ED can be very noisy. The patient with ASD can be very sensitive to sound, as well as smell. Factoring in the anxiety a patient may face upon receiving a diagnosis and the pain and discomfort of the medical or psychiatric problem, the whole experience can be overstimulating and frightening. The environment of the ED is even more challenging for a person on the autism spectrum. Emergency providers, particularly emergency nurses, can adjust workflow and situational factors to make the experience more tolerable for the patient with ASD. A quick reference for ED staff and paramedics is available from the Autism Society (Autism Society, 2011). A nurse must apprehend the reality of the patient with ASD by trying to see the ED through the eyes of a person with autism. A typical ED room is, at minimum, confusing to a person with limited or no language skills, resistance to change, aversion to loud noise and the inability to interpret social cues (see Figures 12.1 & 12.2).

In addition to the many reasons any person may arrive at the ED for treatment, some reasons are specific to the patient with ASD. Therefore, the ED nurse must integrate routine ED care with special considerations for ASD. Knowing that the patient has ASD can provide clues to explain a chief complaint. The emergency nurse can adapt and modify his or her plan of care for a patient based on this knowledge. Exhibit 12.1 provides some examples of situations in which an emergency nurse may encounter a patient with ASD.

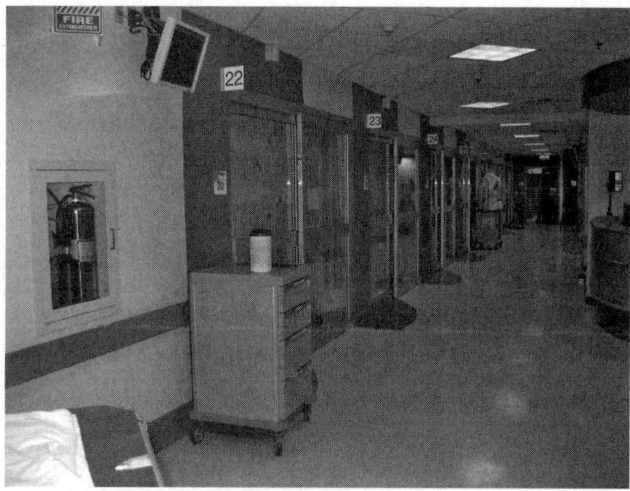

FIGURE 12.1 ■ The view of a hallway in a typical ED. There are several visual distractions that may lead to confusion and fear on the part of a patient with ASD.

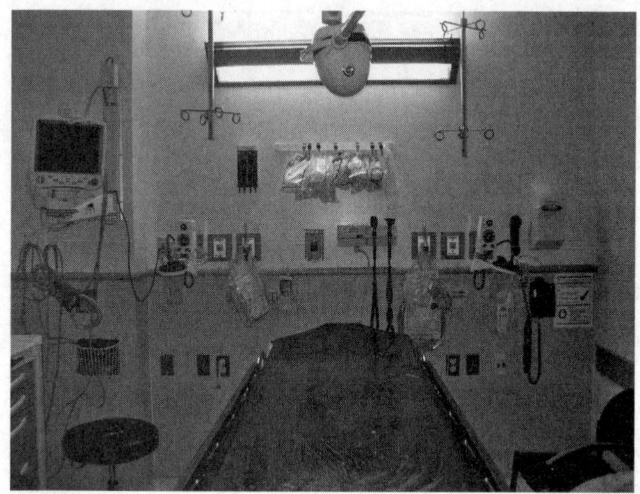

FIGURE 12.2 ■ The view of a typical holding room in an ED. There are several visual distractions and objects that may cause distress or anxiety for a patient with ASD.

A VISIT TO THE EMERGENCY DEPARTMENT: TRAUMATIC INJURY

CASE–INITIAL PRESENTATION

It is a Friday afternoon in the Emergency Department. At 4 p.m., emergency medical services (EMS) arrives with Charlie Emerson, a 40-year-old male who was in an automobile crash. Mr. Emerson is approximately 6 feet tall and appears overweight. Mr. Emerson was sitting in the passenger seat when the car he was in collided with another car at an

(*Continued*)

CASE–INITIAL PRESENTATION (Continued)

intersection when that car ran through a stop sign. EMS reports they found Mr. Emerson sitting in the car awake and alert. The airbags in the car deployed. They report having difficulty getting a history from Mr. Emerson as to what happened. He could not tell the staff if he hit his head or lost consciousness during the accident. He keeps repeating that his neck is sore. This is all he has said since they arrived. Cervical spine protection was initiated at the scene of the accident, and Mr. Emerson arrived with a cervical collar in place and is lying flat on a backboard. He is having difficulty lying still on the board.

When asked if Mr. Emerson had any medical history, EMS stated that his sister was driving the car and was also coming to the ED for evaluation. Before they left the scene, the sister told EMS that Mr. Emerson is autistic. She gave to the EMS a card with emergency contact information for Mr. Emerson's family members and health care providers.

EXHIBIT 12.1

Possible Reasons People with ASD Could Visit the Emergency Department

- General medical issues or issues related to comorbidities associated with ASD
- Injury
    - Resulting from disregard for safety or alterations in perception
        - Running into traffic
        - Injury from climbing acts/jumping
    - Self-injury
- Drowning (Some patients with ASD have a strong affinity for water.)
- Seizures
- Evaluation to rule out intoxication or psychosis (Situation could have started out with police being called.)
- Escalation crisis
- Abuse/neglect

Based on Kelble (2009).

Initial Encounter

The first person to encounter a patient who comes to the ED for treatment is most often the triage nurse. The purpose of emergency triage is to perform an initial evaluation of each patient who arrives to the ED and determine the acuity of their problem. The triage nurse aims to ensure patient safety by sorting patients who need to be seen and evaluated right away from patients who can wait longer before being seen. A brief history of the present complaint is taken, as well as information about past medical and surgical history, current medications, and allergies. A set of vital signs are also taken to aid in assessment. For a patient who walks into the ED, this process is usually completed in a small office close to the waiting area. A patient who arrives via ambulance may be sent to this area or may be placed immediately in a treatment room with the process completed at the bedside.

To keep up with the flow of patients coming into the ED, the goal is to complete the triage process quickly, usually in less than 5 minutes. Triage nurses are skilled at rapidly determining the level of care that patients need. While this benefits the majority of patients in the ED, some patients may feel rushed and overwhelmed at how quickly the process takes place. Nurses working in triage might benefit from having basic knowledge of ASD and how to modify their approach to these patients to ensure their comfort and safety. Special considerations need to be taken when triaging patients with ASD. Moving too quickly can overwhelm the patient, which will make the process more difficult and time-consuming. For example, the triage nurse must recognize that simply entering a crowded, noisy waiting room may trigger anxiety and/or difficult behaviors in an autistic patient. Sensory overload and increased anxiety might cause a person with autism to respond with self injury or aggressive behaviors toward the hospital staff, or hospital equipment. The triage nurse can help by moving the patient and their caregiver to a quiet area to complete the triage process (Center for Autism and Related Disabilities, 2010). Exhibit 12.2 provides questions that should be asked during the triage process to assess the level of acuity of each patient. The challenge for the ED nurse is to adapt these fundamental questions to the developmental age and communication style of the patient with ASD. Nurses must understand autism to provide safe and appropriate care (Olejnik, 2004; Volkmar et al., 1999).

Reaction to Behaviors

Without the information of an ASD diagnosis, a nurse may react inappropriately to the patient's behavior. A lack of personal familiarity with individuals who have a disability may cause an ED nurse to feel professionally awkward and uncertain when providing emergency care and assistance. Common reactions to individuals with disabilities include fear, embarrassment, or pity. Awareness of the core features of ASD improves the nurse's ability to notice the nuances of behavior that may suggest a developmental disability.

Recognizing the Patient Has ASD when It Is Not Disclosed

When encountering the patient with ASD, emergency nurses will need to alter their approach. On many occasions, a patient may arrive to the ED for evaluation without a family member, friend, or caregiver. One example is if a patient with ASD was in a car accident and the family caregiver, perhaps an elderly parent, was also injured and is unable to provide support or information in the ED. A second passenger may also be taken to a different facility. A quick assessment using a screening tool for ASD can be extremely useful to the nurse who may not have adequate data on health history when the patient arrives.

A patient on the autism spectrum may indirectly disclose that they have ASD. On initial presentation, nurses can look for MedicAlert bracelets, necklaces, or ankle bands that state the patient has ASD. The patient may have an identification card sewn into his or her clothing or in a wallet. While all patients with ASD are unique and have variations in symptoms, an understanding of core and associated features is beneficial, especially when a diagnosis is not disclosed. See Exhibit 12.3 for a list of behaviors that could indicate ASD to the ED Nurse.

If the nurse suspects that a patient may have ASD, the safest course of action is to begin by approaching the patient as if he or she is on the spectrum. Approaching the patient the way the nurse normally does might cause the situation to deteriorate and could possibly escalate the patient's distress. An example of this can be as simple as applying a blood-pressure cuff while taking vital signs. Typically this is done while the nurse is talking to the patient

EXHIBIT 12.2

Behaviors That Could Indicate ASD to the Emergency Department Nurse

Impairment in Social Interaction

Poor eye contact: Looking down, making and losing eye contact almost immediately, staring elsewhere

Lack of facial expression: Flat affect, or an expression that may be inappropriate for the situation

Differences in body posture: Shrugged shoulders, leaning in one direction or another, instability

Gestures to regulate social interaction: Hand-flapping or other repetitive gestures used as a method of self-soothing

Impairment in Communication

Nonverbal communication only: Pointing at objects or pictures, nodding or shaking the head

Inability to sustain a conversation: Nonresponsive when addressed directly, unwilling to respond, or will respond initially and become easily distracted or anxious

Repeating words or phrases: Answering the same question over and over, even if a new question has been asked

Restricted Patterns of Behavior

Inflexible adherence to routines or rituals: Inability to adapt to hospital environment, insistence upon following typical "home regimen"

Abnormal preoccupations or patterns of interest: Obsessing over a piece of equipment, a particular staff member, or a question posed to the patient

Stereotyped and repetitive motor movements (e.g., hand-flapping or twisting, whole-body movements)

Persistent preoccupation with parts of objects (e.g., fixated on flashing light or spinning wheel)

without a large amount of preparation or explanation. However, many patients with ASD do not respond well to being touched or have extreme reactions to certain textures or sounds, such as Velcro®. Do not presume that the patient has previously had a blood-pressure reading and remembers the sensation. The nurse will need to explain to the patient what is happening and prepare him or her for what the cuff will feel like when it is applied and measuring the blood pressure. Some patients with ASD may need to be distracted completely during this ordinarily routine procedure. If the nurse begins by using strategies tailored to the person with ASD, and the patient does not need them, the nurse can then go back to the usual approach (American Academy of Child and Adolescent Psychiatry, 1999; Kelble, 2009). The nurse must also remember that all patients with ASD are unique, and strategies that work for one patient may not work for all patients. It is vital that each interaction is carefully considered

EXHIBIT 12.3

Methods for Approaching a Patient with ASD

- Be patient when communicating. Speak and move slowly.
- Use simple phrases and ask one question at a time.
- Avoid using medical terminology.
- Allow extra time for the patient to respond after you ask a question.
- Use calming body language.
- Give the patient personal space.
- Allow the patient to touch and hold medical equipment when possible.
- Expect minimal eye contact.
- Inform the patient before touching or moving him or her.
- Involve family or caregivers, when present.
- Unless the person is causing injury or damaging property, do not stop repetitive behaviors.
- Avoid touching if possible. If you must have physical contact with the individual, explain in simple terms what you are going to do and why. Try saying, "I want to help you, but I [explanation of procedure]."
- Gently persuade or remove the person from the dangerous situation. Offer an alternative to the dangerous action. Be aware that if the person is anxious, there is a risk he or she could bolt without warning.
- Use a communication board if possible, and allow time for processing of information before responses are given.
- Avoid making assumptions about alcohol or drug use.
- Use the least-invasive technique possible to ensure the individual's safety.

and evaluated for effectiveness by observing the patient's reaction. In anticipation of seeing a patient with ASD, the ED nurses should keep a list of support professionals who may be contacted to provide immediate consultation, including a social worker, child or adult psychiatrist, behavioral therapist, and occupational therapist. Exhibit 12.4 lists some general rules to apply when approaching a patient who has ASD.

Room Placement in the ED

When possible, the nurse should place the patient with ASD in a private room in a quiet area of the ED. Due to the sensitivity to light common in patients with ASD, dimming the lights may be necessary. Removing pictures or posters from the wall can also aid in reducing stimuli. Many patient rooms in the ED contain numerous supplies and pieces of equipment that could pose a threat to the safety of the patient, their family, and ED staff. Removing equipment that is not needed can help to reduce visual stimulation, distractions, and sources of harm. Have bumpers available to place on the bed or stretcher to prevent injury. Keep staff

EXHIBIT 12.4

Key Questions to Ask the Patient and/or the Caregiver during Triage

- When did you start to have [the problem, e.g., bad feelings, pain]? Be specific.
- What was your/the patient doing when [the problem] started?
- Has there been any change in behavior?
  - If behavior has changed, what is usual behavior compared to now?
- Has anything helped or made you/the patient feel better?
- Does anything make you/the patient feel worse?
- Do you/does the patient have any medical, surgical, or psychological history?
- Are you/is the patient on any medications?
- Are you/is the patient, allergic to any medications?
- How does the patient prefer to communicate?
- Are there any strategies that have worked in the past when you/the patient have/has been in the ED?
- Are you/is the patient in pain? Use scales appropriate to the developmental age and language of the patient.

Additional Triage Questions for Trauma Patients[a]

- What was the mechanism of injury?
- Was there a major acceleration or deceleration injury?
- Are there any signs of bleeding or bruising?
- For auto accidents:
  - Was the patient wearing a seatbelt?
  - Did the airbags deploy?
- For head/neck injury
  - Did the patient strike his or her head?
  - Did the patient lose consciousness?
  - Are there any changes in vision or sensitivity to light?
  - Is the patient having difficulty breathing or swallowing?
  - Is there any hoarseness
- Is the patient having any numbness or tingling?

[a]Adapted from Emergency Nurses Association (2007).

consistent throughout the stay and control the number of people and professionals who are permitted to approach the patient. Assigning the patient to a primary nurse who will be working for the next several hours might increase comfort and help to establish a trusting therapeutic rapport.

CASE–ASSESSMENT AND CARE

The charge nurse finds out he likes to be called "Charlie." She notes this information on his chart. She places him in a private room, away from any entrance or exit to the ED and away from the main nurse's station, where it tends to be noisy and hectic. There is a smaller nurse's station near Charlie's room where his nurse can observe him continually and monitor activities. Before Charlie is placed in the room, the charge nurse asks another staff member to assess the room for safety. A large supply cart is removed and placed outside the room.

While they are waiting for the room to be ready, the charge nurse introduces herself and the primary nurse to Charlie. Neither nurse touches him during this process, because they observe that his is rocking and holding his body, which indicates a response to increased stress. The nurses take care to move Charlie into a room quickly, because of the noise and activity level at the main nurse's station. The charge nurse says to Charlie:

> Hi Charlie, my name is Amanda. I am one of the nurses in the Emergency Department. You are here because you were in a car accident and need special care. We are going to take good care of you. We have a quiet room ready for you. You can wait there for the doctors and nurses. They will visit you soon [shows him a clock and writes down the time]. Would you like a blanket to hold? I know it hurts to lie still on the board, but it is important you stay still until we can make sure your bones are okay. Someone is calling your mom right now and she will be here soon. If you need any help we will be right here with you. You are doing a great. This is Anna. Anna is going to be your nurse while you are here.
>
> Charlie does not answer or make eye contact. The nurse does not force Charlie to respond, because she knows this behavior is characteristic of ASD.

BEST PRACTICES: NURSING CARE INITIAL ASSESSMENT

All patients presenting to the ED have an initial evaluation during which a nurse assesses the acuity of the complaint and collects background information. Obtaining this information can be difficult when there are impairments in communication and social interaction associated with ASD. If the patient arrives with a family member or other caregiver, the nurse should involve this person in the triage process of gathering accurate, comprehensive information.

Caregiver Involvement

The caregiver becomes a member of the ED team (Gabriel & Gluck, 1972) and has valuable information about the patient's medical history and medications. Involving the caregiver at the beginning of the triage process helps the nurse in many ways. Family caregivers or friends can advise the staff on how to interact with the patient, including how the patient communicates and what strategies will work for patient care, including monitoring, procedures, and diagnostic tests. Involving the caregiver early in the process can improve patient comfort and cooperation with treatments in the ED. The family member or caregiver might bring objects that help the patient stay calm and focused. The caregiver can also inform the team of strategies that have worked in the past and elements of the patient's history that can lead to the final diagnosis. If the patient must wait to be taken to a treatment room, being in the waiting room can be very difficult. If at all possible, the patient and caregiver should wait in a quiet area.

The importance of involving the patient's caregiver throughout the patient's visit to the ED is one of the most important factors for success for the patient and the health care team. Caregivers provide valuable insight into patient's likes and dislikes, and how the patient communicates and responds to medical treatments. A patient also knows and trusts his or her caregivers. Involving the caregiver in parts of the assessment, including applying medical equipment such as blood-pressure cuffs or leads for the cardiac monitor, prevents avoidable anxiety. Involving the caregiver can also help alleviate the caregiver's anxiety and build trust between the caregiver and the provider (Gurney, McPheeters, & Davis, 2006).

If a Caregiver Is Not Present

Communication about the patient's history will be more difficult if there is no caregiver present to assist in obtaining information. A useful method to communicate with nonverbal patients is the picture-exchange communication system (PECS; Ganz and Simpson, 2004). This is a collection of pictures, usually kept in a book, that can be used to communicate with others nonverbally. Autistic children and adults that use this system will take the book with them so they can communicate wherever they are (Ganz and Simpson, 2004). In an extreme emergency, and especially if the family member or caregiver is not present, PECS will not arrive with the patient. The nurses can still use pictures to communicate with the patient. Emergency nurses may want to consider having a set of pictures available in their departments to facilitate communication with nonverbal patients, including patients with autism.

Another option if the caregiver is unavailable is to contact the patient's primary health care provider for health information about the patient. The nurse might consult with the primary physician, for example, to formulate a plan of care consistent with the care being provided outside of the ED.

Co-occurring Health Problems

Other health problems may co-occur with autisms. The nurse might need this information to properly assess the patient's complaint and assign an acuity level during triage (Ghaziuddin, Tsai, & Ghaziuddin, 1992; Leyfer, Folstein, & Bacalman, 2006; Seltzer, Krauss, Shattuck, Orsmond, Swe, & Lord, 2003). Co-occurring conditions can have an effect on how symptoms present in the patient, and knowledge of them is essential for a differential diagnosis. These are listed in Exhibit 12.5.

In situations involving trauma, the patient may need spinal immobilization. This can be uncomfortable for any patient. Spinal immobilization, involves wearing a cervical collar and laying flat on a backboard. It can be particularly difficult for the patient with ASD. Because movement is contraindicated, the patient who communicates nonverbally could have difficulty describing or even identifying the location of the injury or where he or she is experiencing pain. If the patient unable to speak, the nurse will not be able to obtain an accurate history and must proceed cautiously. Appropriate triage can be made only if there is accurate assessment of the severity of the condition.

EXHIBIT 12.5

Coexisting Conditions in Patients with ASD

- Seizure disorders (affect 30% of patients with ASD)
- Sleep disturbances
- Pica
- Gastrointestinal disorders (affect 70% of patients with ASD)
    - Abnormal stool
    - Constipation
    - Vomiting
    - Abdominal pain
- Sensory abnormalities
- Self-injury
- Psychiatric conditions
    - Anxiety
    - Depression
    - Obsessive–compulsive disorder
    - Psychosis

Based on De Bruin, Ferdinand, & Meester (2007); Ghaziuddin, Tsai, & Ghaziuddin (1992); Levy et al. (2010); Leyfer et al. (2006); Simonoff, Pickles, Charman, Chandler, Loucas, & Baird (2008).

CASE–TRIAGE

Anna, Charlie's primary nurse, works on completing the triage process at the bedside. She uses information received during the report from EMS providers as part of her history. Charlie is not responding to questions but is saying "My neck," repeatedly. He remains on the backboard with the cervical collar in place.

Part of the triage assessment is to take vital signs. Charlie is informed of the process step by step, with Anna using basic words and pictures before placing the arm cuff. After taking his vital signs, Anna works quickly to document a triage note. The charge nurse spoke with Charlie's mother on the phone and obtained information about his medical history, medications, and allergies, and his methods of communication. Charlie's mother said that Charlie has been to an ED before for abdominal pain and has some familiarity with the hospital environment. She said one of the best things that happened during that visit was that Charlie's physical exam was completed once and only by a few essential personnel, rather than a large team. She also said he likes classical music and that providers can communicate with him verbally. She said she will bring his headphones and disc player to the ED.

(*Continued*)

CASE–TRIAGE (Continued)

Anna tells Charlie his mother is on her way to the ED and turns the television on to a classical channel offered by the hospital. She documents the following triage note:

> Patient is a 40-year-old male presenting to ED for evaluation of neck pain following a motor vehicle collision. Patient was sitting in the passenger side of the vehicle when it was struck by another car. Airbags deployed. Unsure if patient lost consciousness. Patient is currently awake and alert, complaining of neck pain. Spinal precautions maintained. No signs of bleeding or bruising. Patient has poor eye contact and is not responding to questions. Mother reports this is normal for the patient and is on her way to the ED. Vital signs: T: 98.2; BP: 110/77; P: 90; R: 22; Sp02: 99% on room air. Past medical history, from telephone contact with mother, ASD, seizures, gastroesophageal reflux disease, depression. Medications: valproic acid, sertraline, melatonin, ranitidine. Allergies: penicillin: anaphylaxis.

Physical Assessment and History Taking

Completing a physical assessment on a patient with ASD involves many stimuli that cause discomfort. Performing a collaborative assessment during the completion of a physical examination in the ED can help the nurse to reduce the number of times the patient is disturbed. Assessments should be completed with as few providers as possible present. Emergency nurses should organize members of the health care team to perform the physical assessment and history, while also assuring the maintenance of patient comfort and the avoidance of patient escalation. Key factors for success in the examination of a patient with ASD are listed in Exhibit 12.6.

Participation of Support Personnel

Support personnel should leave the patient room during the history and physical assessment. These providers can remain outside the room in order to be available in the case assistance is needed, especially if there is concern that the patient could escalate. While many providers, especially in teaching hospitals, would like to help and also gain experience with patients with ASD, the nurse must advocate for a reduction in personnel present for the comfort of the patient. Too many providers in the room can hinder attempts to provide care (Blake, 2010; Grubenhoff, Kirkwood, Gao, Deakyne, & Wathen, 2010; Kelble, 2009). The ED physician and ED nurse can both be in the room for the history and physical exam. Afterward, they can report findings to other members of the team.

Approaches to History Taking

If the patient with ASD can answer yes or no questions with words, nods, or pointing, he or she will be able to participate in some portions of the health history. If the patient is not able to communicate, the nurse's approach to taking the history will be similar to taking a pediatric patient's history from a parent. In contrast to the triage history, at this time the nurse will take an in-depth history. While taking an in-depth history, the nurse has more time to adapt the questions to the language and developmental level of the patient. It is most important to sort out the information that might have a direct effect on delivery and evaluation of care, including prior medical, surgical, and psychiatric history; current medications and allergies; and review of body systems.

EXHIBIT 12.6

Key Factors for Success during the ED Evaluation

- Involve caregivers.
  - Have the caregiver apply equipment (e.g., blood-pressure cuff) or position the patient for physical examination.
- Consult with primary health care providers.
  - Call the patient's primary provider for additional history and collaboration regarding a treatment plan.
- Remove unnecessary personnel.
  - Avoid sensory overload by minimizing the number of personnel in the patient's room.
- Cluster assessments.
  - Prevent overstimulation by clustering activity in smaller doses.
- Allow the patient to explore the environment and equipment that will be used.
  - Let the patient touch your stethoscope before you listen to his or her lungs.
- Be aware of sensory sensitivities to light, sound, touch, and pain.
  - Reduce noise and bright lights.
- Communicate with the patient before acting.
  - Before palpating the abdomen, tell the patient what you are going to do.
- Maintain a calm demeanor and clear approach.
  - To help keep the patient relaxed, try to avoid appearing flustered or nervous.

Approach to the Physical Assessment

After it has been decided which members of the team will participate in the physical assessment, this group will develop a plan for how to approach the patient. The team will prioritize which systems are most important to assess as related to the patient complaint, in case the exam has to be stopped prematurely due to patient overstimulation or lack of cooperation. Providers will need to be flexible with these patients and careful to move at a pace that the patient can tolerate. As with the triage, caregivers can be involved in this process. The caregiver can play a part in helping the team to plan the order of assessment that the patient will tolerate, as well as providing insight into strategies that have worked in the past. The caregiver can help communicate with the patient what is happening and suggest what type of reward will motivate the patient to cooperate with the assessment.

CASE–PHYSICAL ASSESSMENT

Charlie's mother arrives to the ED approximately 15 minutes after Charlie arrived. Anna reports to her what has transpired since Charlie has arrived at the ED. Before they enter

(*Continued*)

CASE–PHYSICAL ASSESSMENT (Continued)

the room, she explains to Charlie's mother that he is on spinal precautions and that they are waiting to perform an exam to clear him to come off of the spinal board. She explains they will need the mother's help with the physical examination and quickly finds the physician so that they can remove Charlie from the board and improve his comfort. She finds a nursing colleague to help her and the physician. The physician explains the process of log-rolling Charlie's body and removing the board, and explains that while Charlie is on his side, he will examine his spinal column to determine if it is safe for the spinal precautions to be discontinued. He emphasizes the importance of Charlie staying still while this examination is completed. Charlie's mother says she understands and they enter the room. Charlie appears calm with his mother present. She tells them they are going to roll him to the side to take the board out from under him and that he has to stay still. The nurse and doctor carefully observe Charlie for signs of an increase in pain during the examination of his spinal column. The process is completed without difficulty and Charlie is cleared from spinal precautions. Charlie's mother rewards him for cooperating by giving him a new baseball card.

Anna and the physician start taking Charlie's history by asking his mother questions. Charlie's sister had just picked him up from a day program he participates in and was bringing him home when the accident occurred. The nurse tells his mother what happened in the car accident. Charlie's mother asks him if he is having any pain. He vocalizes and grasps his head and neck with an open hand indicating pain. It is uncertain whether Charlie hit his head during the collision. When his mother asks if he hit his head, he says "I don't know."

Since Charlie's mother was not present during the collision, and the report was given by the EMS personnel who was at the scene, they move on to obtaining information about Charlie's medical and surgical history. Charlie has a history of seizures, gastroesophageal reflux disease, and depression. His medications and allergies are listed on the triage note. He has not had any surgeries. He was diagnosed with autism at the age of 5 years. His mother states Charlie is rarely verbal. He is able to feed and dress himself but is otherwise needs help with his activities of daily living. He can perform some activities for recreation but needs extensive prompting. Charlie loves baseball. His mother says his whole room is decorated with a baseball theme. Charlie collects baseball cards and enjoys watching baseball on television. His caregivers use baseball cards as a reward system for good behavior. This system is often used when he visits his primary-care providers to help incentivize cooperation. He has sensitivities to loud noise and to being touched, but his mother reports that if the touch is announced, he is usually okay. If he feels overwhelmed, Charlie attempts to run away, sometimes injuring those in his path. Charlie's mother tells the health care team that a secret to success is clustering care and allowing him to have breaks, and telling him what they are going to do before they proceed. This information is placed in the front of the chart, and as an alert in the electronic medical record.

Based on the history obtained, the physician and nurse decide to examine Charlie's head, eyes, ears, nose, and throat, along with his cardiovascular, respiratory, integumentary, and musculoskeletal systems. Charlie's mother is present. The physician and nurse ask permission prior to touching Charlie and speak in basic terms when telling him what they are going to do, avoiding using any medical terminology. Charlie tolerates the assessment without any problems.

Key medical and behavioral issues to continually monitor are also placed on the chart. Medical issues are seizures, depression, and multiple medications. Other issues are noise sensitivity, aversion to touch, self-care deficits, and flight risk during stress. A nurse might use baseball cards, television, and classical music for positive reinforcement.

BEST PRACTICES: DIAGNOSTIC TESTING AND PROCEDURES

Performing diagnostic testing or procedures on a patient with ASD requires a great deal of preplanning to ensure both patient and staff safety and patient comfort. The emergency nurse plays an important part in facilitating planning for tests and procedures and advocating for the patient. Performing tests and procedures on a patient with ASD will likely take longer than usual. Nurses should ensure tasks are completed for other patients before beginning a procedure on a patient with ASD, and may need another nurse to cover his or her assignment until the procedure is completed. Factors to consider when planning for such procedures are listed in Exhibit 12.7.

When planning for tests and procedures, the emergency nurse will need to consider what is involved in the test. For example, a computerized tomography (CT) scan will require the patient to lie flat and still for period of about 2 minutes, while the test is completed. Magnetic resonance imaging may be more difficult in terms of compliance, because the patient must lie still for several minutes, sometimes 30 to 45 minutes, and will be in a much smaller space. This may be impossible without sedation for the patient with autism. If the patient cannot tolerate the test, the nurse may explore with other members of the health care team selecting an alternative method of evaluation. Providers may also consider deferring treatments or tests that are not immediately necessary to treat life-threatening problems (Blake, 2010; Coury, Jones, Klatka, Winklosky, & Perrin, 2009; Kelble, 2009; Souders, 2010; Souders, Freeman, DePaul, & Levy, 2002). It is important to remember that medical treatments for patients with ASD who have a life-threatening emergency are no different than those for any other patient. For example, if a patient presents with cardiac arrest, then CPR, early defibrillation, and early access to care are to be performed, regardless of whether or not the patient has ASD, and treatments takes precedence over behavioral issues. Sedation may be required.

Several patients presenting to the ED require phlebotomy. This invasive procedure can cause anxiety. If the patient makes a sudden movement during the procedure, the nurse risks a

EXHIBIT 12.7

FACTORS TO CONSIDER WHEN PLANNING FOR A PROCEDURE

- Developmental age of the person with ASD
- What the procedure entails
- What equipment is needed
- How many people will need to assist
- How long the procedure takes
- Whether pain medications, sedation, or restraint will be needed
- Sensory profile of patient
- Personal space
- Attention span
- Family involvement
- Communication with other departments (radiology, phlebotomy, etc.)

Adapted from Souders (2010).

needlestick injury. If the patient is not restrained, he or she may become violent and hit a provider in response to pain. Some patients may not be able to tolerate the pressure of a tourniquet or seeing the equipment needed for phlebotomy. The nurse can apply a topical anesthetic to help decrease the pain of the needle. Several staff may be needed to hold the patient's extremities while the procedure is completed. This form of restraint may be extremely distressing and should be used only if no other options are available. A similar process will need to take place if the patient has a laceration and requires sutures. Members of the team should be experts in the procedure they are performing. If possible, one should employ the fastest and most experienced member of the team.

Sedation and Pain Medications

The use of sedation is recommended for extreme cases of agitation. The patient with ASD is at risk for having a paradoxical reaction to benzodiazepines. Risks of extrapyramidal reactions exist with the administration of haloperidol. Diphenhydramine by mouth can be effective and is well tolerated by most patients (Blake, 2010; Kelble, 2009). Shah and colleagues (2009) recommended oral ketamine combined with midazolam for deep sedation if a child, for example, is extremely difficult to manage. This sedative has also been used for burn patients with autism (Allison & Smith, 1998). In all cases of sedation, an anesthesiologist must be immediately available to make a determination of the safety, drug interactions, and possible adverse reactions to the medication. The patient with ASD may not have relief from pain with standard dosages of pain medications and may have abnormal reactions to medications usually prescribed in the ED. The ED nurse and physician must work with the pharmacist, anesthesiologist, and family caregiver, if possible, to develop and adjust the plan for pain management.

CASE–DIAGNOSTIC TESTING

After his physical exam is completed and considering the history obtained, the team decides Charlie will need to have some additional testing. The physician orders a CT scan of Charlie's head and some blood work. The team also determines that Charlie should have an IV placed and orders IV medication for pain. Anna discusses the plan with Charlie's mother, who said Charlie had a CT scan before when he was being evaluated for seizures. He has also had blood drawn, but he becomes anxious when he sees needles and may try to run away.

Based on Charlie's past experiences in the hospital having blood drawn and his tendency to run away when overstimulated, Anna formulates a plan for drawing blood and obtaining IV access. She feels confident in her experience with this procedure and decides she will be the provider to perform it. Charlie is approximately 6 feet tall and 220 pounds. Anna believes she will need help holding down Charlie's arms and legs during the procedure, so she asks the charge nurse to find people to help. Anna gathers the equipment needed to insert an IV and draw blood. She plans on accomplishing this with only one attempt. She will insert the IV and draw blood from the IV site to prevent additional discomfort from a second stick. She brings the equipment into the room on a tray covered by a drape so Charlie cannot see it.

Charlie's mother prepares Charlie for the procedure. Five staff members enter the room and Anna introduces them to Charlie. Charlie's mother says she will give him a

(*Continued*)

CASE–DIAGNOSTIC TESTING (Continued)

reward when Anna is finished and tells him he has to stay still. Charlie appears anxious and begins to rock. Anna applies a topical anesthetic. Charlie's mother holds one of his hands while the staff hold Charlie's arms and legs. Anna applies the tourniquet, locates a vein and inserts the IV. Charlie yells out in pain but otherwise does not move. Anna and Charlie's mother praise him for letting Anna insert the IV, and his mother gives him a baseball card for his free hand. Anna draws blood from the site and then administers pain medication.

After the IV has been inserted and Charlie has been medicated for pain, Anna wraps the IV in gauze in an effort to prevent it being pulled out, and gives Charlie another baseball card. The plan is for him to have a CT of his head. Because of the possibility of head injury and the need to monitor his mental status, sedation is not advised in this situation. In developing a plan for the CT scan, Anna is relieved that the entire test will only take 2 minutes and that it is not loud inside the CT scanner. Though she does not anticipate difficulty in getting the CT scan completed, she recommends Charlie's mother travel to CT with him. Charlie is reassured he will get a break after the CT is completed and will be able to listen to music in his room.

In the section on the physical exam and history, we advised removing unnecessary personnel, however when an invasive procedure is being performed, we advise the inclusion of several personnel in the room. In the case of a procedure such as inserting an IV line, having the extra staff in the room to ensure the safety of staff and patient outweighs reducing personnel for the patient's emotional comfort. Staff must be vigilant to avoid personal harm and be prepared to restrain a violent patient with soft wraps, if necessary.

Differential Diagnosis

As in the triage assessment, nurses have to take into consideration common co-occurring conditions related to ASD when forming a diagnosis. When establishing a diagnosis, a nurse must also be sure to rule out life-threatening causes of symptoms and behaviors and avoid attributing the behavior to the patient having ASD. Caregivers and those who know the patient well will be vital sources of information on what is abnormal.

SPECIAL ISSUES

Managing Escalation and Meltdowns

Escalation is an involuntary increase in behaviors similar to a tantrum and can include screaming, biting, swearing, kicking, punching, and other violent gestures. These behaviors occur in response to stress and can also include self-injury. As the behavior escalates, it can be referred to as a "meltdown." Managing escalation is one of the most important skills ED nurses can learn as they work with patients with ASD. Sometimes nurses are able to anticipate an escalation, while at other times the meltdown may occur without warning (Kelble, 2009).

The AUTISM approach is recommended for managing meltdowns (Debbaudt and Rothman, 2001). This approach assigns an action for every letter in the word "autism," with each action recommending how to best manage or even prevent a meltdown. The AUTISM Approach is as follows:

A: Approach in a quiet, nonthreatening manner

U: Understand touching may create an unexpected reaction

T: Talk in moderate, calm, relaxed voice

I: Instructions and communication should be simple and direct

S: Seek indicators to reevaluate the situation

M: Maintain safe distance

Nurses might be able to control these encounters by redirecting the patient through slow and simple instructions or distracting his or her attention with a favorite object, interest, or activity. In Charlie's case, music was effective.

The Use of Restraints

The use of restraints is recommended only as a last resort, when other methods have failed and physical harm to self or others is likely. By placing a patient with ASD in restraints, the nurse might compromise any trust that has been built and place the patient at risk for negative outcomes, including death (Blake, 2010; LeBel et al., 2004). Many special-interest groups, including the Autism National Committee (2010), advocate for the elimination of restraints for people with autism.

Abuse and Neglect

Abuse and neglect encompass many situations in which a parent, guardian, or caregiver fails to provide for the health and well-being of their charge. Abusive acts perpetrated by caregivers have negative effects on the physical, psychological, or developmental well-being of an individual. Categories include physical abuse, sexual abuse, medical neglect, neglect, and psychological abuse (Giardino, 2003).

The Child Abuse Prevention and Treatment Act

Each state may have slightly different statutes on abuse prevention and mistreatment, but all are based on the Child Abuse Prevention and Treatment Act (U.S. Department of Health and Human Services,1996). This law was enacted by the U.S. Legislature to ensure that child victims of abuse and neglect can receive a comprehensive approach to treatment through state resources to integrate multiple agencies, such as social services, legal aid, and mental health and education providers.

If a patient with ASD presents with any physical injury or signs of neglect, the patient should be assessed for the possibility of maltreatment. Nurses and physicians in the ED work as a team to determine if there is evidence of physical neglect, purposeful trauma, or abuse. If abuse cannot be ruled out, social work should be consulted. The Fourth National Incidence Study (NIS-4) group defined physical abuse as a form of maltreatment, in which an injury is inflicted on the person by a caregiver via various nonaccidental means, including hitting with a hand, stick, strap, or other object; punching; kicking; shaking; throwing; burning; stabbing; or choking to the extent that demonstrable harm results (U.S. Department of Health and Human Services, 2009).

Sexual abuse is the deliberate exposure of child or adult to sexual activity, such that a person is forced or talked into sex or sexual activities by another. Such abuse includes touching (fondling), sexual intercourse, oral sex, pornography, and other sexual activity.

Prevalence of Abuse and ASD

Children with mental impairments and developmental disabilities are at increased risk of physical and sexual abuse (Westcott & Jones, 1999). Sullivan and Knutson (2000) reported that 31% of children in a city in the midwest had a record of being maltreated, compared with 9% of other children. Reports of risks for abuse and neglect among hospitalized children were also elevated (Sullivan, Knutson, Scanlan, & Cork, 1997).

Hershkowitz, Lamb, and Horowitz (2007) reported that children with disabilities are more likely to be victims of abuse than neurotypical peers. In a study of the maltreatment of children with disabilities, Hymel and Jenny (1996) reported that adolescents have the highest rate of sexual assault in the United States and disabled adolescents have 1.75 times the rate of abuse seen in nondisabled adolescents. Adolescents with developmental delay, or cognitive disability that is considered mild, are at particular risk for date and acquaintance rape (Quint, 1999).

Several authors have offered reasons for this increased risk of sexual abuse, which include long-term dependency on caregivers, a tendency toward unquestioning compliance, lack of knowledge about sex or sexuality and sexual abuse, and poor communication skills. They also suggested that insecure attachment between mother and child due to early separation from the mother, the disappointment of having an impaired child, rejection and hostile feelings toward the impaired child, deficits in behaviors that promote attachment, and disappointment due to unrealistic expectations regarding behavior and abilities might increase the risk of physical abuse. While these proposed reasons apply to children, it is conceivable that many of these reasons might apply to adults with autism and their guardians (Ammerman, Hersen, Van Hesselt, Lubetsky, & Sieck, 1994; Howlin & Clements, 1995).

Cook, Kieffer, Charak, and Leventhal (1993) reported a case of an adolescent who reported being physically abused by a staff member after being admitted to the hospital. Psychiatric evaluation revealed posttraumatic stress disorder (PTSD) including symbolic anxiety and repetition of the trauma. Therefore, a diagnosis of PTSD should be considered in children or adults with autistic disorder and other developmental disorders who have experienced physical and sexual abuse.

In a recent review of records from a Comprehensive Community Mental Health Services for Children and their Families program, investigators showed that caregivers reported that 18.5% of children with autism had been physically abused and 16.6% had been sexually abused. Physically abused children had engaged in sexual acting out or abusive behavior, had made a suicide attempt, or had conduct-related or academic problems more often than those who were not abused. Sexually abused children more likely had engaged in sexual acting out or abusive behavior, suicidal or other self-injurious behavior, had run away from home, or had a psychiatric hospitalization. In adjusted multivariate models, the relationship between sexual abuse and sexual acting out, running away from home, and suicidal attempts persisted (Mandell, Walrath, Manteuffel, Sgro, & Pinto-Martin, 2005).

Neglect

Perkins and Wolkind presented six case histories of children admitted to a psychiatric inpatient unit at a tertiary referral center because of concerns about poor functioning and possible emotional abuse. On initial assessment, the children appeared to be not functioning well and the impression was confirmed that their emotional needs were not being met by their parents. This form of neglect may be easily overlooked and considered secondary to physical neglect or abuse (Perkins & Wolkind, 1991).

Nursing Care when Suspecting Abuse

The nurse's responsibility in dealing with mistreatment essentially comprises identification of the victim and family's or caregiver's needs specific to the maltreatment and provision of appropriate services. The nurse in the ED should recall the above statistics when a person with ASD is admitted with old and new injuries that could be associated with maltreatment. Do not assume self-injury is the cause. Due to poor social and communication skills, people with ASD might be at particular risk of physical and sexual abuse (Howlin & Clements, 1995).

Understanding the developmental level and abilities of the person is essential in determining if the history provided by the parent or caregiver is a possible or plausible explanation for the injury. Once the full extent of the injury is determined, based on physical examination and laboratory workup, the nurse can further assess the plausibility of the explanation offered by the parent or caregiver. A history that is implausible based on what a child at that level is capable of doing should raise a high degree of concern for possible maltreatment.

Each form of injury as a result of physical abuse has its own set of biomechanics and pathophysiology. Whenever a person with ASD is injured, a complete history of the circumstances surrounding the injury is essential. Basic questions explore the temporality and circumstances of the injury such as: What was the date and time of the injury and when was it first noted? Where did the injury occur? Who witnessed the injury? What was happening prior to the injury? What did the person do after the injury? What did the caregiver do after the injury? How long after the injury did the caregiver wait until seeking care for the person with ASD? Ask the basic question: "Do you feel safe where you live?"

Physical abuse is often an ongoing pattern of unsafe care, therefore, performing a thorough head-to-toe examination is essential in order to find other areas of either current or previous injury (Giardino & Giardino, 2003a, 2010). The past medical history should be examined for evidence of previous trauma and hospitalizations, as well as for the source of health care and developmental and social aspects of the child's life (Giardino & Giardino, 2003b).

Physical indicators that should raise the nurse's suspicion of maltreatment include the following: injury pattern inconsistent with the history provided, multiple injuries/multiple types of injuries, injuries at various stages of healing. Fractures that raise a high degree of suspicion for inflicted injury include metaphyseal fractures; multiple, bilateral, differently aged posterior rib and scapular fractures; multiple and complex skull fractures. Burn patterns that may suggest physical maltreatment include forced-immersion burn pattern with sharp stocking and glove demarcation and sparing of flexed protected areas; splash/spill burn patterns not consistent with history or developmental level; and cigarette burns.

Additionally, other aspects of the burn physical examination that should raise the nurse's concern for possible abuse include incompatible history and physical examination; developmental level; bilateral or mirror image burns; localized burns to genitals, buttocks, and perineum (especially at toilet-training stage); evidence for excessive delay in seeking treatment; and the presence of other forms of injury. Patterns of bruising that raise the concern of possible abuse are those on multiple areas of the body beyond bony prominences; markings resembling objects, grab marks, slap marks, human bites, and loop marks (Giardino, Brown, & Giardino, 2003).

Finally, nurses are mandated reporters of abuse in every state and the District of Columbia. Nurses must understand reporting laws in their specific states, the circumstances under which one reports abuse or neglect, and to whom the report should be presented (O'Toole, O'Toole, Webster, & Lucal, 1996).

CASE–MEDICAL DECISION MAKING

Charlie's laboratory and CT results return and show no abnormalities. The team decides to admit him overnight for monitoring. Since they are unsure of head injury or loss of consciousness during the car accident, they think he should be monitored for symptoms of concussion.

PREPARING FOR TRANSITIONS

Following evaluation and diagnosis in the ED, the team makes a decision about the patient disposition. A patient is generally admitted to the inpatient units, discharged home, or transferred to an outside facility. All transitions in care will require communication with the receiving area to ensure continuity of care and facilitate preparation of staff and the physical environment in order to meet the patient's and family's needs. The transferring nurse should discuss the complexity of care with the receiving nurse and provide all necessary information, including past history, reason for the visit, current assessment, and plan of care. The ED nurse might wish to verify that the receiving unit is prepared to accommodate the special needs of the patient, before beginning the transfer. For ASD patients, strategies for working with the patient, necessary environmental modifications, and triggers for meltdown should be reported. Keeping key information related to ASD on the front of the patient's hospital record will remind all health care providers that special needs must be continually addressed.

Discharge to Home

If a patient is discharged home, he or she is instructed to follow up with their primary provider. Communication will need to take place between the ED and the primary provider to ensure that all caregivers (formal and informal) are aware of the plan and can arrange for a follow-up evaluation. The emergency nurse can work with other health care providers and formal caregivers to make sure discharge instructions are clear and others are aware of warning signs that the patient should return for reevaluation. Some patients might be discharged to independent living, group homes, or other settings, and need arrangements for home health care. The emergency nurse can facilitate these arrangements before the patient is discharged.

Admission and Transfer

A patient being admitted to the hospital or transferred to an outside facility will require the nurse to report to the receiving area about the patient assessment and plan of care. The nurse can help ensure a smooth transition by informing receiving staff of the patient's sensory issues, preferences, methods of communication, and successful strategies that have worked throughout the visit. He or she can also advise the facility of changes that might need to be made to the physical environment in the patient's room. Systematic communication among the nursing staff during transfer is important in any patient transition, but especially important for patients with ASD, who often have difficulty dealing with change.

CASE–TRANSFER TO INPATIENT FLOOR

Charlie receives a bed assignment on the medical unit. Anna makes sure he is assigned a private room. She calls the nurse to report. In addition to the triage note, her report is as follows:

> It is unknown whether Mr. Emerson lost consciousness, so he is being admitted for observation to rule out concussion. His CT scan was negative, and he had labs drawn that were all normal. He is allergic to penicillin and takes ranitidine, valproic acid, and sertraline. Charlie's primary caregiver is his mother, but he also attends a day program. His mother is here with him. He understands verbal communication but does not often respond. He cooperates best with procedures when he is informed beforehand what will happen. He does not like physical contact if it is unannounced. If he is overstimulated, he may run away or hit others. This has not happened in the ED, but his mother said he has a history of this behavior. He loves baseball and will do what his mother asks if she rewards him with something baseball-related. He also likes to listen to classical music or his disc player and headphones. I would turn the lights down in his room so it is not too bright for him and have the classical music station on the TV. He is listening to that now and seems to like it. You'll also want to remove any equipment from the room that isn't necessary.
>
> Anna goes on to tell the nurse about her physical assessment of Charlie and when he was last medicated for pain. Charlie is transported out of the ED at 7 p.m.

SUMMARY

The emergency nurse plays a pivotal role in the management of patients with ASD in the ED. Working together with the patient, family, and health care team, the nurse ensures patient safety and comfort while they are being evaluated and treated for the emergency. Knowledge of ASD and its common characteristics is invaluable in caring for these patients; however, emergency nurses must recognize that each of these patients is unique and he or she will need to modify the approach depending on the patient. Knowledge of patient behaviors, preferences, and tendencies, as well as successful methods that have worked in prior visits, will contribute to best-practices nursing care in the ED. If the ED admission is managed thoughtfully, the patient's experience will begin as a therapeutic encounter and will set the example for subsequent contacts with health services providers. With increased knowledge of ASD, nurses can lead other members of the health care team as more patients with ASD reach adult age and present for emergency care.

REFERENCES

Allison, K. P., & Smith, G. (1998). Burn management in a patient with autism. *Burns*, *24*, 484–486.

American Academy of Child and Adolescent Psychiatry. (1999). Practice parameters for the assessment and treatment of children, adolescents, and adults with autism and other pervasive developmental disorders. *Journal of the American Academy of Child & Adolescent Psychiatry*, *38*(12), 32s–53s.

Ammerman, R., Hersen, M., Van Hasselt, V., Lubetsky, M., & Sieck, W. (1994). Maltreatment in psychiatrically hospitalized children and adolescents with developmental disabilities: Prevalence and correlates. *Journal of the American Academy of Child & Adolescent Psychiatry*, *33*(4), 567–576.

Autism National Committee. (2010). *Position on restraints.* Retrieved from http://www.autcom.org/articles/Position4.html.

Autism Society. (2011). *Autism: Information for paramedics and emergency room staff.* Retrieved from http://support.autism-society.org/site/PageServer?pagename=shop_downloads#medics.

Blake, K. (2010, October). *Autism spectrum disorder: A new generation of complex patients.* Presented at Villanova University Gateway to Innovation and Creativity in Nursing Education Conference, Baltimore, MD.

Center for Autism and Related Disabilities. (2010). *Autism and the hospital emergency room.* Retrieved from http://www.umcard.org/files/CARD_AwarenessBrochures_ER.pdf.

Centers for Disease Control and Prevention. (2009). Prevalence of autism spectrum disorders – Autism and Developmental Disabilities Monitoring Network, United States, 2006. *MMWR*, *58*(SS–10), 1–19.

Cook, E. H., Jr., Kieffer, J. E., Charak, D. A., & Leventhal, B. L. (1993). Autistic disorder and post-traumatic stress disorder. *Journal of the American Academy of Child & Adolescent Psychiatry*, *32*(6), 1292–1294.

Coury, D., Jones, N., Klatka, K., Winklosky, B., & Perrin, J. (2009). Healthcare for children with autism: The Autism Treatment Network. *Current Opinion in Pediatrics*, *21*(6), 828–832.

Debbaudt, D., & Rothman, D. (2001). Contact with individuals with autism: Effective resolutions. *FBI Law Enforcement Bulletin*, *70*(4), 20–24.

deBruin, E. I., Ferdinand, R. F., & Meester, S. (2007). High rates of psychiatric comorbidity in PDD-NOS. *Journal of Autism and Developmental Disorders*, *37*, 877–886.

Emergency Nurses Association. (2007). *Trauma nursing core course: Provider manual* (6 ed.). Des Plaines, IL: Author.

Gabriel, H. P., & Gluck, R. (1972). Management of an autistic child undergoing open heart surgery. *Pediatrics*, *51*(2), 251–253.

Ganz, J., & Simpson, R. (2004). Effects on communicative requesting and speech development of the picture exchange communication system in children with characteristics of autism. *Journal of Autism & Developmental Disorders*, *34*(4), 395–409.

Ghaziuddin, M., Tsai, L., & Ghaziuddin, N. (1992). Comorbidity of autistic disorder in children and adolescents. *European Child and Adolescent Psychiatry*, *1*(4), 209–213.

Giardino, E. R. (2003). The problem of child abuse and neglect. In E. R. Giardino, & A. P. Giardino (Eds.), *Nursing approach to the evaluation of child maltreatment* (pp. 1–16). St. Louis, MO: G.W. Medical Publishing.

Giardino, E. R., Brown, K. M., & Giardino, A. P. (2003). The physical examination in the evaluation of suspected child maltreatment: Physical abuse and sexual abuse examinations. In E. R. Giardino, & A. P. Giardino (Eds.), *Nursing approach to the evaluation of child maltreatment* (pp. 69–136). St. Louis, MO: G.W. Medical Publishing.

Giardino, E. R., & Giardino, A. P. (2003a). Multidisciplinary teamwork issues related to child sexual abuse. In A. P. Giardino, E. Datner, & J. Asher (Eds.), *Sexual assault victimization across the life span: A clinical guide* (pp. 173–188). St. Louis, MO: G.W. Medical Publishing.

Giardino, E. R., & Giardino, A. P. (2003b). *Nursing approach to the evaluation of child maltreatment.* St. Louis, MO: G.W. Medical Publishing.

Giardino, A., Lyn, M. A., & Giardino, E. R. (Eds.) (2010). *A practical guide to the evaluation of child physical abuse and neglect* (2 ed.). New York: Springer.

Grubenhoff, J. A., Kirkwood, M., Gao, D., Deakyne, S., & Wathen, J. (2010). Evaluation of the standardized assessment of concussion in a pediatric emergency department. *Pediatrics*, *126*(4), 688–695.

Gurney, J. G., McPheeters, M. L., & Davis, M. M. (2006). Parental report of health conditions and health care use among children with and without autism. *Archives of Pediatric and Adolescent Medicine*, *160*, 825–830.

Hershkowitz, I., Lamb, M. E., & Horowitz, D. (2007). Victimization of children with disabilities. *American Journal of Orthopsychiatry*, *77*(4), 629–635.

Howlin, P., & Clements, J. (1995). Is it possible to assess the impact of abuse on children with pervasive developmental disorders? *Journal of Autism and Developmental Disorders*, *25*(4), 337–354.

Hymel, K. P., & Jenny, C. (1996). Child sexual abuse. *Pediatric Review*, *17*, 236–249, quiz 249–250.

Kelble, D. (2009). *It's all about them: Autism preparedness for EMS professionals.* Retrieved from http://www.autismems.net/media/Handout.pdf.

LeBel, J., Stromberg, N., Duckworth, K., Kerzner, J., Goldstein, R., Weeks, M., ... Sudders, M. (2004). Child and adolescent inpatient restraint reduction: A state initiative to promote strength-based care. *Child and Adolescent Psychiatry*, *43*(1), 37–45.

Levy, S. E., Giarelli, E., Lee, L., Schieve, L. A., Kirby, R. S., Cunniff, C., ... Rice, C. E. (2010). Autism spectrum disorder and concurrent developmental, psychiatric, medical conditions among children in multiple populations of the United States. *Journal of Developmental and Behavioral Pediatrics, 31*(4), 267–275.

Leyfer, O. T., Folstein, S. E., Bacalman, S., Davis, N., Dinh, E., Morgan, J., Tager-Flusberg, H., & Lainhart, J. (2006). Comorbid psychiatric disorders in children with autism: Interview development and rates of disorders. *Journal of Autism and Developmental Disorders, 36*(7), 849–861.

Mandell, D. S., Walrath, C. M., Manteuffel, B., Sgro, G., & Pinto-Martin, J. A. (2005). The prevalence and correlates of abuse among children with autism served in comprehensive community-based mental health settings. *Child Abuse & Neglect, 29*(12), 1359–1372.

McDermott, S., Zhou, L., & Mann, J. (2008). Injury treatment among children with autism or pervasive developmental disorder. *Journal of Autism & Developmental Disorders, 38*(4), 626–633.

Nelson, D., & Amplo, K. (2009). Care of the autistic patients in the perioperative area. *AORN Journal, 89*(2), 391–397.

Olejnik, L. (2004). Understanding autism: How to appropriately and safely approach, assess and manage autistic patients. *Journal of Emergency Medical Services, 29*(6), 56–61, 64.

O'Toole, A., O'Toole, R., Webster, S., & Lucal, B. (1996). Nurses' diagnostic work on possible physical child abuse. *Public Health Nurse, 13*, 337–344.

Parish, S. L., Moss, K., & Richman, E. L. (2008). Perspectives on health care of adults with developmental disabilities. *Intellectual and Developmental Disabilities, 46*(6), 411–426.

Perkins, M., & Wolkind, S. N. (1991). Asperger's syndrome: Who is being abused? *Archives of Disease in Childhood, 66*(6), 693–695.

Quint, E. H. (1999). Gynecological health care for adolescents with developmental disabilities. *Adolescent Medicine, 10*, 221–229.

Seltzer, M. M., Krauss, M. W., Shattuck, P. T., Orsmond, G., Swe, A., & Lord, C. (2003). The symptoms of autism spectrum disorders in adolescence and adulthood. *Journal of Autism and Developmental Disorders, 33*(6), 565–581.

Shah, S., Shah, S., Apuya, J., Gopalakrishnan, S., & Martin, T. (2009). Combination of oral ketamine and midazolam as a premedication for a severely autistic and compative patient. *Journal of Anesthesia, 23*(1), 126–128.

Simonoff, E., Pickles, A., Charman, T., Chandler, S., Loucas, T., & Baird, G. (2008). Psychiatric disorders in children with autism spectrum disorders: prevalence, comorbidity, and associated factors in a population-derived sample. *Journal of the American Academy of Child &Adolescent Psychiatry, 47*(8), 921–929.

Sobsey, D., Wells, D., Lucardie, R., & Mansell, S. (1995). *Violence and disability: An annotated bibliography.* Baltimore, MD: Brookes Publishing.

Souders, M. (2010, June). *Nursing care of children with autism spectrum disorders: Three case studies.* Presentated at the Clinical Management of Autism Spectrum Disorder Conference, Philadelphia, PA.

Souders, M. C., Freeman, K. G., DePaul, D., & Levy, S. E. (2002). Caring for children and adolescents with autism who require challenging procedures. *Pediatric Nursing, 28*(6), 55–62.

Sullivan, P., & Knutson, J. (2000). Maltreatment and disabilities: A population-based epidemiological study. *Child Abuse & Neglect, 24*(10), 1257–1273.

Sullivan, P., Knutson, J., Scanlan, J., & Cork, P. (1997). Maltreatment of children with disabilities: Family risk factors and prevention implications. *Journal of Child Centered Practice, 4*, 33–46.

U.S. Department of Health and Human Services. (1996). *Child Abuse Prevention and Treatment Act, As Amended* (October 3, 1996). 42 U.S.C. 5106g et seq.P.L. 104-235, October 3, 1996.

U.S. Department of Health, Human Services. (2009). *Abuse, neglect, adoption & foster care research. National incidence study of child abuse and neglect (NIS-4), 2004–2009.* Retrieved from http://www.acf.hhs.gov/programs/opre/abuse_neglect/natl_incid/index.html#reports.

Vessey, J. A. (1988). Care of the hospitalized child with a cognitive developmental delay. *Holistic Nursing Practice, 2*(2), 48–54.

Volkmar, F., Cook, E. H., Jr., Pomeroy, J., Realmuto, G., & Tanguay, P. (1999). Practice parameters for the assessment and treatment of children, adolescents, and adults with autism and other pervasive developmental disorders. *Journal of the American Academy of Child & Adolescent Psychiatry, 38*(12), 32s–53s.

Westcott, H., & Jones, D. (1999). Annotation: The abuse of disabled children. *Journal of Child Psychology & Psychiatry, 40*(4), 497–506.

Cancer Care for Adults With Autism Spectrum Disorder: The Case of Prostate Cancer

13

Ellen Giarelli and Jean Ruttenberg

Responsible cancer care involves comprehensive care across the lifespan that includes primary, secondary, and tertiary prevention strategies. Primary prevention should begin early in life and should include education about a healthy diet that is rich with antioxidants and low in fat. It should include a program of exercise and conscientious avoidance of risk by avoiding carcinogens, excluding tobacco use, and limiting oneself to a moderate intake of alcohol. Secondary prevention includes early identification of precancerous lesions or cancer through a systematic process of routine screenings or enhanced surveillance and diagnostic follow-up in the presence of symptoms. Tertiary prevention is the limitation of morbidity and reduction of mortality as a consequence of a cancer diagnosis. Tertiary prevention is accomplished best through early diagnosis and individualized patient-centered treatments, follow-up care, and rehabilitation. People with autism spectrum disorder (ASD) are at the same risk for cancer as the general population. They may be at increased risk for higher morbidity and mortality as a consequence of inadequate primary and secondary preventive care.

In this chapter, we begin with a discussion of the disparities in cancer incidence among people with disabilities and explore the idea that people with ASD are less likely to receive cancer screening, less likely to benefit from primary prevention, and less likely to maximize their benefit from secondary prevention once diagnosed with cancer. In the case study, we explore circumstances to overcome by a patient with autism to promote wellness, prevent cancer, and intervene early to mitigate morbidity. The prostate cancer overview covers most of the information needed by a person with ASD and his or her family members to make decisions about screening, diagnosis, and treatment.

CANCER IN THE ASD POPULATION

Prostate cancer is the most common malignancy among men of all races and the second leading cause of cancer-specific death in men in the United States (Centers for Disease Control and Prevention, 2006). Approximately 186,000 new cases and 28,000 deaths occur annually. Because ASD is significantly more prevalent in males than females (4:1), prostate cancer is the most common malignancy among people with ASD. The ratio of newly diagnosed cases to prostate cancer deaths shows that although the disease is lethal for some, most men die with, rather than from, their cancers. These statistics translate to a startling number of men with ASD who are at risk for or are living with this cancer and to a conspicuous need to prepare providers to meet the health care needs of this group.

There are no specific data on prostate cancer incidence specifically among people with ASD. However, there are limited data from studies of health disparities among individuals with ASD and cancer incidence among people with intellectual disabilities. In general, adults with developmental disabilities are more likely to lead sedentary lives and to report being in fair or poor health. Additionally, they are seven times more likely than neurotypical adults to report inadequate emotional support (Cooke, 1997; Gilbert, Wilkinson, & Crudgington, 2007; Tuffrey-Wijne, Bernal, Jones, Butler, & Hollins, 2006).

CANCER SCREENING

As individuals with ASD achieve longer life expectancies, suboptimal cancer-screening practices will add to the cancer burden for this population. Approximately 30% of people with ASD have an intellectual disability (ID), and cognitive impairment impacts cancer screening. For example, women with cognitive impairment had lower rates of mammography screening (18%) compared with women with normal cognition (45%; Mehta, Fung, Kistler, Chang, & Walter, 2010). Among people with ID, there are higher rates of brain, testicular, gallbladder, and thyroid cancers, which highlights the importance of screening patients with ASD (Patja, Eero, & Iivanainen, 2001).

Adults with communication disorders have unique issues that affect health care experiences. Negative experiences and avoidance or nonuse of health services are reported, largely due to the lack of a common language with health care providers. This is true for people who are hearing impaired (Steinberg, Wiggins, Barmada, & Sullivan, 2002) and may be equally true for people who have a language-processing disorder, as is seen with ASD.

Some cancer-screening guidelines specify upper-age cutoffs for screening, as a surrogate for life-expectancy, and prostate-specific antigen (PSA)-screening guidelines suggest stopping at age 75 years (U.S. Preventative Services Task Force, 2008). There are no guidelines that specify a type of comorbid condition, such as autism, that would preclude screening. Methta and colleagues (2010) concluded from their study of women with ID that guidelines should explicitly recommend against mammography for these women given the limited life expectancy of women with severe cognitive impairment. With regard to prostate cancer, with the possible exception of a comorbidity of severe cognitive impairment, men with ASD should be offered PSA screening up to age 75 years.

Tyler and colleagues (Tyler, Zyzanski, Panaite, & Council, 2010) surveyed nurses to document health disparities in cancer screening for adults with intellectual and developmental disabilities (including ASD). The perceived barriers to screening (and percent of respondent agreement) were: (1) the individual's behaviors/lack of cooperation interrupts screening (76%); (2) cancer screenings are not prescribed by health care providers (48%); (3) individual is fearful (47%); (4) individual refuses to be screened (41%); (5) individual/family does not understand the benefit (38%); (6) family or guardian refuses to allow screening (26%); (7) individual lacks insurance to pay for preventive care (22%); and (8) transportation is difficult to arrange (19%). All of these barriers to cancer screening are surmountable with appropriate education and support for the health care provider, patient, and family.

Screening for Prostate Cancer

In 2010, the American Cancer Society updated its 2001 guidelines for the early detection of prostate cancer. The guidelines state that men who have at least a 10-year life expectancy should have an opportunity to make an informed decision with their health care provider about whether to be screened for prostate cancer with a digital rectal examination (DRE) or PSA after receiving information about the benefits, risks, and uncertainties (Wolf et al., 2010). Routine screening for prostate cancer includes a DRE, during which the examiner inserts a gloved finger into the rectum to feel for lumps in the prostate, and an evaluation of serum levels of PSA. Prostate-specific antigen is a protein produced by the prostate and an indicator of cellular proliferation in the prostate gland. A prostate that feels abnormal during DRE and/or an elevated PSA level (greater than or equal to 4.0 ng/ml) are both possible indicators of the disease. However, neither test alone or in combination is sufficient to provide a definitive diagnosis of prostate cancer. Many men who have a common, noncancerous condition called benign prostatic hyperplasia (BPH) may also have elevated PSA levels. Therefore, if findings are informative, a biopsy is required to confirm a diagnosis (Presti, 2004).

Prostate Cancer Screening Guidelines

Prostate cancer screening guidelines for men in general and for men with ASD may be based on the following principles:

- Some men with prostate cancer do not need to be treated.
- Compliance with screening will increase if men are told whether they are at high, intermediate, or low risk and are informed accordingly about their need for subsequent screening.
- A diagnosis of prostate cancer is information used to help make decisions, not an indication for immediate treatment.
- There is a balance between the harms and benefits of screening: The ratio between benefits and harms will be maximized if screening focuses on men at highest risk of life-threatening prostate cancer.

When clinicians wrote prostate cancer screening guidelines, they incorporated these principles and suggested ways to act on findings from screening tests. Table 13.1 describes the suggested guidelines practiced at Memorial Sloan-Kettering Hospital in New York for treating a man based on his PSA values (Memorial Sloan-Kettering Cancer Center, 2010). These guidelines can be applied to the care of men with ASD. In addition, the National Comprehensive Cancer Network posted recommendations in 2010 for active surveillance for the

TABLE 13.1 Suggested Guidelines Practiced at Memorial Sloan-Kettering Hospital in New York for Decision Making after PSA Testing

Age range	PSA value	Intervention
All men at age 45 years	PSA greater than or equal to 3 ng/ml	Consider biopsy
	PSA greater than 1 but less than 3 ng/ml	Return for PSA every 2 years
	PSA from 0.65 to 1 ng/ml	Return for PSA at age 50
	PSA less than 0.65 ng/ml	Return for PSA at age 55
For men aged 45 to 59	PSA greater than or equal to 3 ng/ml	Consider biopsy
	PSA greater than 1 but less than 3 ng/ml	Return for PSA every 2 years
	PSA from 0.65 to 1 ng/ml	Return for PSA in 5 years, or at age 60 if age is over 55
	PSA less than 0.65 ng/ml	Return for PSA at age 60
For men aged 60 to 70	PSA greater than or equal to 3 ng/ml	Consider biopsy
	PSA greater than 1 but less than 3 ng/ml	Return for PSA every 2 years
	PSA less than or equal to 1 ng/ml	No further screening
For men aged 71 or older		No further screening

following situations: low-risk men who have life expectance of less than 10 years and very-low-risk men who have a life expectancy of less than 20 years (Mohler, 2010).

Accessing Services

Havercamp, Scandlin, and Roth, (2004) reported significant medical utilization disparities among disabled persons for some breast and cervical cancer screening. We can presume that similar disparities might exist for men at risk for prostate cancer. The patient with ASD and the health care provider are likely to avoid services that require body adjustments or the use of equipment, or that are uncomfortable due to disability, repetitive or restrictive interests, or sensory-processing difficulties. In addition to unique sensory barriers, negative altitudes might reduce the likelihood that adults with ASD will receive recommended preventive screenings. Specific barriers are: lack of accessible transportation, equipment and environment perceived as threatening, difficulty with positioning during procedures, difficulty processing instructions, and the lack of provider knowledge regarding the disability (Nosek & Howland, 1997). For women, provider attitudes may be the most significant barrier oto overcome, as women with disabilities may be considered asexual. Providers may wrongly presume that women do not need regular preventive gynecological care (Becker, Stuifbergen, & Tinkle, 1997; Fine & Asch, 1988). This same misconception may be at work among patients with ASD. In general, the higher the quality of the cancer-screening experience, the more likely the patient will be to participate in routine cancer screening. The quality of the therapeutic relationship between the health care provider and person with ASD will ultimately improve prostate cancer screening, early detection, and effective treatment.

CASE

Nick is a 58-year-old man. He was diagnosed at age 5 with autism cognitive impairment, anxiety, and obsessive behaviors. Additional diagnoses were added as Nick's development progressed. Nick's formal IQ was placed at 70. However, there is a 20-point spread between his verbal IQ and his performance IQ. Although Nick is capable of using words and vocabulary, this does not mean that he possesses functional comprehension of the words or concepts. This discrepancy often leads people interacting with Nick to believe that he understands more than he does. To illustrate the point, Nick could use the word "danger" appropriately, as well as give a dictionary definition of danger. However, in dangerous situations Nick is unable to recognize the danger nor can he produce an appropriate response to an imminent risk.

In his early years, Nick had difficulty being held and making eye contact. He demonstrated sensitivity to many sounds. For example, the sound of a vacuum cleaner or the sound of a siren from a fire or police vehicle was distressing. Later evaluations identified an auditory- and visual-processing abnormality. Nick also had an occupational therapy evaluation at age 8 years. This evaluation described a youngster who had difficulty in fine, gross, and visual motor areas. The assessment also highlighted the many sensory challenges that Nick confronted on a daily basis. Nick reacted negatively to loud, unfamiliar, or unexpected sounds. He also reacted to certain tones and voice qualities. For example, if someone spoke in an excited, agitated, or threatening manner, Nick's reaction took the form of a meltdown. Nick would scream, push people, throw objects, kick furniture, or run away from the source

(*Continued*)

CASE (Continued)

of the noise. These episodes could last up to an hour and put both Nick and parents/staff at risk. Nick also reacted with an extreme fear response to quick or unpredictable movement. Many of Nick's ritualized behaviors, such as repeating specific scripts, functioned to control his environment and to block out noxious stimuli. Over time, Nick used this self-protective coping strategy even when there was no imminent threat.

In his younger years, Nick attended a specialized program for children with ASD. Through training, Nick developed excellent skills in counting, recognition of numbers, letters, and words, and handwriting. Nick's challenges included reading comprehension, inference making, sequencing events, and problem solving. Nick was highly dependent on his teachers to guide and organize him in order for him to successfully complete assignments. In the social competency area, Nick did not play with his peers and could not understand the feelings or perspectives of others, nor could he maintain a reciprocal conversation with children or adults. Nick's panic reaction to his sound sensitivity of fire bells continued throughout his school years and was a source for continuous meltdowns.

Presently, Nick resides in a community-living arrangement (CLA) with two roommates and is supported by staff 24 hours a day. Although Nick's parents are elderly, they still join Nick once a week for dinner at his CLA. Nick has many functional skills. He can groom and dress himself, straighten his bed, vacuum, set the table, make simple sandwiches, heat meals in the microwave, and wash and dry his own dishes. Nick can also do his own laundry, take walks in his neighborhood, make simple purchases, handle his own banking, and take medications with oversight from staff.

His behavioral challenges include his negative reaction (meltdown) when one of his roommates invades his physical space too quickly or makes a loud noise or screams. Nick also reacts to change. For example, he becomes upset when he has not been prepared that a substitute staff person will be coming. Change and newness reflect Nick's developmental disability, which favors consistency and predictability. Nick does not like his routine to change. He expects his meals, television schedule, and outings to follow predictable schedules. If a change occurs, such as the van breaking down and preventing Nick from following his schedule, he usually reacts negatively. The staff has learned to give Nick a lot of alternate plans to account for unanticipated changes. Nick can adjust to most changes if prepared in advance with an alternate suggestion. Nick is encouraged to use his iPod™ during all outings, in case of an unpredictable loud sound or yelling of any kind. The iPod™ functions to both limit the volume of noise and as a distraction for Nick. Visual schedules and notes are used to prepare him for all new events and changes. Nick enjoys dancing, swimming in the pool, playing basketball, and exercising on the treadmill. Nick also keeps a daily journal on the computer. He chronicles the events of each day in copious detail, down to reporting the foods he consumed, what programs he watched on television, and with whom he spoke. Nick also watches his favorite childhood videos—every day—at specific times during the day.

Nick has enjoyed good health, with the exception of a tonsillectomy at age 10 years. Nick suffers from seasonal allergies related to pollen and mold. He takes an over-the-counter medication a week prior to allergy season. The staff has learned that if they wait for symptoms to appear, Nick is at greater risk for meltdowns, given his increased level of irritability and discomfort. In addition, Nick takes lorazepam for treatment of anxiety, carbamazepine to stabilize his mood, and fluvoxamine to treat his obsessive behavior. Nick has been on this combination of medications for most of his adult years. Nick also takes vitamin C and a daily multivitamin.

OVERVIEW OF PROSTATE CANCER

As they age, many men are diagnosed as having prostate cancer, and men often live with the disease for years. In each person with prostate cancer, the disease may manifest itself in different ways. In some men, the disease is aggressive and requires treatment. In other men, it is a slow-growing disease that is unlikely to cause serious problems. The disease can evolve in many ways, thus the need for screening and early identification. With such screening, a large percentage of prostate tumors can be identified early when they are still in the local or regional stages. The survival rate for all stages of prostate cancer combined has increased from 67% to 92% over the past 20 years (American Cancer Society, 2010), primarily because more men are now diagnosed earlier in the course of the disease than in the past.

Risk Factors

Risk factors for prostate cancer are inherited traits, age, race, diet, and exposure to cancer-causing agents in the environment. A family history of prostate cancer may also increase a man's risk of developing the disease, particularly if he has a number of close relatives who were diagnosed with prostate cancer or if any relatives were younger than 60 at the time of diagnosis (Neville, Casey, & Witte, 2004). Inherited predispositions might be responsible for about 5% to 10% of all prostate cancers.

Investigators suggest that a high-fat diet may be the cause of an increased risk of prostate cancer. A diet rich in vegetables, particularly cruciferous vegetables (broccoli, cabbage, cauliflower, kale, collard and mustard greens, horseradish, kohlrabi, Brussels sprouts, broccoli rabe, radishes, turnips, rutabagas, and watercress) is associated with a reduced risk (Kristal et al., 2010; Thompson, Ankerst, & Tangen, 2010).

For reasons that are not clearly described, African American men are twice as likely as White men to develop prostate cancer. Incidence rates are lower among Asian and Native American men (Thompson et al., 2010). A man's risk of developing prostate cancer increases with age. The disease can occur at any age, but it is most often found in men older than 50, and more than 75% of tumors are found in men over age 65 years. Nick has several risk factors (Reid & Hamdy, 2008).

Symptoms

Many men with prostate cancer experience no symptoms; the first indication that they may have the disease may be an abnormal finding on a routine screening exam. Other noticeable symptoms include: frequent urination or an inability to urinate; difficulty starting or holding back urine; pain or stiffness in the lower back, hips, or upper thighs; and painful ejaculation or trouble having an erection. Because these symptoms may be associated with other conditions, including BPH, a patient must report the symptoms and seek medical attention (Scher & Heller, 2000; National Comprehensive Cancer Network, 2009).

CASE–CONTINUED

During a quarterly checkup with a physician who had been treating Nick for many years, staff raised a concern about recent extended periods Nick was spending in the bathroom.

(*Continued*)

CASE (Continued)

On more than one occasion Nick told staff that he "couldn't go." His physician recommended blood work for a PSA check and attempted a prostate exam. Nick became extremely agitated, making an examination impossible. A member of the staff explained to his physician that Nick's reaction probably stemmed from years of sexuality training, during which he learned that he should not allow anyone to touch him in his private area. Due to Nick's concrete thinking, he was incapable of understanding that under certain circumstances this was permissible. Staff might have been able to prepare him in advance for this exception had they known that his physician was going to perform this examination.

Assessment during first visits also provides information for follow-up appointments. For example, How much time may be needed for each procedure? How will "success" be measured?

What does each person want to accomplish for the visit? What accommodations will be needed? How will the patient access support services? (See Raposa, 2009). Table 13.2 lists some sensory barriers to accessing services.

Diagnosis

If a man has an elevated PSA level and/or his digital rectal exam is abnormal, his physician will likely suggest a biopsy to microscopically examine prostate tissue samples. A biopsy can be performed in a urologist's office with a transrectal ultrasound probe or it can be performed under general anesthesia if a patient cannot cooperate during the procedure. At least 1 hour is needed for patient preparation and sample collection (a minimum of ten tissue samples).

Diagnosticians will characterize the aggressiveness of prostate cancer using the Gleason grading system, which provides an estimate of the cancer's potential to progress and metastasize. This system is used by clinicians around the world and is based on glandular architecture, which can be divided into five patterns of growth (also known as grades) with different levels of differentiation (Gleason, 1992). The Gleason grade is used to compare tissue samples with normal prostate cells. The higher the Gleason score, the greater the risk of metastasis. A tumor with a cellular structure close to normal is not likely to be aggressively malignant, while a tumor with cells that have little resemblance to normal prostate cells is more likely to be aggressive and spread outside the prostate and will receive a high Gleason score (greater than or equal to 7). Treatment is usually recommended for high-grade cancers, while observation may be recommended for low-grade

TABLE 13.2 ■ Variables in Oncologist's or Office or during Radiotherapy that may Affect Sensory Processing and Regulation

Environmental variable	Affect or sensory system
Chemotherapeutic medications	Olfactory, taste
Alcohol	Olfactory, touch
Sphygmomanometer	Tactile, touch proprioception
Water usage	Auditory processing/hearing, touch
Radiotherapy table movement, positioning	Vestibular: motion
Gloves, instruments, syringe, textures of fabrics	Touch
Lighting	Visual
Physical examination	Touch, olfactory

cancers, especially when the patient is elderly and has other medical conditions that place him at increased medical risk (National Comprehensive Cancer Network, 2009).

Depending on the findings of the DRE, PSA level, biopsy, and Gleason score, some imaging tests may be performed to evaluate the extent of tumor growth and spread (Reid & Hamdy, 2008). These tests may include:

- Magnetic resonance imaging (MRI) using an endorectal or surface coil to assess the extent of the tumor in the prostate and surrounding tissues;
- Computerized tomography (CT) scans or radionuclide bone scans to see if the disease has spread to lymph nodes, organs, or bones; and
- Positron emission test (PET), a technique to assess particular features of the tumor's biology, such as its responsiveness to hormonal therapy.

CASE–CONTINUED

Nick's PSA test was positive, indicating a high likelihood of prostate cancer. The presenting challenge to the medical team was how to provide Nick with the medical treatment his condition warranted, while keeping him emotionally and behaviorally stable. Given that medical environments are complex environments in which time and efficiency have to be considered, the nurse in charge will take the lead role in evaluating and coordinating Nick's care with both the medical professionals and Nick's CLA staff and family. The nurse will begin by contacting the CLA staff and Nick's family to collect information that will prove critical to the development of a successful plan.

The nurse's questions will be structured to ascertain what strategies have worked in the past to support Nick in remaining calm and cooperative during previous procedures and hospital visits. The nurse will simultaneously evaluate the environmental challenges that the new medical setting will present to Nick. In order to accomplish this, the nurse will walk through every room that Nick will encounter during his stay. The nurse will carefully note possible obstacles such as lighting, sound, movement patterns, odors, people, and equipment. The nurse will list each challenge, marking those that can be modified or adapted in order to address Nick's special needs. The nurse will also list those obstacles that cannot be adapted. After doing so, the nurse will contact Nick's network of staff and family to problem-solve strategies to prepare Nick for those events or environments that cannot be modified. Together they will discuss strategies such as role playing, use of Nick's iPod™ to reduce irritating sounds, having familiar people accompany him, learning and practicing calming strategies in advance of the scheduled procedure, having familiar objects around, using a weighted blanket to keep him calm and secure, and using visual supports to prepare him for unfamiliar environments, events, equipment, and personnel.

After a team evaluation of Nick's lab and pathology results, the team concludes that he is a candidate for prostatectomy.

Prostate Cancer Treatments

When a patient is diagnosed with prostate cancer, his disease is categorized into one of several clinical stages (Egevad, Allsbrook, & Epstein, 2005; Scher & Heller, 2000). Treatment is designed to either cure the disease or slow its progression, depending on the staging of the individual patient's disease. Not all prostate cancers are equally aggressive.

Watchful Waiting

Men who have an elevated or rising PSA or a family history of the disease are at higher risk of developing prostate cancer. These men are watched closely and undergo regular digital rectal examinations and PSA testing. If a patient's prostate cancer is not advanced and is slow growing, he may not need treatment until later in life, or not at all. Watchful waiting is an active and dynamic option for managing disease, and patients with slow-growing cancer may be monitored effectively until the time when the disease becomes active and requires additional treatment (Klotz, 2005; Albertsen, 2008).

Surgery

The overall goal of prostate cancer surgery is to eliminate a patient's cancer completely while preserving normal urinary and sexual function. To treat prostate cancer, surgeons generally remove the prostate (a procedure called radical prostatectomy) as well as some tissue surrounding it, and often remove a sample of the lymph nodes in nearby tissue to determine whether the cancer has spread beyond the prostate. Seventy-five percent of men treated with surgery will never have a recurrence of their cancer (Stephenson et al., 2005). Nick is a candidate for this surgery.

A radical prostatectomy can be performed using either traditional "open" surgery or a minimally invasive procedure known as laparoscopic radical prostatectomy. Through the laparoscopic and robotic-assisted laparoscopic approach, the surgeon performs a prostatectomy using specialized tools inserted through tiny incisions in the pelvic area. The general advantages of this approach are reduced blood loss, quicker recovery, and a better cosmetic result. Minimally invasive surgery using laparoscopy may be used to treat prostate cancer (Rodriguez & Pow-Sang, 2007).

Salvage Surgery

Salvage treatment refers to treatment after failure of radiation therapy. Salvage treatment options vary widely for men with local recurrence of prostate cancer after radiation therapy. Options include continued observation; immediate, continuous, or intermittent hormonal therapy; or further local therapy with radiofrequency thermal ablation, high-intensity focused ultrasonography (known as HIFU), salvage cryoablation, salvage brachytherapy, or salvage radical prostatectomy. Of these treatments, only salvage radical prostatectomy has been shown to eliminate cancer for 10 years or more (Stephenson & Eastham, 2005). Candidates for salvage prostatectomy should be otherwise healthy, with a life expectancy of greater than 10 years, and should have a cancer that was initially curable with radical prostatectomy (Rodriguez & Pow-Sang, 2007). The chance for a cure is greater when the cancer is confined to the prostate.

CASE–CONTINUED

The nurse will then meet with the various medical and ancillary staff that Nick will encounter during his procedure to provide information on who Nick is and what exceptional accommodations will be necessary. Most of the team has little or no information on autism and what they might expect. The nurse will patiently diffuse the myths by giving

(*Continued*)

CASE (Continued)

accurate information about autism and specific details that best describe Nick's brand of autism. Each mini-team will help to prepare for Nick and failure-proof his stay. The nurse will be the liaison for the teams in order to provide everyone with information on ow other teams will be proceeding. This will be both educational to staff and will provide continuity. The nurse will recommend that Nick's procedure should be the first procedure of the day. This will reduce wait time for Nick and limit the number of people he will encounter. The nurse will have the CLA staff give Nick a small dose of relaxation medication prior to his leaving for the hospital. The same person will obtain permissions, releases, and information pertaining to consents in advance of his arrival. Nick will go straight to the room where the nurse will prepare him for his procedure. The nurse will ensure that the room does not have frightening equipment, if possible, and will allow favored staff and parents to accompany him.

Counseling on Choice of Treatment

With the exception of watchful waiting, all treatment options are associated with side effects that can affect quality of life (Bill-Axelson et al., 2005). A given side effect may occur with a certain frequency; however, patients may report different and varying degrees of bother from a side effect. Some side effects will improve or worsen over time but this is difficult or impossible to predict. A treatment decision based only on the frequency of side effects is ill informed. In Nick's case, treatment counseling must factor in his behavioral characteristics, especially his need for consistency and predictability. His long-standing journaling may be employed to engage him in tracking his symptoms and changes in side effects. Nick should be encouraged and supported in efforts to identify ways to maintain a high quality of life.

One of the most important ethical issues in cancer care is assuring the patient is fully informed of treatment options and outcomes. Informed consent is not merely a legal technicality, but a duty. Patients with ASD and cognitive impairment are considered vulnerable, and additional consideration must be given to assess competence prior to medical treatment (Bernat, 2004). Surrogate decision making may be necessary. Informed decision making relies on accurate information that is age and developmentally appropriate. However, cancer educational materials have not been developed for patients in this unique cohort. Cancer information tailored to meet the specific needs of people with ASD is a top priority (O'Regan & Drummond, 2008).

Nick has the right to be treated with dignity and respect. Although Nick is of the age to provide consent, he does not possess the capability to truly make an informed decision. It is important to have a family member or someone who knows him best present during teaching and counseling; one who understands the quality-of-life issues that are at stake. The nurse can simplify written information and describe the procedures well in advance of the event. Nick will be able to think about what will happen and talk about it with trusted family or staff members. Whenever possible, a nurse should give people with ASD the opportunity to consider risks and benefits of any procedure. When options are explained, a visual support should be used. For example, if surgery will eliminate Nick's ability to achieve an erection through masturbation, the nurse may use an images of the act with a large "X" through it.

CASE–CONTINUED

The nurse can prepare medical staff with a set of simple recommendations: ensure that Nick has a positive experience by using a calm, steady approach and avoiding any quick movement or loud hurried voice; use as few words as necessary to communicate with each other; and use simple words with Nick. Nick will have the use of the iPod if the nurse cannot limit noise/sound levels in the environment. The nurse and CLA staff will have reviewed with Nick pictures of the rooms and medical staff he will encounter. The CLA staff will also practice with Nick putting on his hospital gown. These role-playing sessions will be done in a playful manner. The CLA staff will also practice several calming strategies. When Nick gets nervous they will teach him to count numbers up to 100 with his eyes closed. This calming strategy will be introduced to Nick in a gentle, quiet voice, avoiding any tone of demand and will be practiced over a 2-week period.

During Nick's hospital stay, staff and parents should be on hand to provide continuity for Nick and to function as interpreters between Nick and hospital staff. Much of the advanced planning will be focused on keeping Nick emotionally and behaviorally stable during his hospitalization. Points that will be addressed by the nurse include keeping Nick calm, controlling noise and activity, providing Nick with as much routine consistency and familiarity as possible, controlling the number of hospital staff interacting with Nick, and developing an emergency strategy in case Nick becomes highly agitated.

Based on the results of this advance planning, Nick will be placed in a single room, because this limits noise and activity levels. His hospital room door will remain closed and lighting in his room will be kept low. When possible, the nurse will turn off beeping signals on equipment. Equipment will be out of Nick's reach. Arm or leg restraints will not be used, because these may cause Nick to panic and possibly become aggressive. Relaxation medication and antianxiety medication will be available as needed to address such situations. The nurse in charge will coordinate Nick's medications for treatment of his cancer, pain management, and mental health issues with all physicians. The nurse will also share with his doctors Nick's medication history and his unique reactions to medications, as compared to the general population. A profile book will also be available with Nick's chart. This book will provide a description of his behaviors, sensitivities, triggers, calming needs, and interaction preferences. The nurse will encourage hospital staff to read this prior to seeing Nick.

Once Nick is conscious and able to eat, menus will be preselected by CLA staff and family who are intimately familiar with Nick's preferences. A visual schedule will be coordinated between the CLA staff and the nurse. This schedule will visually provide Nick with the order of daily events, such as blood pressure checks and mealtimes. Specific times will not be attached to these schedules as Nick would then expect events to occur exactly at those times. Additionally, CLA staff and family members will have pre-determined visiting hours. The CLA staff will assist Nick in participating in enjoyable activities similar to those he experiences at his residence. The purpose of familiar staff and routine will be to maintain a level of consistency and security for Nick, all of which are designed to keep Nick occupied and emotionally stable.

CLA staff and family members will not overlap their hospital visits, as Nick may perceive this as confusing. Visiting separately will provide Nick with much-needed coverage and activity. Staff and visitors will be instructed not to discuss Nick's medical condition, behaviors, or future needs while Nick is present. Additionally, visitors and staff are to

(*Continued*)

CASE (Continued)

keep their emotions calm and regulated at all times while in Nick's company. In the past, Nick internalized the tension and emotional state of those around him. The nurse will orchestrate an emergency plan in advance for Nick. It will provide a standard protocol for managing meltdown behavior. This protocol will include recommending that staff anticipate and observe Nick's emotional states closely in order to prevent escalation. However, if Nick does become agitated staff should remain calm, limit talking, touching, or restraining Nick, as well as keeping their body actions calm and modulated. Staff may not necessarily prevent an event, but supporting Nick in this manner will increase the chance of Nick limiting the duration of the meltdown, as well as maintaining his trust and goodwill toward staff.

Managing the Side Effects of Surgery

Patients who undergo surgery or radiation therapy or who have used hormone therapies for advanced disease may experience sexual and/or urinary dysfunction and infertility. Careful preoperative preparation is the first step to effective postoperative management. Preparation of Nick may use concepts used to prepare children with cognitive developmental delay for a similar experience (Vessey, 1988). Prepare the patient with procedure information, including the sights and sounds of the operating room, holding still for preoperative injections, the use of a mask for anesthesia, tubes or lines after surgery, the temperature of the operating room, and the use of hospital gowns and paper foot-coverings. Postoperatively, Nick may resume self-stimulating behaviors as a source of comfort. These should be allowed, as long as they do not significantly interfere with treatments. Unacceptable appearance and slowing down of routine care are not reasons to prevent Nick's self-soothing behaviors.

Urinary incontinence: Urinary incontinence is one possible consequence of surgery, and patients tend to regard incontinence as the most significant potential side effect after radical prostatectomy. This side effect will require patient education about its nature and impact. It is not an all-or-nothing occurrence, and many patients only have leakage during stress. Postoperative urinary incontinence usually resolves within a few months of surgery and is treated with pelvic floor exercises. However, about 5% to 10% of all men will have permanent mild stress incontinence, in which a small amount of urine passes during coughing, laughing, or exercising. This condition can be treated with a regimen of pelvic floor exercises alone, but can also be treated with an injection of bulking agents, such as collagen, a male bulbourethral sling, or in severe cases, an artificial urinary sphincter (Hu & Wallner, 1998; Talcott et al., 1998). See Table 13.3 for key messages to guide patient education.

As with other learned accomplishments and procedures, the team, lead by the nurse, may be able to teach pelvic floor exercises to Nick. Most individuals with ASD are fairly clumsy, with a decreased awareness of external and internal sensations and their precise locations. Therefore, even if Nick was able to perform the exercise, it might not be in a form that would produce the desired outcome. Other patients with ASD may be less disabled, and like people who have been required to hold their urine or bowel movements temporarily, may already understand the physical feeling created during the exercise. To prepare for postoperative care, the more cognitively able patient may learn that this feeling can be recreated and practiced on a schedule and that it has definite benefits to his health and well-being. For any patient with ASD, the procedure should be introduced by the nurse via modeling and video as part of his daily exercise routine (Bacon, Giovannucci, Testa, & Kawachi, 2001; Herr, 1994).

TABLE 13.3 ■ Key Messages on Prostate Cancer to Assist Patients and Caregivers with Decision Making Regarding Prostate Cancer Screening and Treatment Options

Main message	Strategies for person with ASD
Prostate cancer is an important concern for all men	Emphasize that men with ASD have the same health problems as other men and all men need to guard their health.
Screening with the PSA blood test alone or with both PSA and DRE detects cancer at an earlier stage than if no screening is performed	Focus on the patient's interests and quality of life and the intent of health care providers to help the patient maintain regular activities.
Prostate cancer screening may be associated with a reduction in the risk of dying from prostate cancer; however, evidence is conflicting, and experts disagree about the value of screening	Emphasize that health care providers require these tests of all adult men and they are done to help men stay healthy.
For men whose prostate cancer is detected by screening, it is currently not possible to predict which men are likely to benefit from treatment. Some men who are treated may avoid death and disability from prostate cancer. Others who are treated would have died of unrelated causes before their cancer became serious enough to effect their health or shorten their lives.	Consider the possibility that persistent pain or physical discomfort might occur and how this might impact the patient's routine and irritability.
Depending on the treatment selected, treatment of prostate cancer can lead to urinary, bowel, sexual, and other health problems. These problems may be significant or minimal, permanent or temporary.	Consider the specific impact treatment side effects will have on the patient. Tell him about the possible side effects using words that are familiar to him such as "pee" or "poop" or how erectile dysfunction may affect his practice of "playing with his penis" (masturbation).
The PSA and DRE may have false-positive or false-negative results, meaning men without cancer may have abnormal results and undergo unnecessary additional testing, and clinically significant cancers may be missed. False-positive results can lead to sustained anxiety about prostate cancer risk.	Consider how the patient has reacted in the past to situations that are out of his control. Remind him that some tests are required for all men.
Abnormal results from screening with the PSA and DRE require prostate biopsies to determine whether the abnormal findings are cancer. Biopsies can be painful, may lead to complications such as infection or bleeding, and can miss clinically significant cancer	Use visuals and calendars to prepare him for all tests. Prepare him well in advance and carefully, again using words that he uses himself. Avoid technical terms or words such as "cutting" or "knife." Words such as "stitches, needles, stretcher, IV, armboard, etc." may be completely unfamiliar to him in the context of health care.
Not all men whose prostate cancer is detected through screening require immediate treatment, but they may require periodic blood tests and prostate biopsies to determine the need for future treatment	Do not presume that the patient remembers the details of previous visits. Prepare him with the same care as was done for the first visit.

(*Continued*)

TABLE 13.3 ■ *Continued*

Main message	Strategies for person with ASD
In helping men to reach a decision based on their personal values, once they understand the uncertainties, risks, and potential benefits, it can be helpful to provide reasons why some men decide for or against screening. For example:	If there are complications from a procedure, use visuals when possible and explain to the patient in highly concrete, clear terms what will be done for the complication. For example, "This is how we will treat bleeding."
1. A man who chooses to be screened/tested might place a higher value on finding a cancer early, might be willing to be treated without definitive expectation of benefit, and might be willing to risk injury to urinary, sexual, and/or bowel function.	Tell the patient how his quality of life or ability to do usual things will be affected.
2. A man who chooses not to be screened/ tested might place a higher value on avoiding the potential harms of screening and treatment, such as anxiety or risk of injury, sexual, and/or bowel function.	Tell the patient how his quality of life or ability to do usual things will be affected.
Other	Bundle tests in as few visits as possible Follow each health care visit with his choice of activity, so he will associate the encounter with a reward. For example, a favorite food or visit to a favorite place.

Erectile dysfunction: A patient's expectation for sexual functioning after any form of therapy must be addressed. Like incontinence, erectile dysfunction is more common after surgery than after radiation and can improve during the year following prostatectomy (Catalona, Carvalhal, Mager, & Smith, 1999). Erectile dysfunction may occur when the nerves running along the two sides of the prostate that control the blood flow to the penis are injured during the operation (Han & Catalona, 2010). Recovery of full erections may take as long as 3 years after the operation. The nurse and caregiver/guardian must carefully evaluate these options before offering them to Nick. Because the nerves responsible for erections are close to the prostate, one or both of these nerves sometimes must be removed to ensure that the cancer is completely eliminated. These nerves may be replaced in some cases by nerve-graft surgery. About one-half of patients who have had nerve grafts on both sides of the prostate recover their ability to have erections and another one-fourth recover their ability to have partial erections (Catalona, Roehl, & Antenor, 2002; Heyman & Rosner, 1996; Jakobsson, Hallberg, & Lowen, 2000). Men are encouraged to use prescription drugs, penile injections, or other devices to assist with erections soon after the operation.

Radiation Therapy

Radiation is used to treat prostate cancer with high-energy rays delivered by external beam (similar to an X-ray) or brachytherapy (implanted radioactive seeds) (Coleman, 2010).

External beam: High radiation therapy doses are associated with lower PSA levels and much lower rates of positive biopsies 3 years after the completion of therapy, and with new techniques, radiation therapists can deliver higher doses with fewer side effects (Christodouleas, Fox, Song, & DeWeese, 2010). Intensity-modulated radiation therapy (IMRT) may be used. This technique using computerized tomography creates a 3D image of the prostate from multiple scans and uses this image and moveable leaves, similar to the lens on a camera, to shape the radiation beam precisely to the contours of the prostate. The beam delivers high doses of radiation to prostate tissues, while sparing surrounding organs and reducing the risk of injury to healthy tissues. Prior to radiation treatment, three small "markers," which can be visualized during the delivery of each treatment, are embedded within the prostate (Coleman, 2010).

In general, outpatient IMRT treatments are given daily, Monday through Friday, for a period of 9 to 10 weeks. Side effects include frequent urination and urgency of urination. These effects often are relieved with medications and gradually resolve a few months after treatments. However, late effects are possible, such as permanent impotence and occasional rectal bleeding and a risk of chronic irritation of the bladder, resulting in problems with urination (Lee, Moughan, Owen, & Zelefsky, 2003). This schedule might significantly impact the routine of a person with ASD.

Brachytherapy: In brachytherapy, radioactive seeds implanted into the prostate can deliver high doses of radiation directly to the tumor. In this outpatient procedure, physicians use ultrasound images of the prostate to determine the most effective placement of the seeds, which are permanently implanted in the prostate through thin needles. The seeds are small (about the size of sesame seeds), cause little or no discomfort, and their radioactivity diminishes over time. Brachytherapy can be as effective as surgery in treating men with low-grade, early-stage prostate cancer (Nag, Beyer, Friedland, Grimm, & Nath, 1999). Possible side effects include impotence, urinary urgency and frequency, and occasional rectal discomfort (Reis, Netto, Reinato, Thiel, & Zani, 2004).

Systemic and hormonal therapies: Some prostate cancer patients have a form of the disease that is aggressive or has a high risk of metastasis. Combination therapy is an alternative. Treatment usually includes hormonal therapy and/or chemotherapy, often in combination with radiation or surgery (Aragon-Ching, Williams, & Gulley, 2007).

A patient whose prostate cancer has spread beyond the prostate or has recurred after treatment may receive hormonal therapy. Testosterone can stimulate the growth of prostate cancer cells; therefore, treatments aim to reduce levels of testosterone by removing the source of male hormones (Armas et al., 1994; Reuter, 1997). This can be done by orchiectomy (removing the testicles) or with drugs that reduce the body's testosterone production. Potential side effects of hormone therapy include reduced or absent feelings of sexual desire, impotence, weakness, fatigue, loss of muscle mass, growth of breast tissue, and hot flashes. The nurse should warn the patient and guardians about the symptoms that might result from treatment.

Chemotherapy

Chemotherapy is usually reserved for patients whose prostate cancer has spread outside of the gland and for whom hormone therapy is not an option or has not been effective. With chemotherapy for prostate cancer, a multimodal approach can prolong patients' lives, reduce pain from bone metastases, and enhance overall quality of life. This treatment is reserved for men with a high-risk recurrent disease defined as a PSA greater than 2 ng/ml and a PSA doubling time less than 8 months with an original Gleason score of greater than 7

(Smoot & Dawson, 2004). The benefits of chemotherapy for advanced prostate cancer are comparable to the benefits seen in patients with other advanced solid tumors who receive chemotherapy. Two classes of antineoplastics are vinka alkaloids (such as vinblastine) and taxanes. The taxanes are an active class of antineoplastics used for advanced prostate cancer. The agent now considered the standard of care for prostate cancer patients is docetaxel (Taxotere). Another chemotherapeutic agent commonly prescribed is paclitaxel. Both paclitaxel and docetaxel may be combined with estramustine, which is a complex of an estradiol phosphate derivative linked to a nonnitrogen mustard molecule (alkylating agent; Dahmani et al., 2010; Dreicer, 2005; Freter & Perry, 2008).

Bone-Protecting Treatments

The most common site of distant spread of prostate cancer is the bones. Most symptoms of advanced prostate cancer are caused by the presence of disease in the bone (Campbell et al., 2010). These symptoms can be reduced with zoledronic acid, which can slow the spread of disease, reduce the development of bone pain, inhibit bone fractures, and have other beneficial effects. Zoledronic acid is most commonly given to patients whose cancer is no longer responding to hormones. It may also be given to prevent bone thinning and weakening that results from hormonal treatments (Campbell et al., 2010).

Rising PSA after Primary Therapy

As a result of widespread PSA testing, men whose prostate cancer is confined to the prostate now make up the largest group of prostate cancer patients. Their disease may be curable with therapy directed solely at the prostate. Physicians and nurses will need to continue to monitor such patients. Men whose PSA levels rise after treatment are the second largest segment of the prostate cancer population. For these patients, therapy is directed toward preventing the disease from progressing to the point that it is detectable on a scan or by physical examination, or from becoming symptomatic. Because prostate cancer can be slow-growing and can have a prolonged natural history, many patients in this clinical state live a long life (Droz et al., 2010; Mohler et al., 2010).

Patients with rising PSA levels have unique clinical needs. For some, the rising PSA represents the first evidence that the cancer is no longer confined to the prostate, the prostate bed, or even the pelvis, but has become a systemic problem (i.e. metastasized). A rising PSA may also signify persistent local disease. For men with persistent local disease, therapeutic approaches may include observation alone or further treatments. Men with systemic disease have choices. For those at high risk, aggressive therapies may be warranted. For others, watchful waiting may be the best approach. Treatment must be tailored to the specific patient. Despite advances in the management of advanced prostate cancer, many patients ultimately develop progressive pain, wasting (cachexia/anorexia), and fatigue (Penson, Rossignol, Sartor, Scardino, & Abenhaim, 2008).

CASE–CONTINUED

Nick will probably require follow-up, outpatient treatment such as chemotherapy or radiation, for his cancer. Therefore, arrangements will be made for Nick to visit that hospital

(*Continued*)

CASE (Continued)

department where his outpatient treatment will occur prior to his release. The CLA staff and the nurse in charge will accompany Nick on these visits. They will show Nick around and introduce him to the environment, people, and equipment. Those accompanying Nick will also bring with them something that Nick likes for the radiation staff to give to Nick when he leaves. This will be done to help Nick make a positive association with the outpatient department and the staff. When Nick returns to his CLA, staff will also review visuals (pictures) with him that depict the routine and procedures that will occur during his daily outpatient treatment visits. The CLA staff will also plan for Nick to purchase one of his favorite snacks at a local store after each outpatient visit. On the most recent visit, Nick complains of pain.

BEST PRACTICES NURSING CARE

By the time a person with ASD reaches adulthood, his or her patterns, in terms of abilities preferences, interests, and motivations are critical to planning for therapeutic communications. Health care planning must take into account the particular environments to which the adults will be brought. Environments can be modified, often in very minimal ways, to accommodate the individual's communication and behavioral strengths and challenges. Adults with ASD suffer chronic emotional stress as a consequence of their uneven mental profile of strengths and weakness. They may continually struggle to interface successfully with other people due to inherent deficits in social processing skills. Their mental health problems are related to their inability to fit in with society and social institutions.

A diagnosis of cancer can have a profound psychological impact on patients with ASD and their caregivers. It is documented that people in the general population suffer existential crises, anxiety, and depression from the cancer diagnosis (Tuffrey-Wijne et al., 2006). People who are psychologically fragile from a diagnosis of a developmental disability are at greater risk to suffer increased emotional distress. Additionally, such individuals may be denied certain choices in their care by well-intentioned caregivers who wish to avoid outbursts and additional distress (Foster, 2006).

Language and Communication

The principle areas of deficit that are likely to interfere with a satisfactory therapeutic relationship are language, communication, and social skills. Fewer than 10% of autistic individuals have language skills approximating those of neurotypical patients (Lord & O'Neill, 1983). The current adult population with autism may not have been diagnosed until later in life. Because of the older average age of the patient with prostate cancer, the nurse may expect that an autistic adult probably did not receive intensive language and communication therapy as a child.

Echolalia

Although this is not present in Nick, adults with autism may echo words and sentences they have heard. This may be done immediately after hearing the words or days later. The echolalia may be exact or modified by changes in sentence structure. Echolalia can be extremely problematic during clinical encounters, especially those that are brief and likely to have an instructional focus. Consider the postoperative encounter during which a patient is being instructed on how to use the nurse call button or the importance of postoperative deep breathing. The autistic adult may use echolalic phrases that they do not understand. This may cause a nurse to overestimate their ability to comprehend and follow instructions. Echolalia may sometimes have a purpose that, if understood by the nurse, may assist in the delivery of care. For example, an adult with autism may have memorized and use the phrase "play it again, Sam" in an almost appropriate way, which implies he did not hear or understand. Also, an adult who loudly repeats phrases from television shows or distant voices to himself may need to be placed in a private room. However, this decision should be weighed carefully, as it denies the patient's very real need for company and emotional support. If the adult patient with ASD has complicated fantasies and echolalia, these may appear to the uneducated eye as signs of hallucinations or psychotic breaks with reality. This may be a unique risk immediately after surgery, when the patient is coming out of anesthesia.

Except for a few of the more highly functioning individuals, adults with autism will have some deficit in comprehension. This will become most conspicuous when the nurse communicates abstract ideas. Adults with autism generally think quite literally and may not understand the inferences in statements such as "short and sweet" or "keep it down." Therefore, the nurse should endeavor to be as concrete as possible when communicating with the adult with ASD. If abstract or complex ideas are warranted, photographs and simple pictures or phrases are more effective. Even common gestures, such as an index finger to the lip to ask for quiet, may not be understood.

The adult with autism may have a difficult time processing faces. The nurse may work with the patient for several days, successfully establishing a level of trust, only to find that upon returning from several days off, a new hairstyle, absence of a name tag, or different colored scrubs results in the patient resuming the behaviors manifest during the first encounter.

Challenging Behaviors

People with ASD may not be capable of cooperating fully during complex procedures or invasive procedures, such as a prostate exam, and as many as 50% to 77% may be frightened or uncooperative during such procedures (Marshall, Sheller, Williams, Manci, & Cowan, 2007). Some may require general anesthesia in order to accomplish the exam (Klein & Nowak, 1999).

Organic Conditions

In addition to the known history of meltdowns in Nick, aggression or "meltdowns" may be associated with acute medical conditions, such as injury, colds, flu, or sore throat. In addition to environmental factors, meltdowns may be a response to pain or discomfort from severe congestion. A history of aggression may reveal that the meltdown behavior has been effective in securing attention or solitude or other desired events or objects, such as food. Meltdowns may also occur when the autistic person wants to avoid or escape a certain person or situation. This scenario may occur when Nick is expected to comply with some hospital routines or medical procedures that are painful, uncomfortable, or simply new and frightening. These situations may be so aversive or frustrating that outbursts may be Nick's only means of escape or control. The best approach is to capitalize on what has worked in the past for the patient and be prepared to use multiple alternatives and positive reinforcement. Even during relatively brief therapeutic encounters, the nurse must explore ways to provide Nick with alternative ways to achieve comfort.

Pain Management

Depending on the level of cognitive impairment and deficits in communication, caregivers such as the CLA staff can assess pain by proxy and compare current behaviors to baseline behaviors prior to surgery. Pain is an internal, subjective experience that cannot be directly assessed. In persons with limited capacity for self-reporting, pain must be evaluated through the observation of behaviors that may overlap with other physical problems. This is especially true for the individual with sensory-processing difficulties. Pain may be mistaken for hunger, thirst, over or understimulation, anxiety, or depression (Feldt, Warne, & Ryden, 1998; Wynne, Ling, & Remsburg, 2000). The only clues may be nonverbal indicators, including grimacing, furrowing of the brow, squinting, rapid blinking, nose wrinkling, and restlessness. Pain may be suspected if there is a change in agitation, increased withdrawal, increased aggression, or a different kind of aggressiveness.(McCracken & Iverson, 2001; Wick, 2007) A consultation with the pharmacist is necessary when medicating Nick for pain, because of the high likelihood of adverse reactions due to polypharmacy (Lacasse, 2011). Potential toxicities may be unpredictable in a person who has a neurodevelopmental disorder. Therefore, best-practices nursing care includes constant observation during initial pharmacotherapy.

Pain Assessment

Pain assessment of cognitively impaired patients requires careful observation. Try to avoid facial-expression scales, as these may be confusing to individuals with ASD, who have difficulty interpreting the meaning of what they see. Whatever tool is selected should be practiced well in advance of any procedure or stressful medical situation. The nurse should be aware that even with preparation, individuals with ASD may decompensate under stressful situations and may not be able to cooperate or communicate appropriately. Therefore, understanding the person's unique way of demonstrating pain will be critical. Both the patient's family members and staff should describe how the patient has historically behaved when experiencing pain. Many individuals with ASD become irritable, noncompliant, and even aggressive when experiencing pain without being able to communicate what is happening in their bodies.

Pain assessment does not require a verbal response from patients with ASD. By pointing, a patient may provide the necessary information without the need to interpret complex messages. A tool that has a color meter for pain can be used effectively with adults. The nurse may associate levels of pain with three to five colors ranging from light green to medium yellow to fire orange. Underneath the colors, pain arrows become larger and bolder in size and darkness. The color gradations are wide enough to allow the patient to point to one without touching the next color. The patient with ASD can point to the color that best describe his/her level of pain.

Another tool may use five different size circles or other shapes ranging from small to very large with the word "pain" written inside the circle. Big is a concept that would be easily understood by people with ASD. The visual is simple, and the bigger shape represents the bigger pain. Nick would only have to point to one of the shapes that best described his pain level. Meaningful communication is the first communication mode to be affected for individuals with ASD under stressful situations. Both tools are visual and do not require Nick to speak.

The other important tool to train Nick to is that of knowing where he is experiencing pain in his body. His family and the staff at the residence should know whether Nick is capable of understanding and communicating where in his body it hurts. Nick would be capable of indicating by pointing to general areas of his body, but may not be able to tell more specifically where he feels pain (see Exhibits 13.1 and 13.2).

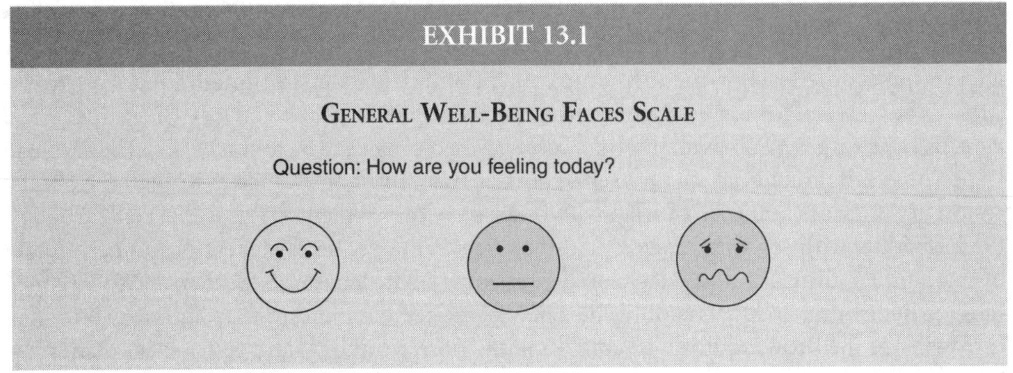

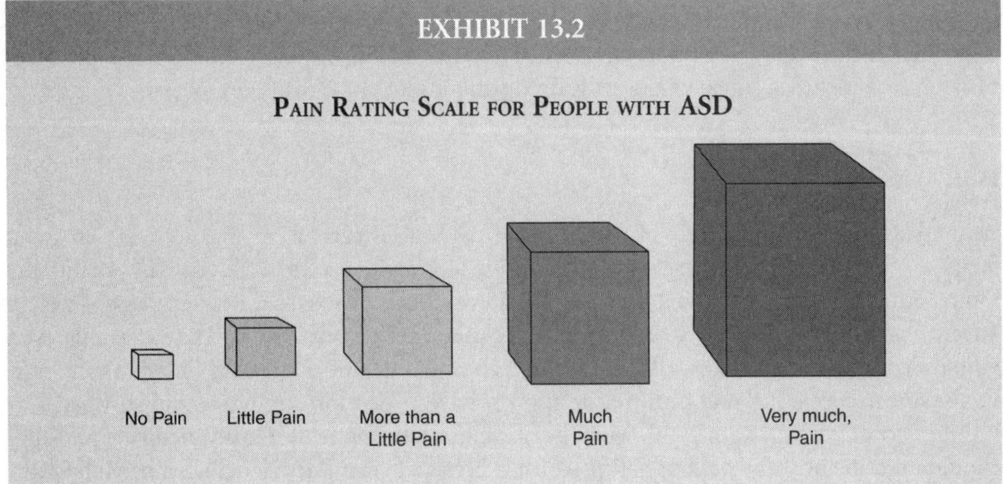

Another important point is to be sure everyone who works with Nick understands what word Nick uses to indicate pain. If Nick understands and uses the word "hurt" versus pain, then everyone who deals with Nick should be using this term instead of the term "pain." This would also apply to descriptions of any assessment tools. If Nick only understands or uses the term "hurt," then the assessment tool for pain should reflect his preference.

Self-reporting tasks, such as rating pain, will be compromised in the presence of cognitive impairments. Self-reporting tasks require an understanding of the request, the ability to recall pain events in a given time frame, and the ability to interpret experiences of noxious stimuli (Buffum, Hutt, Chang, Craine, & Snow, 2007). For Nick, the nurse may have more success anchoring his subjective pain using a visual analogue scale that rates pain linearly with words, rather than pictures on a 10-point scale. This may be more useful than the popular "Faces" pain rating scale, as the person with ASD may be less capable of identifying with facial expressions indicating feelings. Herr and colleagues published a systematic review of 10 behavioral scales, along with details, critiques, and the actual scales, online (Herr, Bjoro, & Decker, 2007). A very simple "Faces" scale may be easily created by the nurse, free hand, and used to identify general well-being. See Exhibits 13.1 and 13.2.

SUMMARY

A nurse may improve Nick's medical prognosis and emotional stability through careful, integrated planning with individuals who care for him. Medical interventions, such as hospitalizations, are times of great change and stress for typical individuals. For individuals with autism or individuals with cognitive challenges, medical events can prove traumatic. Integrated advanced planning can reduce the use of invasive and costly procedures for individuals with highly specialized needs. Nurses and other professionals in the medical community can make an enormous contribution to individuals such as Nick and ensure positive medical outcomes for them by gaining a better understanding of their unique characteristics and needs.

The first step to improving cancer care is overcoming the barriers to screening. Interventions for improving screening should center first on the education of the person with ASD and his/her family and caregivers and health care providers. Second, transportation must be available and easy to secure. Third, the costs of screening must be evaluated and reduced if possible, through improved insurance coverage that includes transportation to facilities. Tyler and colleagues (2010) recommended that procedures be modified to include sedation, desensitization, testing at home, and better coordination of services to include tracking of screening.

In conclusion, exemplary care of Nick is personal and patient-centered. It integrates best-practices nursing with knowledge of ASD by using a team approach to decision making. It engages family members, if possible, and caregivers in all phases of pre- and post-operative care. A perspective that aims for "no surprises" has the best chance of assuring success for the patient and the staff. By working with the strengths and special abilities of the patient, and within the limitations of the health care environment, the entire experience can be minimally distressing and maximally accommodating. On the trajectory of cancer care, people with ASD need accurate, tailored information and continuous emotional and psychological support.

REFERENCES

Albertsen, P. (2008). Should men with low-risk, localized prostate cancer choose active surveillance or undergo a robotic prostatectomy? *Current Urology Reports, 9*(1), 1–2

American Cancer Society. (2010). *Cancer Facts and Figures, 2010*. Atlanta, GA: Author.

Aragon-Ching, J. B., Williams, K. M., & Gulley, J. L. (2007). Impact of androgen-deprivation therapy on the immune system: Implications for combination therapy of prostate cancer. *Frontiers in Bioscience, 12*, 4957–4971.

Armas, O. A., Aprikian, A. G., Melamed, J., Cordon-Cardo, C., Cohen, D. W., Erlandson, R., Fair, W. R., & Reuter, V. (1994). Clinical and pathobiological effects of neoadjuvant total androgen ablation therapy on clinically localized prostatic adenocarcinoma. *American Journal of Surgical Pathology, 18*(10), 979–991.

Bacon, C. G., Giovannucci, E., Testa, M., & Kawachi, I. (2001). The impact of cancer treatment on quality of life outcomes for patients with localized prostate cancer. *Journal of Urology, 166*(5), 1804–1810.

Becker, H., Stuifbergen, A., & Tinkle, M. (1997). Reproductive health care experiences of women with physical disabilities: A qualitative study. *Archives of Physical Medicine and Rehabilitation, 78*(12), S26–33.

Bernat, J. L. (2004). Ethical issues in the perioperative management of neurologic patients. *Neurologic Clinics of North America, 22*, 457–471.

Bill-Axelson, A., Holmberg, L., Ruutu, M., Garmo, H., Stark, J. R., ... Busch, C. SPCG-4 Investigators (2005). Radical prostatectomy versus watchful waiting in early prostate cancer. *New England Journal of Medicine, 352*, 1977–1984.

Buffum, M. D., Hutt, E., Chang, V. T., Craine, M. H., & Snow, L. (2007). Cognitive impairment and pain management: Review of issues and challenges. *Journal of Rehabilitation Research and Development, 44*(2), 325–330.

Campbell, S. C., Bhoopalam, N., Moritz, T. E., Pandya, M., Iyer, P., Vanveldhuizen, P., . . . Reda, D. J. (2010). The use of zoledronic acid in men receiving androgen deprivation therapy for prostate cancer with severe osteopenia or osteoporosis. *Urology, 75*(5), 1138–1143.

Catalona, J. W., Carvalhal, G. F., Mager, D. E., & Smith, D. S. (1999). Potency, continence, and complication rates in 1870 consecutive radical retropubic prostatectomies. *Journal of Urology, 162*(2), 433–438.

Catalona, J. W., Roehl, K. A., & Antenor, J. A. (2002). Potency, continence, complications, and survival analysis in 3,032 consecutive radical retropubic prostatectomies. *Journal of Urology, 164*(suppl 4), 625.

Centers for Disease Control and Prevention. (2006). *United States cancer statistics: Top ten cancers in the United States.* Retrieved from http://apps.nccd.cedc.gov/uscs/toptencancers.aspx

Christodouleas, J., Fox, J., Song, D., & DeWeese, T. (2010). Basic terms and concepts of radiation. In L. M. Su (Ed.), *Early diagnosis and treatment of cancer series: Prostate cancer* (pp. 159–176). Philadelphia, PA: Saunders/Elsevier.

Coleman, A. M. (2010). Treatment procedures. In C. M. Washington & D. Leaver (Eds.), *Principles and practice of radiation therapy* (3rd ed., pp. 158–179). St. Louis, MO: Elsevier Mosby.

Cooke, L. B. (1997). Cancer and learning disability. *Journal of Intellectual Disability 41*(4), 312–316.

Dahmani, A., de Plater, L., Guyader, C., Fontaine, J. J., Berniard, A., Assayag, F., . . . Decaudin, D. (2010). A preclinical therapeutic schedule optimizing docetaxel plus estramustine administration in prostate cancer. *Anti-Cancer Drugs, 21*(10), 927–931.

Dreicer, R. (2005). Management of the patient with androgen-independent metastatic prostate cancer. In E. A. Klein (Ed.), *Management of prostate cancer* (2 ed., pp. 579–606). Totowa, NJ: Humana Press.

Droz, J. P., Balducci, L., Bolla, M., Emberton, M., Fitzpatrick, J. M., Joniau, S., . . . Sternberg, C. N. (2010). Management of prostate cancer in older men: Recommendations of a working group of the International Society of Geriatric Oncology. *BJU International, 106*(4), 462–469.

Egevad, L., Allsbrook, W. C., Jr., & Epstein, J. I. (2005). Current practice of Gleason grading among genitourinary pathologists. *Human Pathology, 36*, 5–9.

Feldt, K. S., Warne, M. A., & Ryden, M. B. (1998). Examining pain in aggressive cognitively impaired older adults. *Journal of Gerontology Nursing, 24*(11), 14–22.

Fine, M., & Asch, A. (1988). *Women with disabilities: Essays in psychology, culture and politics.* Philadelphia, PA: Temple University Press.

Foster, J. (2006). End of life care: Making choices. *Learning Disability Practice, 9*(7), 18–22.

Freter, C. E., & Perry, M. C. (2008). Principles of chemotherapy. In M. C. Perry (Ed.), *The chemotherapy source book* (4th ed., pp. 30–36). Philadelphia, PA: Lippincott Williams & Wilkins.

Gilbert, T., Wilkinson, T., & Crudginton, S. (2007). Supporting people with intellectual disability in the cancer journey: The "living with cancer" communication pack. *European Journal of Oncology Nursing, 11*(4), 357–361.

Gleason, D. F. (1992). Histological grading of prostate cancer: A perspective. *Human Pathology, 23*(3), 273–279.

Han, M., & Catalona, J. W. (Eds.) (2010). *Open radical retropubic prostatectomy: Techniques and outcomes.* Philadelphia, PA: Saunders/Elsevier.

Havercamp, S. M., Scandlin, D., & Roth, M. (2004). Health disparities among adults with developmental disabilities, adults with other disabilities, and adults not reporting disability in North Carolina. *Public Health Reports, 119*(4), 418–426.

Herr, H. W. (1994). Quality of life of incontinent men after radical prostatectomy. *Journal of Urology, 151*(3), 652–654.

Herr, K., Bjoro, K., & Decker, S. (2007). State of the art review of tools for assessment of pain in nonverbal older adults. *Project Overview.* Retrieved from http://prc.coh.org/pain-noa.htm

Heyman, E. N., & Rosner, T. T. (1996). Prostate cancer: An intimate view from patients and wives. *Urologic Nursing, 16*(2), 37–44.

Hu, K., & Wallner, K. (1998). Urinary incontinence in patients who have a TURP/TUIP following prostate brachytherapy. *International Journal of Radiation Oncology, Biology and Physics, 40*, 783–786.

Jackobsson, L., Hallberg, I. R., & Loven, L. (2000). Experiences of micturition problems, indwelling catheter treatment and sexual life consequences in men with prostate cancer. *Journal of Advanced Nursing, 31*(1), 59–67.

Klein, U., & Nowak, A. J. (1999). Characteristics of patients with autistic disorder presenting for dental treatment: A survey and chart review. *Specialty Care in Dentistry, 19*(5), 200–207.

Klotz, L. (2005). Active surveillance for prostate cancer: For whom? *Journal of Clinical Oncology, 23*, 8165–8169.

Kristal, A. R., Arnold, K. B., Neuhouser, M. L., Goodman, P., Platz, E. A., Albanes, D., & Thompson, I. (2010). Diet, supplement use, and prostate cancer risk: Results from the prostate cancer prevention trial. *American Journal of Epidemiology, 172*(5), 566–577.

Lacasse, C. (2011). Polypharmacy and symptom management in older adults. *Clinical Journal of Oncology Nursing, 15*(1), 27–30.

Lee, W. R., Moughan, J., Owen, J. B., & Zelefsky, M. J. (2003). The 1999 patterns of care study of radiotherapy in localized prostate carcinoma: A comprehensive survey of prostate brachytherapy in the United States. *Cancer, 98*, 1987–1994.

Lord, C., & O'Neill, P. J. (1983). Language and communication needs of adolescents and adults. In E. Schopler, & G. B. Mesibov (Eds.), *Autism in adolescents and adults* (pp. 57–77). New York, NY: Plenum.

Marshall, J., Sheller, B., Williams, B. J., Manci, L., & Cowan, C. (2007). Cooperation predictors for dental patients with autism. *Pediatric Dentistry, 29*(5), 369–376.

McCracken, L. M., & Iverson, G. L. (2001). Predicting complaints of impaired cognitive functioning in patients with chronic pain. *Journal of Pain and Symptom Management, 21*, 392–396.

Mehta, K. M., Fung, K. Z., Kistler, C. E., Chang, A., & Walter, L. C. (2010). Impact of cognitive impairment on screening mammography use in older U.S. women. *American Journal of Public Health, 100*(10), 1917–1923.

Memorial Sloan-Kettering Cancer Center. (2010). *Prostate cancer*. Retrieved from http://www.mskcc.org/mskcc/html/403.cfm

Mohler, J., Bahnson, R. R., Boston, B., Busby, J. E., D'Amico, A., Eastham, J. A., ... Walsh, P. C. (2010). NCCN clinical practice guidelines in oncology: Prostate cancer. *Journal of the National Comprehensive Cancer Network, 8*(2), 162–200.

Nag, S., Beyer, D., Friedland, J., Grimm, P., & Nath, R. (1999). American Brachytherapy Society recommendations for transperineal permanent brachytherapy of prostate cancer. *International Journal of Radiation Oncology, Biology, and Physics, 44*, 789–799.

National Comprehensive Cancer Network. (2009). *NCCN clinical practical guidelines in oncology: prostate cancer [v.2.2009]*. Retrieved March 1, 2012 from http://www.nccn.org/professionals/physician_gls/pdf/prostate.pdf

Neville, P. J., Casey, G., & Witte, J. S. (2004). Hereditary prostate cancer and genetic risk. In E. A. Klein (Ed.), *Management of prostate cancer* (pp. 57–69). Totowa, NJ: Humana Press.

Nosek, M. A., & Howland, C. A. (1997). Breast and cervical cancer screening among women with physical disability. *Archives of Physical Medicine and Rehabilitation, 78*(1), S–39.

O'Regan, P., & Drummond, E. (2008). Cancer information needs of people with intellectual disability: A review of the literature. *European Journal of Oncology Nursing, 12*, 142–147.

Patja, K., Eero, P., & Iivanainen, M. (2001). Cancer incidence among people with intellectual disability. *Journal of Intellectual Disability Research, 45*(4), 300–307.

Penson, D. F., Rossignol, M., Sartor, A. O., Scardino, P. T., & Abenhaim, L. L. (2008). Prostate cancer: Epidemiology and health-related quality of life. *Urology, 72*(suppl 6), S3–11.

Presti, J. (2004). Current trends in biopsy techniques. In E. A. Klein (Ed.), *Management of prostate cancer* (pp. 143–158). Totowa, NJ: Humana Press.

Raposa, K. A. (2009). Behavioral management for patients with intellectual and developmental disorders. *Dental Clinics of North America, 53*(2), 359–373.

Reid, S. V., & Hamdy, F. C. (2008). Epidemiology, pathology, and pathogenesis. In V. H. Nargund, D. Raghavan, & H. M. Sandler (Eds.), *Urological oncology* (pp. 451–469). London: Springer.

Reis, F., Netto, N. J., Jr., Reinato, J. A., Thiel, M., & Zani, E. (2004). The impact of prostatectomy and brachytherapy in patients with localized prostate cancer. *International Urology and Nephrology, 36*(2), 187–190.

Reuter, V. E. (1997). Pathological changes in benign and malignant prostatic tissue following androgen deprivation therapy. *Urology, 49*, 16–22.

Rodrigues, A., & Pow-Sang, J. M. (2007). Urologic oncology. In M. S. Sable, V. K. Sondak, & J. J. Sussman (Eds.), *Surgical foundations: Essentials of surgical oncology* (pp. 387–401). Philadelphia: Elsevier Mosby.

Scher, H. I., & Heller, G. (2000). Clinical states in prostate cancer: Toward a dynamic model of disease progression. *Urology, 55*(3), 323–327.

Smoot, J., & Dawson, N. A. (2004). When to refer a patient with prostate cancer to a medical oncologist. In E. A. Klein (Ed.), *Management of prostate cancer* (2 ed., pp. 553–560). Totowa, NJ: Humana Press.

Steinberg, A. G., Wiggins, E. A., Barmada, C. H., & Sullivan, V. J. (2002). Deaf women: Experiences and perceptions of health care system access. *Journal of Women's Health, 11*, 729–741.

Stephenson, A. J., & Eastham, J. A. (2005). Role of salvage radical prostatectomy for recurrent prostate cancer after radiation therapy. *Journal of Clinical Oncology, 23*(32), 8198–8203.

Stephenson, A. J., Scardino, P. T., Eastham, J. A., Bianco, F. J. J., Dotan, Z. A., DiBlasio, C. J., ... Kattan, M. W. (2005). Postoperative nomogram predicting the 10–year probability of prostate cancer recurrence after radical prostatectomy. *Journal of Clinical Oncology, 23*(28), 7005–7012.

Talcott, J. A., Rieker, P., Clark, J. A., Propert, K. J., Weeks, J. C., Beard, C. J., … Kantoff, P. W. (1998). Patient reported symptoms after primary therapy for early prostate cancer: Results of a prospective cohort study. *Journal of Clinical Oncology, 16*, 275–283.

Thompson, I. M., Ankerst, D. P., & Tangen, C. M. (2010). Prostate-specific antigen, risk factors, and prostate cancer: Confounders nestled in an enigma. *Journal of the National Cancer Institute, 102*(17), 1299–1301.

Tuffrey-Wijne, I., Bernal, J., Jones, A., Butler, G., & Hollins, S. (2006). People with intellectual disabilities and their need for cancer information. *European Journal of Oncology Nursing, 11*, 182–188.

Tyler, C. V., Zyzanski, S. J., Panaite, V., & Council, L. (2010). Nursing perspectives on cancer screening in adults with intellectual and other developmental disabilities. *Intellectual and Developmental Disabilities, 48*(4), 271–277.

U.S. Preventative Services Task Force. (2008). Screening for prostate cancer: US Preventative Services Task Force recommendations statement. *Annals of Internal Medicine, 149*(3), 185–191.

Vessey, J. A. (1988). Care of the hospitalized child with a cognitive developmental delay. *Holistic Nursing Practice, 2*(2), 48–54.

Wick, J. Y. (2007). Pain in a special population: The cognitively impaired. *Pharmacy Times*, 1–4.

Wolf, A. M., Wender, R. C., Etzioni, R. B., Thompson, I. M., D'Amico, A. V., & Volk, R. J., … American Cancer Society Prostate Cancer Advisory Committee (2010). American Cancer Society guidelines for the early detection of prostate cancer: Update 2010. *CA Cancer Journal for Clinicians, 60*, 70–98.

Wynne, C. F., Ling, S. M., & Remsburg, R. (2000). Comparison of pain assessment instruemnts in cognitively intact and cognitively impaired nursing home residents. *Geriatric Nursing, 21*(1), 20–23.

III Discussion Questions

CHAPTER 10

1. What role could the high school nurse play in helping students transition successfully into the community? Develop a nursing care plan to demonstrate your understanding of this role. What interventions could the school have put in place earlier that would have eased Daryl's senior year transitions?
2. Why is it important to individualize the nursing plan of care? What steps are needed to complete a personalized nursing plan of care for an adolescent or young adult with an autistic spectrum disorder (ASD)?
3. What is the benefit of using naturalistic teaching strategies in the education of a student with ASD?
4. Briefly explain the rationale for each of the steps to a successful transition. What roadblocks might be encountered if these principles are not implemented?
5. How might sensory issues impact a person's ability to function successfully in the workplace? What could be done to support an individual with these difficulties?
6. What is a nurse's role in addressing personal sexual questions that a student with ASD may pose?

CHAPTER 11

1. What are the ethical issues related to pregnancy and childbearing in individuals with ASD?
2. How should routine prenatal care be modified for individuals with Asperger's syndrome (AS)?
3. Prepare a plan of care for a pregnant woman with AS who has developed pregnancy-induced hypertension 8 weeks prior to her due date.
4. During a preconception office visit, how can the advanced practice nurse (APN) best guide a woman with a diagnosis of AS to prepare herself for childbearing?
5. Considering the social deficits related to AS, discuss whether a women with AS can adequately care for her newborn infant.
6. Q.L. is a 35-year-old woman with 3 pregnancies and 2 live births presenting for prenatal care at 8 weeks gestation. After a year of evaluation, her 28-month-old son has just been given a formal diagnosis of an ASD. During the diagnostic process for her son, she learned she has AS. As the APN caring for Q.L., discuss the implications of this information and some approaches to tailor her care to meet the her needs and those of her family.

7. Translating research into practice, discuss at least four specific strategies to tailor nursing care for the woman with AS during labor and delivery.

CHAPTER 12

1. A patient arrives in the Emergency Department (ED) with spinal precautions intact. He was cooperative with the precautions until he was removed from the board. What could the nurse do if a patient with ASD needed to be on spinal precautions and could not tolerate it?
2. How can involving the family or home caregiver improve the quality of care provided to patients with ASD in the ED?
3. You are transferring a patient with ASD from the ED to an inpatient unit. Prepare a transfer plan of care.
4. You are the nurse for a patient in the ED and a radiology technician approaches you and asks that a patient be restrained so they can get an X-ray of his chest. What do you do?

CHAPTER 13

1. Describe potential side effects of anesthesia and propose nursing actions to manage them.
2. Outline specific instructions that you would give to the different health care team members pre- and post-prostate surgery.
3. Apply techniques of applied behavioral analysis to promote compliance with respiratory treatments post-prostatectomy.
4. A patient with ASD is in cardiac arrest. How does the treatment differ?

ADDITIONAL CASES FOR PRACTICE

CASE III.1

Maureen is a 39-year-old female living in a group home. She was diagnosed with AS at age 15 years. Maureen has an extensive vocabulary and is fluent in labeling objects. However, she is unable to participate in reciprocal conversation. She talks at people and in no way moderates conversation based on the response of others. She has marked difficulty in the context of social interaction that demands reflexivity. Maureen demands sameness, and this affects every aspect of her life, from eating the same foods to self-care activities to ordering the content of a conversation. She is obsessed with astronomy and the solar system. She presents to the nurse practitioner for a routine history and physical exam. She has never had a cervical smear to screen for cervical cancer, and there is no history of regular breast examinations. While listening to her ordered description of her life events while growing up, you hear her say her twin sister and mother had the same surgery for cancer.
Describe your comprehensive plan of care.

YouTube Video Clips: Late Adolescence—Communication

Teen Author Talks about Her Autism and Books, Nov 2007

Summary:

A teen author talks about her autism, her horses, and two fantasy books she has published.

Length of clip: 6:11 min.

Link: http://www.youtube.com/watch?v=oA6hcUZNjdI

Discussion Questions

1. Discuss the ways that Alea's autism has been an asset to her.
2. Describe the therapeutic relationship Alea has with her horses. What sort of benefits do you think animals can offer for teenagers with autism?
3. What are your thoughts on the subject matter of Alea's books? Discuss the potential pros and cons of special interests in fantasy for teenagers with autism.
4. Discuss ways that special interest can be integrated with medical treatment plans.

Autism Education Trust–Helen's film.mov

Summary:

Helen is a high school student on the autism spectrum who uses communication aides. She made this video to describe her likes, dislikes, and everyday challenges and successes at her school.

Length of clip 5:37 min.

Link: http://www.youtube.com/watch?v=twGDm5Be_iQ

Discussion Questions

1. Describe different emotions and interests that Helen is able to communicate without words. What do you notice in her body language?
2. You are given this video prior to admitting Helen for a preoperative workup for an appendectomy. Describe alternative methods of communicating that might help during the therapeutic encounter.
3. How would you use this information to prepare the staff and patient for postoperative care?
4. Discuss the benefits of speech therapy for autistic people. Identify different techniques that are utilized and discuss what might work well for Helen.

YouTube Video Clips: Late Adolescence—Socialization

Asperger Dating Video

Summary:

A song about a mechanical man looking for a robot girl.

Length of clip 2:48 min.

Link: http://www.youtube.com/watch?v=d1yOEfB1Rjw& feature=related

Discussion Questions

1. What is the mechanical man saying about himself?
2. Identify the particular challenges that adolescents on the autism spectrum might face when seeking companionship and intimacy.
3. List the strategies for discussing sexual health with adolescents with AS. Would you show this video? Why or why not?

Asperger's Documentary–My Crazy Life. Part 1 of 3

Summary:

An introduction to Reuben, a teenager with AS and a very high IQ.

Length of clip 8:06 min.

Link: http://www.youtube.com/watch?v=q_PBVxGEEY4

Discussion Questions

1. Image that Reuben is brought to the ED after sustaining a head injury after an automobile accident. How would you assess cognitive status and the potential effect of a concussion on emotions? How would you explain this kind of injury? Anticipate Reuben's emotional reaction.
2. What are your thoughts on his relationships with inanimate objects?
3. What do you see as the benefits of providing a formal diagnosis of autism?
4. Create a set of questions that you would ask during an intake health history.

YouTube Video Clips: Late Adolescence—Ritualistic/Repetitive Movements

Asperger's Documentary–My Crazy Life. Part 2 of 3

Summary:

Second part of a documentary about Reuben, a high-IQ teenager with AS. In this clip, Reuben tries to negotiate the grocery store and conducts interviews with his mother and his friend. He also experiments with sports and his looks in order to fit in.

Length of clip: 7:56 min.

Link: http://www.youtube.com/watch?v=UviCfQC8Uzk& feature=related

Discussion Questions

1. What is Reuben most interested in achieving though his questioning of others?
2. List the potential benefits and drawbacks of "getting stuck in a groove" and thinking of one thing only for Reuben. Discuss how this might help or hinder him in his life.
3. Rueben makes a good point in this video, that some things are much more socially acceptable as an object of obsession than others. What are your thoughts on this issue? What makes Reuben's interest in neurology different from his friend's interest in Manchester United?
4. How would you translate aspects of this interest to other health-related topics to develop a lifelong plan for health promotion?

Dressed and Out the Door with Severe Autism

Summary:

Family helping a young man with severe autism to get dressed.

Length of clip 4:23 min.

Link: http://www.youtube.com/watch?v=AcINQS0g5us

Discussion Questions

1. Getting dressed can be a metaphor for becoming socially acceptable. Discuss the ways that this young man must be "dressed" for public life. Can you apply this to your practice environment?
2. What changes in James' behavior did you notice with the music therapy? How might music therapy be useful in a clinical setting?
3. Explain the functional purpose of self-destructive/injurious behavior. What do you think you would try to do if one of your autistic patients was repeatedly striking himself as James does in this video? What did his mother try?
4. Design a best-practices approach for your practice area, for a patient with ASD who is exhibiting self-injurious behavior.
5. The blue tube his mother places on his neck in the video is called a "vibration tube" and can help to curb mild episodes of self-abuse. Make a list of other tools (not restraints) that may be useful for autistic patients who are self-injurious.
6. Explain the difference between sensory-seeking and sensory-avoiding behaviors. Can James' behavior be sensory seeking *or* sensory avoiding?

YouTube Video Clips: Adults—Communication

Body Language

Summary:

A woman with ASD shares insight about various body language challenges.

Length of clip: 10:12 min.

Link: http://www.youtube.com/watch?v=mCW5HnNsDd8&feature=related

Discussion Questions

1. Describe the "typical" or "classic" body language symptoms that people associate with autism.
2. Describe the less typical symptoms of autism that she mentions in this video.
3. The video talks about avoiding eye contact, especially when uncomfortable. Discuss what you can do to make your patients with autism more comfortable in the hospital or outpatient setting?
4. If you observed some of the behaviors she describes in one of your adult patients, problem solve a strategy for communication that would allow you to take a comprehensive health history and perform a physical exam.

In My Language

Summary:

This video is "a strong statement on the existence and value of many different kinds of thinking and interaction."

Length of clip 8:37 min.

Link: http://www.youtube.com/watch?v=JnylM1hI2jc

Discussion Questions

1. What assumptions did you make about the person's behaviors during the first segment of the video?
2. Discuss alternative means of communication that you can offer to help better understand both your nonverbal and verbal patients?
3. Based on this video, how do you now define effective communication and language?
4. Discuss how you would determine if a patient is competent to make medical decisions? List your criteria for competence when considering patients on the autism spectrum.

Successful Adults with Autism

Summary:

The work experience of a 42-year-old man with autism.

Length of clip: 2:35 min (the video continues, but is only relevant up to 2:35).

Link: http://www.youtube.com/watch?v=0z1-MWb2hFQ&feature=related

Discussion Questions

1. Analyze the communication style used by Bob's boss to give him directions at the beginning of the clip. List the elements that make it effective.
2. Discuss the techniques you observe the therapists using to communicate with the clients. How could you apply these strategies to nursing care of autistic adults?
3. What criteria would you use to assess whether or not an adult with autism and comorbid medical conditions is capable of living independently?

YouTube Video Clips: Adults—Socialization

Adult Life Skills Program (ALSP) for People with Autism

Summary:

Suggestions for developing social skills.

Length of clip: 5.12 min.

Link: http://www.youtube.com/watch?v=QC0Tdlug_4o

Discussion Questions

1. Summarize the social problems among adults with ASD.

2. Describe an approach to a functional assessment and predict antecedents of behavior problems.
3. What impact might these behaviors have on his ability to work effectively with his coworkers?
4. Propose a health promotion plan to mitigate stress associated with the diagnosis of ASD, including ways to modify the environment.
5. Design a nursing staff in-service educational program on caring for adults with ASD who wish to seek employment.
6. You are a nurse manager and have observed that an employee is having difficulty socializing, exhibiting symptoms similar to those described in the clip. How would you approach assessment? What strategies would you use to manage the situation?

Autism–ANTM–Heather

Summary:

Clips from the popular television series *America's Next Top Model* portraying a contestant, Heather, who has mild AS, and her interactions with the other contestants.

Length of clip: 9:42 min.

Link: http://www.youtube.com/watch?v=ZWArtIXY5WA& feature=related

Discussion Questions

1. Summarize your impressions of the portrayal of AS in the public media.
2. How does popular culture affect the way health care providers interact with patients?
3. Analyze the way that Heather is portrayed on this video clip. Which aspects of AS do the editors choose to focus on?
4. *America's Next Top Model* is one example a competitive environment. Consider the special needs of people with AS in a competitive work environment; should they be afforded any special evaluation criteria? Should they be mandated to disclose their diagnosis to their potential employers?
5. Contestants made comments about Heather. If a colleague made similar comments about a patient, how would you address these comments?

Temple Grandin (Trailer)

Summary:

Trailer for an HBO biopic on Temple Grandin, an autistic savant with visual-spatial memory abilities.

Length of clip: 1:52 min.

Link: http://www.youtube.com/watch?v=cpkN0JdXRpM

Discussion Questions

1. Describe what you notice about the way that Temple Grandin introduces herself and interacts with people. How does it differ from what is considered "normal"?

2. What would be your reaction if a patient introduced/described herself to you in a similar way.
3. In the clip Temple Grandin is asked if she can "bring everything she sees to her mind?" She responds, "Sure, can't you?" Discuss strategies you can come up with to understand an autistic person's point of view.
4. Translate Temple Grandin's coping behaviors to recommendations for patients during clinical encounters.

YouTube Video Clips: Adults—Repetitive Movements

Autism–Repetitive Behaviors Like Rocking and Flapping

Summary:

Video depicting repetitive behaviors in response to stress.

Length of clip 3:59 min.

Link: http://www.youtube.com/watch?v=f15JexiQt4U

Discussion Questions

1. Define "normal" and "abnormal" repetitive behaviors.
2. What are they, and do you exhibit them more in times of stress? In which situations do you notice yourself performing these behaviors?
3. Explain the value of applied behavioral analysis for repetitive behaviors. Do you think behavior modification therapy is helpful or necessary for autistic people who exhibit repetitive behaviors?
4. Discuss your thoughts on assuring successful therapeutic encounters when a patient has ritualistic/repetitive movement disorder. List the factors in the workplace that could be barriers to success for a person with "abnormal" stress behaviors?
5. Describe situational factors in your practice area that may lead to an abnormal stress response.

Sensory Overload Simulation

Summary:

Clip produced by a person with autism designed to simulate the experience of having sensory overload.

Length of clip 3:33 min.

Link: http://www.youtube.com/watch?v=BPDTEuotHe0&feature=related

Discussion Questions

1. Describe your emotional, psychological, and physical reactions when the video clip got louder. Explain human biological responses to sensory overload.
2. List the aspects of the hospital environment that you think could be difficult for an adult on the autism spectrum.
3. Propose ways to modify the hospital environment to reduce sensory overload for adults with ASD.

4. Describe different warning signs or behaviors that indicate that a person with autism is becoming overwhelmed.
5. Identify interventions that might be helpful when a person with autism is overstimulated.
6. How would you approach the care of a patient who requires additional stimulation (sensory seeking).

Bob Drakope: (Episode 2) Autistic Man Stimming

Summary:

Animation showing a confrontation between a man and a woman.

Length of clip: 1:46 min.

Link: http://www.youtube.com/watch?v=j-sjg33nnXc

Discussion Questions

1. Discuss what the video is trying to depict.
2. Tweet the main message.
3. Contrast types of "stimming" or repetitive movements that are seen as socially acceptable with types of movements that are not accepted in society. List the repetitive movements you see that are accepted in adults.
4. Elaborate on the different ways actions may be understood or interpreted from the point of view of the man, the woman, and outside observers.
5. What do you think about the woman's comment that he cannot have autism because he can talk? List some common misconceptions about autism that you have heard in the public and in the health care arena.
6. Propose five questions to ask during a clinical assessment to help you correctly interpret the behavior of an autistic person.

Introduction: Older Years and End of Life

IV

Marcia R. Gardner

Comprehensive and person-centered care of clients with autism spectrum disorder (ASD) requires an approach that integrates knowledge of biophysical and genetic underpinnings, the epidemiology of ASD, evidence-based therapeutics and behavioral and physical treatment modalities, developmental science, and nursing science, among others, with an authentic appreciation of unique individual and family characteristics. However, care for this population is still incomplete, unless such knowledge is complemented by an appreciation of family struggles, understanding of future planning and transition issues, use of ethical principles and models, and facility with formal and informal community programs, structures, and systems of care for developmentally disabled people and their families. The population of elderly individuals and the population of elderly individuals with autism continues to grow. There are an estimated 641,000 people over the age of sixty years with a developmental disability (Simmons-Romano, 2011). The life expectancy for an individual with a developmental disability is approaching that of the general population of older adults (Tyler & Noritz, 2009). Clinicians working with older adults will need to expand their skills and knowledge repertoires in order to assess and manage the scope of problems of older adulthood, which are complicated by ASD.

Much more research attention needs to be directed toward the aging population of people with ASD, as the evidence base for practice is not well developed. Models for community-based services, transition planning, long-term care, and chronic illness management need development, expansion, and refining. As the population of people with ASD grows and ages, the dissemination and use of best-practice strategies and models to facilitate engagement of autonomy, assisted capacity, and shared decision making by individuals with ASD, especially in end-of-life care, becomes even more crucial. Hospice services will need to be adapted to the unique characteristics of people with ASD. Pain assessment instruments and interventions need to be further tested in this population, so that pain in acute, chronic, and end-of-life contexts can be recognized and quickly alleviated.

To fill gaps in our current health care system with respect to services for an increasingly older group of people with autism, more clinicians at all levels of care need to be educated about best practices in assessment and treatment of people with ASD. Models to facilitate access to clinicians with targeted skills need to be refined, and greater numbers and higher quality of day programs, group homes and long-term care facilities, and other specialized services must be available. Case management models specific to older adults with autism are also needed, considering the interaction of ASD with the aging process and the resultant, potentially complex health conditions they may have.

Of course, in an era of increasing health care costs and decreasing fiscal resources, it may be very challenging to make the case that such services are equally important as services for other diseases, disorders, and conditions. It will require advocacy and quick action emerging from the fundamental ethical standard of our discipline, as articulated in the *Code for Nurses* (American Nurses Association, 2001), to ensure the best quality of care possible for all persons. Nurses who know the family challenges, clinical dilemmas, service gaps, and struggles of patients are primed to represent the needs of this population in clinical practice and in the funding and policy arenas. As Mason, Leavitt, and Chaffee (2007) have written, "The values that nursing embodies can shape not just policies, but how those policies are developed" (p. 6).

To this end, section IV of this book offers readers a broad perspective on aging adults with autism. In Chapter 14, care for an older individual with autism is addressed by integrating theoretical perspectives on the aging process, physiology, pharmacotherapeutics and dynamics of aging, health promotion needs of older adults, along with evidence-based strategies to provide appropriate, autism-specific care for a highly vulnerable population. Chapter 15, which discusses future planning and decision making, focuses on aging caregivers of adults with ASD. This chapter establishes a framework for important decisions, such as responsibility for caregiving, access to services, and selection of a place of residence, that relatives or other invested persons must make when all members of the family of an individual with ASD are growing older. The chapter reviews the surprising geographic (state-level) variability in services available for older adults with ASD. Finally, Chapter 16 describes the ethical context for end-of-life decision making and care in this population. The foundation of this chapter is a discussion of ethical frameworks, approaches, and basic ethical principles relevant to the care of individuals with autism in general, but especially at the end of life. Best-practice strategies for care are examined using the exemplar case of an older individual with autism dying of brain cancer.

REFERENCES

American Nurses Association. (2001). Code of ethics for nurses with interpretive statements. Retrieved from http://nursingworld.org/MainMenuCategories/EthicsStandards/CodeofEthicsforNurses/Code-of-Ethics.aspx

Mason, D. J., Leavitt, J. K., & Chaffee, M. W. (2007). Policy and politics: A framework for action. In D. J. Mason, J. K. Leavitt, & M. W. Chaffee (Eds.), *Policy and politics in nursing and health care* (5 ed., pp. 1–16). St. Louis, MO: Saunders/Elsevier.

Simmons-Romano, M. (2011). Elderly individuals with developmental disabilities and the office visit. *Clinical Geriatrics, 19*(5), 52–56.

Tyler, C. V., & Noritz, G. (2009). Healthcare issues in aging adults with intellectual and other developmental disabilities. *Clinical Geriatrics, 17*(8), 30–35. Retrieved from http://www.clinicalgeriatrics.com/articles/Healthcare-Issues-Aging-Adults-with-Intellectual-and-Other-Developmental-Disabilities

Evidence-Based Care of the Older Client With Autism

14

Debi A. Schuhow and Tamara L. Zurakowski

The population of the world is aging rapidly. Additional numbers of older adults will stress health care, economic, and government systems and agencies already struggling to provide necessary services (United Nations, 2009). As more persons with ASD reach older adulthood, nurses and other health care professionals will be on the front lines; knowledge and skills to address the challenges of successful aging and the unique aspects of aging on the autism spectrum will be essential. Nurses who work with this aggregate of people (and almost all will) must be proficient practitioners, working in all domains of patient care: physiological, psychosocial, family and caregiver support, and community outreach. This chapter discusses changes associated with the aging process and will consider the way these changes interact with physiological, social, and emotional aspects of autism spectrum disorder (ASD). Nurses who accept the challenge of providing excellent care to older adults with ASD will find that all of their skills are utilized and will know the satisfaction of fulfilling the needs of a very vulnerable segment of society.

BACKGROUND

There are an increasing number of people being diagnosed with ASD, due to the broadening of its definition; nurses can expect to encounter this cohort of the population in all settings in which they practice. Autism spectrum disorder is a lifelong condition (Levy, Mandell, & Schultz, 2009), yet is rarely diagnosed in the older population, due to difficulties in obtaining a developmental history (van Niekirk et al., 2010).

The Adult Psychiatric Morbidity Survey in England (McManus, Meltzer, Brugha, Bebbington, & Jenkins, 2009) determined that the prevalence of ASD remained consistent across all age groups. The U.S. Census Bureau projects a doubling of the 2000 U.S. population over 65 years of age by 2030 (Vincent & Velkoff, 2010). Heller, Janicki, Hammel, and Factor (2002) projected that there will be 1.9 million people with ASD by the year 2020. Juxtaposing these data with the current prevalence rate of ASD in children, it is probable that there will be about 700,000 older adults with ASD in the United States by 2030.

Co-occurring Intellectual Disabilities among the Elderly

Intellectual disabilities (IDs) in ASD have been reported in ranges of 40% to 70% (Bertrand et al., 2001; Fombonne, 1999). Although the life expectancy of those with IDs remains lower than that of the general population (Patja, Iivanainen, Vesala, Oksanen, & Ruoppila, 2000), it is increasing. Aging is accompanied by physiological changes in normal function, including important changes in the metabolism of medications that are commonly used by persons with ASD. Cognitive changes, such as a decrease in short-term memory and alterations in learning process, are common in old age, and will be superimposed on the IDs of persons with ASD. Furthermore, chronic conditions that are common in older adults, such as osteoarthritis and hypertension, may require the person with ASD to manage mobility changes or complex medication regimens. These changes result in the need to adapt daily activities, which are made more difficult by the characteristics of ASD. Pharmacological adjuncts for managing daily life, such as anxiolytics, may not be safe as the person with ASD reaches older age and might be discontinued due to adverse effects; a coping resource is then removed.

Problems with Diagnosing the Elderly ASD Patient

The accuracy of epidemiological studies in this population continues to be skewed by the variety of methodologies used, lack of agreement on how ASD should be defined, and the likelihood that older adults with ASD remain invisible to formal health care providers and thus are not identified. The population of aging individuals with ASD will need comprehensive health care, and providers will need to be knowledgeable and competent in their care. While there is an expanding body of research in adults with ASD, there is a dearth of research on adults greater than 60 years of age who have ASD (James, Mukaetova-Ladinska, Reichelt, Briel, & Scully, 2006; Totsika, Felce, Kerr, & Hastings, 2010).

Multiple factors, such as comorbidities, level of function, social support, preexisting intellectual disability (ID), institutionalization, and lifestyle disabilities all interact with normal age-related changes, which need to be addressed in the nursing care of the older adult with ASD. Nurses are well-poised to develop the individualized plans of care needed by this population, as little is known about how ASD will affect any given individual over his or her lifetime (Holmes, 1998).

Comprehensive Lifelong Care

In addition to the United States, other countries are contemplating a continuum of care across the lifespan of individuals with ASD. For example, the Autism Management Advisory Team of Nova Scotia in Canada is in the process of gathering support for centers that are designed to house all services in one central location and to provide these services across the lifespan (Casey, 2010). Kerins, Price, Broadhurst, and Gaynor (2010) related that more of the developmentally disabled population reside in nursing homes for longer periods prior to their death and are admitted to a nursing home earlier than the general population.

CASE

Mr. Smith is a 76-year-old man with coronary artery disease, gastroesophageal reflux disease (GERD), hypertension, osteoarthritis of both hips and knees, and ASD. He was diagnosed with epilepsy, but had been without seizure activity for 6 years. Mr. Smith is 5 feet, 8 inches tall, of medium build, and walks without assistive devices. His current list of medications is noted in Exhibit 14.1.

He resides in a group home and has recently been diagnosed with Alzheimer's disease (AD). The care staff has noted that he is having more difficulty managing his activities of daily living and is more resistant to accepting help with them. There has also been an increase in head-banging behavior, particularly on first rising in the morning and after

(*Continued*)

CASE (Continued)

physical activities. Mr. Smith's oral intake has decreased over the past few weeks, and he has been particularly unwilling to eat his usual favorite, saltwater taffy. Mr. Smith's last physical examination was 1 month ago, and laboratory data are listed here and in Exhibit 14.1.

Mr. Smith is 5 feet 8 inches tall; weight is 140 pounds. He has lost 6 pounds since his previous exam, 6 months ago. His blood pressure is 140/88 mmHg, with heart rate 96 and regular. Based on the physical exam, and laboratory results, Mr. Smith's physician increased his phenytoin from 100 mg, po, tid, to 100 mg, po, qid, increased his simvastatin from 20 mg daily to 40 mg daily, and asked the care staff to make sure Mr. Smith's fluid intake is at least 1.5 liters per day.

EXHIBIT 14.1

CASE DATA FOR MR. SMITH

Current Medications

- Omeprazole, 20 mg, by mouth, at bedtime
- Amlodipine, 10 mg, by mouth, daily
- Hydrochlorothiazide, 12.5 mg, by mouth, daily
- Simvastatin, 40 mg, by mouth, daily
- Acetaminophen, 1000 mg, by mouth, as needed
- Phenytoin, 100 mg, by mouth, four times per day

Laboratory Data

- Serum phenytoin level: 7 μg/ml (therapeutic level: 10 to 20 μg/ml)
- Hemoglobin: 12.8 g/dl (normal: 13.5 to 16.5 g/dl)
- Hematocrit: 38% (normal: 41% to 50%)
- Red blood cells: 4.8×10^6/ml (normal: 4.5 to 5.5×10^6/ml)
- White blood cells: 5200/ml (normal: 5000 to 10,000/ml)
- Platelets: 137,000 (normal: 100,000–450,000)
- Glucose: 112 mg/dl (normal: fasting 70 to 110 mg/dl)
- Potassium: 4.6 mEq/l (normal: 3.5 to 5.0 mEq/l)
- Sodium: 138 mEq/l (normal: 135 to 145 mEq/l)
- Blood urea nitrogen: 45 mg/dl (normal: 7 to 20 mg/dl)
- Creatinine: 1.9 mg/dl (normal: 0.6 to 1.2 mg/dl)
- GFR: 29.5 ml/min (normal > 100 ml/min)
- Total cholesterol: 230 mg/dl (desirable: <200 mg/dl)

(*Continued*)

EXHIBIT 14.1 (Continued)

- Low-density lipoproteins: 180 mg/dl (desirable: <130 mg/dl)
- High-density lipoproteins: 56 mg/dl (desirable: >40 mg/dl)

MANIFESTATIONS OF ASD IN OLDER ADULTS

There is limited literature about the manifestations of ASD in the older adult. The physiological changes of normal aging, along with the typical behavioral trajectory of ASD across the lifespan will influence both the manifestations of ASD in older adults and their care. Refer to Exhibit 14.2 for a summary of age-related physiological changes.

The paucity of literature on older adults with ASD makes planning for the needs of this aggregate difficult. There is some evidence that the behavioral manifestations of ASD lessen with age. Esbensen, Seltzer, Lam, and Bodfish (2006) reported that restrictive and repetitive behaviors were less frequent and less severe among older individuals with ASD then their younger counterparts. Totsika and colleagues (2010) conducted a study on those with IDs and autism and found that behavior problems were less prevalent when compared to their younger counterparts. Jacobson, Sutton, and Janicki (1985) reported that prolonged institutionalization can accelerate the aging process, as can lifestyle-induced disabilities.

Assessment of Complex Symptoms in the Elderly

A high rate of comorbid conditions have been reported in those with ASD (Gillberg & Billstedt, 2000). Older adults are more likely to have multiple comorbidities that exacerbate, supersede, or mask ASD behavioral characteristics. Autism spectrum disorder can be misdiagnosed in the older adult because of the similarities among symptoms of ASD and other common disorders, such as dementia or depression. The nursing assessment of the older client with ASD should include a baseline assessment of past "setting events" (Carr & Smith, 1995). Setting events are incidents or situations that precipitate a behavioral outburst or maladaptive response by the person with ASD. Medical conditions may be setting events, particularly if they cause discomfort, such as pain from osteoarthritis or GERD. The nurse should ask prior caregivers about medical conditions that the older client with ASD experiences and associated behaviors.

Identification of these medical conditions and subsequent behaviors can help the nurse assess Mr. Smith for symptoms he is not able to express and/or recognize. Older adults with ASD presenting with functional decline often have other treatable conditions (Chicoine, McGuire & Rubin, 1999; Evenhuis, 1997, 1999; Thorpe, 1999); health status changes should not be peremptorily attributed to "behavior issues" or dementia. Mr. Smith's decreased functional status, resistance to care, decreased appetite, and increased head-banging *might* be manifestations of ASD and the new AD diagnosis. They can also be indications of acute illness or an exacerbation of one of his chronic conditions. It is crucial that Mr. Smith be thoroughly assessed for new-onset health problems and offered appropriate treatment.

Associated Chronic Conditions

Common physiological conditions in the older adult with ASD include epilepsy, GERD, hypothyroidism, osteoporosis, sensory impairments, enuresis, tuberous sclerosis, and sleep

EXHIBIT 14.2

Selected Physiological Changes Associated with Aging[a]

Cognitive and Psychological

- Slower rate for learning new material
- Decreased ability to multi-task
- Mild short term memory and recall impairment

Sleep

- Decreased deep sleep, increased light sleep
- Total need for hours of sleep remains stable

Skin

- Loss of elasticity and tensile strength
- Dermis becomes thinner, less subcutaneous fat
- Decreased number of sweat glands

Sensory Function

- Fewer taste buds, less saliva production
- Fewer rods and cones in retina of eye
- Loss of elasticity in lens, more difficulty with accommodation
- Thickening of lens, more difficulty with glare
- Drier cerumen in ear canal
- Loss of hearing in higher frequency sounds
- Decreased sense of smell
- Decreased tactile sensation and acute pain perception

Cardiovascular Function

- Loss of elasticity of arteries and veins
- Increased likelihood of cardiac arrhythmias
- Baroreceptors slow to respond to changes in blood pressure
- Decreased ability to increase cardiac output

Respiratory Function

- Decreased forced respiratory capacity
- Tidal volume remains constant
- Less effective respiratory-protective mechanisms such as cough, ciliary activity

Genitourinary Function

- Kidneys produce more urine at night than during the day
- Decreased glomerular filtration rate
- Decreased bladder capacity, less ability to sense bladder fullness

(*Continued*)

EXHIBIT 14.2 (Continued)

- Sexual response takes more time

Musculoskeletal Function

- Bone mineral density decreases
- Muscle fibers weaken

Endocrine Function

- Decreased thyroid function and basal metabolic rate
- Increased resistance to insulin, less insulin produced

Gastrointestinal Function

- Longer gastric emptying time
- Liver less effective at detoxifying blood
- Slower absorption of nutrients from gut

Hematologic Function

- Slower production of red blood cells
- Increased likelihood of vitamin B12 deficiency

Neurological Function

- Longer reaction time
- Increased sensitivity to chronic pain
- Decreased sense of balance

Immune Function

- Decreased fever response
- Increased autoimmune function
- Decreased T cell production and function
- Delayed inflammation response

[a]Data from Tabloski (2010).

disturbances. Psychiatric comorbid conditions include anxiety disorders, depression, dementia, and delirium by definition, is time-limited and not chronic. See Table 14.1 for a list of these conditions.

Epilepsy

A study conducted by Shavelle, Strauss, and Pickett (2001) found that seizures were a major source of mortality in those with autism, compared with the general population. Epilepsy has a higher prevalence, contributes to a higher mortality and morbidity rate, is more severe, and has a lower remission rate in older individuals with IDs, compared with the general population (Morgan, Baxter, & Kerr, 2003).

Nearly 70% of people with ASD also have an ID (Matson & Rivet, 2008). A survey of community-dwelling adults with IDs conducted by Matthews, Weston, Baxter, Felce, and

TABLE 14.1 ■ Common Chronic Health Conditions in Older Adults with ASD

Physical	Behavioral
Epilepsy	Sleep disturbances
GERD	Anxiety disorders
Hypothyroidism	Depression
Osteoporosis	Dementia
Enuresis	Delirium
Tuberous sclerosis	
Vision and hearing impairments	

Kerr (2008) reported a wide variety of epilepsy types in this population. This same study found that those with epilepsy had a significantly lower ability to adapt, a higher level of challenging behaviors, and a higher representation of the triad of impairments that define ASD: social interaction deficits, impaired social communication, and restricted behavior pattern. Those with a later onset of epilepsy had a better prognosis than those whose epilepsy began in childhood.

Mr. Smith has epilepsy and has been seizure-free for 6 years. Although his laboratory work indicated his phenytoin level was subtherapeutic, there has been no report of recent seizure activity. It is important to evaluate the individual's response to medications and not consider only the laboratory data. In Mr. Smith's case, the "subtherapeutic" phenytoin level might not have been problematic, since he has not had seizures. It is also possible that his phenytoin level was on a decline and that he might have seized in the near future. Careful observation and close communication with the group home staff are important in maintaining Mr. Smith's neurological health.

GERD

Galli-Carminati, Chavet, and Deriaz (2006) conducted a study on adults with and without PDD (mean age: 35; SD = 12). The Mantel-Haenszel test confirmed a significant association between PDD and gastrointestinal disorders, such as gastritis, esophagitis, GERD with esophagitis, heartburn, dyspepsia, intestinal malabsorption, and duodenal ulcer. Constipation and/or diarrhea are common complaints of those with ASD. Gastroesophageal reflux disease is the most common physiological comorbidity in those with ASD and in those who have an ID (National Health Service [NHS] Health Scotland, 2004) and places this population at increased risk for complications, such as an esophageal stricture/stenosis or bleeding from GERD.

Age-related changes place these individuals at further risk, due to delayed gastric emptying, decreased upper esophageal sphincter pressure and prolonged relaxation of the sphincter, longer reflux episodes with impaired clearance of refluxed materials, and the need for more acid suppression in order to achieve healing (Linton, 2007a). Mr. Smith has a diagnosis of GERD and is taking the proton pump inhibitor omeprazole. There are two important symptoms that require further nursing assessment: the increased head-banging in the morning and his avoidance of saltwater taffy. Some patients experience a worsening of GERD symptoms when lying flat, and Mr. Smith's morning head-banging might be a sign that he is experiencing increased heartburn (or is more aware of it, after being in bed all night). Furthermore, some patients with GERD have mouth pain that makes chewing unpleasant. Mr. Smith's symptoms should be brought to the attention of his primary-care provider for possible referral to a gastroenterologist.

Hypothyroidism and Other Endocrine Problems

Morgan, Roy, and Chance (2003) reported an increased prevalence of hypothyroidism in those with autism. Clinical manifestations of hypothyroidism can mimic psychiatric disturbances, and its classic symptoms, found in the younger population, are frequently absent from the older population (Linton, Hooter, & Elmers, 2007). Age-related changes in the thyroid do not affect function, but there is an increased incidence of hypothyroidism in older persons (Linton et al., 2007).

Mr. Smith has recently been diagnosed with AD. Assessment of thyroid function is an important part of the clinical evaluation for the diagnosis of AD, as hypothyroidism can mimic dementia. There is no clear evidence that supports screening for hypothyroidism in asymptomatic older adults (Karlin, Weintraub, & Chopra, 2004). However, the nurse should monitor the older adult patient for signs of thyroid dysfunction so that appropriate tests can be conducted in a timely manner.

Another common endocrine dysfunction in older adults is diabetes mellitus type 2 (DM type 2). The serum level of glycosylated hemoglobin (HgbA1c) is an effective screening test for DM type 2 (Ackermann et al., 2011). Mr. Smith has slightly elevated fasting blood glucose (112 mg/dl), and follow-up is warranted. If his HgbA1c does not meet the current criteria of 6.5% for a diagnosis of DM type 2, but is above 5.7%, it is appropriate to implement strategies to decrease risks for DM and cardiovascular disease (Ackermann, Cheng, Williamson, & Gregg, 2011).

Osteoporosis

Older adults who have an ID (NHS Health Scotland, 2004) or take anticonvulsants on a routine basis (Phillips, 1998) are at an elevated risk for osteoporosis. With aging, the rate of bone resorption begins to exceed the rate of bone formation, with resultant bone loss. The majority of this bone loss is in the trabecular bone, which places the older adult with ASD at risk for vertebral compression fractures, Colles' fractures, and femoral neck fractures. Decreased vitamin D intake and reduced sun exposure also accelerate osteoclast activity, leading to increased bone resorption (Linton, 2007c). The nurse should suspect osteoporosis if the older adult with ASD suffers from a low-impact fracture.

Mr. Smith is at risk of poor bone health because of long-term use of phenytoin, diagnosis of ASD, and advanced age. The role of vitamin D in bone health has been very prominent in the literature over the past few years, but the needs of older men have not been addressed in most of the studies (Orwoll et al., 2009). Nearly three-fourths of older men have vitamin D levels that are classified as insufficient. Older men who engaged in outdoor work, such as yard work, and who took at least 400 IU of vitamin D per day, were at lower risk for vitamin D insufficiency. Adults who are over the age of 70 should take 1200 mg of calcium and 800 IU of vitamin D per day (Ross, Taylor, Yaktine, & Del Valle, 2011). Exercise is an important health-promotion activity with benefits for bone health, among others (Nelson et al., 2007). The American College of Sports Medicine and American Heart Association recommend that older adults engage in 30 minutes of daily, moderate activity, as well as stretching and balance exercises.

Sensory Impairments

Older adults with ASD and IDs have a high rate of sensory impairments (NHS Health Scotland, 2004). The sense organs also undergo age-related changes, compounding difficulties for these older individuals with ASD. The aging eye contains many fewer rods and cones than are found in the younger adult's eye, with concomitant losses in color vision and visual acuity and increased need for contrast and ambient lighting (Salvi, Akhtar, & Currie, 2006).

Older adults with ASD might benefit from more lighting, particularly nonglare lightbulbs, with up to four times the wattage that younger adults need. For example, if you are comfortable with a 25-watt light bulb, consider using a 100-watt bulb for elders with ASD. Visual acuity can be enhanced by using black ink on light yellow paper in a large font. Colors such as blue and green might be very difficult for the older adult to differentiate, and this should be considered when providing visual stimulation. Furthermore, the development of cataracts is almost ubiquitous in elders, causing blurring of vision, increased glare, and decreased ability to accommodate. Small details might not be detectable, further decreasing the level of sensory stimulation available to the older adult.

Hearing is also affected by normal aging, with losses in the ability to detect both low- and high-frequency sounds. The result is that the older adult is not unable to hear volume, but is unable to interpret what is heard, because critical speech sounds are missing (Liu & Yan, 2007). The sibilant consonants (s, th, f, ph) and short vowels are the most difficult to discern, because they are high-frequency sounds. Hearing aids are not always helpful and might be too annoying for the older adult with ASD. Environmental management, including decreasing background noise and using sound-absorbing flooring, might be helpful. People who interact with the older adult should raise the volume of their speaking voices slightly.

Enuresis

Tanguay (2010) reported an increased risk of enuresis in people with ASD; incontinence is also more common (Felce et al., 2008). Age-related changes, such as the weakening of the bladder muscles, decreased force of urinary stream, decreased bladder capacity, increased urinary frequency, and the decreased ability to postpone voiding (Linton, 2007b), all contribute to the condition of urinary incontinence or retention in the older adult.

Benign prostatic hyperplasia (BPH) affects nearly three-fourths of men over the age of 60 (Wei, Calhoun, & Jacobsen, 2007) and is a common cause of urinary symptoms. Nocturia is a very common symptom of BPH. Urinary changes can also be associated with prostate cancer. As he is over the age of 75, with no previous evidence of prostate malignancy, Mr. Smith does not need to be screened for prostate cancer (United States Preventive Services Task Force, 2008).

Mr. Smith takes a diuretic (hydrochlorothiazide) that has a half-life in excess of 6 hours, so he will experience diuresis for at least that long. The combined effects of possible BPH, hydrochlorothiazide, and normal aging put Mr. Smith at very high risk for incontinence and enuresis. Scheduled voiding might help decrease episodes of incontinence, and the timing of hydrochlorothiazide administration should take Mr. Smith's daily activities into consideration.

Tuberous Sclerosis

Autism spectrum disorder and tuberous sclerosis are frequently found together (Numis, Major, Montenegro, Muzykewicz, Pulsifer, & Thiele, 2011). Lesions can appear in the brain, kidney, retina, heart, or lung, in addition to the skin (Schwartz, Fernandez, Kotulska, & Jozwiak, 2007). Forty to fifty percent of those with tuberous sclerosis meet the criteria of ASD (Wiznitzer, 2004). Kidney failure is the most common reason for death in persons with tuberous sclerosis who are more than 30 years of age. About 75% to 100% of those who have ASD and tuberous sclerosis have a history of a seizure disorder with onset in the first years of life (Wiznitzer, 2004) leading to a poor prognostic outlook. However, older adults with milder forms of tuberous sclerosis can reach 60 years of age or greater.

Mr. Smith has glomerular filtration rate (GFR) of 29.5 ml/min, consistent with stage IV chronic kidney disease (CKD). His personal medical history of hypertension might have contributed to the CKD, or the kidney damage might be related to other causes, such as tuberous sclerosis. Regardless of the cause, the nurse must consider his decreased GFR when administering medications. Many medications, including cardiovascular drugs, many antibiotics, and gastrointestinal preparations, require dose adjustments when the GFR is below 50 ml/min (Hassan, Al-Ramahi, Aziz, & Ghazili, 2009). In one setting, over one-half of inpatients who required a dose adjustment because of impaired renal function were prescribed inappropriately (Hassan et al., 2009). Pharmacists and pharmacologists are extremely helpful allies for nurses who work with patient populations with CKD.

Sleep Disturbances

Older adults with ASD can have impaired sleep patterns. The most common sleep difficulties are impaired sleep latency, early morning awakening, irregular sleep–wake cycle, and parasomnias (Ivaneko & Johnson, 2010). These can coexist with normal changes in sleep that come with advancing age, such as lighter sleep, increased time spent in the transition between wakefulness and sleep, decreased time spent in restorative sleep (Millsap, 2007) and normal changes in neurotransmitters (Gibson & Farrell, 2004).

Mr. Smith has not had any reports of sleep disturbance, but he does display other indicators of possible pain. Body pain is a common cause of disturbed sleep in older adults, and osteoarthritis is a frequent etiology for this type of pain (Wilcox et al., 2000). He should be monitored for restless sleep or frequent awakenings and offered appropriate analgesia.

Anxiety Disorder

The prevalence of anxiety disorder in the older adult population is estimated to be 10.2% to 15%, and older adults with ASD have an additional risk (Hybels & Blazer, 2003; Lauderdale & Sheikh, 2003). Social anxiety disorder, obsessive–compulsive disorder (OCD), and panic disorder (Tanguay, 2010) are also more common in adults with autism than in those without ASD. These risks are compounded by the presence of an ID (Ramirez & Lukenbill, 2007). Older adults with ASD can present with stereotypical behaviors that are not usually attributed to anxiety. However, such behaviors can reflect anxious feelings and thoughts (Dosen, 2005). Panic disorder (Hybels & Blazer, 2003) and late-life onset of OCD are relatively uncommon, but there might be a past history of these disorders in the older adult with ASD. Obsessions and compulsions in older persons tend to be focused on somatic symptoms (Linton et al., 2007). Differentiation of OCD and ASD can be facilitated by determining if the repetitive behavior/compulsion is perceived as comforting (van Niekirk et al, 2010).

Depression

Adults with ASD are at increased risk for depression as they age (Ghaziuddin, Ghaziuddin, & Greden, 2002). In addition to this risk, age-related changes put them at risk for depression. These changes include decreased serotonin levels, increased breakdown of serotonin and dopamine by monoamine oxidase B, elevated glucocorticoid levels, changes in the hypothalamic–pituitary–adrenal axis, loss of dendritic spines, decreased growth hormone production, decreased metabolism of neurotransmitters, and changes in the number of receptor sites

EXHIBIT 14.3

Symptoms of Depression in Older Adults[a]

- Sleep disturbance with daytime fatigue
- Psychomotor retardation (slowing of thought and activity)
- Apathy and anhedonia (inability to enjoy usually pleasant activities)
- Complaints of memory impairment
- Decreased executive function
- Mood may NOT be depressed

[a]Data from Fiske, Wetherell, & Gatz (2009).

(Carroll & Linton, 2007). Given that polypharmacy is common in older adults, iatrogenic causes of depression must also be considered (Dhondt, Beekman, Deeg, & vanTillburg, 2002). Depression in older adults tends to be multifactorial, and often is associated with losses of loved ones, functional decline, social isolation, multiple medical comorbidities, and disability (Bruce, 2002; Carroll & Linton, 2007).

The use of depression-screening tools, such as the Geriatric Depression Scale and the Cornell Scale for Depression in Dementia (Alexopoulos, Robert, Robert, & Shamoain, 1988), must be tailored for use with the adult with ASD. The Glasgow Depression Scale for People with a Learning Disability (Cuthill, Espie, & Cooper, 2003) shows promise for depression-screening in those older adults with ASD who also have an ID. See Exhibit 14.3 for a summary of indicators of depression in older adults.

Increased Risk for Depression

Higher-functioning adults with ASD have increased social awareness and intelligence when compared with others with ASD (Capps, Sigman, & Yirmya 1995; Tantam, 2000; Wing, 1981). Sterling, Dawson, Estes, and Greenson (2008) found that those with less social impairment and higher cognitive ability were more likely to report depressive symptoms; these factors are postulated to increase depression risks in individuals with ASD. Lainhart and Folstein (1994), Shtayermman (2008), and Wing (1981) have noted that adults with ASD can have suicidal ideations and make suicide attempts. Nurses should carefully assess individuals with ASD, particularly those taking antidepressant medications, for self-injurious behaviors or suicidal ideation, as these can be side effects of the drugs. Exhibit 14.4 summarizes warning signs for suicide in older adults, to be considered in conjunction with an understanding of the communication and behavior patterns of individuals with ASD.

Dementia

Dementia is defined as a progressive syndrome involving loss of cognitive function and memory that impedes the functions of daily living. Level of consciousness is not affected until late in the disease process (Kane, Ouslander, & Abrass, 2004). Only 6% to 7% of elders have dementing illnesses (van der Flier & Scheltens, 2005), but nearly 38% of those aged 90 and over have dementia (Plassman et al., 2007). Older adults with IDs have a higher prevalence rate (Strydom, Shoostari, Lee, et al., 2010). The average time from diagnosis of dementia to death from dementia is 7 to 10 years, depending upon the type of dementia (van der Flier & Scheltens, 2005).

EXHIBIT 14.4

WARNING SIGNS OF SUICIDE IN OLDER ADULTS[a]

Personal history of depression or other affective health disorder
Giving away money or possessions
Hoarding medications
Deterioration in personal hygiene or social interaction
Lack of interest in food or eating
Relocation
Loss of a person important to the individual
Dramatic change in health or functional status
Lack of social support or social connectedness
Use of alcohol or drugs

[a]Data from Mitty and Flores (2008).

Cognitive decline is *not* a normal change of aging, although elders might have a benign slowing of response rate and difficulty accessing information (Millsap, 2007). A 6% to 11% decrease in brain weight is seen in some healthy elders, but there is considerable "overlap" in neuron function, and the remaining neurons can compensate for the lost ones (Timiras & Maletta, 2007). Normal aging does involve changes in levels of neurotransmitters, which can lead to slight losses in memory (Gibson & Farrell, 2004). Some of the age-related decreases in neurons and neurotransmitters can be delayed, inhibited, or even reversed in some cases. There is evidence that appropriate cognitive stimulation is important throughout the lifespan and might delay the onset of dementias (Plassman, Williams, Burke, Holsinger, & Benjamin, 2010).

Those with IDs, and possibly those with ASD, frequently develop dementia as they age (NHS Health Scotland, 2004), and older adults who have a history of inadequately treated seizures are at higher risk for impaired cognitive function (Aldenkamp, 1997). All changes in cognitive ability, however, must be thoroughly investigated for reversible causes before a diagnosis of dementia is confirmed.

There are many different causes of dementia, with AD being the most common etiology. Vascular dementia (VaD) is the next most prevalent dementia, followed by dementia with Lewy bodies, (frontotemporal or Pick's dementia (FTD), and dementias related to specific diseases, such as Parkinson's disease or AIDS (Grossman, Bergmann, & Parker, 2006). Each dementia has a unique pathophysiology and early manifestation, but all involve destruction of brain tissue. As yet, there is no conclusive evidence to support a direct link between ASD and one type of dementia.

Predictors of AD applied to ASD: Older adults with AD have increased quantities of abnormal proteins on the cerebral cortex, which are arranged in a characteristic "plaques and tangles" pattern (Grossman et al., 2006). Many of the risk factors for cardiovascular disease, such as elevated blood pressure, hyperlipidemia, and sedentary lifestyle, are predictors for the development of AD (Launer, 2007). The cardinal symptom of AD is memory impairment, which might be difficult to detect in older adults with IDs, but remains the most common presenting symptom in the population (Strydom et al., 2010). Changes in functional ability or personality might also be observed early in the course of AD in elders with ID. Behavioral and emotional changes with the onset of AD are fairly common in older adults without ID, but appear to be less common in older adults with ID. Epilepsy and AD share several chemical and physical changes in the brain (Noebels, 2011)—a finding that is significant for persons with ASD, as epilepsy is a common comorbidity.

Vascular dementia is similar to stroke, in that a blood vessel is damaged, and the tissues beyond it receive no oxygenation. Chronic hypertension and diabetes mellitus, particularly when poorly controlled, put an older adult at higher risk for developing VaD, because of the level of damage caused to the microvasculature. The degree of cognitive impairment and behavioral manifestations are dependent upon the area of the brain that is affected by ischemia. Cognitive deficits might not be apparent until several infarcts have occurred and damaged a large area of the brain. As subsequent infarcts happen, more deficits might appear. The deficits in VaD tend to be sudden, with periods of no change, unlike those in AD, which are gradual.

Nursing care when dementia co-occurs: Older adults with both ASD and FTD might be the most challenging to work with, because the loss of social skills that is the hallmark of FTD compound the baseline social impairments in ASD. Persons with FTD become increasingly antisocial and disinhibited, often times using crude language and sexual acting out; they are also unconcerned about the needs of others (Grossman et al., 2006). Furthermore, patients with FTD might manifest compulsive oral behaviors, such as overeating, sucking on objects, or eating nonfoods. Unfortunately, there are few treatment options for FTD, and mostly are used to control problematic behavior. Cooper (1999) reported that older adults with dementia in addition to an ID had a greater number of physical problems than older adults without ID.

Aylward, Burt, Thorpe, Lai, and Dalton (1997) recommended following the criteria and procedures identified by the Working Group for the Establishment of Criteria for the Diagnosis of Dementia in Individuals with Intellectual Disability, with the caveat that criteria and procedures were developed based on the collective experience of experts in the field. The working group recommended that individuals with an ID have a thorough baseline assessment before the age of 50 (age 40 for Down syndrome), and periodic assessment every 1 to 5 years thereafter, so that changes can be detected. A caregiver who is familiar with the individual should participate in the process, in order to obtain the most accurate information about the person being tested. A single screening test has not yet been validated, and current practice includes an extensive battery of tests (Pyo, Curtis, Curtis, & Markwell, 2009; Exhibit 14.5).

Delirium

Delirium is a disorder that is distinct from dementia. It has a specific constellation of signs and symptoms. Manifestations of delirium have a sudden onset; timely recognition and treatment is important so that the condition does not become chronic (Shawler, 2010). Diagnostic criteria include changes in cognition and consciousness that cannot be explained by an existing diagnosis of dementia (American Psychiatric Association, 2000). Mental status changes are often accompanied by changes in attention and misperception of environmental stimuli. For example, a patient with delirium might view a polka dot pattern on wallpaper as insects crawling up the wall. The patient might not be able to focus attention on a simple task. Delirium can also involve sleep cycle disturbances, agitation, or hyperactivity. Table 14.2 compares manifestations of typical aging, dementia, delirium, and ASD.

EXHIBIT 14.5

COMPONENTS OF TEST BATTERY FOR THE DIAGNOSIS OF DEMENTIA IN INDIVIDUALS WITH IDs[a]

Dementia Scale for Mentally Retarded Persons (administered to caregiver)
Dementia Scale for Down Syndrome (administered to caregiver)
Reiss Screen for Maladaptive Behavior (administered to caregiver)
Scales of Independent Behavior (administered to caregiver)
AAMR Adaptive Behavior Scale/Residential and Community (administered to caregiver)
Stress Index (administered to caregiver)
Test for Severe Impairment
Stanford-Binet Sentences
Fuld (modified)
Spatial Recognition Scan
Autobiographical Memory
Boston Naming Test
McCarthy Verbal Fluency
Simple Commands
Purdue Pegboard
Developmental Test of Visual Motor Integration

[a] See Burt and Aylward (2000) for further detail.

Risk factors for delirium: Risk factors for delirium in older adults include dementia or other underlying cognitive impairment, multiple medical comorbidities, functional impairments, vision/hearing impairment, chronic renal insufficiency, and depression (Inouye, 2003). In some cases, delirium might be due to a single cause, but most often the cause of delirium is multifactorial. Precipitating factors for delirium include medications, infection, immobilization (therapeutic and nontherapeutic), dehydration, malnutrition, electrolyte disorders, metabolic disorders, iatrogenic events, and any changes in health status (Inouye, 2003; Roche, 2003; Tullman & Dracup, 2000).

Older adults tend to have lower basal temperatures and often do not produce fevers, even in response to overwhelming infection (Hoshino, Tamura, Nakazawa, & Koyama, 2007), but might develop delirium as the presenting sign. Fever in elders is defined as a rise of 2 °F (1.1 °C) over baseline, or repeated findings of oral temperature ≥99 °F (37.2 °C) or rectal temperature ≥99.5 °F (37.5 °C). Even with these adjusted diagnostic criteria, only about 55% of elders in nursing homes (the most physically frail) ever demonstrate any fever with infections (Bentley et al., 2001). A combination of fewer antigen-specific antibodies, less effective thermoregulation by the central nervous system, less responsiveness of the hypothalamus, and a decreased production of endogenous pyrogens is related to the absence of fever in elders with infections.

Once factors that contribute to delirium are addressed, the symptoms begin to recede. Interventions that help reorient the older adult with delirium—adequate hydration and sleep, mobility, use of eyeglasses and hearing aids, and therapeutic activities—all contribute to resolution of delirium (Inouye, Bogardus, Williams, Leo-Summers, & Agostino, 2003) (Exhibit 14.6).

TABLE 14.2 ■ Manifestations of Usual Aging, Dementia, Delirium, and ASD

	Usual aging	Dementia	Delirium	ASD
Typical behaviors	Mild short-term memory loss; mild decrease in overall cognitive function (thinking, orientation, comprehension, calculation, learning capacity, language, judgment); tremendous variation among individuals	Multiple cognitive domains affected (memory, thinking, orientation, comprehension, calculation, learning capacity, language, judgment)	Fluctuation in mental status and level of consciousness, with changes in attention	Impairment in social skill, difficulty interpreting environment, impaired control of behavior
Onset	45 to 54 years of age	Prevalence increases with age, greater prevalence over age 85	More common in people over 70 years of age	Early childhood
Trajectory	Very gradual decline	Gradual decline	Acute, rapid onset	Lifelong patterns of behavior
Associated events	Better preserved function in those with more education	Multiple etiologies, some dementias are related to other diagnoses (e.g. Parkinson's disease, AIDS)	Acute illness, addition of new medications, physical trauma	Stressful or painful events may trigger behavioral response.
Resolution	None—chronic condition	Terminal disease, life expectancy after diagnosis about 10 years	Delirium usually clears once underlying condition is treated; cognition may remain impaired for up to several months.	Behavior usually abates when irritating stimulus is removed.
Interventions	Suggest memory aids, such as writing notes, using calendars or electronic timers.	Minimize environmental demands, simplify daily routines.	Identify exact timeline of events, reorient patient, ensure use of glasses, hearing aids, clocks.	Identify circumstances that lead to behavioral outburst; avoid triggers.

Adapted from Ardila (2007); Reilly, Rodriguez, Lamy, & Neils-Strunjas (2010); Savva et al. (2009); van Niekirk et al. (2010).

The Confusion Assessment Method (Inouye et al., 1990) is an observational instrument that is widely used to detect delirium. It requires accurate observation of the patient's behavior, but does not require the patient's cooperation. It is an appropriate instrument to use with older adults with ASD, because of the emphasis on observation, and does not require the older adult to answer questions or perform activities. The Confusion Assessment Method is available online (http://consultgerirn.org/resources).

CASE–CONTINUED

Mr. Smith's new diagnosis of AD is unlikely to change his usual care needs at this time. As the disease progresses, he will require more assistance with instrumental activities of daily living, then with activities of daily living. It is important for the nurse to anticipate Mr. Smith's functional decline, but to refrain from overloading Mr. Smith and his caregivers with information (Duffy, 2010). Any abrupt changes in mental status should be thoroughly investigated as possible indications of infection or other new-onset physiological disturbances.

EXHIBIT 14.6

Interventions for the Person with Delirium[a]

- Frequent reorientation to place, time, and activities of care
- Adequate hydration
- Adequate sleep
  - Protect the individual from interruptions in sleep.
  - Schedule care activities to minimize sleep disruptions.
  - Minimize use of lights during sleep time.
  - Maintain a quiet environment during sleep time.
  - Maintain a comfortable ambient temperature during sleep time.
- Ensure that the individual's eyeglasses and hearing devices, if any, are in good working order, and are used.
- Frequent ambulation or other permitted mobility
- Therapeutic activities, such as card games or social interaction

[a]Data from Inouye et al. (2003).

MEDICATIONS FOR ASD IN THE OLDER ADULT POPULATION

While no single medicine has been shown to be effective in ameliorating the core deficits in autism, there is evidence that medication can help those with autism through reduction of aggressive behaviors, hyperactivity, repetitive behaviors, self-injurious behaviors, inattention, and sleep disorders (Findling, Maxwell & Wiznitzer, 1997; King & Bostic, 2006; Kwok, 2003; McDougle et al., 1998; Tanguay, 2010). It should be noted that the available research on the use of medications in the person with ASD is compromised due to small sample sizes, failure to control for maturation effects, and brief treatment duration (Broadstock, Doughty, & Eggleston, 2007).

Existing research on the use of medications in people with ASD is for the most part focused on the pediatric and adolescent populations. As individuals with ASD age, the number of medications prescribed for their treatment appears to trend upward, but this evidence is based on a sample ranging from 10 to 48 years of age (Esbensen, Greenberg, Seltzer, & Aman, 2010). Refer to Table 3.4 for a summary of medications used in the population of individuals with ASD.

Antipsychotics

Risperidone is the most heavily researched atypical antipsychotic used in the behavioral treatment of children with ASD. In a double-blind, randomized, controlled trial of adults with autism and pervasive developmental disorders, only risperidone was found to control aggressive behaviors (McDougle et al., 1998). In addition, it is the only drug approved by the U.S. Food and Drug Administration to treat ASD in children. However, all atypical antipsychotics carry a black box warning of the increased risk of death in the older population, and their use should be restricted to situations in which the benefits of controlling difficult behavior clearly outweigh the risks of using the medication.

Stimulants

Methylphenidate and atomoxetine have been used to treat distractibility, hyperactivity, excitability, concentration deficits, and task completion, as well as decreased attention in children with ASD (Lecavalier, 2006). Stimulants are less likely to be to be tolerated in older adults, especially considering the prevalence of cardiac comorbidities in this population. Age-related changes in the heart, particularly the increased prevalence of arrhythmias, make central nervous system stimulants problematic (Semla, Beizer, & Higbee, 2007). Stimulants are associated with fatal arrhythmias, including tachycardia, myocardial infarction, angina pectoris, and hypertension. These adverse effects are more likely in individuals with preexisting cardiac disease or structural changes in the heart. Both are prevalent among older adults.

Antidepressants

Antidepressants have been successfully used in the treatment of depressed mood, sleep disturbances, self-injurious behavior, psychomotor agitation, weight loss, reduced communication, tearfulness, and loss of interest in individuals with ASD (Perry, Marston, Hinder, Munden, & Roy, 2001). Selective serotonin reuptake inhibitors (SSRIs) are the most widely used antidepressants in those with ASD. Many SSRIs have caused increased hyperactivity and irritability, in addition to insomnia, in children and adolescents (Floyd & McIntosh, 2009).

Alpha Agonists

Clonidine and guanfacine are used to treat hyperactivity, impulsivity, and irritability in children with ASD (Elder & D'Alessandro, 2009). These might be safer options in the older adult with ASD. However, if these are used, the nurse will need to monitor patients closely for sedation and/or hypotension.

Anticonvulsants

The nurse can expect to monitor patients diagnosed with ASD and seizure disorder for seizure manifestations, as well as for therapeutic and side effects of anticonvulsant medications. Hollander et al., (2006) conducted a double-blind trial and reported a reduction in repetitive behaviors, instability, and aggression associated with ASD in the pediatric population when divalproex was used. Nurses should be familiar with conditions associated with anticonvulsant use in older adults. These include neurocognitive changes; osteoporosis with chronic use; osteomalacia (phenytoin); gingival hyperplasia (phenytoin); and cerebellar atrophy (phenytoin; Phillips, 1998; Tyler and Noritz; 2009).

Nurses should recognize that the use of antiepileptic drugs in the elderly is associated with an increased risk of fractures (Jette, Lix, Metge, et al., 2011). Individuals living in institutional settings have an increased prevalence of specific fracture types: femoral neck, intertrochanteric, ankle, and proximal humerus (Desai, Ribbans, & Taylor, 1996). Valproic acid is the only antiepileptic drug that is not associated with an increased risk of fracture in the older population (Jette et al., 2011).

There are multiple potential drug interactions associated with anticonvulsant use; a thorough knowledge of these drugs is crucial for the nurse who cares for the older client with ASD and epilepsy. Use of carbamazepine can lead to elevated levels of macrolide antibiotics (azithromycin, capreomycin, clarithromycin, clindamycin, dactinomycin, erythromycin, kanamycin, mithramycin, streptomycin, tobramycin, and vancomycin) and increased risk for toxic effects of the antibiotics. Depakote can interact with carbapenem antibiotics (ertapenem, imipenem, and meropenem), leading to decreased seizure and/or behavior control. Risks are further exacerbated by the older adult's lower rate of drug absorption, and altered drug distribution and metabolism (Linton, 2007c).

Older adults have age-related decreases in ability to concentrate urine and limit excretion of water, sodium, potassium, and acid (Linton, 2007b). Elderly individuals taking carbamazepine and oxcarbazepine are at further risk for hyponatremia secondary to Syndrome of Inappropriate Antidiuretic Hormone Hypersecretion. Antidepressants with the least potential for altering antiepileptic drug metabolism include: citalopram, escitalopram, venlafaxine, duloxetine, and mirtazapine (Levy & Collins, 2007).

Age-related Changes in Pharmacokinetics and Pharmacodynamics

The aging process affects many processes involved in the kinetics and dynamics of drug therapy. It is important to remember that aging occurs in a heterogeneous fashion, and no two people will experience these age-related changes at the same rate or in the same pattern. The liver, along with the kidneys, plays a major role in the excretion of medications. Chronic renal disease is caused by irreversible age-related and disease-related damage to the kidney and affects nearly 30% of elders (Carter, O'Riordan, Eaglestone, Delaney, & Lamb, 2008). A reasonably accurate estimate of the GFR in older adults might be made using the Cockcroft-Gault equation. Changes in the immune system of the elderly are of particular concern when infection sets in (Faulkner, Cox, & Williamson, 2005). Macrolides do not concentrate well in elders, but penicillin, ceftriaxone, sulfonamides, and clindamycin might have concentrations higher than in younger adults. Longer courses of antiinfectives might be needed to adequately treat infections in the older adult with ASD (Table 14.3).

Polypharmacy

The intersection of aging, multiple health problems, and more successful medication therapies has made polypharmacy a fact of life for all older adults. One study found that older adults were using, on average, drugs from 3.8 different therapeutic categories. Cardiovascular, central nervous system, and hormone (e.g., thyroid) therapies were the most common drug categories (Linton, Garber, Fagan, & Peterson, 2007). Individual patients were prescribed an average of 6.1 medications across these categories. This study did not find unnecessary prescriptions or frivolous prescribing patterns. Kuijpers et al. (2008) reported that 43% of older

TABLE 14.3 ■ Age-related Changes That Affect Pharmacokinetics and Pharmacodynamics

Change	Physiological consequence	Pharmacotherapeutic consequence
Decreased gastric and intestinal mobility	Medication remains in GI system longer	Delayed onset of action
Decreased subcutaneous fat, flattened junction between dermis and epidermis, increased fragility of capillaries	Medication does not transfer well through skin	Transdermal medications may be less effective
Decreased lean muscle mass	Medication is not optimally absorbed	Intramuscular medications may be less effective
Decreased cardiac output	Medication is not equally dispersed throughout body	Delayed onset of action
Increased total percent of body fat	Fat-soluble medications remain in body longer	Longer period of action of medications such as diazepam
Decreased total percent of body water	Water-soluble medications achieve higher serum concentrations	Increased activity of medications such as oxycodone, atenolol, captopril
Decreased level of total body protein	Protein-binding drugs circulate more freely	Increased therapeutic action of medications such as phenytoin
Decreased liver function	Medications are not metabolized as effectively	Prolonged period of activity for medications
Decreased kidney function	Medications are not metabolized as effectively	Prolonged period of activity for medications
Altered immune function	Antiinfectives reach lower concentrations	Different classes of antiinfectives require adjustments in dose and length of treatment

Based on Baumann (2007); Faulkner et al. (2005); Galban, Maderwald, Stock, & Ladd (2007); Phillips & Powley (2007); Singh, (2005); Timiras & Luxenberg (2007).

adults, taking at least five medications, were *underprescribed* by an average of 1.4 medically indicated drugs.

One of the major concerns in polypharmacy is the increased likelihood of drug interactions (Viktil, Blix, Moger, & Reikvam, 2006). The relationship between the number of medications and number of drug-related problems is linear. Each additional medication increases the risk of an adverse effect. Nurses should vigilantly monitor for adverse effects any time a new medication is added to the regimen of an older adult with ASD. When assessing a new symptom or complaint, the nurse should consider whether polypharmacy and related drug interactions and/or adverse effects might be contributing factors.

Mr. Smith is taking six medications, about the average for older Americans. Phenytoin, important for his epilepsy, interacts with a number of Mr. Smith's other medications (Micromedex, 2011). Phenytoin can increase the metabolism of acetaminophen, decreasing the length of time the acetaminophen provides analgesia, and also increasing the likelihood of acetaminophen toxicity. The omeprazole Mr. Smith takes for GERD increases the probability of phenytoin toxicity, a real concern because, as noted in the case above, the physician just increased Mr. Smith's phenytoin dose. Phenytoin can also decrease the effectiveness of simvastatin in lowering Mr. Smith's cholesterol. Close monitoring of Mr. Smith's status and laboratory values, particularly when medication doses are changed or new medications are added, is essential.

BEST PRACTICES: PLAN OF CARE

The older adult with ASD requires expert nursing care, with particular emphasis on communication, work with the family and caregivers, and managing the environment of the older adult. Persons with ASD might not be able to communicate their own needs, therefore the nurse must be vigilant for subtle indications that care is needed.

Communication Strategies

Given that individuals with autism have difficulty communicating, their symptoms, concerns, and illnesses can present atypically and can be challenging to identify. Accurate assessment begins with effective communication. With all interactions, the nurse should use communication strategies with which the individual is already familiar. Family members or caregivers are typically knowledgeable about effective communication approaches and patterns; the nurse should start there.

Communication strategies successfully used in children with ASD might be adapted for elderly patients. These include the picture-exchange communication system (PECS; Bondy & Frost, 1994); discrete trial teaching (Wolf, Risley, & Mees, 1964); developmental individual differences relationship–based approach (DIR; Wieder & Greenspan, 2001); relationship development intervention (Gutstein & Sheely, 2002); sensory integration training (Ayers & Robbins, 2004); and social communication, emotional regulation, and transactional support treatment (SCERTS; Prizant, Wetherby, Rubin, Laurent, & Rydell, 2006). These use visual supports as a major communication element. Research evidence for each of these approaches varies; several aspects of the SCERTS model meet Level 1 and 2 strength of evidence criteria (Melnyk & Fineout-Overholt, 2011). However, the current cohort of older people is more likely to have used sign language or imitative gestures as a form of verbal communication.

Initiating the Communication

Communication with the older adult who has ASD should be conducted in a calm, concise, and economic fashion, with minimal facial expression and few distractions, so that the individual has adequate time to process what is being communicated. Interacting first with the caregiver can provide the older adult with ASD time to adjust to the nurse's presence (Aylott, 2010). Nurses should remember that people with ASD might not recognize or be able to interpret facial expressions or other nonverbal communications. Individuals with ASD tend to interpret words literally. Nurses should be careful to use concrete statements and visual methods, such as pictures (Williams, 1996). It is important to understand that an older adult with ASD might communicate through behavior. Aggression or other dysfunctional behavior can be related to stresses, such as trauma (Focht-New, Bard, Clements, & Milliken, 2008). Appropriate communication strategies are critical to incorporate into care of older adults with ASD, as they engage the health system more frequently than younger individuals, due to chronic disease states and conditions that become more prevalent with age.

Pain Management in the Elderly

Assessment and care of older adults with ASD must incorporate a careful history that includes discussion of usual patterns of behavior. This will help the clinician recognize deviations that indicate changing health status (Holmes, 1998). For example, medical conditions that cause pain or discomfort can precipitate recurrence or intensification of self-injurious behaviors (Bosch, Van Dyke, Milligan Smith, & Poulton, 1997). From a retrospective chart review, Bosch and colleagues (1997) found that self-injurious behavior decreased by 86% when an undiagnosed medical condition known to cause pain or discomfort was treated. Carr and Owen-DeShryver (2007) determined that older individuals with ASD who did not feel well were more likely to exhibit serious problem behaviors.

Assessment of pain can be a challenge in older adults with ASD, because they might be unable to express their experiences of pain or other problems. Conditions such as postseizure pain or exacerbations of GERD symptoms can serve as setting events for behavior changes (Bottos & Chambers, 2006). The nurse can take a proactive approach in addressing pain by being alert for common manifestations of pain in those with ASD, such as head-banging, hitting or biting oneself, or throwing oneself against hard objects (Bosch et al., 1997). Nurses can also be proactive in identifying and treating pain by asking caregivers about typical pain-related behaviors seen in the older adult (Baldridge & Andrasik, 2010). Refer to Exhibits 13.1 and 13.2 for examples.

Health Promotion

Health problems associated with smoking, alcohol, and illegal drug use are uncommon in individuals with ID (NHS Health Scotland, 2004). We do not know the prevalence among elders with ASD. However, the literature illustrates that that those with IDs have less involvement in health promotion activities, receive less preventive care, have poorer diets, and are more obese than the general population (Beange & Durvasula, 2001; Ouellette-Kuntz, 2005).

Nurses in all practice roles should seek to optimize physical health. Advanced practice nurses have a unique opportunity to reduce health risks in the older adult. Hahn and Aronow (2005) conducted comprehensive geriatric risk assessments on 70 adults (age range of 20 to 65 years) with developmental disabilities and were able to reduce health risks in their pilot study. Felce and colleagues (2008) reported that the number of new

EXHIBIT 14.7

Common Physical Problems That May Lead to Behavioral Consequences

Cerumen impaction
Decreased visual acuity; not using eyeglasses
Hearing impairment; not using assistive hearing devices
Constipation
Indigestion, particularly as related to GERD
Untreated pain
Painful gums, if taking phenytoin

needs identified at subsequent health visits was similar to the number of problems identified at an initial visit. Cooper (1999) reported that older adults with IDs have a higher rate of physical disorders. As with all individuals with developmental disabilities, psychobehavioral changes or exacerbation of behavioral problems might be related to unrecognized physiological problems or illness. Before initiating a referral for psychiatric or other services, nurses should be aware of common factors and conditions that might contribute to difficulties. Close attention to conditions such as earwax impaction, vision and hearing impairment, or constipation will be more significant in this population, given their already limited social, communicative, and practical abilities (Exhibit 14.7). Nurses must take an active role in assessing for these conditions on a regular basis, and particularly when there are changes in the older adult's (with ASD) health status.

Nurses should also assess for interpersonal violence as part of routine visits. Individuals with developmental disorders are at 4 to 10 times greater risk for interpersonal violence than those without disabilities (Focht-New et al., 2008). Some older adults with ASD might have been traumatized in the past (e.g., bullying, financial exploitation, physical and/or sexual abuse, or rape). The inability to read nonverbal cues might place individuals with ASD at risk for sexual assault (Attwood, 1998). Nurses should be sensitive to these possibilities and carefully assess history, current status, and risks for interpersonal violence or exploitation.

Environment

Nursing care should include a focus on elimination of environmental factors that are barriers to effective care and on facilitation of an environment that will support the individual's most effective functioning and achievement of highest potential.

Individuals with autism have difficulty when the environment overwhelms their senses and capability to adapt. Gerland (2000) described this as a heightened sense of awareness. Nurses should exploit the knowledge caregivers or family members have about usual patterns of older adults with ASD, especially about their reactions to new experiences and environments, and about strategies and "best practices" that minimize distress. The nurse can use this information to prepare the health care environment to meet the individual's needs. For example, if possible, include a preappointment medical office visit to prepare an older adult with ASD for the medical appointment experience. Include exposure to the place and staff and demonstrate the sequence of expected activities. Photographs of the setting and the sequence of activities can also be used (Aylott, 2010). For example, show photographs that illustrate meeting the nurse, entering the room, having blood pressure taken, opening mouth and saying "ah."

Modifying the Environment for the Elder

Examination rooms or other health care settings should be as quiet as possible, and modified with minimal equipment/furniture in the immediate environment, screening of equipment so that it is out of sight, and use of incandescent lighting. During any health care encounter, minimize extraneous conversations and decrease the number of caregivers with whom the older adult with ASD has to interact. Nurses who are responsible for the milieu of a unit might find the Snöezelen approach to be useful. Lotan and Gold (2009) reported improvement in maladaptive behaviors in those with IDs when using this approach. Ensuring that the unit has a quiet room and/or that the office has a separate waiting room are other ways in which the nurse can modify the environment to accommodate the needs of an older adult with ASD.

There is limited evidence about the functioning of older adults with ASD. However, data reported by Graetz (2010) demonstrate that 58% need assistance with instrumental activities of daily living and a large majority, 84%, need assistance with activities of daily living. Hahn and Aronow (2005) reported similar findings. Nurses might be directly assisting older adults with ASD or educating family caregivers or aides who assist with their daily care about health needs, specialized treatments and medications, safety considerations in the home or long-term care setting, or diet management, among others. A concrete daily schedule should be incorporated into the care of older adults with ASD to facilitate comprehension of the sequence of the day and allow them to predict what will happen next. Consulting with caregivers and/or family members will help the nurse to determine strategies or techniques that have worked in the past so that these can be incorporated into the plan of care.

Safety: Older adults are at an increased risk for falls due to age-related diminished muscle mass and resultant decreased muscle strength. Additional risk factors for fall-related injuries in the developmentally disabled population include ambulatory status and seizures occurring monthly (Hsiech, Heller, & Miller, 2001). In general, falls in the older adult population are associated with higher mortality and morbidity rates (Lach & Smith, 2007). Falls are the leading cause of death due to injury in the population of developmentally disabled individuals older than 65 years of age (Hsiech et al., 2001).

All older adults with ASD should receive an assessment of risk for falling, including the following elements: evaluation of gait and balance, medications, muscle coordination, vision, and cardiovascular status (Lach & Smith, 2007). Nurses can use the Timed Up and Go Test by Podsiadlo & Richardson (1991) to assess balance and functional mobility as part of the assessment. Remember that exercise is also an important health promotion and injury prevention strategy. Increased muscle strength, stamina, balance, and flexibility all decrease the risk for falls. Appropriate lighting supports safe ambulation. Incandescent lighting and nonglare surfaces are best, as glare can literally blind older adults with ASD, due to age-related changes. Red lights should be used at night to enhance visual adaption as individuals move from dark to light environments.

Interpersonal environment: A quiet and unhurried physical and "interpersonal" environment that is consistent, structured, and predictable can help to prevent increased anxiety and allow the person with autism more time to process what their senses are telling them. Touch should be used judiciously, as it has been reported that some people with ASD perceive touch as painful or overwhelming.

If problematic behaviors or withdrawal are noted, the nurse should quickly assess the environment to decrease stimuli, including noise, light, movement, and personnel. The nurse should also consider the effects of changes in schedules or structures upon which the older adult with ASD depends. An adult psychiatric clinical nurse specialist/nurse practitioner might provide group therapy for older adults with ASD, with a focus on reading social cues and reduction of intrusiveness. Cognitive behavior therapy, accommodating ASD-related information-processing differences, has been proposed as a therapeutic model to use in adults with ASD (Gaus, 2011).

Nurses have a great deal of control over the health care milieu and should take a proactive approach to ensure that it is appropriate for the individual, that changes are introduced gradually, and that the client's typical schedule, pattern, and structure are adhered to by other health care professionals and care providers. Keeping to a schedule, working with the person's strengths and interests, introducing changes gradually, communicating in a concrete fashion, providing feedback, ensuring opportunities for physical activity, and offering unconditional positive regard are aspects of environmental control that might support the older adult with ASD at home and in health care settings.

Intimacy

Health care professionals should not assume that older adults with ASD have no interest in sexual or intimate relations with others. Higher-functioning individuals with ASD might marry and/or have long-term relationships. Renty and Roeyers (2007) reported that males with ASD who marry supportive spouses have higher-quality relationships then those who do not marry supportive spouses. Research, however, is lacking on the phenomenon of sexuality in the older adult with ASD. Stokes, Newton, and Kaur (2007) reported that adolescents and young adults with ASD were likely to engage in inappropriate courting behaviors, focus attention on celebrities, strangers, colleagues, and ex-partners, and pursue their targets for longer periods of time. Although findings from this study cannot be generalized to the older population, nurses should be aware of these behaviors, and might care for clients or patients who have demonstrated these behaviors in the past. Additional research is needed.

Strategies to address loneliness need to be modified in this population. There is little research-based evidence about loneliness or peer interactions in older adults with ASD. Koenig and Levine (2011) reported that individuals with ASD do not find social interaction to be a mechanism for sharing thoughts and emotions, but rather for sharing activities. The nurse should consider these needs when working with older adults with ASD and their families.

Engaging and Supporting Families

Family caregivers are important and valued members of the health care team (Phelps, Hodgson, McCammon, & Lamson, 2009) and are often the greatest experts in the care of their family members with autism. It is critical to impress on family members that their input is needed, so that accurate and timely intervention can take place. Nursing assessment should include evaluation of the social context in which older individuals with autism function; interventions should be geared toward family support and toward strengthening and expanding the primary caregiver's support and social networks (Renty & Roeyers, 2007). Caregivers of individuals with ASD often function as their own care coordinators and case managers, in addition to providing more direct care (Carbone, Behl, Azor, & Murphy, 2010). These roles can be highly time consuming. Their efforts should be respected and valued. Caring for an individual with a lifelong developmental disability is difficult, even when the individual's level of functioning is high. Nurses should not assume that the care of a higher-functioning adult with ASD is less challenging and/or stressful (Moreno, 1992).

The nurse can promote family engagement in the older adult's care by being cognizant of the need for "future planning"—that concept in which arrangements are made for who will serve as the caregiver and surrogate decision maker as the older client with ASD outlives his or her caregivers (see Chapter 15). Caregivers of the older adults with ASD might experience financial strain as they provide care and pay for services; this directly impacts their psychosocial well-being (Phelps et al., 2009). Nurses need to be sensitive to family and caregiver financial resources when planning for care, making referrals, and recommending interventions and health promotion strategies for an individual with ASD. Families should be linked with local community services and, of course, state services, such as departments of developmental disabilities, federal programs such as Medicare, and advocacy groups at the local and state level. Families might need to be referred for counseling or to social services.

Nurses can play pivotal roles in the establishment of formal and informal networks in which caregivers of older adults with ASD find support from one another. There is a growing movement for peer support programs for caregivers to help each other as they navigate the health care system. Mentoring one another can help caregivers cope with their own experiences (Turnbull, Blue-Banning, Turbiville, & Park, 1999). The nurse can serve as a liaison between the caregiver of the older client with ASD and peer support systems. Nurse leaders can design processes and/or programs to link experienced and inexperienced caregivers for mutual sharing and problem solving. McCabe (2008) conducted a qualitative study of caregivers' perceptions about meeting other caregivers who had similar challenges. Themes identified included the perception that one learned from other caregivers and the sense of emotional support experienced when caregivers shared their experiences with one another.

Making a decision to place an older adult with ASD in a long-term care setting can be difficult for family members. The nurse can help by providing referrals to appropriate facilities, acting as a liaison between long-term care and other health care settings, acknowledging difficulties, and offering support and opportunities to express feelings. Most family members continue contact with their loved ones once they have been placed in long-term care (Krauss, Seltzer, & Jacobson, 2005) and nurses in long-term care settings are likely to interact with family members. Long-term care nurses and advanced practice nurses should cultivate supportive relationships and open communication with families of their older residents with ASD, so that information necessary for the most individualized and effective care can be exchanged. Older adults with ASD who lack supportive family members will rely on their nurses to advocate for appropriate heath care and services. Considering the difficulties that most individuals with ASD have with changes to routines or environment, any transitions to new caregivers should occur slowly, with sensitivity and patience.

Advocacy in the Health Care Delivery System

Older adults with ASD experience barriers in accessing necessary health care services, especially when there are concomitant IDs (Carbone et al., 2010; NHS Health Scotland, 2004). This is particularly concerning, given that they experience greater health needs than the general population of older adults (Beange, McElduff, & Baker, 1995; Kapell et al., 1998; Wilson & Haire, 1990). Case management is critical, as older clients with ASD will have complex needs requiring multidisciplinary expertise (Walsh, Kastner, & Criscione, 1997). Lack of effective case management has been found to contribute to the mortality of those with developmental disorders in long-term care facilities (Kerins et al., 2010). Carbone and colleagues (2010) found that parents of individuals with ASD reported unmet needs in the following areas: extended visits with the health provider, care coordination, and interdisciplinary collaboration. Nurses will need to be effective care managers with a collaborative approach to achieve the best outcomes for this population.

Nurse leaders can collaborate with other disciplines to design processes that support extended visits with physicians and other providers, effective care coordination, and family involvement, such as that found within a medical home. Medical homes with fluid boundaries between the primary care providers, such as physicians or advanced practice nurses, family members, mental health providers, staff, social workers, and supported employment personnel, would decrease the perception of a "unsupportive system" by family members and/or caregivers of this population (Woodgate, Ateah, & Secco, 2008).

It is important to involve older adults with ASD in their own care. Their wishes can be respected by utilizing the concept of assisted autonomy. The nurse can advocate for the client's involvement, even when others assume that the older adult cannot understand or does not have preferences regarding care. The American Association of Intellectual and Developmental Disabilities (AAIDD) developed a guide to consent, outlining the informed consent process for health care, sexual activity, and residential options (Dinerstein, Herr, & O'Sullivan, 1999). A quantitative study conducted by Hurlbutt and Chalmers (2002) found that high-functioning adults with autism want their preferences honored and consider themselves to be experts on autism. Nurses can take the lead by translating medical and other health care information into "pictorial language" or by using other visual supports to help older adults with ASD understand or consent to medical procedures.

End-of-Life Considerations

Studies show that people with disabilities rate their quality of life as high as that of the general population. Life-sustaining treatment for people with disabilities such as ASD should not be summarily rejected, and care must be taken so that health care providers do not accelerate end-of-life care due to their own biases (Savage, Ast, Bess, Castrogiovanni, & Conway, 2010). While there is little end-of-life research related to older adults on the autism spectrum, the literature on end-of-life care in the older adult with IDs can offer some guidance. Savage et al. (2010) identified barriers in end-of-life care for those with IDs that nurses are well-poised to address: case management and care coordination, knowledge of unique abilities, needs, preferences, responses to change, and effective communication with the individual.

Assessment of end-of-life preferences and end-of-life decision-making capacity is important for both the older individual with ASD and his or her family. Savage et al. (2010) proposed two instruments that can be adapted to assess decision-making capacity in this population: the Mac Arthur Competence Assessment Tool for Treatment (Grisso and Applebaum, 1998) and Aid to Capacity Evaluation (Etchells, Darzins, Silberfield, et al., 1999). The booklet *Five Wishes* (Aging with Dignity, n.d.) can be used as a tool to elicit the end-of-life preferences of the older adult with ASD.

Older adults with ASD might not be able to specifically articulate advance directives or preferences. Nurses should advocate for individuals' preferences related to end-of-life care. Advocacy should begin before the person with ASD is facing the end of life, and involves assisting individuals and family members to consider end-of-life issues, and helping them identify preferences and wishes. In the case above, the nurse should initiate discussions related to advance directives before Mr. Smith becomes terminally ill. The *Five Wishes* approach might help Mr. Smith review his support system, identify his likes and dislikes, and participate in making important decisions about his future care. Refer to Chapter 16 for additional discussion of end-of-life issues for individuals with ASD.

SUMMARY

Individuals with ASD enter older age with life histories, accumulated experiences, and the health problems common in the population of adults with ASD. Aging brings physical changes, such as decreased physical strength and flexibility, and physiological changes, such as decreased renal and cardiac function. As individuals with ASD move beyond middle age, they are as susceptible as other elders to common age-related diseases and infirmities. Older adults with ASD, however, may not be able to directly communicate their needs, and the nurse must be vigilant for subtle clues that indicate discomfort or potential disability.

Judicious adaptations in the environment, and increased health surveillance, can lead to a satisfying old age for those on the autism spectrum.

REFERENCES

Ackermann, R. T., Cheng, Y. J., Williamson, D. F., & Gregg, E. W. (2011). Identifying adults at high risk for diabetes and cardiovascular disease using hemoglobin A1c: National Health and Nutrition Examination Survey 2005–2006. *American Journal of Preventive Medicine, 40*, 11–17.

Aging with Dignity. (n.d.) *Five wishes.* Retrieved from http://www.agingwithdignity.org/catalog/nonprintpdf/Five_Wishes_MyWishes_Final.pdf

Aldenkamp, A. P. (1997). Effect of seizures and epileptiform discharges on cognitive function. *Epilepsia, 38*(S1), S52–S55.

Alexopoulos, G. S., Robert, C. A., Robert, C. Y., & Shamoain, C. A. (1988). Cornell scale for depression in dementia. *Biological Psychiatry, 23*, 271–284.

American Psychiatric Association. (2000). *Diagnostic and statistical manual of mental disorders* (4 ed., text revision). Arlington, VA: Author.

Ardila, A. (2007). Normal aging increases cognitive heterogeneity: Analysis of WAIS-III scores across age. *Archives of Clinical Neurology, 22*, 1003–1011.

Attwood, T. (1998). *Asperger's syndrome: A guide for parents and professionals.* London: Jessica Kingsley.

Ayers, A. J., & Robbins, J. (2004). *Sensory integration and the child: Understanding the hidden sensory disorders* (25 anniv. ed.). Los Angeles, CA: Western Psychological Services.

Aylott, J. (2010). Improving access to health and social care for people with autism. *Nursing Standard, 24*, 47–56.

Aylward, E. H., Burt, D. B., Thorpe, L. U., Lai, F., & Dalton, A. (1997). Diagnosis of dementia in individuals with intellectual disability. *Journal of Intellectual Disability Research, 41*, 152–164.

Baldridge, K. H., & Andrasik, F. (2010). Pain assessment in people with intellectual or developmental disabilities. *American Journal of Nursing, 110*(12), 28–35.

Baumann, L. (2007). Skin ageing and its treatment. *Journal of Pathology, 11*, 241–251.

Beange, H., & Durvasula, S. (2001). Health inequalities in people with intellectual disability: Strategies for improvement. *Health Promotion Journal of Australia, 11*, 27–31.

Beange, H., McElduff, A., & Baker, W. (1995). Medical disorders of adults with mental retardation: A population study. *American Journal of Mental Retardation, 99*, 595–604.

Bentley, D. W., Bradley, S., High, K., Schoenbaum, S., Taler, G., & Yoshikawa, T. (2001). Practice guidelines for evaluation of fever and infection in long-term care facilities. *Journal of the American Geriatrics Society, 49*, 210–222.

Bertrand, J., Mars, A., Boyle, C., Bove, F., Yeargin-Allsup, M., & Decoulte, P. (2001). Prevalence of autism in Brick Township, New Jersey: Investigation. *Pediatrics, 108*, 1155–1161.

Bondy, A. S., & Frost, L. A. (1994). The Picture Exchange Communication System. *Focus on Autistic Behavior, 9*, 1–19.

Bosch, J., Van Dyke, D. C., Milligan Smith, S., & Poulton, S. (1997). Role of medical conditions in exacerbating self-injurious behaviors: An exploratory study. *Mental Retardation, 35*, 124–130.

Bottos, S., & Chambers, C. T. (2006). The epidemiology of pain in developmental disabilities. In T. F. Oberlander, & F. J. Symons (Eds.), *Pain in children and adults with developmental disabilities.* (pp. 67–87). Baltimore, MD: Paul H. Brookes.

Broadstock, M., Doughty, C., & Eggleston, M. (2007). Systematic review of the effectiveness of pharmacological treatments for adolescents and adults with autism spectrum disorder. *Autism, 11*, 335–348.

Bruce, M. L. (2002). Psychosocial risk factors for depressive disorders in late life. *Biological Psychiatry, 52*(3), 175–184.

Burt, D. B., & Aylward, E. H. (2000). Test battery for the diagnosis of dementia in individuals with intellectual disability. *Journal of Intellectual Disability Research, 44*(2), 175–180.

Capps, L., Sigman, M., & Yirmya, N. (1995). Self-competence and emotional understanding in high functioning children with autism. *Development and Psychopathology, 7*, 137–149.

Carbone, P. S., Behl, D. D., Azor, V., & Murphy, N. (2010). The medical home for children with autism spectrum disorders: Parent and pediatrician perspectives. *Journal of Developmental Disorders, 40*, 317–324.

Carr, E. G., & Owen-Deshryver, J. S. (2007). Physical illness, pain, and problem behavior in minimally verbal people with developmental disabilities. *Journal of Autism and Developmental Disabilities, 37*, 413–424.

Carr, E. G., & Smith, C. E. (1995). Biological setting events for self-injury. *Mental Retardation and Developmental Disabilities Research Reviews, 1*, 94–98.

Carroll, D. W., & Linton, A. (2007). Age-related psychological changes. In A. Linton, & H. Lach (Eds.), *Matteson's and McConnell's gerontological nursing: Concepts and practice* (pp. 631–684). St. Louis, MO: Elsevier.

Carter, J. L., O'Riordan, S. E., Eaglestone, G. L., Delaney, M. B., & Lamb, E. J. (2008). Chronic kidney disease prevalence in a UK residential care home population. *Nephrology, Dialysis, and Transplant, 23,* 1257–1264.

Casey, Q. (2010). Nova Scotia contemplates a continuum of coordinated, lifetime care for autism patients. *Canadian Medical Association Journal, 182,* SE433–SE434.

Chicoine, B., McGuire, D., & Rubin, S. S. (1999). Specialty clinic perspectives. In M. P. Janicki, & A. J. Dalton (Eds.), *Dementia, aging, and intellectual disabilities: A handbook* (pp. 278–293). Philadelphia, PA: Taylor & Francis.

Cooper, S. A. (1999). The relationship between psychiatric and physical health in elderly people with intellectual disability. *Journal of Intellectual Disability Research, 43,* 54–60.

Cuthill, F. M., Espie, C. A., & Cooper, S. A. (2003). Development and psychometric properties of the Glasgow Depression Scale for people with a learning disability. *British Journal of Psychiatry, 182,* 347–353.

Desai, K. B., Ribbans, W. J., & Taylor, G. J. (1996). Incidence of five common fracture types in an institutional epileptic population. *Injury, 27,* 97–100.

Dhondt, T. D., Beekman, A. T., Deeg, D. J., & vanTillburg, W. (2002). Iatrogenic depression in the elderly. Results from a community-based study in the Netherlands. *Social Psychiatry and Psychiatric Epidemiology, 37,* 393–398.

Dinerstein, R. D., Herr, S. S., & O'Sullivan, J. L. (Eds.) (1999). *A guide to consent.* Washington, DC: American Association on Mental Retardation.

Dosen, A. (2005). Applying the developmental perspective in the psychiatric assessment and diagnosis of persons with intellectual disability. *Journal of Psychology and Psychiatry, 41,* 407–417.

Duffy, E. G. (2010). The neurologic system. In P. A. Tabloski, *Gerontological nursing* (2 ed., pp. 735–782). Upper Saddle River, NJ: Pearson.

Esbensen, A. J., Greenberg, J. S., Seltzer, M. M., & Aman, M. G. (2009). A longitudinal investigation of psychotropic and non-psychotropic medication use among adolescents and adults with autism spectrum disorders. *Journal of Autism and Developmental Disorders, 39,* 1339–1349.

Esbensen, A. J., Seltzer, M. M., Lam, K. S. L., & Bodfish, J. W. (2009). Age-related differences in restricted repetitive behaviors in autism spectrum disorder. *Journal of Autism and Developmental Disorders, 39,* 57–66.

Evenhuis, H. M. (1997). Medical aspects of aging in a population with intellectual disability: III. Mobility, internal conditions and cancer. *Journal of Intellectual Disability Research, 41,* 8–18.

Evenhuis, H. M. (1999). Associated medical aspects. In M. P. Janicki, & A. J. Dalton (Eds.), *Dementia, aging, and intellectual disabilities: A handbook* (pp. 103–118). Philadelphia, PA: Brunner-Mazel.

Faulkner, C. M., Cox, H. L., & Williamson, J. C. (2005). Unique aspects of antimicrobial use in older adults. *Clinics in Infectious Disease, 40,* 997–1004.

Felce, D., Baxter, H., Lowe, K., Dunstan, F., Houston, H., Jones, G., Felce, J., & Kerr, M. (2008). The impact of repeated health checks for adults with intellectual disabilities. *Journal of Applied Research in Intellectual Disabilities, 21,* 585–596.

Findling, R., Maxwell, K., & Wizniter, M. (1997). An open clinical trial of risperdone monotherapy in young children with autistic disorders. *Psychopharmacology Bulletin, 33,* 155–159.

Fiske, A., Wetherell, J. L., & Gatz, M. (2009). Depression in older adults. *Annual Review of Clinical Psychology, 5,* 363–389.

Floyd, E. F., & McIntosh, D. E. (2009). Current practices in psychopharmacology for children and adolescents with autism spectrum disorders. *Psychology in the Schools, 46*(9), 905–909.

Focht-New, G., Bard, B., Clements, P. T., & Milliken, T. F. (2008). Persons with developmental disability exposed to interpersonal violence and crime. *Perspectives in Psychiatric Care, 44,* 89–98.

Fombonne, E. (1999). The epidemiology of autism: A review. *Psychological Medicine, 29,* 769–786.

Galban, C. J., Maderwald, S., Stock, F., & Ladd, M. E. (2007). Age–related changes in skeletal muscle as detected by diffusion tension magnetic resonance imaging. *Journals of Gerontology: Medical Sciences, 62A,* 453–458.

Galli-Carminati, G., Chavet, I., & Deriaz, N. (2006). Prevalence of gastrointestinal disorder in adult clients with pervasive development disorders. *Journal of Intellectual Disability Research, 50,* 711–718.

Gaus, V. L. (2011). Adult Asperger syndrome and the utility of cognitive-behavioral therapy. *Journal of Contemporary Psychotherapy, 41,* 47–56.

Gerland, G. (2000). *Finding out about Asperger Syndrome, high functioning autism and PDD.* Philadelphia: Jessica Kingsley Publishers, LTD.

Ghaziuddin, M., Ghaziuddin, N., & Greden, J. (2002). Depression in persons with autism: Implications for research and clinical care. *Journal of Autism and Developmental Disorders, 32,* 299–306.

Gibson, S. J., & Farrell, M. (2004). A review of age differences in the neurophysiology of nociception and the perceptual experience of pain. *Clinical Journal of Pain, 20*, 227–239.

Gillberg, C., & Billstedt, E. (2000). Autism and Asperger syndrome: Coexistence with other clinical disorders. *Actas Psychiatrica Scandinavica, 102*, 321–330.

Graetz, J. E. (2010). Autism grows up: Opportunities for adults with autism. *Disability and Society, 25*, 33–47.

Grisso, T., & Appelbaum, P. (1998). *MacArthur Competence Assessment Tool for Treatment (MacCAT-T)*. Sarasota, FL: Professional Resource Press/Professional Resource Exchange.

Grossman, H., Bergmann, C., & Parker, S. (2006). Dementia: A brief review. *Mount Sinai Journal of Medicine, 73*, 985–992.

Gutstein, S., & Sheely, R. (2002). *Relationship Development Intervention with young children: Social and emotional development activities for Asperger's, Autism, PDD and NLD.* London: Jessica Kingsley.

Hahn, J. E., & Aronow, H. U. (2005). A pilot of a gerontological advanced practice nurse preventive intervention. *Journal of Applied Research in Intellectual Disabilities, 18*, 131–142.

Hassan, Y., Al-Ramahi, R. J., Aziz, N. A., & Ghazali, R. (2009). Impact of a renal drug dosing service on dose adjustment in hospitalized patients with chronic kidney disease. *The Annals of Pharmacotherapy, 43*, 1598–1605.

Heller, T., Janicki, M. D., Hamell, J., & Factor, A. (2002). *Promoting healthy aging, family support, and age-friendly communities for persons with aging with developmental disabilities.* Chicago: The Rehabilitation Research and Training Center on Aging with Developmental Disabilities, Department of Disability and Human Development, University of Illinois at Chicago.

Holmes, D. L. (1998). *Autism through the lifespan: The Eden model.* Bethesda, MD: Woodbine House.

Hoshino, A., Tamura, J., Nakazawa, M., & Koyama, H. (2007). Middle-aged and elderly outpatients show lower body temperature responses than the young, even with the same C-reactive protein levels. *Journal of International Medical Research, 35*, 329–337.

Hsiech, K., Heller., T., & Miller, A. B. (2001). Risk factors for injuries and falls among adults with developmental disabilities. *Journal of Intellectual Disability Research, 45*, 76–82.

Hurlbutt, K., & Chalmers, L. (2002). Adults with autism speak out: perceptions of their life experiences. *Focus on Autism and Other Developmental Disabilities, 17*, 103–111.

Hybels, C. F., & Blazer, D. G. (2003). Epidemiology of late-life mental disorders. *Clinics in Geriatric Medicine, 19*(4), 663–696.

Inouye, S. K. (2003). Delirium. In C. K. Cassel (Ed.), *Geriatric medicine: An evidence-based approach* (pp. 1113–1122). New York: Springer Publishing.

Inouye, S. K., Bogardus, S. T., Williams, C. S., Leo-Summers, L., & Agostino, L. V. (2003). The role of adherence on the effectiveness of nonpharmacological interventions: Evidence from the Delirium Prevention Trial. *Archives of Internal Medicine, 63*, 958–964.

Inouye, S. K., van Dyck, C., Alessi, C., Balkin, S., Siegal, A. P., & Horwitz, R. (1990). Clarifying confusion: The confusion assessment method. *Annals of Internal Medicine, 113*(12), 941–948.

Ivaneko, A., & Johnson, K. P. (2010). Sleep disorders. In M. K. Dulcan (Ed.), *Dulcan's textbook of child and adolescent psychiatry* (pp. 299–324). Arlington, VA: American Psychiatric Association.

Jacobson, J., Sutton, M., & Janicki, M. (1985). Demography and characteristics of aging and aged mentally retarded persons. In M. Janicki, & H. Wishiewski (Eds.), *Aging and developmental disabilities: Issues and approaches* (pp. 95–131). Baltimore, MD: Paul H. Brookes.

James, I. A., Mukaetova-Ladinska, E., Reichelt, R., Briel, R., & Scully, A. (2006). Diagnosing Asperger's syndrome in the elderly: A series of case presentations. *International Journal of Geriatric Psychiatry, 21*, 951–960.

Jette, N., Lix, L. M., Metge, C. J., Prior, H. J., McChesney, J., & Leslie, W. D. (2011). Association of antiepileptic drugs with nontraumatic fractures: A population-based analysis. *Archives of Neurology, 68*, 107–112.

Kane, R. L., Ouslander, J. G., & Abrass, I. B. (2004). *Essentials of clinical geriatrics* (5 ed.). New York: McGraw-Hill.

Kapell, D., Nightingale, B., Rodriquez, A., Lee, J. H., Zigman, W. B., & Schupf, N. (1998). Prevalence of chronic medical conditions in adults with mental retardation: A comparison with general population. *Mental Retardation, 36*, 269–279.

Karlin, N. J., Weintraub, N., & Chopra, I. J. (2004). Current controversies in endocrinology: Screening of asymptomatic elderly for subclinical hypothyroidism. *Journal of the American Medical Directors Association, 5*, 333–336.

Kerins, G. J., Price, L. C., Broadhurst, A., & Gaynor, C. M. (2010). A pilot study analyzing mortality of adults with developmental disabilities residing in nursing homes in Connecticut. *Journal of Policy and Practice in Intellectual Disabilities, 7*, 177–181.

King, B. H., & Bostic, J. Q. (2006). An update on pharmacologic treatments of autism spectrum disorders. *Child and Adolescent Psychiatric Clinics of North America, 15*, 161–175.

Koenig, K., & Levine, K. (2011). Psychotherapy for individuals with autism spectrum disorders. *Journal of Contemporary Psychotherapy, 41*, 29–36.

Krauss, M. W., Seltzer, M. M., & Jacobson, H. T. (2005). Adults with autism living at home or in non-family settings: Positive and negative aspects of residential status. *Journal of Intellectual Disability Research, 49*(2), 111–124.

Kuijpers, M. A. J., van Marum, R. J., Egberts, A. C. G., Jansen, P. A. F., and the Old People Drugs & Dysregulations Study Group (2008). Relationship between polypharmacy and underprescribing. *British Journal of Clinical Pharmacology, 65*, 130–133.

Kwok, H. W. M. (2003). Psychopharmacology in autism spectrum disorders. *Current Opinion in Psychiatry, 16*, 529–534.

Lach, H. W., & Smith, C. M. (2007). Assessment: Focus on function. In A. D. Linton, & H. Lach (Eds.), *Matteson's & McConnell's gerontological nursing: Concepts and practice* (pp. 25–51). St. Louis, MO: Elsevier.

Lainhart, J. E., & Folstein, S. E. (1994). Affective disorders in people with autism: A review of published cases. *Journal of Autism and Developmental Disorders, 24*, 587–601.

Lauderdale, S. A., & Sheikh, J. I. (2003). Anxiety disorders in older adults. *Clinics in Geriatric Medicine, 19*(4), 721–741.

Launer, L. J. (2007). Next steps in Alzheimer's disease research: Interaction between epidemiology and basic science. *Current Alzheimer's Research, 4*, 141–143.

Lecavalier, L. (2006). Behavioral and emotional problems in young people with pervasive developmental disorders: Relative prevalence, effects of subject characteristics, and empirical classification. *Journal of Autism and Developmental Disorders, 36*, 1101–1114.

Levy, R. H., & Collins, C. (2007). Risk and predictability of drug interactions in the elderly. *International Review of Neurobiology, 81*, 235–251.

Levy, S. E., Mandell, D. S., & Schultz, R. T. (2009). Autism. *Lancet, 374*, 1627–1638.

Linton, A., Garber, M., Fagan, N. K., & Peterson, M. R. (2007). Examination of multiple medication use among TRICARE beneficiaries aged 65 years and older. *Journal of Managed Care Pharmacy, 13*, 155–162.

Linton, A. D. (2007a). Gastrointestinal system. In A. D. Linton, & H. Lach (Eds.), *Matteson's and McConnell's gerontological nursing: Concepts and practice* (pp. 442–483). St. Louis, MO: Elsevier.

Linton, A. D. (2007b). Genitourinary system. In A. D. Linton, & H. Lach (Eds.), *Matteson's and McConnell's gerontological nursing: Concepts and practice* (3 ed.) (pp. 484–524). St. Louis, MO: Elsevier.

Linton, A. D. (2007c). Pharmacological considerations. In A. D. Linton, & H. Lach (Eds.), *Matteson's and McConnell's gerontological nursing: Concepts and practice* (pp. 138–168). St. Louis, MO: Elsevier.

Linton, A. D., Hooter, L. J., & Elmers, C. R. (2007). Endocrine system. In A. D. Linton, & H. Lach (Eds.), *Matteson's and McConnell's Gerontological nursing: Concepts and practice* (pp. 525–571). St. Louis, MO: Elsevier.

Liu, X. Z., & Yan, D. (2007). Ageing and hearing loss. *Journal of Pathology, 211*(2), 188–197.

Lotan, M., & Gold, C. (2009). Meta-analysis of the effectiveness of individual intervention in the controlled multisensory environment (Snoezelen) for individuals with intellectual disability. *Journal of Intellectual and Developmental Disability, 34*, 207–215.

Matson, J. L., & Rivet, T. T. (2008). Characteristics of challenging behaviours in adults with autistic disorder, PDD-NOS, and intellectual disability. *Journal of Intellectual and Developmental Disability, 33*, 323–329.

Matthews, T., Weston, N., Baxter, H., Felce, D., & Kerr, M. (2008). A general practice-based prevalence study of epilepsy among adults with intellectual disabilities and of its association with psychiatric disorder, behaviour disturbance and carer stress. *Journal of Intellectual Disability Research, 52*(2), 163–173.

McCabe, H. (2008). The importance of parent-to-parent support among families of children with autism in the People's Republic of China. *International Journal of Disability, Development, and Education, 55*(4), 303–314.

McDougle, C. J., Holmes, J. P., Carlson, T. C., Pelton, G. H., Cohen, D. J., & Price, L. H. (1998). A double-blind, placebo-controlled study of risperdone in adults with autistic disorder and other pervasive developmental disorders. *Archives of General Psychiatry, 55*, 633–641.

McManus, S., Meltzer, H., Brugha, T. S., Bebbington, P. E., & Jenkins, R. (2009). *Adult psychiatric morbidity in England, 2007: Results of a household survey*. London: The NHS Centre for Health and Social Care.

Melnyk, B. M., & Fineout-Overholt, E. (2011). Making the case for evidence-based practice 2e. In B. M. Melnyk, & E. Fineout-Overholt, *Evidence-based practice in nursing and healthcare: A guide to best practice.* Philadelphia, PA: Lippincott, Williams & Wilkins.

Micromedex. (2011). Phenytoin. New York: Thompson Reuters. Retrieved from http://www.thompsonhc.com

Millsap, P. (2007). Neurological system. In A. D. Linton, & H. Lach (Eds.), *Matteson's and McConnell's gerontological nursing: Concepts and practice* (pp. 406–441). St. Louis, MO: Elsevier.

Mitty, E., & Flores, S. (2008). Suicide in late life. *Geriatric Nursing, 29*(3), 160–165.

Moreno, S. (1992). A parent's view of more able people with autism. In E. Schopler, & G. B. Mesibov (Eds.), *High functioning individuals with autism* (pp. 91–103). New York: Plenum.

Morgan, C. L., Baxter, H., & Kerr, M. P. (2003). Prevalence of epilepsy and associated health service utilization and mortality among patients with intellectual disability. *American Journal on Mental Retardation, 108*, 293–300.

Morgan, C. N., Roy, M., & Chance, P. (2003). Psychiatric comorbidity and medication use on autism: A community survey. *The Psychiatrist, 27*, 378–381.

National Health Service Health Scotland (2004). *Health needs assessment report. People with learning disabilities in Scotland.* Glasgow: Author.

Nelson, M. E., Rejeski, W. J., Blair, S. N., Duncan, P. W., Judge, J. O., King, A. C., . . . Casteneda-Sceppa, C. (2007). Physical activity and public health: Recommendation from the American College of Sports Medicine and the American Heart Association. *Circulation: Journal of the American Heart Association, 116*, 1094–1106.

Noebels, J. (2011). A perfect storm: Converging paths of epilepsy and Alzheimer's dementia intersect in the hippocampal formation. *Epilepsia, 52* (suppl. 1), 39–46.

Numis, A. L., Major, P., Montenegro, M. A., Muzykewicz, D. A., Pulsifer, M. B., & Thiele, E. A. (2011). Identification of risk factors for autism spectrum disorders in tuberous sclerosis complex. *Neurology, 76*, 981–987.

Orwoll, E., Neilson, C. M., Marshall, L. M., Lambert, L., Holton, K. F., Hoffman, A. R., . . . Osteoporotic Fractures in Men (MrOS) Study Group (2009). Vitamin D deficiency in older men. *Journal of Clinical Endocrinology & Metabolism, 94*, 1214–1222.

Ouellette-Kuntz, H. (2005). Understanding health disparities and inequities faced by individuals with intellectual disabilities. *Journal of Applied Research in Intellectual Disabilities, 18*(2), 113–121.

Patja, K., Iivanainen, M., Vesala, H., Oksanen, H., & Ruoppila, I. (2000). Life expectancy of people with intellectual disability: A 35 year follow-up study. *Journal of Intellectual Disability Research, 44*(5), 591–600.

Perry, D. W., Marston, G. M., Hinder, S. A. J., Munden, A. C., & Roy, A. (2001). The phenomenology of depressive illness in people with a learning disability and autism. *Autism, 5*, 265–275.

Phelps, K. W., Hodgson, J. L., McCammon, S. L., & Lamson, A. L. (2009). Caring for an individual with autism disorder: A qualitative analysis. *Journal of Intellectual & Developmental Disorders, 34*, 27–35.

Phillips, J. (1998). Complications of anticonvulsants and ketogenic diets. In J. Biller (Ed.), *Iatrogenic neurology* (pp. 397–414). Boston, MA: Butterworth-Heinemann.

Phillips, R. J., & Powley, T. L. (2007). Innervation of the gastrointestinal tract: Pattern of aging. *Autonomic Neuroscience: Basic Clinics, 136*, 1–19.

Plassman, B. L., Langa, K. M., Fisher, G. G., Heeringa, S. G., Weir, D. R., Ofstedal, M. B., . . . Wallace, R. B. (2007). Prevalence of dementia in the United States: The Aging, Demographics, and Memory Study. *Neuroepidemiology, 29*, 125–132.

Plassman, B. L., Williams, J. W., Burke, J. R., Holsinger, T., & Benjamin, S. (2010). Systematic review: Factors associated with risk for and possible prevention of cognitive decline in later life. *Annals of Internal Medicine, 153*, 182–193.

Podsiadlo, D., & Richardson, S. (1991). The Timed Up and Go: A test of basic functional mobility for frail elderly persons. *Journal of American Geriatrics, 39*, 142–148.

Prizant, B., Wetherby, A., Rubin, E., Laurent, A., & Rydell, P. (2006). *The SCERTS Model: A comprehensive educational approach for children with Autism Spectrum Disorders.* Baltimore, MD: Paul H. Brookes.

Pyo, G., Curtis, K., Curits, R., & Markwell, S. (2009). A validity study of the Working Group's Orientation Test for individuals with moderate to severe intellectual disability. *Journal of Intellectual Disability Research, 53*(9), 780–786.

Ramirez, S. Z., & Lukenbill, J. F. (2007). Development of the fear survey for adults with mental retardation. *Research in Developmental Disabilities, 28*, 225–237.

Reilly, J., Rodriguez, A. D., Lamy, M., & Neils-Strunjas, J. (2010). Cognition, language, and clinical pathological features of non-Alzheimer's dementias: An overview. *Journal of Communication Disorders, 43*, 438–452.

Renty, J., & Roeyers, H. (2007). Individual and marital adaptation in men with autism spectrum disorder and their spouses: The role of social support and coping strategies. *Journal of Autism and Developmental Disorders, 37*, 1247–1255.

Roche, V. (2003). Etiology and management of delirum. *American Journal of Medical Science, 325*, 20–30.

Ross, A. C., Taylor, C. L., Yaktine, A. L., & Del Valle, H. B. (Eds.) (2011). *Dietary reference intakes for calcium and vitamin D: The Institute of Medicine report.* Washington, DC: National Academies Press.

Salvi, S. M., Akhtar, S., & Currie, Z. (2006). Ageing changes in the eye. *Postgraduate Medical Journal, 82*, 581–587.

Savage, T. A., Ast, K., Bess, R., Castrogiovanni, M., & Conway, P. (2010). Supports and resources for older adults. In S. L. Friedman, & Dt. T. Helm (Eds.), *End of life care for children and adults with intellectual disabilities* (pp. 313–328). Washington, DC: American Association on Intellectual and Developmental Disabilities.

Savva, G. M., Wharton, S. B., Ince, P. G., Foster, G., Matthews, F. E., & Brayne, C. (2009). Age, neuropathology, and dementia. *New England Journal of Medicine, 360*, 2302–2309.

Schwartz, R. A., Fernandez, G., Kotulska, K., & Jozwiak, S. (2007). Tuberous sclerosis complex: Advances in diagnosis, genetics, and management. *Journal of the American Academy of Dermatology, 57*, 189–202.

Semla, T. P., Beizer, J. L., & Higbee, M. D. (2007). *Geriatric dosage handbook: Including clinical recommendations and monitoring guidelines* (12 ed.). Hudson, OH: Lexi-Comp.

Shawler, C. (2010). Assessing and maintaining mental health in older adults. *Nursing Clinics of North America, 45*(4), 635–650.

Shavelle, R. M., Strauss, D. J., & Pickett, J. (2001). Causes of death in autism. *Journal of Autism and Developmental Disorders, 31*, 569–576.

Shtayermman, O. (2008). Suicidal ideation and co-morbid disorders in adolescents and young adults diagnosed with Asperger's Syndrome: A population at risk. *Journal of Human Behavior in the Social Environment, 18*, 301–328.

Singh, B. N. (2005). A quantitative approach to probe the dependence and correlation of food-effect with aqueous solubility, dose/solubility ratio, and partition coefficient (Log P) for orally active drugs administered as immediate-release formulations. *Drug Development Research, 65*, 55–75.

Sterling, L., Dawson, G., Estes, A., & Greenson, J. (2008). Characteristics associated with presence of depressive symptoms in adults with autism spectrum disorder. *Journal of Autism and Developmental Disorders, 38*, 1011–1018.

Stokes, M., Newton, N., & Kaur, A. (2007). Stalking, and social and romantic functioning among adolescents and adults with autism spectrum disorder. *Journal of Autism and Developmental Disorders, 37*, 1969–1986.

Strydom, A., Shoostari, S., Lee, V., Raykar, V., Torr, J., Tsiouris, J., . . . & Maaskant, M. (2010). Dementia in older adults with intellectual disabilities—Epidemiology, presentation, and diagnosis. *Journal of Policy and Practice in Intellectual Disabilities, 7*(2), 96–110.

Tabloski, P. (2010). *Gerontological nursing* (2 ed.). Upper Saddle River, NJ: Pearson.

Tanguay, P. (2010). Autism spectrum disorders. In M. K. Dulcan (Ed.), *Dulcan's textbook of child and adolescent psychiatry* (pp. 79–88). Arlington, VA: American Psychiatric Association.

Tantam, D. (2000). Psychological disorder in adolescents and adults with Asperger syndrome. *Autism, 4*(1), 47.

Thorpe, L. (1999). Psychiatric disorders. In M. P. Janicki, & A. J. Dalton (Eds.), *Dementia, ageing, and intellectual disabilities: A handbook* (pp. 217–230). Philadelphia, PA: Brunner-Mazel.

Timiras, M. L., & Luxenberg, J. S. (2007). Pharmacology and drug management in the elderly. In P. S. Timiras (Ed.), *Physiological basis of aging and geriatrics* (4 ed., pp. 355–361). New York: Informa Healthcare.

Timiras, P. S., & Maletta, G. J. (2007). The nervous system: Structural, biochemical, metabolic, and circulatory changes. In P. Timiras (Ed.), *Physiologic basis of aging* (4 ed., pp. 71–87), New York: Informa Healthcare.

Totsika, V., Felce, D., Kerr, M., & Hastings, R. P. (2010). Behavior problems, psychiatric symptoms, and quality of life for older adults with intellectual disability with and without autism. *Journal of Autism and Developmental Disorders, 40*, 1171–1178.

Tullman, D. F., & Dracup, K. (2000). Creating a healing environment for elders. *AACN Clinical Issues, 11*, 34–50.

Turnbull, A. P., Blue-Banning, M., Turbiville, V., & Park, J. (1999). From parent education to partnership education: A call for a transformed focus. *Topics in Early Childhood Special Education, 19*, 164–172.

Tyler, C. V., Jr., & Noritz, G. (2009). Healthcare issues in aging adults with intellectual and other developmental disabilities. *Clinical Geriatrics, 17*, 30–35.

United Nations (2009). *World population prospects, 2008 revision*. New York: Author.

United States Preventive Services Task Force (2008). Screening for prostate cancer: U. S. Preventive Services Task Force Recommendations. *Annals of Internal Medicine, 149*, 185–191.

van der Flier, W. M., & Scheltens, P. (2005). Epidemiology and risk factors of dementia. *Journal of Neurology, Neurosurgery, and Psychiatry, 76*(suppl. 5), v2–v7.

van Niekirk, M. E., Groen, W., Vissers, C., van Driel-deJong, D., Kan, C. C., & Oude Voushaar, R. C. (2010). Diagnosing autism spectrum disorders in elderly people. *International Psychogeriatrics, 23*, 1–11.

Viktil, K. K., Blix, H. S., Moger, T. A., & Reikvam, A. (2006). Polypharmacy as commonly defined is an indicator of limited value in the assessment of drug-related problems. *British Journal of Clinical Pharmacology, 63*, 187–195.

Vincent, G. K., & Velkoff, V. A. (2010). *The next four decades: The older population in the United States, 2010–2050* (U.S. Census Bureau Current Population Reports, P25-1138). Washington, DC: U.S. Census Bureau.

Walsh, K. K., Kastner, T., & Criscione, T. (1997). Characteristics of hospitalizations for people with developmental disabilities: utilization, costs, and impact of care coordination. *American Journal on Mental Retardation, 100*, 505–520.

Wei, J. T., Calhoun, E. A., & Jacobsen, S. J. (2007). Benign prostatic hyperplasia. In M. S. Litwin, & C. S. Saigal (Eds.), *Urological diseases in America: US Department of Health and Human Services, Public Health Service, National Institutes of Health, National Institute of Diabetes and Digestive and Kidney Diseases* (pp. 43–70). Washington, DC: U.S. Government Printing Office (NIH Publication No. 07-5512).

Wieder, S., & Greenspan, S. (2001). The DIR (Developmental, Individual-Difference, Relationship-Based) approach to assessment and intervention planning. *Bulletin of ZERO TO THREE: National Center for Infants, Toddlers, and Families, 21*(4), 11–19.

Wilcox, S., Brenes, G., Levine, D., Sevick, M. A., Shumaker, S. A., & Craven, T. (2000). Factors related to sleep disturbance in older adults experiencing knee pain or knee pain with radiographic evidence of knee osteoarthritis. *Journal of the American Geriatrics Society, 48*, 1241–1251.

Williams, D. (1996). *Autism: An inside-out approach.* London: Jessica Kingsley.

Wilson, D., & Haire, A. (1990). Health care screening for people with mental handicap living in the community. *British Medical Journal, 301*, 1379–1381.

Wing, L. (1981). Asperger's syndrome: A clinical account. *Psychological Medicine, 11*, 115–129.

Wiznitzer, M. (2004). Autism and tuberous sclerosis. *Journal of Child Neurology, 19*, 675–679.

Wolf, M. M., Risley, T. R., & Mees., H. (1964). Application of operant conditioning procedures to behavior problems of an autistic child. *Behavior Research and Therapy, 1*, 305–312.

Woodgate, R. L., Ateah, C., & Secco, L. (2008). Living in a world of our own: The experience of parents who have a child with autism. *Qualitative Health Research, 18*, 1075–1083.

Wong, D. L., & Baker, C. M. (1988). Pain in children: Comparison of assessment scales. *Pediatric Nursing, 14*, 9–17.

15 The Nurse's Role in Managing Transitions and Future Planning for Aging Adults With Autism and Their Families

Kathleen M. Fischer and Justin D. Peterson

Aging individuals with autism spectrum disorder (ASD) are at risk for experiencing difficulties in accessing needed services and quality health care. Currently, little attention is being directed to programs for health prevention and promotion that might support improvements for "aging in place" or growing old where one lives—that is, in an individual's own community. A number of factors contribute to disparities in health status, access, and quality of care for adults, including race, gender, lower socioeconomic status, geographic proximity to health care providers, increasing age, and having a disability (Perkins & Moran, 2010; Rubin & Crocker, 2006). The risk of experiencing poor health is enhanced by increasing age and membership in a vulnerable population, while health promotion and prevention programs specifically targeted to older adults with lifelong disabilities are limited (Beirne-Smith, Ittenbach, & Patton, 2002; Parish, Seltzer, Greenberg, & Floyd, 2004; Perkins & Moran, 2010).

Research on the aging process of adults with ASD is scarce, even though this is a chronic, lifelong condition. Research rarely extends beyond childhood or adolescence (Seltzer, Krauss, Orsmond, & Vestal, 2001). Few studies focus on how families, parents, and siblings are affected by and manage the challenge of lifelong responsibility for a child with ASD. For example, Ann Turnbull, the past president of the American Association of Intellectual and Developmental Disabilities, described her experiences, including the influences on siblings, of parenting a child with an intellectual disability (Turnbull, 2004). She stated that helping her son with an intellectual disability develop skills for independence and helping her two younger daughters manage their concerns and fears about their brother's behaviors during adolescence should have been addressed as parenting priorities. Yet, as Dr. Turnbull explained, fitting all of this into her life as a working mother at that time would have been difficult, even though she was an expert on developmental disabilities (Turnbull, 2004).

Seltzer and colleagues (2001) observed that older parents can be haunted by the legacy of self-blame for their child's disorder, which has yet to be replaced with accurate, evidence-based information regarding parenting and role demands from the life course perspective (Seltzer et al., 2001). Studies of siblings of individuals with ASD and other developmental disabilities suggest that ambivalence can define the sibling relationship (Orsmond & Seltzer, 2007; Rubin & Crocker, 2006). Nurses should be attentive to family needs surrounding the challenges of managing care for a family member with autism. Furthermore, nurses should anticipate the spoken or unspoken question of, "Who will take care of the family member with autism after Mom dies?" This question looms large for parents *and* siblings in these families.

Hopefully, change will occur in concert with the increasing prevalence of this disorder, better education about ASD, and the general movement to focus on quality of life and lifespan outcomes (Perkins & Moran, 2010). While we are learning more about ASD in general, we have limited population-based evidence about the aging process and its impacts for those with ASD and their families. We clearly need to learn from all stakeholders, including individuals with ASD, parents, siblings, caregivers, and community members. Until very recently, ASD research has focused almost exclusively on children and adolescents. However, with the assumption that those with ASD will have a normal lifespan, such a limited focus excludes most of the people affected by this disorder, that is, adults (Murphy, Beecham, Craig, & Ecker, 2011). Research is needed to identify the changes that accompany aging in ASD in anticipation of needed support systems and additional resources (Totsika, Felce, Kerr, & Hastings, 2010). The goal of this chapter is to assist nurses in appreciating the impact of aging on the individual with autism, parents/caregiver, family, and community. We also explore the nurse's role in partnering with each stakeholder to create a healthier future. Nurses and other professionals need to be knowledgeable about community, health, and educational resources for individuals with autism to support the entire family throughout the lifespan.

CASE

Jacob is 45 years old and has an unspecified ASD. Although he lives with his 71-year-old mother, Jacob is considered to be a high-functioning individual. He does have a sister, who lives with her husband and two teenage daughters in a neighboring state, although he rarely sees them. Jacob's social network is limited to his mother and her only brother. He takes one psychotropic medication: a selective serotonin reuptake inhibitor for depression.

Jacob works at the local ballpark stadium, where he helps guests find their seats. Jacob enjoys the organization of the seating system and the repetitive pattern of concession stands and restrooms. Within his first few weeks of work, Jacob had memorized the entire seating plan and locations of common fan destinations. Jacob can get overwhelmed by crowds and noise. Therefore, he is often moved to a quieter or emptier place prior to the start of each game and is closely monitored. Despite this, others appreciate him for his eagerness and dedication to his job, and he has missed very few shifts in the past 10 years.

At home, Jacob can handle most daily tasks, but he lacks the ability to manage his own fiscal affairs in any way. He can spend hours a day working on his favorite hobby: crossword puzzles. He becomes flustered with changes in plans or environment or when things do not go his way. When Jacob discovered that his uncle moved his puzzle while cleaning, he threw the plate he had been carrying, flipped a table over, and stormed into his room, where he stayed for almost 2 days. His mom worried that the aggressive tendencies he experienced in late adolescence were returning. His aggressive behavior at age 19 included hitting and choking a person in a sheltered workshop, resulting in his expulsion from the only adult program in their community.

Recently, Jacob spotted a stray dog outside his bedroom window and refused to sleep in his own bed, as he is afraid of dogs. Instead, he insisted on staying in his mother's bedroom. Jacob was not able to tell his mother that he was afraid of the dog outside, as he struggles to answer open-ended questions. When she tried after a few days to coerce him to sleep in his own bed, he became upset and pushed his mother on his way out of the room. She fell and suffered a broken hip, which resulted in hospitalization and home care convalescence. Jacob says he is deeply sorry, but it is not clear whether he fully realizes the implications of his actions. An emergency institutional placement will be necessary

(*Continued*)

CASE (Continued)

unless his sister, uncle, or another caregiver is available and willing to stay with him at home. His mother worries that she will not be able to continue to watch over Jacob; she has concerns, in addition to those surrounding her already declining health, that his behaviors create safety and health risks for her. At the same time, she worries about what is next for her son, as no conversation with Jacob, his sibling, or any other family member about what might happen in the future has ever taken place.

Assessment of Jacob and the Family Context

Jacob's case illustrates some common characteristics of ASD, including the inability to manage finances, a preference for routines or sameness, obsessive behavioral tendencies, heightened sensitivity to environmental stimuli, communication difficulties, medical problems, behavioral problems, a limited social sphere, caregiver issues, and the eventual need for change in residential status.

Jacob's mother had been becoming increasingly worried about her ability to care for her son; when the altercation between the two resulted in the mother's broken hip, her concerns were justified. Both Jacob and his mother are in need of significant help and support. Jacob's mother can no longer care for him, but Jacob cannot care for himself. She recognizes that there are no family members or friends who can accept or even help alleviate the burden of caring for her son. Jacob's mother is frightened by the thought of Jacob's future, as he is the "love of her life." This case also highlights the missing "crucial conversation" about what is next for Jacob, and the need for an intervention by a nurse to encourage this discussion. However, the nurse needs to be proactive and have these "crucial conversations" with family members before a crisis point.

PUBLIC EXEMPLAR

While Jacob's case is hypothetical, his experience is to an extent mirrored in over one million individuals with autism in the United States. One of the most recognized individuals living with autism, Dr. Temple Grandin, is an advocate for autism and is passionate about the welfare of animals. In 2010, she was the subject of an award-winning HBO movie *Temple Grandin*, which portrayed her unique challenges with autism and her intense interest in, and perception of, animal behavior. The movie depicts many common characteristics of autism, such as hypersensitivity to noise and other sensory stimuli, focused interests, atypical communication, and deficits in social skills. Dr. Grandin's story illustrates the way an individual with autism can succeed when supported by family and educators. She was able to translate a set of unusual behaviors and interests into assets, which culminated in her designing more humane animal-handling facilities and equipment. Considered both a national and international expert in this area, Dr. Grandin was awarded a fellowship in the American Society of Animal Science in 2010 (see also Grandin, 2011). It is impossible to know if Dr. Grandin might have reached the same level of achievement had her family followed the expert advice of the day and agreed to institutionalization, as was recommended upon her being diagnosed with autism as a young child (Luce, 2010).

For health professionals, as well as families, this story offers an example of an individual who was able to effectively harness her interests and make a meaningful societal contribution despite the challenges associated with an ASD. In the case above, Jacob also benefits from the support of family and employers who understand his patterns, are able to interpret his behaviors, and can help him to use his skills to make a contribution at the ballpark. Health care professionals are challenged to recognize ability, not "dis-ability"; this philosophy has become an important statement of strength for many individuals and families living with a disability.

NEEDS OF INDIVIDUALS AGING WITH AUTISM

We know little about the evolving needs of those with ASD as they age. Arthritis, diabetes, heart disease, and hypertension are examples of common chronic illnesses that can accompany aging and that can lead to complex and difficult health management issues for our community-dwelling seniors. As illustrated by Jacob's case, aging individuals with autism might be on psychoactive medications that can have a number of side effects. They might also have limited interpersonal skills that make it difficult to properly access the health care system and supportive programs. In other words, elders need support to manage changing health care needs if they are to maintain independence. It is likely that aging individuals with autism might experience this need even more acutely.

While evidence about aging and autism in community settings is just beginning to emerge, some of the important nursing roles are clear: The skill of advocacy and care, or case management, will be crucial, whether the nurse meets the individual with ASD in primary care, during hospitalization, or in the community. The essential components of nursing practice for this population of community-based elders with autism are: an understanding of the social context, that is, where and with whom the individual resides; expert assessment skills, education and health teaching; health and wellness promotion; and an appreciation of community systems to facilitate the journey through the myriad layers of the health care system. In addition, the nurse is expected to be knowledgeable about federal, state, and local programs available to support self-directed and successful aging for individuals with ASD in the communities where they live.

LIFE STAGES

A number of responses are possible when parents receive the diagnosis that their child has a developmental disability such as ASD. Reactions include relief that a diagnosis is known, intense stress and fear regarding the meaning of the diagnosis, concern over their ability to deal with such a situation, grief for the child they had hoped to have, and the need to develop adaptation strategies for the child they actually have (Pelchat & Lefebvre, 2004; Rubin & Crocker, 2006; Turnbull, 2004). The nurse's role in supporting a family at this early stage centers on reducing stress. This includes active listening, establishing a relationship with the family based on trust, and providing appropriate education and referrals to supportive professionals, agencies, and programs. Next, the family will need to establish a new reality that includes a child with an ASD. They are assisted in this process when the nurse demonstrates mutual recognition and offers support in the development of parenting competencies for a child with special needs.

The nurse should be acutely aware that this challenging transition has consequences for the entire family system and needs to be knowledgeable about existing programs and services for referral. Early interventions for the child and family are critical and need to be established in order for optimal outcomes to be realized (Rubin & Crocker, 2006). As we learned from our case example, ASD varies widely in symptom presentation and is characterized by impairments in communication, social interactions, limited interests, and restricted repetitive stereotyped behaviors (American Psychiatric Association, 2000), with social difficulty being a hallmark of the disorder. Therefore, interventions that benefit families and children with ASD include specialized psychosocial and educational programs that target the behavioral, communication, educational, and social needs of the individual child.

Education and Skills Development

In 1997, the Individuals with Disabilities Education Act (IDEA) was amended versus enacted, mandating and entitling special needs children to receive special services and educational accommodations. Education is provided without cost and must involve the "least restrictive environment" possible for the child and adolescent (American Academy of Child and Adolescent Psychiatry, 2008). Federal law requires that an individualized transition plan (ITP) and an individualized education plan (IEP) be created by the school in conjunction with the student and family. The Individuals with Disabilities Education Improvement Act of 2004 mandates that public schools provide services supporting the transition from school to work; these should appear in the student's IEP by the time the student is age 16. These services include vocational training, guidance related to possibilities for postsecondary education, and help in obtaining adult services. Before the student leaves the school system, a vocational rehabilitation counselor, whose focus is the goal of helping the individual obtain and maintain employment, must participate in the ITP (Rubin & Crocker, 2006). This is the case with Jacob, who was assisted by these laws to find meaningful work at the local ballpark as he transitioned to adulthood.

Individuals with disabilities can continue their public education through age 21, but special services end at graduation from the public education system (Rubin & Crocker, 2006). Not all will be as fortunate as Jacob in terms of functional skills and transition to employment. Many individuals and families struggle with the question "What happens next?" as the person "ages out" of the educational system and alternative support services are needed.

A nurse's holistic approach to this family situation requires knowledge of supportive services and agencies. Adolescents and young adults with ASD should be encouraged to participate in age-appropriate community recreation programs to help develop strategies that will enable them to avoid social isolation and encourage the formation of friendships across the lifespan. In addition, the nurse must appreciate that support of the entire family is ongoing throughout the life cycle and will need to be reevaluated at different developmental stages and transitions. Figure 15.1 summarizes nursing roles at transition points such as diagnosis, developmental change, or aging out of the education system.

Adulthood and Aging

Early cognitive and behavioral interventions, as described above, must support an individual's self-care, social, and communication skills, because a cure for ASD does not exist. In fact, researchers debate whether the neurodevelopmental abnormalities and core diagnostic symptoms detected early in life with autism persist, change, or are helpful in predicting outcomes in later life (Murphy et al., 2011; Rapin & Tuchman, 2008; Shattuck et al., 2007). Some suggest that symptoms continue, but are muted (Rapin & Tuchman, 2008), while others report a persistence of symptoms into adulthood (Shattuck et al., 2007; Totsika et al., 2010). Clearly, we need more research to address this debate, so that appropriate services and programs can be made available to meet the needs of individuals aging with autism.

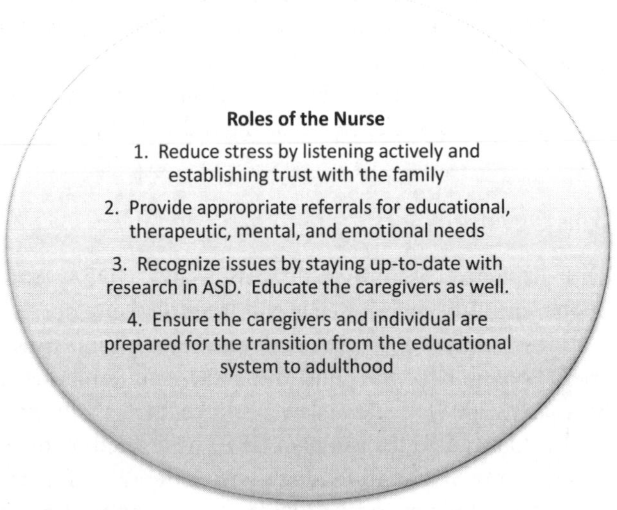

Roles of the Nurse

1. Reduce stress by listening actively and establishing trust with the family
2. Provide appropriate referrals for educational, therapeutic, mental, and emotional needs
3. Recognize issues by staying up-to-date with research in ASD. Educate the caregivers as well.
4. Ensure the caregivers and individual are prepared for the transition from the educational system to adulthood

FIGURE 15.1 ■ Nursing roles at transition points.

For example, we do not know if impaired social interaction and reciprocity, a core symptom of ASD, improves with age, behavioral training programs, education about ASD, or some combination of the above. Socialization challenges, recreational activities, and peer relationships were explored in a study of 235 adolescents and adults with autism living at home (Orsmond, Krauss, & Seltzer, 2004). The prevalence of peer relationships, friendships, and participation in social and recreational activities were all low in this sample. Almost 50% of the sample had no peer relationships outside previously arranged settings (e.g., school, work, or other arranged social groups). The researchers point out that they do not know whether individuals with ASD want or are even motivated to form friendships, or whether their findings suggest a lack of interest in the social world (Orsmond et al., 2004). More research in these areas is needed.

Autism has been described as a symptom of atypical development of the immature brain (Rapin & Tuchman, 2008), and ongoing developmental changes in brain function and structure have been reported throughout childhood and adolescence. Researchers also have reported that as adults, individuals with ASD no longer have a significantly larger overall brain volume but have anatomical and functional abnormalities in the frontal lobe, basal ganglia, and limbic systems of the brain, based on evidence from magnetic resonance imaging (Murphy et al., 2011). Theories of age-related, specific anatomical abnormalities in autism are being studied, and uncertainty exists as to whether these changes are at the genetic, molecular, synaptic, cellular, and/or circuit levels of the brain (Courchesne, Campbell, & Solso, 2010). One of the most common manifestations of a disturbance in the brain are seizures, which occur in approximately 20% to 35% of children with ASD (Rubin & Crocker, 2006). The two peak periods of seizure onset are early childhood and adolescence and are often accompanied by behavioral regression (Rubin & Crocker, 2006).

Currently, researchers continue to support behavioral diagnosis of ASD. Autism spectrum disorder is associated with a high prevalence of co-occurring psychiatric disorders requiring treatment (Murphy et al., 2011). Difficulty in the social skills realm can lead to inadequate social interactions (Courchesne et al., 2010) and can cause difficulties in managing stress and frustration, as illustrated by Jacob's case.

Pharmacotherapeutic agents are used to treat psychiatric comorbidities and assist with behavior management in the population of people with autism. In a longitudinal study of medication use in 286 adolescents and adults with ASD, researchers found increases in both the number of medications taken and the proportion of individuals taking these medications (Esbensen, Greenberg, Seltzer, & Aman, 2009). The proportion of individuals taking medications increased from 70% to 81% at completion of the study, which took place over a $4\frac{1}{2}$-year period. Medications addressed in this study included both psychotropic (e.g., antipsychotics, antidepressants, anxiolytics, sedative-hypnotics, and CNS stimulants) and nonpsychotropic (e.g., anticonvulsants, antihypertensives, and diabetes, thyroid, and gastrointestinal medications) agents. The researchers conclude that adolescents and adults with ASD are highly medicated and likely to increase medication usage as they age.

Nurses caring for individuals with autism should be familiar with the indications and side effects of these agents to ensure their patients are appropriately and closely monitored for both therapeutic effect and side effects. In addition, use of psychotropic medications coupled with reduced interpersonal skills adds complexity to the plan of care. The care of individuals with ASD can include multiple providers for both ASD- and age-related health concerns, creating greater challenges in navigating the health care system. Nurses need to pay attention to this potential cumulative effect to ensure appropriate care is provided and needed services and programs are accessed and utilized (see Exhibit 15.1).

The Aging Family

Successful aging occurs in a social environment or community in which adaptation to life changes are facilitated by the family or community members. This process involves promotion of optimal physical and mental health. Preventing disease and disability; maintaining optimum physical and cognitive functioning; and maintaining engagement in daily life activities are all components of successful aging (Rubin & Crocker, 2006). Individuals with ASD might live in a number of diverse community settings, including: the family home, a nursing home, an adult family or foster care, supported and independent living arrangements, licensed intermediate care facilities, group homes, and other congregate-living facilities managed within the elder network (Rubin & Crocker, 2006).

EXHIBIT 15.1

Considerations for Care of an Aging Individual with ASD

- Some symptoms may diminish in adulthood, but many symptoms will likely persist.
- Peer relationships remain limited in the adult population, but there is debate whether this should be a cause for concern.
- Overall brain size becomes relatively similar to size in nonautistic adults. There appear to be anatomical and functional abnormalities in the frontal lobe, basal ganglia, and limbic system of brains of individuals with autism.
- Medication use is likely to increase with age, both for mental and physical health.
- The combination of ASD and age-related health concerns can create challenges in navigating the health care system.

Support for the aging individual with ASD is provided formally through government-sponsored professional services or informally by family members or caregivers. Sixty percent of Americans with developmental disabilities live with their families (Parish et al., 2004), making informal family caregivers the largest group of caregivers for individuals with developmental disabilities.

Aging Caregivers and Future Planning Issues

A growing concern for the informal family caregiver system includes the aging of both the individual with ASD and his or her primary caregiver or parent. Parents or caregivers often avoid talking about who will care for their adult child with a disability when they can no longer provide services or die. Many parents cannot imagine that any one person will be able to provide the love and care that they have for their son or daughter. Some assume that a sibling or close relative will step into the caregiving role, without ever asking if that is even desired or possible. Some realize that there is no one else, and they worry about the quality of residential or institutional placement, the lack of staff, resources, long waiting lists, and long distances to travel to see their son or daughter.

Regardless, it is important that these "crucial conversations" occur for the care and well-being of all, as emergency placements in crisis situations, such as illness or death of a parent, are becoming more frequent. The main aspects of "future" planning that need to be addressed are "succession" planning (i.e., determining the next caregiver, legal planning for financial and/or residential concerns). Future planning-related questions the nurse/case manager should consider and bring to the family's attention are summarized in Figure 15.2. Having built and nurtured a trust-based relationship with a family, the nurse has an important role in engaging both the individual with autism and the primary caregiver in such a "crucial conversation."

RESOURCES FOR FAMILIES

Planning needs for individuals with ASD will vary. In Jacob's case, emergency housing and caregiver needs occurred when his mother sustained a hip fracture and was no longer able to care for her son. Jacob's situation, unfortunately, is not uncommon. Several state governments have recognized the need for services for individuals with ASD in the aging and disabled population. However, the services, funds, resources, policies, and plans vary greatly

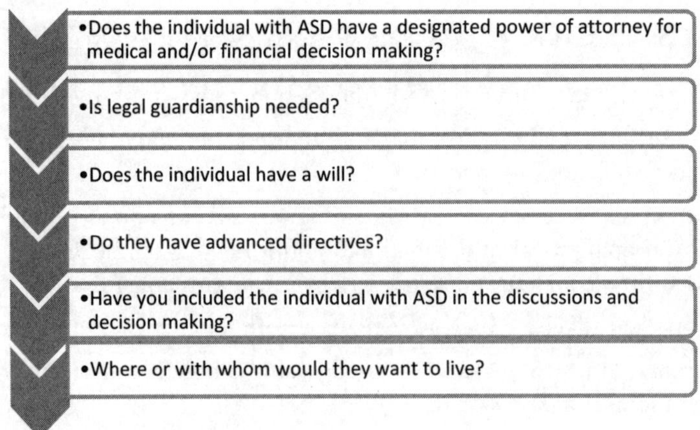

FIGURE 15.2 ■ Critical questions related to future planning.

from state to state. Depending on where Jacob and his mother reside, they might be eligible for a great deal of help from state services. Nurses providing care for either Jacob or his mother need to be aware of the variety of resources and services to support healthy aging in the community, particularly for individuals like Jacob who have a developmental disability.

To illustrate the significant variation in state-based programs for this population, services and resources in three states were reviewed. We consider what might happen and what resources would be available for Jacob if he lived in the states of Connecticut, Wyoming, and Arizona.

CASE UNFOLDING IN CONNECTICUT

In Connecticut, Jacob and his mother would have access to a fairly new program called the Autism Spectrum Disorders Pilot Program, which was developed in 2006 for adults with ASD without intellectual disability. It is less common to see a state-level program specifically addressing this variant of ASD, since only 25% of those with ASD will have normal or near-normal intelligence (Rubin & Crocker, 2006). Three years prior to 2006, the Connecticut Department of Developmental Services had established the Focus Team on Aging to address supportive and assistive living services for aging individuals; this would also be a resource for Jacob's mother when she tries to find residential placement for her son. After calling a representative and completing the application process, Jacob's mother is thrilled to find that he has been accepted for the program.

A case manager takes on Jacob's case right away. This person works full-time for autistic program members. The case manager assesses Jacob's specific needs and develops a unique plan of action for him based on the assessment. Some services are utilized by Jacob right away. He has the opportunity to meet with a job coach, who ensures Jacob's employment continues to go smoothly. Jacob also meets with a life skills coach and community mentor, both of whom will ensure that Jacob can continue to function in his daily activities without the assistance of his mother. Respite care is provided for his mother, as she has been in desperate need of a break from her caregiving role. Finally, Jacob receives an electronic device for the personal emergency response system, just in case he has an accident in which he needs immediate medical help.

In addition to the direct services Jacob receives, he has access to numerous consultation services. Jacob and his life skills coach met with a dietitian, from whom he receives a customized and easy to follow schedule for meal preparations. He also sees an autism spectrum disorder specialist and a behavior management specialist, both provided by the program. Previously, Jacob had relied on his mother to set up his appointments, but Jacob's case manager and coaches help him develop his own network. Each individual in the network offers services to enhance a different aspect of Jacob's life, as his mother transitions out of the caregiver role.

Another scenario might unfold for Jacob and his mother if they lived in Wyoming. The care of Jacob is reviewed below.

CASE UNFOLDING IN WYOMING

Jacob and his family enjoy the quiet life they live, but the lack of community resources has become an increasing issue for their family. Jacob's uncle, who visits frequently, lives almost

(*Continued*)

CASE UNFOLDING IN WYOMING (Continued)

one half-hour away in a neighboring town. Many of the services Jacob has needed have required his mother drive him to and from appointments. Jacob's mother applies for services under the Developmental Disabilities Division. Jacob is given limited access to service, as he does not have intellectual disability, which is the focus of the program in Wyoming. He is assigned a case manager, but there is no funding currently available for these services for Jacob. He is put on a waiting list, with no time frame provided.

While browsing through the department's website, Jacob's mother comes across a program involving the collaboration of a few states, including Wyoming, called AT4ALL, (https://www.wy.at4all.com/items/ItemSearch.aspx), which promotes independence by providing assistive technology for individuals with disabilities. Most are items of used medical equipment, such as wheelchairs, walkers, and adjustable tables, as well as technological equipment, such as televisions and computers. Almost all pieces of equipment are on loan, free of charge, for several years or more. These might be useful for Jacob and his family. His mother plans to use the grab-bar in her bathroom while she recuperates from her hip surgery and has decided to donate a leg brace leftover from when Jacob fractured his leg years ago.

Jacob and his mother found the loaned products to be of great help. They also plan to inquire about self-directed services, in which individuals and family decide which services best meet individual needs, including residential or day habilitation and supported living. These services include housecleaning; assistance with health issues; medications and medical services; aid with managing personal financial affairs; help with building and maintaining interpersonal relationships; and 24-hour emergency service. These are offered to the developmentally disabled population on a limited basis as funds are available. Services may also include supported employment; respite care; personal, environmental, and skilled nursing; specialized equipment; access to a dietician; and/or occupational, physical, and speech therapy, as needed.

CASE UNFOLDING IN ARIZONA

If this family lived in Arizona, they would need to contact the Division of Developmental Disabilities, which offers myriad services to eligible individuals with autism (among other disabled individuals). There are two different types of services for the aging adult. One service is the Arizona Long Term Care System (ALTCS), a federally funded Medicaid program designed for individuals like Jacob, who will possibly need decades of support. The second is support planning and services for developmentally disabled people, which is provided directly from the state.

If Jacob is accepted into the ALTCS, he will be provided with a health plan to cover a wide host of medical services, such as doctor's visits, prescriptions, hospital services, transportation to and from appointments, dental care, vision exams, specialist care, and more. In addition, he will be assigned to a case manager, who will schedule a number of services, including hospice care, assisted living, home-delivered meals, adult day care, health services, and access to a nursing facility. If Jacob is eligible to receive benefits only from the state support-planning and services program, he will not be enrolled in the health plan to pay for the numerous medical services and related costs listed above. He might receive such

(*Continued*)

CASE UNFOLDING IN ARIZONA (Continued)

services as attendant care, respite care, transportation, some therapies, and a home health aide. The services and supports are based on individual eligibility, as well as availability of funds and resources. Jacob's mother, however, is optimistic, as she believes help is coming for her son very soon.

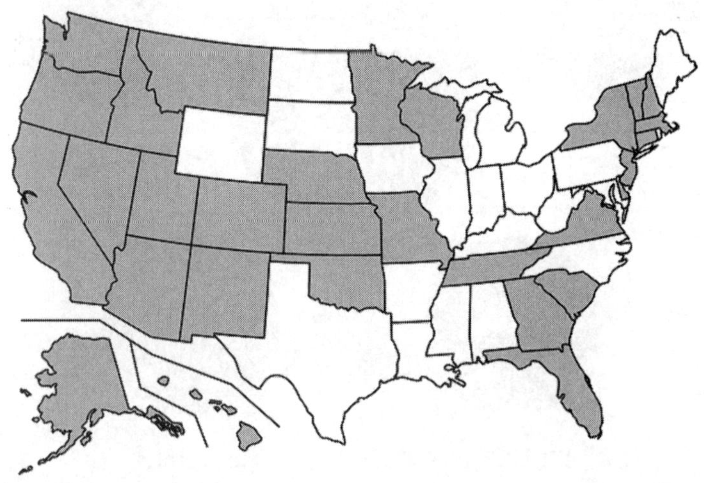

FIGURE 15.3 ■ States with easily searchable resources for autism-specific needs. Key: Shaded states have services easily located via the Internet. *Source:* http://en.wikipedia.org/wiki/File:Blank_US_map_borders.svg

Summary Points

While these three states are highlighted due to different or unique autism-specific resources or programs provided, professional staff working with families of adults with ASD, and families themselves, can have more or less difficulty locating appropriate, autism-specific, adult-focused resources in their localities. Internet searches for adult ASD-related services are useful if these services make their information available online. In addition, there is variability in the types and scope of such services available across the United States. Figure 15.3 maps the states where resources were easily identified using the Internet. We are not suggesting that resources specific for individuals with ASD do not exist in the unshaded states on the map, but rather that the diagram shows areas of the country in which these types of resources were readily available. To identify these, we first located the state website listing services for the intellectually disabled and next checked for specific resources or links to autism. This diagram also serves to illustrate challenges some families will face when trying to locate support for their sons or daughters with ASD.

BEST PRACTICES: CARE AND CASE MANAGEMENT

A case manager is assigned to help the individual with ASD navigate and access the various services and programs offered by the respective states. In addition to the more typical care management and care coordination roles in health care, nurses might also assume such

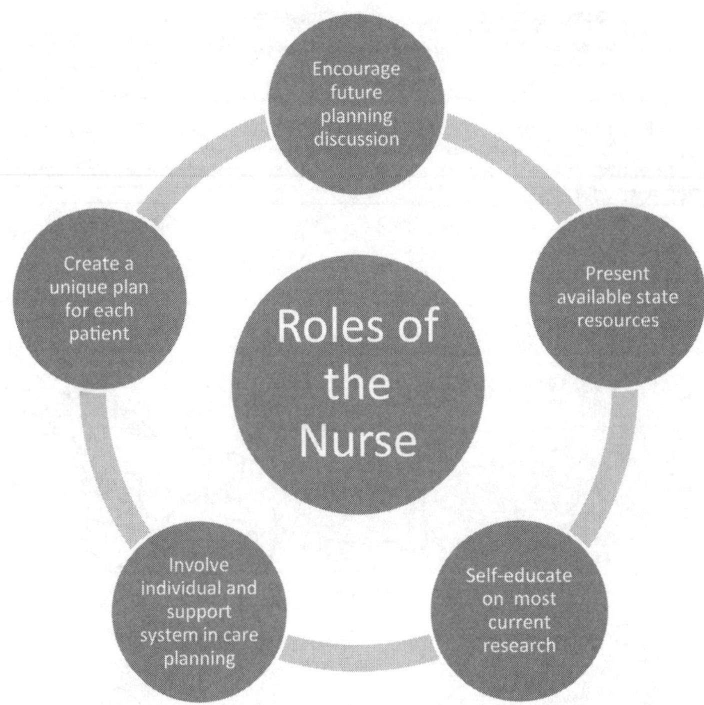

FIGURE 15.4 ■ Care management roles.

case management roles, particularly in community and home settings. A crucial step in the care and case management processes is to conduct a thorough needs assessment, which serves as a tool for planning, monitoring, and evaluating interventions and services available for the individual with ASD. We know that individuals and families can experience additional difficulties that are not specifically associated with the core symptoms of ASD. Such unmet needs also require specific attention, as they are associated with lower levels of quality of life (Renty & Roeyers, 2006). Comprehensive assessment of strengths and needs of the individual and family is very important.

Nurses may be ideal case managers. The role of the nurse as described throughout this chapter also involves establishing relationships with both the individual with autism and the family. Relationships are built on mutual trust and openness and will help ensure that when it is time to make difficult future planning decisions or to manage difficult transitions, the individual, parent caregiver, and nurse will be able to do so in a mutually supportive, trust-based environment. Importantly, the individual with ASD needs to be included at all levels of the discussion to the full extent of his or her ability. See Figure 15.4 for a schematic representation of the roles for nurses in ASD care.

SUMMARY

Considering the increased life expectancy of individuals with ASD and the aging of their caregivers, it is vital that future planning be integrated as a standard component of any plan of care. Decisions should not be delayed, particularly when the individuals with autism are adults and their caregivers are also growing older. Consideration of future needs and related decisions should ideally begin when the family is young. First and foremost, families and caregivers must formulate a plan for a transition of care in the event that the caregiver can no longer provide it. Second, caregivers must become aware of resources available in their states for individuals with ASD. Even if services are not needed immediately, the family should formally request these services in advance, because waiting lists and limited financing for such programs are common. Finally, caregivers must recognize that needs of individuals with ASD are continually evolving as they progress through life. Staying on top of needs is simply not enough; they must continually plan for tomorrow, anticipating problems they will inevitably face. The nurse plays a vital part in educating families about these issues, as well as about the resources and services that are available. Nurses should acknowledge issues and bring them to family members' attention, help to facilitate discussion about the future needs of the person with autism, identify appropriate services, make referrals, and assist families in accessing the needed services and programs.

Despite the variation in services offered and funds available in different states, all U.S. states have passed legislation related to funding and services for individuals with developmental disabilities. Some, like Connecticut, have targeted services for individuals on the autism spectrum. Developmental disability services offered in most states across the country include case management, individualized plans of care, care facilities, respite services, and various day services. Other commonly available services include transportation, emergency response, 24-hour assistance, residential living, medical services, and financial and employment assistance services. Since these services might have limited funding, it is wise to encourage families to apply for them before an accident, incident, or critical need occurs. There is an urgent need for all families with aging developmentally disabled family members to plan for future care, because the current caregiver situations will not be permanent.

REFERENCES

American Academy on Child and Adolescent Psychiatry. (2008). *Services in school for children with special needs fact-sheet: What parents need to know* (No. 83). Washington, DC: Author.

American Psychiatric Association. (2000). *Diagnostic and statistical manual of mental disorders, Text revision (DSM-IV-TR)*. Washington, DC: Author.

Beirne-Smith, M., Ittenbach, R., & Patton, J. (2002). *Mental retardation* (6 ed.). Columbus, OH: Merrill Prentice Hall.

Courchesne, E., Campbell, K., & Solso, S. (2011). Brain growth across the life span in autism: Age-specific changes in anatomical pathology. *Brain Research, 1380*, 138–145.

Esbensen, A. E., Greenberg, J. S., Seltzer, M. M., & Aman, M. G. (2009). A longitudinal investigation of psychotropic and non-psychotropic medication use among adolescents and adults with autism spectrum disorders. *Journal of Autism and Developmental Disorders, 39*, 1339–1349.

Grandin, T. (2011). Official website. http://www.templegrandin.com/templehome.html

Individuals with Disabilities Education Improvement Act, PL 108–446, 20 U.S.C. § 1400 *et seq.* (2004).

Individuals with Disabilities Education Act Amendments of 1997. (Public Law 105–17). Retrieved from http://www2.ed.gov/offices/OSERS/Policy/IDEA/index.html

Luce, J. (2010, May 9) World renowned autistic advocate Temple Grandin's mother to tell the family story. *Daily Kos.* Retrieved from http://www.dailykos.com/story/2010/5/9/124943/7452

Murphy, D. G. M., Beecham, J., Craig, M., & Ecker, C. (2011). Autism in adults: New biological findings and their translational implications to the cost of clinical services. *Brain Research*, 1380, 22–33. doi:10.1016/jbrainres.2010.10.042

Orsmond, G. I., Krauss, M. W., & Seltzer, M. M. (2004). Peer relationships and social and recreational activities among adolescents and adults with autism. *Journal of Autism and Developmental Disorders, 34*(3), 245–256.

Orsmond, G. I., & Seltzer, M. M. (2007). Siblings of individuals with autism or Down syndrome: Effects on adult lives. *Journal of Intellectual Disability Research, 51*(9), 682–696.

Parish, S. L., Seltzer, M. M, Greenberg, J. S., & Floyd, F. (2004). Economic implications of caregiving at midlife: Comparing parents with and without children who have developmental disabilities. *Mental Retardation, 42*(6), 413–426.

Pelchat, D., & Lefebvre, H. (2004). A holistic intervention programme for families with a child with a disability. *Journal of Advanced Nursing, 48*, 124–131.

Perkins, E. A., & Moran, J. A. (2010). Aging adults with intellectual disabilities. *Journal of the American Medical Association, 304*(1), 91–92.

Rapin, I., & Tuchman, R. F. (2008). Autism: Definition, neurobiology, screening, diagnosis. *Pediatric Clinics of North America, 55*(5), 1129–1146.

Renty, J. O., & Roeyers, H. (2006). Quality of life in high-functioning adults with autism spectrum disorder. *Autism, 10*, 511–524.

Rubin, I. L., & Crocker, A. C. (2006). *Medical care for children & adults with developmental disabilities* (2 ed.). Baltimore, MD: Paul H. Brookes.

Seltzer, M. M., Krauss, M. W., Orsmond, G. I., & Vestal, C. (2001). Families of adolescents and adults with autism: Uncharted territory. In L. M. Glidden (Ed.), *International review of research on mental retardation* (*Vol. 23*, pp. 267–294). San Diego, CA: Academic.

Shattuck, P. T., Seltzer, M. M., Greenberg, J. S., Orsmond, G. I., Bolt, D., Kring, S., Lounds, J., & Lord, K. (2007). Change in autism symptoms and maladaptive behaviors in adolescents and adults with an autism spectrum disorder. *Journal of Autism and Developmental Disorders, 37*, 1735–1747.

Totsika, V., Felce, D., Kerr, M., & Hastings, R. (2010). Behavior problems, psychiatric symptoms, and quality of life for older adults with intellectual disability with and without autism. *Journal of Autism and Developmental Disorders.* doi: 10.1007/s10803-010-0975-1

Turnbull, A. P. (2004). President's address 2004: "Wearing two hats": Morphed perspectives on family quality of life. *Mental Retardation, 42*(5), 383–399.

Ethical Issues in the Care of Individuals With Autism Spectrum Disorder in the Family and the Community: Hearing the Voice of the Person With Autism at the End of Life

16

Margaret J. Hegge

Ethical issues are present in the care of individuals with autism spectrum disorders (ASD) across the lifespan. Family and formal caregivers face difficult decisions about the aggressiveness of treatment options, the extent of the person's capacity to make reasoned decisions, and the level of support necessary for optimal development. Nurses often find themselves working with families in times of vulnerability and turmoil, when ethical decisions are required.

Optimal outcomes from these decisions are possible when the process involves parents, teachers, health care professionals, and other care providers. Collaborative decision making is particularly challenging and poignant as the pace of co-occurring disorders accelerates and the individual with autism is nearing the end of life. These times are fraught with cumulative stress and unpredictability that can uncover unresolved family conflicts that might impede mutual ethical decision making (Kramer, Kavanaugh, Trentham-Dietz, Walsh, & Yonker, 2010). Nurses working with individuals on the autism spectrum and their families need a thorough understanding of ethical principles as a foundation for making decisions in difficult situations. In this chapter, a case study of an adult with autism and terminal cancer illustrates the ethical and clinical considerations at end of life in the context of the family.

PATIENT-CENTERED CARE

Diagnosis and treatment of individuals with ASD have evolved significantly over the past decade. Early identification and diagnosis of children with ASD has enabled clinicians to employ interventions that increase the functional capacity of affected people across the lifespan. Caregivers welcome recent advances as they attempt to shape the behavior of their affected relatives, increase social interactions, and improve functional ability (A. Keating, personal communication, October 25, 2010). Previously, individuals with functional impairments might have been marginalized or discriminated against as a result of social and communication impairments, diminished functional capabilities, and atypical behavior (Vehmas, 2004). Preconceptions of a person's ability might frame the nurse's approach to caring for people with autism, and might result in communication that bypasses or circumvents the patient (Stein, 2007), particularly at the end of life. In the past, health care providers relied on a paternalistic model of care, in which health care providers made decisions they believed were in the best interests of patients. Such a model did not support the notion of mutual decision making (Stein, 2007). If health care providers considered a person to be incapable of developing deep personal relationships and that person's quality of life was considered less desirable, then decisions about end-of-life care might be made more quickly (Vehmas, 2004). The presence of significant functional impairments and communication impediments used to be adequate justification for withholding or withdrawing lifesaving medical treatment (Vehmas, 2004). In addition, when quality of life slipped below a perceived threshold, decisions about care might have been made based on the view that this type of life had less value (Vehmas, 2004). These decisions might be discriminatory against those with cognitive or verbal disabilities.

The concept of person-centered planning should underlie all discussions in the care of people with ASD (Kingsbury, 2004). Those with ASD should be directly involved in designing, modifying, and evaluating their own care as much as possible (Ghaziuddin, 2005; Kingsbury, 2004). Person-centered care is particularly needed when the person with ASD is dying—when ethical issues compound the complexity of many health care decisions.

National guidelines for quality end-of-life care combined with national interprofessional education and a growing body of research findings have improved care for those with life-limiting illnesses, particularly cancer. An expert panel synthesized western research literature related to end-of-life outcomes. Drawing from 95 systematic reviews, 134 intervention studies, and 682 observational studies, the panel concluded that palliative care has been most successfully melded into oncology care. Several interventions for cancer pain and depression have been found to be effective, while interventions for dyspnea and dementia are less robust (Agency for Healthcare Research and Quality [AHRQ], 2004). Resources related to end-of-life care for providers are readily accessible. Recognition of providers who specialize in palliative care is another step toward full integration of this important aspect of health care (Grant, Elk, Ferrell, Morrison, & von Gunten, 2009).

RESEARCH ON END-OF-LIFE CARE FOR THOSE WITH AUTISM

There is a growing body of research literature related to end-of-life care for persons with intellectual disabilities, but few studies focus specifically on autism (Barnard, Harvey, Potter, & Prior, 2001; Tuffrey-Wijne, Hogg, & Curfs, 2007). Evidence from the literature on intellectual disabilities can inform the nurse's approach to individuals with autism, because there are similarities in terms of family and caregiver issues, cognitive and communication barriers, and other factors. Most end-of-life research related to intellectual disability has been descriptive in nature, with a focus on assessment of pain and symptoms, informed consent, and decision making. Studies, for the most part, used retrospective case review, focus group, and interview methods to describe end-of-life phenomena. Findings suggest that helpful interventions in end-of-life care for this population include enabling persons with intellectual disabilities to live out their final days in their own environments, engaging them in familiar activities, and promoting a person-centered approach in collaboration with other health care providers and the family (King, Janicki, Kissinger, & Lash, 2005; Tuffrey-Wijne et al., 2007). Primary caregivers in these studies benefited from education, support, and respite care (Tuffrey-Wijne et al., 2007). Access to such services depends on many factors, including location, social and fiscal resources; urban areas might be more likely than rural areas to offer these services.

Case reports related to prolonging end-of-life treatment of individuals with intellectual disabilities have highlighted certain barriers to appropriate care. Such reports suggest that providers might hesitate to directly elicit the preferences related to withdrawal of treatment because of the threat of litigation alleging medical negligence or discrimination. The right or preference to refuse or withdraw treatment might be recognized, but not discussed directly, and thus futile care might be extended when such preferences are not raised up by the patient or family (Tuffrey-Wijne et al., 2007).

CASE–CLAYTON HAS CANCER

Clayton is a 54-year-old man with autism. He has an older sister, Dorothy, and a younger brother, Ted. Dorothy has been his major support system since their parents passed away. Ted resented the family attention devoted to Clayton, was embarrassed by his behavior in public, and quickly left home after high school, moving far away, with only rare trips home for funerals and weddings. He recalls several occasions when friends would taunt him about his weird brother. He has chosen to distance himself from Clayton because of guilt, leaving all decisions to his sister. While Dorothy is the major decision maker, no legal guardianship has been established.

Clayton lives in a basement apartment of Dorothy's home. He eats his meals with Dorothy and her husband Hank. Dorothy manages his finances and legal matters. Clayton does not work, loves to listen to classical music on his headphones, and reads the Encyclopedia Britannica daily, working his way from volume A to Z. He is currently in the D volume. Clayton's verbal speech is limited to two- to three-word phrases indicating his requests for food, need for assistance, toileting needs, and other simple commands. He uses picture cards for more complex communication. He has learned to use a magnetic alphabet to spell out his requests.

Clayton has headaches that have increased in frequency and duration over a period of weeks. This prompted a visit to his doctor. During this visit, the family met Susan, a nurse practitioner and case manager, who accompanied Dorothy and Clayton through the series of diagnostic tests needed to confirm a diagnosis. Multiple scans and tests are conducted with great difficulty and distress, given Clayton's aversion to physical touch and unfamiliar environments. Clayton is diagnosed with an inoperable metastatic brain tumor. Following the doctor's disclosure of this diagnosis, Susan spends an hour with Dorothy and Clayton explaining the disease, the likely options for treatment, and the most probable course of the symptoms over the next few months. She makes an appointment with the oncologist and asks if they would like her to go with them to this visit to help clarify the options and plan the next steps. Dorothy welcomes her presence and Clayton nods his agreement.

The oncologist offers a choice of cancer treatment: chemotherapy, radiation, chemotherapy plus radiation, or foregoing any further treatment. He emphasized that in any case, this is a terminal illness with possibly less than 6 months life expectancy. The oncologist suggests that they think about these options, determine what would be best for Clayton, and return for a second visit after having decided a course of treatment. Educational materials are offered to Clayton, who refuses to take them. Dorothy picks them up as she escorts Clayton to the exit. Following the brief visit with the oncologist, Susan reviews treatment options with Clayton and his sister, outlining costs, benefits, and side effects of each. Dorothy calls Ted to convey the diagnosis and need for family decisions about Clayton. Ted reluctantly agrees to fly home to participate in decision making. Dorothy wrestles with multiple concerns:

- To what extent does Clayton understand his condition and its implications?
- Does he want to be the key decision maker regarding his treatment? Does he want Dorothy to make these decisions, as she has in the past?
- Which treatment options are most desirable, from his viewpoint?

(*Continued*)

CASE–CONTINUED (Continued)

- How would he tolerate side effects of chemotherapy and/or radiation?
- How can we determine if he is in pain, has needs, or if comfort measures are working?
- How would he like to spend his last days?
- Would he tolerate a move from home to another setting, such as hospital or hospice?
- How does he understand death? What kind of a death experience would he prefer?

Dorothy is struggling with the anguish of a momentous decision that will impact Clayton's quality of life and her own commitment to care for him to the end. She realizes that the illness might create significant disorientation for Clayton. His typical coping behaviors might become ineffective; he might suffer. Dorothy wants to elicit Clayton's preferences and needs to allow as much independence as he chooses. She does not want to leave him alone in a health care system that might not accommodate his special needs. She does not want to disrupt his familiar routines but recognizes that treatments might disrupt the predictable daily structure of their lives. Dorothy's inclination is to forego all treatment and allow Clayton to do that which he loves living out his days in familiar surroundings. Ted insists that everything possible be done to treat the cancer. He is adamant that Clayton should live as long as possible, for whatever the cost. This conflict deepens over the following days.

Both Dorothy and Ted wish to know what Clayton wants, but communication about such complex issues is very difficult, considering his language and interaction deficits. It is difficult to determine what, and how much, he understands about his diagnosis and possible treatments. Ted cannot imagine "throwing in the towel, doing nothing, and letting the disease run its natural course." He states he would "never just give up like that" and insists aggressive treatment is preferable. Dorothy, on the other hand, imagines treatment side effects that would disrupt Clayton's daily routines.

ETHICAL GUIDANCE FOR END-OF-LIFE CARE

The next section contains a discussion of the major conceptual frameworks, approaches, and principles used to analyze ethical issues and to consider related clinical decisions for end-of-life complexities in collaboration with individuals with ASD and their families. These ethics perspectives help nurses, families, caregivers, and other involved parties resolve ethical conflicts and support clinical decisions that respect the preferences, needs, and uniqueness of individuals with ASD. These will be used in analysis of the chapter's unfolding case study.

Frameworks and Approaches to Ethical Decisions

Ethical frameworks are differentiated from ethical approaches by their origins. Ethical frameworks are built around principles of biomedical ethics. These frameworks derive from the two traditional but opposing philosophical perspectives of deontology (duty-based) ethics and teleology (outcome-based) ethics. Ethical approaches are more contemporary lenses through which to view situations. Virtue-based approaches capture the intention or

TABLE 16.1 ■ Ethical Frameworks, Approaches, and Principles

Ethical frameworks	Ethical approaches	Ethical principles
• Duty-based framework • Outcome-based framework	• Virtue-based • Ethics of caring	• Respect for persons • Autonomy • Beneficence • Nonmaleficence • Justice

motivation of the decision maker, relying on wisdom, discernment, humility, or other character traits. The ethic of caring approach evolved from a feminist perspective that emphasizes relationships of mutual trust as the driving force for making ethical decisions. These approaches are not opposing, and can be used together to understand ethically challenging clinical situations. Table 16.1 lists the ethical frameworks, approaches, and principles considered in clinical care of individuals with an ASD.

Duty-based Framework

Duty-based ethics emanate from a deontological philosophy first postulated by Immanuel Kant. Use of this highly rational model demands strict adherence to a set of moral imperatives, such as: do not lie, kill, steal, or harm others. This obligation-based model holds that people should always be treated as ends in themselves, never as means to the ends of another. A categorical imperative is the centerpiece of this framework, requiring the person as decision maker to consider the impact of the proposed action. The decision maker should ask, if the action were adopted as a universal mandate, would it be right for everyone in all circumstances through all time? Limitations of this framework are its rigidity and disregard for decisional consequences (Beauchamp & Childress, 2008). For example, a provider might strongly believe that every patient deserves the truth, regardless of consequences. Such a provider might be compelled by this *duty* to confront a patient with ASD with his or her impending death in frank terms that might significantly frighten him or her.

Outcome-based Framework

Teleology is an outcome-based ethical model, first described by John Stuart Mill and Jeremy Bentham in England. Anticipated consequences or outcomes drive decisions in this framework. Desired outcomes revolve around welfare, happiness, and best interests. An extension of this theory is utilitarianism, which is concerned with creating the greatest good for the greatest number or the largest benefit for the most people. One difficulty with this theory is that consequences are difficult if not impossible to predict (Beauchamp & Childress, 2008). For example, a provider caring for a patient with ASD who is dying at home might believe that this situation creates undue hardships on the family caregiver (consequence) and does not improve the quality of the patient's life. The provider might recommend quick transfer to inpatient hospice care, despite family or individual preferences for home care, in order to create the greatest good for the most people.

Virtue-based Approach

A virtue is an enduring character trait that matures over time. These positive attributes orient a person toward compassion, humility, trustworthiness, integrity, and conscientiousness

(Beauchamp & Childress, 2008). Other virtues include courage, wisdom, and generosity. A person with a virtue-based ethic derives decisions from these inner motivations, rather than from any external rules, duties, or considerations of consequences. Character development drives this ethical framework. A drawback of this framework is the potential corruptibility of human nature. Under stress or with other pressures, a person might choose expedience or comfort over virtue (Vehmas, 2004, p. 219). A virtuous health professional would act from the intention of compassion to ensure that the person with ASD and his family experience the greatest quality of life possible within the remaining days of life.

The Ethic of Caring

The ethic of caring is a philosophical, feminist perspective that focuses on the meaning of relationships, quality of life, and support for the vulnerable through human presence (Watson, 2006). This framework was derived from the work of Noddings (2003) and emphasizes the primacy of human relationships, nurturance, and the existential encounter. This perspective offers an alternative to impartial duty- or justice-based calculations. The model is depicted as concentric circles that capture the central obligation of caring for another. The internal or closest circle involves those capable of reciprocating; the next involves those within close proximity to the individual, and next, distant others in need. Responsibility for others diminishes as proximity decreases, moving progressively from caring for, to caring about, others (Noddings, 2003). The concentric circles can be interpreted as the layers at which different intensities or purposes of caring occur in different contexts (Noddings, 2003). For health professionals, the duty to patients creates an immediate intimacy through a caring relationship. Thus, the stranger (patient) moves to the center of the concentric circle, becoming the one-cared-for by the professional, but without expectation of reciprocity. This framework calls for individualized care tailored to the expressed needs, values, and priorities of the patient and family. The ethic of care is a nimble approach that emphasizes the presence of the nurse in relationship with the patient and family in the development of mutual goals for quality of life. In this model, value is placed on mutual respect, compassion, fidelity, and emotional investment (Penticuff, 2006). A limitation of this model is its intuitive, fluid nature, which is challenging to describe in measurable or quantifiable terms.

Ethical Principles

A basic moral norm in our society is the *respect for persons* (Beauchamp and Childress, 2008). The American Nurses Association (ANA) Code of Ethics for Nurses places respect for persons in the very forefront of all other ethical considerations, and states, "The nurse, in all professional relationships, practices with compassion and respect for the inherent dignity, worth and uniqueness of every individual, unrestricted by considerations of social or economic status, personal attributes, or the nature of health problems" (ANA, 2001, p. 7). By virtue of being human, every person deserves respect, regardless of disability, cognitive capacity, or approaching death (ANA, 2001, provision 1.3).

Autonomy is the self-determination of the patient. The ANA Code of Ethics calls for nurses to respect patients' autonomy, supporting and facilitating patients' decisions, even when these differ from their own preferences (ANA, 2001). Autonomy might be too narrowly defined by the current bioethics community. A dying person does not approach the final days of life as a lone logical decision maker, bravely facing his own demise and simply adhering to his or her advance directives (Robert Wood Johnson Foundation, 2006). Studies have shown that people progressing through terminal illnesses do not cling to their autonomous decisions about the plan of care, but instead turn to family members to make new decisions on their behalf as the complexities of the disease and its treatment demand (RWJF, 2005).

Beneficence is the intention to do what is best for patients, moving them toward a better quality of life (Beauchamp & Childress, 2008). "Beneficence has been generally understood as saving a life whenever possible; withdrawing treatments when unwanted; and alleviating suffering, especially when cure is not possible" (Byock, 2004, p. 13). This amounts to avoiding, minimizing, or terminating services when they no longer alleviate symptoms or promote optimal functional status (Byock, 2004). This is a rather narrow view of beneficence. Acting in the patient's best interests should also take into account the well-being of the person and the personal and spiritual growth that can occur at the end of life (Byock, 2004).

Beneficence in the extreme is *paternalism*, where a provider assumes he or she knows what is best for the patient, regardless of patient or family preferences. A somewhat derogatory term, paternalism often conveys a power differential in which a more powerful person imposes his or her will on a person with less capacity to ensure that person's safety (Beauchamp & Childress, 2008).

Nonmaleficence is the intention to avoid harm, alleviate suffering or remove harm (Beauchamp & Childress, 2008). Harms might encompass depriving a person of due rights, causing offense, incapacitating the person, inflicting pain or suffering, or ending a person's life (Beauchamp & Childress, 2008). Harming someone else through negligence or incompetence is unacceptable under this principle. At times, inflicting a temporary harm might result in lesser harm later, as in the case of chemotherapy to diminish a tumor. Treatment decisions, therefore, can involve weighing the short-term harm with the long-term benefits of less harm later (Beauchamp & Childress, 2008).

Justice is defined as the fair, equitable, appropriate treatment based on what is owed to people (Beauchamp & Childress, 2008). *Distributive justice* is a concept that requires fair use of society's resources, using a rationale of societal norms, rights, and responsibilities (Beauchamp & Childress, 2008). Decisions about allocation of scarce organs for transplant to thousands of qualified candidates on a waiting list are made using the principle of distributive justice. Decisions about allocation of the federal health care budget by balancing competing proposals are also made through a distributive justice framework using public justifications.

A striking *injustice* in ASD care involved racial and ethnic disparities in diagnosis, with significantly more White children diagnosed correctly with ASD. African Americans have often been diagnosed at least 2 years later than White children. Delayed or missed ASD diagnoses result in delays in treatment and can contribute to lifelong neurobehavioral deficits (Mandell et al., 2009). Native American children might be misdiagnosed with ASD when their apparent verbal delays or perceived disability might be due to cultural differences in language development (A. Keating, personal communication, October 25, 2010).

Ethical Principles Applied to the Case

Dorothy is attempting to support Clayton's *autonomy*, despite his inability to express his desires. As the surrogate decision maker, she is using the *best interests standard* to make decisions. Dorothy clearly wants the best quality of life for Clayton that is possible at this point (*beneficence*). Dorothy is considering the harm that might result from side effects or a physical move into a hospice unit, which would greatly disrupt his daily routine, causing him distress—the principle of *nonmaleficence*. She uses the principle of *justice* to weigh costs of each option to determine the best use of family funds and insurance combined with Medicaid resources. After the emotionally charged reunion with Clayton, Ted is struggling with guilt and remorse, which color his perception of the current situation. Ted believes he knows what is best for Clayton and wishes to pursue aggressive treatment for him. That would be his own preference if he were similarly ill. He does not explore Clayton's preferences for treatment and assumes he knows what is most appropriate. He is acting from the perspective of *paternalism.*

Health Care Professional's Ethical Perspective

A nurse practicing from a *virtue-based ethic* would be compassionate, honest, and loyal to Clayton and his caregiver. This framework does not specify a plan of action; the plan would evolve from the virtues of the nurse as they play out in the situation. A nurse practicing from a *duty-based ethic* would uphold ethical principles, regardless of consequences. In the deontological context, based on the principle of justice, the nurse's duty is to ensure that Clayton receives medically indicated therapy and nursing care for his cancer, in order to avoid discrimination on the basis of his autism. A nurse practicing from an *outcome-based ethic* would attempt to predict the consequences of illness and treatment and to avoid interventions that would diminish Clayton's quality of life in his remaining months. A nurse practicing from an *ethic of caring* philosophy would work with Dorothy, Ted, and Clayton to delve deeply into the existential reality, help to elicit the meaning for each within that new reality, and chart a course for the future that addresses mutual goals for the best quality of life possible, given the situation. The nurse would support Dorothy in her role as advocate for Clayton, key informant about his wishes and major organizer of the plan of care on his behalf.

NURSING ROLES AT DIAGNOSIS AND BEYOND

The time of diagnosis is filled with uncertainty and tension. The family and dying patient are integrally wound together, either or both experiencing loss and grief, which can manifest itself in fractious family dynamics (Byock, 2004). The sense of time running out heightens these tensions (Byock, 2004), and tensions might be complicated by issues related to autism. Family members might find themselves unable to converse together honestly about these complex issues without falling into old traps of blame, guilt, and resentment (Turnbull, 2004). Guilt, shame, fear, and resentment can obstruct decision making related to treatment choices or preferences for care (McCarron & McCallion, 2007; RWJF, 2001). During this difficult time, a nurse might work with the family to help surface these tensions, address them, and facilitate realistic decision making about end-of-life care in the best interests of the patient. Referrals to family therapists, social workers, psychiatric services, or ethics committees might be indicated.

CASE–CONTINUED

To the extent that Clayton is able to participate in decision making, he should participate. An ongoing dialogue will be needed as the disease process progresses. Mutual goals for his care will be developed, refined, and modified as needs change over the course of Clayton's illness. Susan, as his nurse and case manager will help the family anticipate and resolve end-of-life concerns as they arise. Since Dorothy has worked with Clayton throughout

(*Continued*)

CASE (Continued)

his life, she understands his communication patterns and is the best judge of his wishes. Dorothy knows intuitively that there will be unpredictable effects of the disease on Clayton's behavior. She knows he will be afraid, that his routine will be disrupted occasionally, and that the plan of care must be flexible to accommodate his behavioral responses. She also knows her stress level will increase as she tries to keep Clayton comfortable and stable. Susan will work with the entire family to help them prepare for Clayton's needs at the end of life.

The plan of care will involve an ongoing dynamic partnership, with weekly home visits to manage behaviors, adjust medications, and respond to unanticipated symptoms and side effects. Susan will support their exploration of the meaning of this diagnosis/prognosis, and support them in anticipatory grieving, saying goodbye, and dealing with loss (MacLeod & Johnston, 2007).

Family Information and Support Needs

While the initial diagnosis of illness might be delivered by another health care professional, such as an oncologist, nurses are intimately involved with end-of-life diagnoses and care and should help patients and family members to understand the information. The patient, caregiver, and other family members or involved individuals should have accurate information about diagnosis, prognosis, and treatment options, as well as timely referral to appropriate resources. Nurses should verify an accurate understanding of the situation, clarify or correct misunderstandings, and answer questions (American College of Physicians, 2009). The nurse can observe and listen to the family responses, and support family members and significant others in the process of making sense of the diagnosis and related information. Clinicians might help family members determine who else should be told about the diagnosis, as well as how much information others might need to best support the family (American College of Physicians, 2009). The caregiver should be asked about his or her abilities and commitment to care for the ill individual, given the anticipated demands. Needs for support and assistance with care should be assessed, and warning signs of caregiver fatigue, emotional disorders, and need for respite care explored initially and then re-explored with subsequent clinical encounters (American College of Physicians, 2009). The family might need additional training or referrals for counseling or other support services.

Although these factors are important in the care of both terminally ill individuals and their families, further improvements in the approach to such care are still needed. A recent multistate survey of more than 700 nurses explored essential nursing skill sets for care of terminally ill patients. The authors reported that management of patient and caregiver anxiety and depression and use of patient-centered care systems were the primary areas of nursing practice needing additional attention. Findings suggest the need for health care system improvements and additional education to equip nurses with the knowledge and resources necessary for more comprehensive end-of-life care (Reinke et al., 2010).

Decision-making and Consent for Treatment

Decisions about health care can weigh heavily on families, because these often require a good grasp of very complex medical, emotional, and economic issues. Treatment decisions should be guided by informed consent, which assures that decision makers have a full understanding of options for care, risks, benefits, and rights (Goldsmith, Skirton, & Webb, 2008). Effective case management can minimize decision-making burdens on families by streamlining health care processes and bringing information from multiple sources together (Winzelberg, Hanson, & Tulsky, 2005). Family meetings involving the oncologist, nurse case manager, and all providers can help integrate the perspectives of family and health care team, clarify expectations, and keep communication open, so the evolving care plan has the support of all involved.

A discussion of the primary goal of treatment should take place early in the diagnostic process so that all family members can share their perspectives and intentions (Bade, 2008). Discussion should center on any conflicting goals, such as keeping the patient alive as long as possible or allowing a natural death with comfort measures (Bade, 2008). Decisions at the end of life ideally should be made by the individual in collaboration with closest family members (Kleepsies, 2004). Each individual, regardless of decisional capacity, has rights and an interest in making decisions during a terminal illness to the extent capacity allows (Stein, 2007). Few people make these complex decisions at the end of life entirely on their own (Family Caregiver Alliance, 2010b).

Respect for autonomy can collide with the obligation to protect a vulnerable individual from harm (Stein, 2008). The balance between overprotection and underprotection is dynamic, as situations evolve moment by moment, requiring new decisions (Stein, 2008). Collaborative, shared decision making can support the best interests of the patient but might require facilitation by a health care professional, case manager, or counselor. Providers should make every effort to hear and respect the patient's wishes; patients should be asked to identify longevity or comfort as the primary goal, asked what quality of life means to them, and asked what would be the worst choice for them (Winzelberg et al., 2005).

Individuals are presumed capable of autonomy in decision making unless legally determined to be incapable (AHRQ, 2004, 2008). They should be encouraged to communicate their preferences and end-of-life wishes through verbal, nonverbal, textual, pictorial or other means (AHRQ, 2004, 2008). However, since the person with autism is often dependent on family members or caregivers for many activities of daily life, the person's autonomy might not be fully manifested, but instead indirectly pursued by the caregiver (King et al., 2005; Schelly, 2008). For example, people with ASD might have been socialized to rely on adult feedback to guide their behavior, and additionally, often rely on others to adjust the environment to minimize disruptive outbursts and maintain their safety (Hume, Loftin, & Lantz, 2009). Conversely, a caregiver might be uncertain about the treatment preferences or wishes of the individual who is ill (King et al., 2005). As a terminal illness progresses, reassessment is needed. However, with disease progression, an individual with ASD might have increasing difficulty communicating his or her preferences (Diesfeld, 2000).

Assessing Capacity

The capacity for decision making is not simply present or absent, but is dependent on various factors, which can include time of day, concentration on the task at hand, habit, or conditioning (RWJF, 2001). An individual with autism might be competent in some tasks, yet incapable of others. Capacity can be task-specific, so assessment of capacity should include several, different tests (RWJF, 2001). Timing and setting are also key for accurate assessment of capacity for decision making. The individual should be in a distraction-free environment, at the peak time for clear thinking, with no physical symptoms impeding communication or conversation. A familiar individual should be present but silent until the patient requests assistance or intervention. Any commonly used communication supports, such as picture cards, magnetic letters, or computer keyboards, should be provided, along with adequate time for their use, and a familiar staff presence. Assessment focuses on the capacity to express a preference that can be defended by logical reasons and/or the capacity to conceptualize a desired future in light of current diagnosis/prognosis (American College of Physicians, 2009; RWJF, 2001). These facets or abilities are essential for a terminally ill person to exercise true autonomy in the process of informed consent and decision making:

1. Ability to express a choice,
2. Ability to understand information about treatment options,
3. Ability to interpret information about illness and treatment, and
4. Ability to logically weigh treatment options and select the one that best reflects personal values (Kleepsies, 2004).

A recent review of studies on health care informed consent in people with learning disabilities supports the theory that the greater the cognitive and verbal ability of an individual, the greater the capacity to provide authentic consent. Patients also benefit when the provider adapts information to the individual's capacity (Goldsmith, Skirton, & Webb, 2008).

Due to language deficits and limitations in ability to project the future, a person with autism is likely to fall below the threshold of capacity for the complex mental gymnastics required to exercise true autonomy as defined above (Schelly, 2008). If a determination of diminished capacity is made, a surrogate decision maker can be named to act on behalf of the individual with autism. Autonomy should remain a goal, so that decisions support the values, wishes, and life trajectory that the patient has previously expressed in some way. Evidence of the person's wishes can be contextualized in a narrative life story capturing a realistic perspective about the patient (Torke, Alexander, & Lantos, 2008). Such statements as "He was always a fighter" or "He hated going to the doctor" convey preferences—often overlooked in a crisis situation (Torke et al., 2008). Decisions should be made within the context of the current situation and expected disease trajectory (Torke et al., 2008).

The concept of "assisted capacity" promotes the involvement of individuals with diminished capacity, along with family members and health providers, in care planning to the degree that they choose to be involved. Appropriate supports, advocates, and assistance are provided to enable meaningful participation (Stein, 2008). Shared decision making is conducted within the community of care to preserve the best interests of the individual, and to determine and respect the individual's previous life preferences, values, and wishes (Stein, 2008).

End-of-life decisions are not single events, but a series of iterative decision points as the disease process progresses (King et al., 2005). Decisions are needed about personal care, household care, health care, emotional support, supervision, and respite care for the caregiver (Family Caregiver Alliance, 2010a). These complex medical, ethical, legal, and personal considerations weave through family conversations and create additional tensions that can affect daily life, disrupting sleep and the cognitive ability of caregivers and family members to deal logically with them (RWJF, 2007). Outcomes of complex decisions are not always ideal; choices or preferences might be unrealistic or might result in unpredictable consequences. The individual's future is essentially unknowable (Kopelman, 2007). No best decisions or easy answers guarantee benefits when time is limited and health is deteriorating (Kopelman, 2007). Several iterations of a care plan might be needed as the disease and its treatment evolve. Backup plans should be formulated and adapted as needed, with a flexible approach to address rapidly shifting circumstances (Family Caregiver Alliance, 2010a).

Health Care Proxy

A patient might choose a health care proxy who can make decisions on his or her behalf until the choice is revoked or the patient dies (AHRQ, 2008). The proxy is appointed with a formal written authorization, with the patient's full knowledge and voluntary assent, including the right to revoke the proxy if the person is not fulfilling his or her wishes (Lynden, 2010). The proxy makes decisions about diet, recreation, exercise, medications, treatments, procedures, and life-sustaining therapies (Stein, 2007). Decisions should be made within the best interests standard and from a patient-centered perspective (Kopelman, 2007). Given the proxy's knowledge of the patient's values, lifestyle, preferences, and personality, this individual attempts to select the option the patient would choose if he were competent (Torke, Alexander, & Lantos, 2008).

A patient with ASD might need assistance communicating about such complex issues with the proxy, so that wishes are known by the health team, and integrated with the care plan (Agency for Healthcare Research and Quality, 2008). The proxy might need training, counseling, and/or legal direction to make difficult choices about continued life, comfort measures, pain control and communication mechanisms (Kleepsies, 2004; RWJF, 2006). The proxy's substituted judgment is based on the presumption that he or she is choosing options with good will, attempting to respect values and preferences of the person with ASD, and to make life choices that the person with ASD would make if capable of doing so (Torke, Alexander, & Lantos, 2008). Families can also resolve differences of opinion when a third party helps them form a similar substituted judgment based upon the life values and preferences of the patient (Torke Alexander, & Lantos, 2008).

Facilitating Communication about End-of-Life Issues

Conversations about life choices should begin early and continue throughout the course of the terminal illness. These discussions should involve the patient, the caregiver, and any other significant people in the patient's community of concern (Forrester-Jones and Broadhurst, 2007). To facilitate this process and support the autonomy of patients with limited verbal communication skills, nurses should start from the premise that everyone can communicate, given sufficient time and appropriate assistance. Adequate time for processing and responding to information and a distraction-free environment are basic, crucial components of communication with individuals who have verbal communication impairments (RWJF, 2001). Interruptions should be minimized. Everyone involved should be sitting at eye level, to minimize perceptions of power differentials. If the patient has limited verbal communication skills, the nurse should pace the conversation to his or her rhythm of speech (Forrester-Jones & Broadhurst, 2007). Various forms of interaction can be used, from texting to handwriting to nonverbal cues to picture cards, in order to facilitate expression of the individual's preferences for end-of-life care. Only one topic should be discussed at a time to avoid confusion (Forrester-Jones & Broadhurst, 2007).

CASE–CONTINUED

Susan convenes a family meeting with Clayton, Dorothy, and Ted. She begins by asking about concerns about Clayton's condition. She then asks the family to consider their

(*Continued*)

CASE (Continued)

current goals. She asks "What would Clayton want now?" Susan explores the acceptability of home nursing visits for pain management and comfort care. Clayton is asked if the visiting nurse can touch him and he nods yes. He is shown pictures of an indwelling urinary catheter and of intravenous fluid therapy. Susan explains what these are and that they might be needed; Clayton shakes his head, indicating no. Dorothy asks about remedies for some of Clayton's symptoms. Ted begins to cry, and states, "It's just not fair, he has struggled his whole life, and now to suffer like this, it is not fair!" They discuss aggressive treatment to prolong life and comfort care to preserve Clayton's quality of life. Neither Dorothy nor Ted can envision Clayton enduring side effects of aggressive treatment, the rationale for which he would not understand. Ted agrees that such treatment would add to Clayton's suffering, and would not result in a "longer life worth living." Dorothy is relieved about the mutual decision that Clayton will live out his days within his normal routine. Susan introduces the possibility that hospice services might be needed as the end draws near. More complex issues are explored, including what dying might mean to Clayton: separation from family, friends, and community, loss of favorite pastimes, and spiritual concerns. Finally, the discussion addresses preferences for Clayton's remaining weeks of life, such as:

- Where to spend the last weeks of life: They agree that he should be in his apartment with Dorothy as long as possible in order to maintain the daily routine in his structured, stable environment.
- Activities each person has always wanted to do: Ted says he always promised to take Clayton fishing on a nearby lake. Clayton indicates he does want to go fishing with his brother; they begin to plan the day.
- Who should be at the bedside when the patient is dying: Clayton wants Dorothy nearby through the entire process of illness and dying.
- Legacy planning, leaving belongings to loved ones: Clayton agrees to go through his things and mark them so that Dorothy knows to whom they go.

Susan talks about the anticipatory grieving that is already happening. She offers suggestions for life review, reminiscence, and closure, such as the use of photo albums, talking about memorial services, visiting the cemetery where their parents are buried, and making plans for special remembrances to be shared. She asks if their pastor should be contacted to provide spiritual support. The family agrees that this step would be helpful right now. Since Clayton has never attended a funeral, they consider whether he might attend the funeral of an older adult neighbor who recently passed away.

Progression of Illness and Symptom Management

Nurses should help their patients and family members establish clear mutual goals, encouraging questions, and responding immediately with honest, straightforward answers in terms the patient and family can understand (Forrester-Jones & Broadhurst, 2007). These decision points will be revisited as the disease progresses and adjusted accordingly, but should remain tuned to the patient's wishes or caregiver preferences, as based on the caregiver's past experiences with the patient (Rosetti, Ashby, Arndt, Chadwich, & Kasahara, 2008). Nurses should implement realistic plans for symptom assessment, with emphasis on the assessment and management of pain. Pain is a personal subjective experience that cannot be objectively quantified (Herr et al., 2006). When self-reporting of pain is not feasible because of verbal limitations, behavioral cues to distress should be assessed frequently. A baseline behavior assessment should be documented in order to compare and track the trajectory of pain throughout the course of the illness (Herr et al., 2006). The caregiver knows the meaning of behavioral clues better than anyone else and should be relied on to monitor the level of distress of the nonverbal patient (Herr et al., 2006). Behavioral assessment scales such as the Behavioral Pain Scale (Payen et al., 2001) or the Disability Distress Assessment Tool (DisDAT, 2006) might be used. A 10-point rating scale from mild to severe has been developed with progressive behavioral indicators of increasing pain, beginning with happy expression, and progressing to restless squirming, to distorted face, to crying with tremors (P. Pian, personal communication, November 6, 2010). This tool requires direct observation by the nurse with a judgment about the meaning of these behavioral cues. The goal should be pain relief and comfort sufficient to enable the person to enjoy life in usual ways, communicate with loved ones, and spend time doing what he enjoys (Herr et al. 2006). Refer also to Exhibit 13.3 for a sample of a pain scale specific to individuals with ASD.

CASE–PAIN MANAGEMENT

Susan asks Dorothy to describe Clayton's behavior when he is happy, calm, and pain-free. Dorothy responds that Clayton reads or listens to music with no facial expression when he is totally content. Dorothy is then asked to describe Clayton's behavioral signs of discomfort or pain. She reports that Clayton clicks his tongue against his teeth when he is mildly distressed. The greater the distress, the faster his tongue clicks. If pain increases, Clayton rocks from side to side with a facial grimace. When he is in extreme pain, Clayton curls into a fetal position on the floor and pulls at his eyelashes. This has only been observed once, when his wisdom teeth became impacted. Susan constructs a visual pain scale, placing these behavioral clues at the 0, 3, 6, and 9 positions on the scale. Then Susan asks Dorothy about the types of pain relief that work best for Clayton. Dorothy says that for mild distress, Clayton responds well to lower lights, soft classical music, and aspirin. Ibuprofen relieves Clayton's moderate pain. When experiencing pain from wisdom teeth, a visit to the dentist resulted in extractions followed by antibiotics and opioids. Susan inserts these proven pain relief strategies into the pain scale in the appropriate mild, moderate and severe categories and arranges the appropriate prescriptions. She and Dorothy discuss how to track, record, and respond to Clayton's indications of pain using this individualized pain scale.

Pain may be especially difficult to assess in the nonverbal patient with ASD. For Clayton, changes in behavior offer the best clues. Behaviors to assess are facial expressions (unusual or distorted expressions); vocalizations, such as increased outbursts, grunting, or noisy breathing; and body movements, such as increased fidgeting, pacing, rocking, or other self-stimulation. The nurse should also be observing for changes in interpersonal interactions, such as increased withdrawal or aggressiveness. Changes in activity patterns and emotional outbursts may all suggest the pain is out of control and the patient with ASD is experiencing intense difficulty communicating his or her distress (Ferrel, Fine, & Herr, 2010; Herr et al., 2010). For nonverbal patients, an alternative approach consists of administering analgesics and then evaluating behavioral changes related to pain (Herr et al., 2010). Assessment of pain using visual scales is presented in detail in Chapter 13.

QUALITY OF LIFE

Quality of life is the subjective self-perception of well-being that shifts momentarily in response to internal and external factors. Quality-of-life estimations are often critical considerations in end-of-life decisions, but only the person living that life can determine its actual quality. As distressing symptoms escalate, a patient with a terminal illness might experience declining physical well-being, but might transcend discomfort to find greater quality in interpersonal or spiritual dimensions. "In the face of death, people can experience contentment and an ongoing sense of importance, meaning and value in life despite considerable discomfort and profound functional limitations" (Byock, 2004, p. 15). A young person in the peak of health might find any shift in physical stamina unacceptable, while an older person who has adjusted to physical quirks, chronic disease, or moderate discomforts might have a less idealistic view of quality of life. Even individuals who claim that they would not wish to live if quality of life fell below a specified threshold might find this benchmark shifting with disease progression; the previously unacceptable quality of life might become more acceptable. Conversely, individuals might determine that they are ready to withdraw or forego treatment as their disease progresses.

The majority of people with intellectual disabilities rate their quality of life high, even though health care providers would not (Stein, 2007). Gill is quoted as saying "health professionals significantly underestimate the quality of life of persons with disabilities compared with the actual assessments made by persons with disabilities themselves . . . Such pessimistic professional views of life with disability are implicitly conveyed to patients and their families while they are in the midst of decision-making. . . . and are related to professional's views about whether or not to offer life-sustaining treatment options to persons with disabilities" (Gill, 2000). Those with higher levels of adaptive skills have been found to report better quality of life, as they are more engaged with family and community (Diesfeld, 2000; Totsika, Felce, Kerr, & Hastings, 2010). Family members might also judge their relative's quality of life to be lower than the actual quality of life that the person with autism experiences (Vehmas, 2004). Ultimately, quality of life is determined by the perceptions of the individual who is living that life (Schelly, 2008).

Questions about hospitalization, foregoing life-sustaining treatment, withholding or withdrawing nutrition and hydration, and "Do Not Resuscitate" orders often lead to discussions about costs of care and allocation of scarce resources to prolong life in a person whose quality of life is considered by the health care providers as less than ideal. This perspective can devalue the lives of patients with intellectual deficits and create additional concerns related to futile treatments (Stein, 2007). Absent clear and convincing evidence of the desires of people with disabilities to decline life-sustaining procedures, care and treatment should not be withheld or withdrawn unless "death is genuinely imminent and the care or treatment is objectively futile, and would only prolong the dying process" (Center for Human Policy, n.d., e-1).

"Family Quality of Life" involves "conditions where the family's needs are met, and family members enjoy their life together as a family and have a chance to do things which are important to them" (Park et al., 2003, p. 368). In the context of end-of-life care, an important consideration is how to maximize family quality of life in the time remaining (American College of Physicians, 2009). This means intentionally creating activities to add meaning and growth opportunities for dying patients and their families (Byock, 2004). Caregivers might need training, respite care, support groups, and counseling to create and sustain these meaningful activities. Family members of terminally ill individuals frequently adopt a protective stance, intervening between the provider and the patient, and intending to act in the person's best interests (Stein, 2007). Often the patient will be excluded from these conversations. Using the best interests standard, both family and providers should consider the environment that will most likely facilitate well-being for the patient; applying this standard to the question of environment might promote selection of environments that are less restrictive than traditional medical facilities, such as hospitals or other inpatient settings (Diesfeld, 2000).

Palliative Care

When death is imminent, treatment is reframed to a "comfort measure only" emphasis. Ninety percent of people prefer to die at home, yet only 20% do so (Center for Gerontology and Health Care Research, 2000). Palliative care begins with the assumption that life should be lived to its fullest during the normal dying process, that comfort is a focus, and that families should be supported as they cope with caregiving, dying, and grief related to the illness of a loved one. An interdisciplinary team approach is required to meet the physical, emotional, social, and spiritual needs of those experiencing a terminal illness and their families. The goal of palliative care is enhanced quality of life (World Health Organization, 2002). Palliative care is built around partnerships with families to support them in designing, managing, and modifying a plan of care to enhance comfort and minimize pain and anxiety. Palliative care can occur in inpatient or home settings. At home, palliative care includes home visits for environmental assessment, medication management, and family support through the disease process. Interventions are designed to support family decision making, especially during times of unpredictable effects of disease on behavior.

The focus is on improving quality of life across the dying trajectory through anticipation, prevention, and relief of suffering. Functional capacity is optimized through ongoing symptom management, informed by the patient's and family's cultural and spiritual values and practices, which can include complementary and alternative therapies. There is an emphasis on continuity of care throughout the illness and across settings, including hospice services. Practical needs are addressed in a patient/family-centered care approach that offers 24-hour-a-day access to a trusted health care provider. Palliative care provides bereavement support and creates opportunities for growth and healing rituals for the family (National Consensus Project for Quality Palliative Care, 2009). Clinical practice Guidelines for Quality Palliative Care are available free of charge from this website: http://www.nationalconsensusproject.org/AboutGuidelines.asp.

CASE–CONCLUSION

Dorothy calls Susan, sobbing, telling her that Clayton has been inconsolable. He has been writhing in a fetal position on the floor, with a facial grimace and high-pitched whining, for 2 hours. He is grasping his head with both hands. Dorothy has crushed his acetaminophen with codeine in water and tried to administer it, but Clayton will not open his mouth. With Dorothy's permission, Susan calls an ambulance to transport Clayton to the hospital, where he is admitted to the oncology unit under the supervision of the palliative care team. An IV is inserted for administration of morphine. He falls asleep within 15 minutes. Dorothy sleeps in the recliner in Clayton's room so that she can calm him when he awakens in a strange environment. She contacts Ted to inform him of Clayton's hospitalization. Ted lashes out at her, accusing her of not watching him closely enough and allowing

(*Continued*)

CASE (Continued)

his pain to get out of control. Exhausted, Dorothy starts to cry. Susan takes her to a private room and listens. Susan suggests another family conference to talk about what lies ahead and Dorothy agrees. Susan calls Ted, who agrees to a meeting the next day.

Susan sighs, realizing that some family conflicts are deep-seated, beyond her ability to resolve. Clayton's cancer has driven a deeper wedge between Ted and Dorothy at a time when they each need additional support. Clayton remains on the oncology unit for the next 3 weeks. He is kept comfortable with a long acting morphine drip. He uses headphones to listen to classical music and he reads the encyclopedia, having progressed to volume E. He is less alert than he was, but still recognizes Dorothy. Dorothy comes to visit several hours each day, but she is now more rested, as she can sleep through the night. Ted has returned to his home, but Dorothy apprises Ted of Clayton's condition by e-mail. Over the 3 weeks, Ted has not called or returned to visit. As Clayton's condition deteriorates, his morphine dose is increased to keep the pain under control. He gradually slips into a coma and dies peacefully in Dorothy's presence.

CAREGIVER AND SURROGATE DECISION MAKER CONCERNS

The psychological, physical, and financial burdens on family caregivers of individuals with a variety of conditions have been extensively documented in the research literature. A recent retrospective study of caregivers of patients with terminal cancer found that higher caregiver stress was experienced when patient symptoms intensified, quality-of-life diminished, and needs went unmet (O'Hara et al., 2010). While findings from studies in this population cannot be immediately generalized to patients with both ASD and terminal illnesses, it is reasonable to assume that these factors would have similar influences on caregivers of such patients and that support interventions to minimize stress in caregivers through these illness transitions are essential.

Wendler and Rid (2011) conducted a systematic review of 40 studies of 2,854 surrogates and found that surrogate decision makers in end-of-life situations experienced lingering doubt and guilt over their judgments. Stressful though these decisions might have been, surrogates who believed they were actuating their loved one's preferences experienced less of these negative feelings (Wendler & Rid, 2011). Another recent systematic review of more than 129 quantitative studies related to family caregiving at the end of life documented inconsistencies in methods, sample selection, definitions, instruments, and analysis. The authors concluded that clarification of definitions and measures, along with additional research, are needed to build the evidence base for caregiving and palliative care at the end of life (Stajduhar et al., 2010).

Caregiving and ASD

A family used to caring for a healthy individual with autism might have adjusted to the demands of such caregiving. When a terminal illness is diagnosed, the needs of the individual with autism are compounded by pain, symptom control, medical therapies, and unpredictable side effects. These complexities create a marathon of family responsibility, adding to the cumulative stress of caregiving over decades. While the caregiver is used to helping the person with autism transition, improve, and grow, this disease trajectory does not enable such transition, as the inevitable outcome is death (Turnbull, 2004).

The caregiver might wish to provide comfort, but the person with autism might be unable to give or receive comfort, due to a lack of empathy (Kennett, 2002). The person might withdraw further into his or her own world for comfort, predictability, stability, and structure (Davidson, 2007). Sensitivity to touch might be heightened, creating an aversion to personal care (Kennett, 2002) or even a violent response to touch (Davidson, 2007). The caregiver might interpret this as rejection, which adds to the cumulative frustration of caring for an unresponsive patient. Caring for a terminally ill person with autism is time consuming and emotionally draining. Others do not comprehend the intensity of this ongoing responsibility. There is no escape hatch. Uncertainty, pain, fatigue, and financial burdens add layers of stress to a situation already fraught with strain (Family Caregiver Alliance, 2010b).

As the disease progresses, the caregiver assumes increasing responsibility for someone whose capacity to acknowledge caregiving has diminished even further. Criticism from distant family members or others can prompt additional caregiver stress (Family Caregiver Alliance, 2010b). Caregiving can dominate daily life to the exclusion of social contacts and external networks, such as church and work. Family caregivers, like Dorothy, need strong support systems, particularly substitute caregivers to assist with the care of the terminally ill family member with ASD.

The period between diagnosis of terminal illness and the death of a loved one is an emotional and value-laden time, evoking emotions that include guilt, remorse, fear, and confusion (McCarron & McCallion, 2007). This stressful period can also ignite family conflicts that have lain dormant for years (Kramer et al., 2010). Some family members might cling to unrealistic hopes about recovery, and demand that treatments continue (McCarron & McCallion, 2007); others accept the eventuality of death and wish to minimize suffering. "A family wanting to pursue every vanishingly small chance to preserve the life of a relative might reach a different conclusion about what is best, than a family that puts comfort care ahead

TABLE 16.2 ■ End-of-Life Issues in Families of an Individual with ASD

Family of a terminally ill patient	Family of a terminally ill individual with ASD
Hanging on and letting go	Finding methods for communicating and understanding the individual's wishes and preferences
Resolving family issues, reconciliation	Recalling and resolving family issues Addressing caregiving obligations Ensuring support for caregiver Resolving decision-making conflicts
Reminiscence, life review, and closure	Finding methods for the individual to express life highs and lows Identifying strategies to facilitate reminiscence, life review Communicating about preferences for life closure
Pain control and comfort	Recognizing pain cues Responding appropriately to pain Identifying comfort measures Expressing comfort
Unpleasant symptoms (shortness of breath, nausea)	Recognizing symptom cues Responding appropriately to unpleasant symptoms
Spirituality, forgiveness, and hope	Finding ways to communicate about spirituality, hope, and emotion

Based on Ferrell, B., Rhome, A., Paice, J. (2003)

of preserving biological life as long as possible" (Kopelman, 2007, p. 188). Overtreating or prolonging the dying process impairs quality of life (Tuffrey-Wijne et al., 2007), and "Overtreatment can harm, especially when the patient cannot understand the pain or restraints involved in treatment . . ." (Kopelman, 2007, p. 190). Sound end-of-life decisions require a solid understanding of the clinical situation and the ability to integrate and apply the best available information (Kopelman, 2007). Decisions should maximize the person's long-term benefits (beneficence), while minimizing burden (nonmaleficence; Beauchamp & Childress, 2008). A realistic array of options, along with their resource implications, must be weighed together with the patient's values and life plans (Kopelman, 2007). The family must compare burdens/complications of treatment against consequences/complications of nontreatment and compare life before and after treatment versus life in the future without treatment (Kopelman, 2007). When treatment becomes unduly burdensome, with minimal hope of returning to an acceptable quality of life, then new decisions should be made.

NEED FOR FURTHER RESEARCH

Given the limited literature on end-of-life care for individuals with autism, there is a compelling need for research on their lived experiences during this time of vulnerability (Tuffrey-Wijne et al., 2007). Important clinical issues might include pain, pain assessment, symptom management, effectiveness of comfort measures, management of challenging behaviors, and cues to symptoms in the population of terminally ill individuals with ASD. Pain and symptom assessment and management are particularly challenging with nonverbal patients. Research is needed to develop more effective clinical decision-making algorithms for people with ASD in order to manage pain more effectively (Tuffrey-Wijne et al., 2007).

A second research trajectory centers around decisional capacity. Research is needed to develop more finely tuned instruments to assess decisional capacity and to test strategies to support decision-making abilities of people with autism (Stein, 2007, 2008). Studies related to the reliability of proxy decision makers in respecting patient wishes are needed (Koritsas & Iacono, 2009). Since much current family research in this population focuses on burdens, such as stress or family deprivation, a focus on family resilience in this population could elucidate family attributes that contribute to quality of life (Turnbull, 2004). A third research agenda could be developed around the aging process for those with ASD. Longitudinal studies could explore the impact of chronic illness on behavior and adaptation in individuals with ASD (Koritsas & Iacono, 2009). The need for, and acceptability of, support groups for aging people with ASD could also be explored (Totsika, Felce, Kerr, & Hastings, 2010). Finally, end-of-life decision-making studies should explore the challenges of arriving at a proper balance between over- and underprotection of dying patients (Stein, 2008). Such studies might assess provider attitudes about life-sustaining treatment for those with cognitive impairments (Stein, 2007), or advanced care planning (Stein, 2007).

Individuals with ASD as Research Subjects

One of the reasons the literature contains few studies of persons with autism at the end of life is the mandate for human subjects to give informed consent to be included in research studies. Any study involving human subjects must be approved by the institutional review board (IRB) of the sponsoring institution prior to implementing the study (University of California, San Diego, Task Force on Decisional Capacity, 2003). Many studies in the past have been conducted without appropriate protection of vulnerable subjects. Cases of exploitation, manipulation, and even deception of those with decisional impairments are reported in the literature (Noble & Sharav, 2010). Dying patients fit the category of vulnerable research subjects. Those with ASD are classified as vulnerable because of limitations in communicating their understanding of a study and/or consent to participate; vulnerable research subjects require a higher level of protection. Studies involving vulnerable populations might be subject to greater scrutiny by an IRB. For consent to be valid, the person must have sufficient relevant information to make a meaningful decision about participating, including the purposes of the study, the methodology, and the risks and benefits of the study. Another consideration for consent is that the person must voluntarily choose to be involved, free from coercion or duress. In addition, the person must have sufficient capacity to make an autonomous choice about engaging in the study. This capacity is specific to the protocol and the situation (University of California, San Diego, Task Force on Decisional Capacity, 2003). Procedures exist for securing surrogate consent. In any case, the person might withdraw from the study at any point without consequences (University of California, San Diego, Task Force on Decisional Capacity, 2003). Confidentiality of the data must be carefully protected. Participants have a right to request copies of the study findings upon completion (University of California, San Diego, Task Force on Decisional Capacity, 2003). A decision tree for determining capacity to participate in a research study is available online at http://irb.University of California San Diego.edu/DecisionalCapacityAssessment.pdf

WHAT LIES AHEAD?

Increasing numbers of children are being diagnosed with ASD, entering public schools, and seeking health care. While federal funds have been allocated for research on ASD, funding for education and health care for people with ASD has not kept pace with increasing demands. Parents, teachers, and health care providers need training, community resources, and support systems to manage the growing numbers of individuals on the autism spectrum. Typical elementary, secondary, and post-secondary schools are not adequately funded nor necessarily adequately prepared to create environments where these children can flourish; acute and primary health care settings face similar challenges. Massive infusions of resources and continuing education are needed to adequately respond to the needs ahead for care and management of children with ASD (A. Keating, personal communication, October 25, 2010). This is an issue of distributive justice, a key ethical principle.

Given the increasing numbers of adults with ASD, specialized health care services will be increasingly needed, particularly for chronic conditions and in long-term care. Communities have not begun to plan for this eventuality. Society expects family members to care for aging relatives with ASD. The economic and societal burdens of these caregiving responsibilities have not been fully tallied. When parents of an individual with autism dies, the caregiving "baton" is often passed to the siblings, who might not be amenable to accepting this responsibility (Turnbull, 2004). Long-term care facilities have developed environments for dementia patients, but have not adapted care centers for those with ASD, whose special needs are quite different (A. Fielding, personal communication, October 25, 2010). Already, the pipeline of trained caregivers is insufficient for the demand. When the waves of older people with ASD begin to enter long-term care, needing personal services around the clock, the demand for caregivers will only increase. Long-term care staff will also need specialized education to provide high-quality care to people on the autism spectrum.

Ethical issues abound in families caring for those with autism at the end of life. These issues are fraught with emotion and uncertainty that can fuel family conflict (Kramer et al.,

2010). Using appropriate strategies and informed by the ethical frameworks, approaches, and principles, health care professionals can help families make decisions in the best interests of the person with ASD. Given adequate support systems, these times of vulnerability can create moments of meaningful interactions to improve quality of life and create good memories for all family members involved.

REFERENCES

Agency for Health Research and Quality. (2004). *End of life care and outcomes, Report Number 110*, 290-02-0003. Bethesda, MD: Author.

Agency for Healthcare Research and Quality. (2008). *Clinical practice guideline on advance directives: Evidence-based geriatric nursing protocols for best practice.* Hartford Geriatric Center. Retrieved from http://www.guideline.gov/content.aspx?id=12264

American College of Physicians. (2009). *Family caregivers, patients and physicians: Ethical guidance to optimize relationships.* Ethics, Professionalism and Human Rights Committee Position Paper. Philadelphia, PA: Author. Retrieved from http://www.acponline.org/running_practice/ethics/issues/policy/caregivers.pdf

American Nurses Association. (2001). *Code of ethics for nurses with interpretive statements.* Silver Spring, MD: Author.

Bade, P. (2008). Management of gastrointestinal and respiratory symptoms in palliative care. *South Dakota Medicine, Special Edition, 47*(9), 51–3.

Barnard, J., Harvey, V., Potter, D., & Prior, A. (2001). *Ignored or ineligible? The reality for adults with autistic spectrum disorders.* London: National Autistic Society.

Beauchamp, T. L., & Childress, J. F. (2008). *Principles of biomedical ethics* (6 ed.). New York: Oxford University Press.

Byock, I. (2004). The ethics of loving care. *Health Progress, 85*(4), 12–19, 57.

Center for Gerontology and Health Care Research. (2000). *Brown University School of Medicine facts on dying: Policy relevant data on care at the end of life.* Providence, RI: Brown University Medical School. Retrieved from www.chcr.brown.edu/dying/

Center for Human Policy. (n.d.). *A statement of common principles on life-sustaining care and treatment of people with disabilities.* Syracuse, NY: Syracuse University. Available at http://thechp.syr.edu/

Davidson, J. (2007). "In a world of her own": Re-presenting alienation and emotion in the lives and writings of women with autism. *Gender, Place and Culture, 14*(6), 659–677.

Diesfeld, K. (2000). Neither consenting nor protesting: An ethical analysis of a man with autism. *Journal of Medical Ethics, 26*, 27–281.

DisDAT. (2006). *Disability Distress Assessment Tool.* Northumberland, UK: Tyne and Wear NHS Trust and St. Oswald's Hospice.

Family Caregiver Alliance. (2010a). *Fact sheet: Caring for adults with cognitive and memory impairments.* National Center on Caregiving. Retrieved from http://www.caregiver.org/caregiver/jsp/

Family Caregiver Alliance. (2010b). *Fact sheet: Helping families make everyday care choices.* National Center on Caregiving. Retrieved from http://www.caregiver.org/caregiver/jsp/

Ferrell, B. A., Fine, P. G., & Herr, K. A. (2010). Strategies for success: Pharmacologic management of persistent pain in the older adult. *Clinical Advisor*, (October 1), 1–15.

Ferrell, B., Rhome, A., & Paice, J. (2003). *Communication, Module 4. End of Life Nursing Education Consortium.* Washington, DC: City of Hope National Medical Center and American Association of Colleges of Nursing.

Forrester-Jones, V. E., & Broadhurst, S. (2007). *Autism and loss.* Philadelphia, PA: Jessica Kingsley.

Gill, C. J. (2000). Health professional, disability, and assisted suicide: An examination of relevant empirical evidence and reply to Batavia (2000). *Psychology, Public Policy, and Law, 6*, 526–545.

Ghaziuddin, M. (2005). *Mental health aspects of autism and Asperger's syndrome.* London: Jessica Kingsley.

Goldsmith, L., Skirton, H., & Webb, C. (2008). Informed consent to healthcare interventions in people with learning disabilities-an integrative review. *Journal of Advanced Nursing Review Paper, 64*(6), 549–563.

Grant, M., Elk, R., Ferrell, B., Morrison, R. S., & von Gunten, C. F. (2009). Current status of palliative care—clinical implementation, education and research. *CA: A Cancer Journal for Clinicians, 59*(5), 327–335.

Herr, K., Bursch, H., Ersek, M., Miller, L. L., & Swafford, K. (2010). Use of pain-behavioral assessment tools in the nursing home: Expert consensus recommendations for practice. *Journal of Gerontology Nursing, 36*, 18–31.

Herr, K., Coyne, P., Manworren, R., McCaffery, M., Merkel, S., Pelosi-Kelly, J., & Wild, L. (2006). Pain assessment in the nonverbal patient: Position statement with clinical practice recommendations. *Pain Management Nursing, 7*(2), 44–52.

Hume, K., Loftin, R., & Lantz, J. (2009). Increasing independence in autism spectrum disorders: A review of three focused interventions. *Journal of Autism Developmental Disorder, 39*, 1329–1338.

Kennett, J. (2002). Autism, empathy and moral agency. *Philosophical Quarterly, 52*(208), 340–358.

King, A., Janicki, M., Kissinger, K., & Lash, S. (2005). *End of life care for people with developmental disabilities.* Albany, NY: Center for Excellence in Aging Services. Retrieved from http://www.albany.edu/aging/lastpassages/lp-philosophy.htm

Kingsbury, L. A. (2004). Person centered planning in the communication of end of life wishes. *Exceptional Parent, 34*, 44–46.

Kleepsies, P. (2004). *Life and death decisions: Psychological and ethical considerations in end of life care.* Washington, DC: American Psychological Association.

Kopelman, L. (2007). The best interests standard for incompetent or incapacitated persons of all ages. *Journal of Law, Medicine and Ethics, 35*, 187–196.

Koritsas, S., & Iacono, T. (2009). Limitations in life participation and independence due to secondary conditions. *American Journal of Intellectual and Developmental Disabilities, 114*(6), 437–448.

Kramer, B., Kavanaugh, M., Trentham-Dietz, A., Walsh, M., & Yonker, J. (2010). Predictors of family conflict at the end of life: the experience of spouses and adult children of persons with lung cancer. *Gastroenterology, 50*(2), 215–225.

Lynden, M. (2010). *Assessing capacity to execute a health care proxy: A rationale and protocol.* Retrieved from http://www.thefreelibrary.com/_/print/PrintArticle.aspx?id=172169648.

MacLeod, A., & Johnston, P. (2007). Standing out and fitting in: A report on a support group for individuals with Asperger syndrome using a personal account. *British Journal of Special Education, 34*(2), 83–88.

Mandell, D., Wiggins, L., Carpenter, A., Daniels, J., DiGuiseppi, C., Durkin, M., . . . Kirby, R. S. (2009). Racial/ethnic disparities in the identification of children with autism spectrum disorders. *American Journal of Public Health, 99*(3), 493–498.

McCarron, M., & McCallion, P. (2007). End-of-life care challenges for persons with intellectual disability and dementia: Making decisions about tube feeding. *Intellectual and Developmental Disabilities, 45*(2), 128–131.

National Consensus Project for Quality Palliative Care. (2009). *Clinical practice guidelines for quality palliative care* (2 ed.). Pittsburgh, PA: Author.

Noble, J., & Sharav, V. H. (2010). Protecting people with decisional impairments and legal incapacity against biomedical research abuse. *Journal of Disability Policy Studies, 18*(4), 230–244.

Noddings, N. (2003). *Caring: A feminine approach to ethics and moral education* (2 ed.). Berkeley: University of California Press.

O'Hara, R. E., Hull, J. G., Lyons, K. D., Bakitas, M., Hegel, M. T., Li, Z., & Ahlers, T. A. (2010). Impact on caregiver burden of patient-focused palliative care intervention for patients with advanced cancer. *Palliative and Supportive Care, 8*(4), 395–404.

Park, J., Hoffman, L., Marquis, J., Turnbull, A. P., Poston, D., Mannan, H., . . . Nelson, L. L. (2003). Toward assessing family outcomes of service delivery: Validation of a family quality of life survey. *Journal of Intellectual Disability Research, 47*, 367–384.

Payen, J. F., Bru, O., Bosson, J. L., Lagrasta, A., Novel, E., Deschaux, L., . . . Jacquot, C. (2001). Assessing pain in critically ill sedated patients using a behavioral pain scale. *Critical Care Medicine, 29*(12), 2258–2263.

Penticuff, H. (2006). Nursing perspectives on ethics: caring within arm's length. *Tzu Chi Nursing Journal, 5*(5), 65–76.

Reinke, L., Shannon, S. E., Engelberg, R., Dotolo, D., Silvestri, G., & Curtis, J. (2010). Nurses' identification of important yet under-utilized end-of-life care skills for patients with life-limiting or terminal illnesses. *Journal of Palliative Medicine, 13*(6), 753–759.

Robert Wood Johnson Foundation. (2001). *State Initiatives in End-of-Life Care. Issue 12: Caring for Marginalized Groups.* Retrieved from http://www.rwjf.org/pr/product.jsp?id=15763

Robert Wood Johnson Foundation. (2005). *State Initiatives in End-of-Life Care: Issue 23*: Retrieved from http://www.rwjf.org/pr/product.jsp?id=15787

Robert Wood Johnson Foundation. (2006). Thirty-Five Leaders Map the Future of Reform. *State Initiatives in End-of-Life Care: Issue 25*: Retrieved from http://www.rwjf.org/pr/product.jsp?id=15870

Rosetti, Z., Ashby, C., Arndt, K., Chadwich, M., & Kasahara, M. (2008). "I like others to not try to fix me": Agency, independence, and autism. *Intellectual and Developmental Disabilities, 46*(5), 364–375.

Schelly, D. (2008). Problems associated with choice and quality of life for an individual with intellectual disability: A personal assistant's reflexive ethnography. *Disability and Society*, *23*(7), 719–723.

Stajduhar, K., Funk, L., Toye, C., Grande, G., Aoun, S., & Todd, C. (2010). Part 1: Home-based family caregiving at the end of life: a comprehensive review of published quantitative research (1998–2008). *Palliative Medicine*, *24*(6), 573–593.

Stein, G. (2008). Providing palliative care to people with intellectual disabilities: Services, staff knowledge, and challenges. *Journal of Palliative Medicine*, *11*(9), 1241–1248.

Stein, G. (2007). *Advance directives and advance care planning for people with intellectual and physical disabilities.* U.S. Department of Health and Human Services Report. Retrieved from http://aspe.hhs.gov/daltcp/reports/2007/adacp.htm

Torke, A., Alexander, G. C., & Lantos, J. (2008). Substituted judgment: The limitations of autonomy in surrogate decision making. *Journal of General Internal Medicine*, *23*(7), 1514–1518.

Totsika, V., Felce, D., Kerr, M., & Hastings, R. (2010). Behavior problems, psychiatric symptoms, and quality of life for older adults with intellectual disability with and without autism. *Journal of Autism and Developmental Disorders*, *40*, 1171–1178.

Tuffrey-Wijne, I., Hogg, J., & Curfs, L. (2007). End-of-life and palliative care for people with intellectual disabilities who have cancer or other life-limiting illness: A review of the literature and available resources. *Journal of Applied Research in Intellectual Disabilities*, *30*, 331–344.

Turnbull, A. P. (2004). President's address 2004: Wearing two hats: Morphed perspectives on family quality of life. *Mental Retardation*, *42*(5), 383–399.

University of California, San Diego, Task Force on Decisional Capacity (2003). *Procedures for determination of decisional capacity in persons participating in research protocols.* Retrieved from http://irb.University of California San Diego.edu/DecisionalCapacityAssessment.pdf

Vehmas, S. (2004). Ethical analysis of the concept of disability. *Mental Retardation*, *42*(3) 209–222.

Watson, J. (2006). Caring Theory as an ethical guide to administrative and clinical practices. *Journal of Nursing Administration Healthcare Law, Ethics, and Regulation*, *8*(3), 87–93.

Wendler, D., & Rid, A. (2011) Systematic review: The effect on surrogates of making treatment decisions for others. *Annals of Internal Medicine*, *154*(5), 336–346.

Winzelberg, G., Hanson, L., & Tulsky, J. (2005). Beyond autonomy: Diversifying end of life decision making approaches to serve patients and families. *Journal of the American Geriatric Society*, *53*, 1046–1050.

World Health Organization. (2002). *National cancer control programmes: Policies and managerial guidelines.* Geneva, Switzerland: Author.

IV Discussion Questions

CHAPTER 14

1. How would you design the ideal residence for an older person with autism spectrum disorder (ASD)? Would it be a single-family dwelling or a group setting? What architectural features should be included? Should only older adults live there, or adults of various ages? Should only older adults with ASD live there, or any older adult? Give a rationale for your ideas.
2. How might you address Mr. Smith's need for increased oral intake while his gums remain sore?
3. Mr. Smith is having more difficulty managing his activities of daily living (ADLs), and his difficulties are likely to increase as his dementia progresses. People without intellectual disability frequently use notes or other reminders to help maintain independence in ADLs. How can you help Mr. Smith?
4. Design a daily exercise program for Mr. Smith, taking into consideration his osteoarthritis, coronary artery disease, gastroesophageal reflux disease, hypertension, and epilepsy. How will you manage Mr. Smith's pain so that it does not become a barrier to physical exercise?
5. Review Mr. Smith's medication list. Are there medications that you would change or delete? Is there anything that you would add to his medication regimen?

CHAPTER 15

1. At what point is it best for caregivers to discuss future planning for a person with Autism? Is there a "best" or more "ideal" time?
2. Autism is categorized as a disorder, which has a rather negative connotation. Yet, Temple Grandin claims she would not choose to be "cured," if such a treatment existed. She is not alone. Do you think that nurses treat this group with a preconceived notion that this group does not enjoy the same quality of life as nonautistic individuals? How might that affect their treatment?
3. Rather than a "cure," autism treatment involves alleviation of the various problems inherently associated with it. Name three ways a nurse could break the traditional role and assist an individual with ASD with his or her unique needs.

4. Every state has a different policy regarding the resources available to the aging autistic population. What resources are essential for every state to provide for this population? Which resources are admirable but not completely necessary?
5. Should there be more regulation for the resources provided for individuals with ASD in different states? Why or why not?

CHAPTER 16

1. What issues, beyond routine family assessment factors, should the clinician explore with families of individuals with both ASD and terminal illness?
2. How can the nurse integrate understanding of ethical frameworks and principles in the care of individuals with ASD and their families at the end of life?
3. What are the most effective ways a nurse can provide ongoing support to a primary caregiver of a person with ASD?
4. What other support services could alleviate stress and provide resources to a family dealing with a terminally ill person with ASD?
5. What modifications would be needed in an acute-care environment to accommodate the special needs of a person with ASD at the end of life?
6. How could a family meeting be structured to ensure that family members feel empowered to express their biggest fears and most ardent hopes for their family member with ASD at the end of life?

GENERAL QUESTIONS

1. What principles of patient care for younger populations can be applied to the care of a person with ASD at the end of life?
2. Discuss the selection of assessment tools for adults with ASD and interpretation of findings.
3. What are the gaps in care and in community resources for families with adult children with ASD?
4. What strategies can be used to address common concerns of aging parents of adults with ASD?
5. What ethical considerations emerge as parents of individuals with autism become older?

ADDITIONAL CASES FOR PRACTICE

1. Describe possible disparities in diagnosis related to culture and ethnicity
2. How would you design a consent form for research in families with ASD?
3. Discuss/describe the components or process of picture-exchange communication and how it may be applied to a clinical encounter with an elderly person with ASD who: visits the emergency room; undergoes preoperative testing; and is in the outpatient clinic for cast removal.

4. Visit an emergency room, outpatient clinic, adult primary care, or outpatient laboratory and observe for 30 minutes, noting the various obstacles that might be encountered by the child/adolescent/adult with ASD. Discuss/recommend a plan of action to mitigate the obstacles.
5. Write a set of screening questions to ask a parent/caregiver about the best way to interact with the patient in their absence.
6. Develop a script to be used in a practice setting (your choice) to collect personal and behavioral information about a new patient brought in from the long-term facility

Introduction: Putting It All Together—Integrated Care for Individuals With Autism Spectrum Disorder

V

Ellen Giarelli

From elderly people coping with dementia and cardiac disease to young children with asthma, viral infections, and fractures, patients with autism spectrum disorder (ASD) require special care and concern. This last section reviews and summarizes the goal of providing comprehensive care to people with ASD across the spectrum. Successful nursing care of ASD across the lifespan must be accessible, continuous, comprehensive, coordinated, compassionate, and culturally effective. According to the American Academy of Pediatrics (American Academy of Pediatrics, 2002), these are the essential components of health care for children and adolescents, as well as adults.

For the child with ASD, parents are the principle caregivers. For the adult, care should be negotiated among professional health care providers, surrogate caregivers, and the person with ASD. He or she should be able to access such care via public transportation, where available, and trust that there is adequate insurance to cover the cost. Continuous nursing care of ASD ensures that the nurse remains a continuous partner in care, in and out of treatment facilities and across the lifespan, beginning with the diagnosis of ASD or the assessment of characteristic symptoms and continuing through end of life. Comprehensive nursing care is provided after training or advanced education on the specialized needs of this population. Nursing care must range from preventive care to tertiary treatment for co-occurring acute and chronic conditions. Coordination of services and care can be under the purview of nurses, who are uniquely qualified to "see the big picture" and bring providers together for a team approach. The nurse's ability to provide compassionate, culturally effective care will grow as she or he apprehends the reality of the person with ASD and strives to see through that person's eyes to better understand his or her life experience. Assessment tools and educational materials must be available in multiple languages, and plans of care must consider cultural beliefs, customs, and traditions.

PARTNERSHIPS FOR BEST-PRACTICES CARE

Efficient and adequate delivery continues to be a vital issue. Communities are becoming the settings for realizing ideal health care systems. Cotroneo and colleagues (Cotroneo, Purnell, Barnett & Martin, 2004) advised that the development, implementation, and management of community models will require leadership, and nurses have a long history of success in this endeavor. Experts have identified the characteristics of successful community-based health care systems. These characteristics include involving participants in planning, implementing, and evaluating the process, and the use and further development of existing resources. They include interdisciplinary practice and training opportunities for students, faculty, and staff;

links among individuals, families, and communities; and having a vision for a better quality of life (Freudenberg et al., 1995; Kretzmann & McKnight, 1993; Richards, 1995; Sullivan & Kelly, 2001; W. K. Kellogg Foundation, 2002).

One way to realize best-practices care of this population is to form partnerships between schools of nursing and ASD treatment centers. In such partnerships, nursing students will see firsthand how nursing services can augment the effectiveness of a team approach, and behavioral and occupational therapists will observe the unique contributions of professional nursing.

Nurse-managed wellness or primary-care centers are community based and are managed and staffed by registered nurses and advanced practice nurses, such as nurse practitioners (Torrisi & Hansen-Turton, 2005). In a nurse-managed center for people with ASD the nurses would possess advanced clinical education and practice caring for this special population and might provide services for primary-care, as well as health promotion and disease prevention. Students placed at the centers might participate in community-service learning by forming partnerships with community leaders to enrich the experience (Astin & Sax, 1998; Hayes, Haleem, Miller, Miller, & Plowfield, 2005).

In Chapter 17, Bonaduce, van der Veen, and Giarelli discuss the value of partnerships between schools of nursing and autism treatment centers. Using an exemplary program as an illustration, they present strategies for adding an ASD treatment center to the clinical options available to baccalaureate- and master's-level nursing students. They present practical instruction on how to approach and invite partners and how to prepare the staff for the arrival of a cohort of students. Also in this chapter is a summary of an approach to the study of the nursing care of ASD. The authors propose that single-case research might be an ideal methodology for research of service environments. It might be ideal for testing the impact of nursing care on patients' functional outcomes and necessary for advancing nursing expertise. The reader is encouraged to look beyond the descriptions in this chapter to consider the potential value of a nurse-managed wellness center dedicated to meeting the needs of the population of people with ASD across the lifespan.

LEGAL ISSUES

A nurse caring for a person with ASD, especially if that person is older, has additional responsibilities with regard to understanding the laws that protect people with disabilities across services settings. There are special requirements related to ascertaining and confirming guardianship, power of attorney, or other decision-making directives.

A legal guardian is a person who has the legal authority (and the corresponding duty) to care for the personal and property interests of another person, called a ward. Usually, a person has the status of guardian because the ward is incapable of caring for his or her own interests due to infancy, incapacity, or disability. A guardianship is a legal relationship created when a person or institution is named in a will or assigned by the court to take care of minor children or incompetent adults. This agreement is sometimes called a conservatorship. Most states have laws that provide that the parents of a minor child are the legal guardians of that child. In Chapter 18, attorneys Williams and Unumb, expertly outline the legal issues in the care of individuals with ASD, including issues of guardianship, within the context of the family and the community.

Throughout this section, we invite the reader to think differently about the nurse's role in the care of people with ASD. When the reader finishes this book, he or she accepts the responsibility of applying knowledge and experiences as a professional nurse to the care of this special population.

REFERENCES

American Academy of Pediatrics. (2002). Medical home: A policy statement. *Pediatrics, 110*(1), 184–186.

Astin, L., & Sax, A. (1998). How undergraduates are affected by service participation. *Journal of College Student Development, 39*, 251–263.

Cotroneo, M. M., Purnell, J., Barnett, M. C., & Martin, D. C. (2004). Community-academic partnerships. In L. K. Evans, & N. M. Lang (Eds.), *Academic nursing practice: Helping to shape the future of health care* (pp. 219–235). NewYork: Springer Publishing.

Freudenberg, N., Eng, E., Flay, B., Parcel, G., Rogers, T., & Wallerstein, N. (1995). Strengthening individuals and community capacity to prevent disease and promote health: In search of relevant theories and principles. *Health Education Quarterly, 22*(3), 290–306.

Hayes, E., Haleem, D., Miller, J., Miller, M. E., & Plowfield, L. Community service and learning and student engagement. In T. Hansen-Turton, M. E. T. Miller, & P. A. Greiner (Eds), *Nurse-managed wellness centers: Developing and maintaining your center* (pp. 87–97). New York: Springer Publishing.

Kretzmann, J., & McKnight, J. (1993). *Building communities from the inside out: A path toward finding and mobilizing community assets.* Evanston, IL: Northwestern University Institute for Policy Research.

Richards, R. (Ed.). (1995). *Building partnerships: Educating health professionals for the communities they serve.* San Francisco, CA: Jossey-Bass.

Sullivan, M., & Kelly, J. G. (Eds). (2001). *Collaborative research: University and community partnership.* Washington, DC: American Public Health Association.

Torrisi, D. L., & Hansen-Turton, T. (2005). *Community and nurse-managed health centers: Getting them started and keeping them going* (pp. 116–117). New York: Springer Publishing.

W. K. Kellogg Foundation. (2002). *Community participation can improve America's public health system.* Retrieved from http://www.wkkf.org/pubs/health/turningpoint/pub3713.pdf

17 Professional Nursing Partnerships and the Future of Autism Spectrum Disorder Nursing Care

Ellen Giarelli, Judith Bonaduce, and Kristen van der Veen

The role of nurses in the care of people with autism spectrum disorder (ASD) will continue to evolve and expand as the profession responds to the needs of this special population. However, the role of the nurse practitioner can be standardized systematically across states with regard to ASD care. This chapter illustrates how professional nursing education programs can be designed to prepare students to deliver comprehensive and integrated care to patients with ASD, to provide family support, and to construct community outreach programs that aim to ensure the highest quality of care.

CASE MANAGEMENT

Case management has an important role in health care and especially in nursing (White & Hall, 2006). Horst, Werner, and Werner (2000) describe it as a mechanism to optimize the patient's self-care abilities and to effectively use resources. Through case management, we seek to streamline the delivery of complex care. Case management is the opportunity for nurses to demonstrate their roles in multidisciplinary health care teams (Yamamoto & Lucey, 2005). We often use a team approach to ensure cost-efficient services under the leadership of a case manager. The case manager integrates services in a seamless flow from assessment through planning, treatment coordination, monitoring, and evaluation (Oliver, 2003). According to Ling (1999) case management can be limited to one encounter or extend over a lifetime of care.

Care of people with ASD engages the expertise of professionals from medicine; nursing; behavioral and psychological therapy; occupational, speech, and physical therapy; and education. The care of individuals with ASD might be highly complex, and involve multiple health care providers, and extend over a lifetime. An important goal is to incorporate and keep all relevant information intact. Case management, therefore, is the ideal approach to the integrated care of ASD. Moreover, of all these service professions, nursing has been well established as the profession that takes a holistic, comprehensive view of patient care. A nurse manager aims to decrease fragmentation and duplication of care and to enhance quality, cost-effective clinical encounters (American Nurses Credentialing Center, 2005); therefore, a nurse is the ideal ASD case manager.

SCOPE OF NURSING PRACTICE

The scope of nursing practice in the care of people with ASD might include the efficient use of advanced practice nurses as case managers. Payments for services might be "bundled" through the medical home and community-based services, rather than used for episodes and point of services treatments (Fairman, Rowe, Hassmiller, & Shalala, 2011). We can widen the scope of transitional care beyond the movement of the elderly from acute to chronic care (Naylor & Keating, 2008) to include managing an adolescent's transitioning out of secondary education to adulthood and independence. Furthermore, the expanded use of nurse practitioners in managing the needs of adults with ASD is especially viable and supported by the AARP (formerly the American Association of Retired Persons), one of the largest consumer groups in the United States (Laurant et al., 2005).

THE THEORY OF HUMAN CARING

In the theory of human caring (THC), Bevis and Watson attend to the minute-to-minute interactions between the giver and the recipient of care (Bevis & Watson, 2000; Fawcett, 2000). Their theory focuses on the care of individuals, families, and groups (McCance, McKenna, & Boore, 1999) and is applicable to the care of people with ASD and their community of caregivers. The THC takes a holistic approach to the care of this population and complements the practical aspects of case management.

Within the THC, harmony of the mind, body, and soul is accomplished through caring interactions (McCance et al., 1999). Harmony might be achieved by way of the interaction between a mother and a child, the caregiver and the person cared for, and the nurse and the client with ASD. The caring relationship is also extended to the student of nursing and the person with ASD within a community setting that is dedicated to providing educational, support programs or interventions that meet the needs of individuals and families in the community. For an additional perspective on caring in the context of the teacher–student relationship, read Nell Noddings (1984, 1988).

Concepts from the THC can be combined with concepts from integrated care to design a novel approach to nursing care of people with ASD. One might begin this process at the earliest time that children display unusual behaviors or delays in development. At this time, screening for ASD initiates comprehensive lifelong care. Pinto-Martin, Souders, Giarelli, and Levy (2005) reported that "practical application of innovations in screening and diagnostic techniques has lagged far behind the research" (p. 163). Nurses, employed in pediatric primary-care practices are on the front line and are well positioned to perform screening and refer for early diagnosis. Nursing students in clinical placement at primary-care practices are ideally suited to routinely screen for developmental problems. Working under the guidance of a clinical instructor at a community site, nursing students can be prepared to educate family caregivers on developmental milestones, and perform basic screenings, using tools such as the Modified Checklist for Autism in Toddlers (MCHAT; Baron-Cohen et al., 2000) and the Autism Screening Questionnaire (ASQ; Berument, Rutter, Lord, Pickles, & Bailey, 1999).

de Cordova and colleagues (2008) stated there is a need for more opportunities for students to practice evidence-based research. Missal, Schafer, Halm, and Schaffer (2010) described such an opportunity when they reported on a "partnership model" between a university and a health care organization in which nursing students were taught how to search for evidence in the literature, summarize their findings, and then "translate their findings" (Missal et al., 2010, p. 456) into suggestions for their practice. These authors indicated that nursing students in this model acquired the skill of assessing the organizational milieu when attempting to answer research questions posed by their clinical instructors. They were then able to suggest "recommendations for practice change based on the evidence" (Missal et al., 2010, p. 460). This study indicated that nursing students placed at a community site under the guidance of their clinical instructor were able to apply evidence (research)-based recommendations to clinical practice and affect positive change. Leaders in nursing education might form alliances with ASD services organizations in the community, with the intent of combining the unique skills of both sets of professionals to deliver comprehensive care.

A PROTOTYPE FOR THE PLACEMENT OF NURSING STUDENTS IN AN AUTISM TREATMENT CENTER

Webster's (Merriam-Webster, 1983) defined community as "people with common interests living in a particular area or as a group of persons of common interests scattered through a larger society" (p. 267). Viewed from this perspective, a group of individuals affected by ASD, whether patients or family members, might be considered a community that shares common interest and goals. The spirit of the community is well established for ASD, as there are several national and many local support networks (see Exhibit 17.4). In addition to immediate family members, extended family, along with professional caregivers and community advocates might be actively involved in improving the welfare of people with ASD. They are part of this community.

Establishing a Clinical Placement for Students: The Case of Community Nursing of ASD

In the next section, we provide an example of a partnership between a school of nursing and a community-based ASD service provider. The use of a community site for nurse education is an example of the THC model, because the collaboration represents the concept of "caring-in-action" for peer educators, for the nursing students they supervise, and most importantly, for clients who have ASD and their caregivers.

The section begins with a general description of a method used to identify a suitable site for a clinical rotation for senior nursing students enrolled in a community nursing course, and ends with a short discussion of how this method might be utilized to secure a site that serves people with ASD. The case is an exemplar. The process and principles can be applied to any nursing education program and community service agency.

The term "school of nursing" includes any nursing education program preparing graduates with bachelor's level eduation.

Porter-O'Grady (2000) stated that entering into the new millennium "has not just changed what people do—it has changed who we are" (p. 30). Contemporary nursing students have different needs than past nursing students. They learn in different ways and apply knowledge to rapidly evolving clinical scenarios. This necessitates the use of a "whole new script for health service" (p. 31).

Systematic Approach to Selecting a Clinical Site

The acronym CARE stands for: community referral, accessing the site, researching the site, and enacting the site as a clinical rotation site for senior nursing students. The acronym of CARE directs the incorporation of a new community site into the syllabus and is, in addition, derived from the foundational concept within Watson's THC.

Community referrals: The first step in incorporating a new clinical site is the community referral. The best clinical site in an experience-rich institution in which nursing students can practice a range of clinical skills. Referrals for potential sites might be obtained informally by word of mouth, calling the specific site, or by a "cold call." In the first instance, word of mouth, one simply hears from another educator about a wonderful place where it might be possible for students to perform their community clinical rotations, or, perhaps, from an individual at the site itself who would like nursing students to come to the facility. A "cold call" approach is spontaneous and can be highly productive and has a personal touch that might be difficult to refuse.

With regard to placing nurses at ASD treatment centers, the nursing program liaison should explicitly describe the benefits that nursing students bring to a site. The liaison should arrive prepared to describe in detail the role that a nurse might play at the treatment center. It is important that the initial contact end on an optimistic note, with the exchange of contact information and preferably a future appointment for follow-up.

Service providers might directly contact the school of nursing and request to be considered as a clinical site. If this should occur, the contact should be referred directly to the faculty member who will arrange the clinical placement. This is most likely to occur when a school of nursing maintains a stellar reputation and their graduates are respected as professionals.

Accessing the site: The goal of the next step is to conduct an on-site visit that is arranged between the nurse educator seeking the site for student placement and the site representative, who should be able to provide specific information on clinical staff, hours of operation, number of clients, and so on. Visit the agency website (if available) before the physical visit to review their mission and learn staff names and titles. Generate a list of questions that pertain specifically to the nursing care of ASD. Bring a copy of the course syllabus to share, and prepare to match course objectives with potential opportunities. Also, bring a list of equipment or resources needed by the faculty and students to maximize the benefit of the experience for students, staff, and clients. For example, "Does the site have pediatric blood pressure cuffs, thermometers, and exam tables?" All parties should agree that the site can provide sufficient learning experiences for students to accomplish the behavioral objectives of the course, and that clients with ASD will benefit from the interaction with students. The facility should have a room for pre- and postconferencing and consultations. This room should be private and isolated from the patient populations and staff to ensure the confidentiality of the discussions.

A second objective for this meeting is to discuss possible tasks and/or projects that the site might like the students to conduct as part of their community work. At one institution, the director requested that students compile a file of teaching tools on medical issues that the behavioral therapists at that site could bring to the family during a home visit. The nursing students created instructions on evaluating dehydration, heat stroke, and heat stress for use when a client with ASD is nonverbal. At an ASD treatment center for children ages 5 to 10 years, a community nursing student group might conduct a similar project that prepares a list of teaching tools for parents of children with ASD, addressing such issues as managing asthma or allergies at home. Another teaching tool could assist an adolescent in maintaining good hygiene.

Researching the site: At this point in the process, mutual agreement is in place. Both parties have agreed to the students performing a clinical rotation at the specified site. The course syllabus has been shared and discussed and both parties agree that each will benefit from the presence of nursing students at the facility. The nurse educator now has the task of confirming that the legal obligations are met.

Current licensure and/or accreditations for the particular site must be verified and submitted to a designated official in the school of nursing or nursing program who is responsible for generating a formal contract and seeking approval from the State Board of Nursing. This procedure might be similar across states. If not required, it is good practice to verify the licensure of the institution before committing students to work on-site. In Pennsylvania, for example, nursing students are not permitted to have a clinical rotation at an agency until a clinical contract is formally executed and approval of the site has been received from the State Board of Nursing. Generally, any school of nursing can generate the school's standard clinical contract. Each agency should seek legal counsel before the final contract is signed by designated authorities from each institution. A copy of the clinical contract is maintained by the school of nursing and the clinical agency. A school of nursing must also submit to their respective State Board of Nursing for approval. In general, one must allow at least 2 months for the administration of this contractual agreement.

Once the preliminary community referral has been obtained, the site has been accessed and fully researched, and all required appropriate forms are in place, the enactment of the site as a clinical site for nursing students can take place.

Enacting the site: At this point, the nurse educator sends a letter of confirmation of the clinical experience to the agency confirming the dates the students will be on-site, and the clinical instructor's name and contact information. Many facilities also require the names of the students. It is good practice for the clinical instructor to visit the site before the clinical rotation begins. The goal of this preparatory visit is to envision the students' daily movements and interactions with staff, learn the actual layout of the facility, and to meet some of the staff with whom the students will be interacting. If students will be restricted in any way or not have access to any particular files or spaces, then it is important that the clinical instructor know this prior to the students being at the site. The key to a successful clinical rotation is clear, ongoing communication among site personnel and faculty. This rule is essential for ASD nursing care, which is an entirely new practice area for nurses, and the ASD treatment center probably has very little understanding of the role for nurses. See Exhibit 17.1 Sample State Board of Nursing Data Form.

Student orientation: Many clinical agencies require the completion of student orientation materials prior to the clinical rotation. If students are required to sign confidentiality or privacy agreements by the agency or to complete other agency documentation, then the clinical instructor should obtain and have students complete these forms prior to the clinical experience. To ensure an efficient and productive experience and to avoid conflict both for the nursing students and the clinical facility, the clinical instructor should ask logistical questions concerning parking facilities, hours of operation, lockers, use of telephones, places for lunch, and so on. The clinical instructor is responsible for informing students of all important information either prior to or on the first day of clinical, along with emphasizing the impropriety of discussing clients, their diagnosis or care, outside of secured pre- or postconference areas. It is good practice for the instructor to remind students that no client should be identified by name; and they are not permitted to discuss any client via any of the social media, such as Twitter® or Facebook.®

Before the first day of clinical, the clinical instructor is responsible for contacting the students who will be performing their clinical experience at the specified site and supplying them with the name and address of the site, and possibly driving directions and parking instructions or public transportation information, along with the clinical instructor's cell phone number. If students will be making visits to clients in the community, in conjunction

EXHIBIT 17.1

Sample State Board of Nursing Data Form

Name of ALL nursing education programs using facility (include all programs including all out-of-state programs)	Specific clinical area of unit used by students	Average daily patient census on unit(s)/ average # of weekly visits	Average number of students assigned at one time	Faculty-student ratio	Specify schedule		
					Dates of rotation	Time(s) of day	Specific days

Dvlpd: 3/03; Rev: 10/06

Note: For required state board of nursing approval all columns for every program must be completed in detail

with their clinical experience at the site, students will need to know in advance of their clinical rotation that a car is required in order for them to perform clinical at the site. Home visits will gain importance in ASD care, as assessment of the home environment is incorporated into nursing case management plans.

PRACTICAL APPLICATION: AN EXEMPLAR

The purpose of this case study is to examine one initiative by the University of Pennsylvania School of Nursing (UPENN SoN) to develop clinical rotations in coordination with the Center for Autism (CFA) to serve as an exemplar of a clinical partnerships Both institutions are located in Philadelphia, Pennsylvania. The individuals involved in this collaboration were primarily members from the SoN and two staff from the CFA who were targeted as potential collaborators.

Nurse educators at the UPENN SoN became aware of the CFA as a possible clinical site for senior nursing students by word of mouth from another nurse educator who was working in conjunction with the site and performing research on ASD. The director of the ASD program formed an association with both the director and clinical coordinator of the

Pediatric Nurse Practitioner (PNP) Program, as well as with a director of clinical contracts in the Office of Student Information at the SoN. These individuals would oversee the SoN's involvement in the development of this clinical rotation program.

The UPENN SoN established a clinical rotation at the CFA in 2010 in accordance with the steps described in the previous section. Placement began with a master's-level student in the spring of 2011, for one semester.

The CFA

The CFA was founded in 1955, making it the oldest center of its kind in the country. From the outset, the CFA prided itself on improving the evaluation, treatment, and management of ASD. The CFA serves a population of children from preschool to middle adolescence. With a strong understanding that every patient with ASD is unique, the CFA tailors each plan of care based on the person's behavioral problems. Along with that, clinicians at the CFA work to incorporate the suggestions of families and communities into each plan of care (Center for Autism, 2011).

CASE–ESTABLISHING THE RELATIONSHIP WITH THE CFA

The nurse educator made contact and arranged a meeting between the chief executive officer and a social worker of the CFA, along with another educator within the site. The CFA expressed an interest in expanding services to include nursing care. At the meeting, the parties examined the clinical syllabus and agreed that the UPENN SoN and the CFA would benefit mutually. Faculty discussed many possible on-site tasks for the nursing students.

During the initial meeting, parties identified three themes for the collaboration. First, the clinical rotation had to be a hands-on experience, not simply observational in nature. Second, the clinical rotation might be considered a specialty assignment for the Pediatric Nurse Practitioner (PNP) program, similar to past programs in asthma or sports medicine. Last, an eager student–preceptor dyad was the essential factor in making the experience successful.

Selecting a Preceptor

Once the group established that a clinical rotation in the CFA was an appropriate teaching tool for the PNP program, the clinical coordinator contacted the CFA to gauge their willingness to provide an enthusiastic preceptor. Not only did the staff at the CFA view this new collaboration positively, they also were able to identify potential preceptors, including a psychologist, a behavioral therapist, an occupational therapist, and a psychiatrist. Most important was finding a preceptor who was willing and enjoyed teaching, and who was excited about the prospect of working with a master's-level PNP. Ideally, the preceptor would be comfortable giving the student a degree of independence as the clinical experience progressed.

CASE–CONTINUED

After some time, the head of the CFA identified a psychiatrist who could provide the advanced level of training in diagnosing and treating ASD. He showed a willingness to

(*Continued*)

CASE (Continued)

teach and felt strongly that keeping only one student per rotation would best serve the student's learning needs and develop a strong mentoring relationship.

The clinical coordinator for the academic program learned that several students in the PNP program were eligible and interested in participating in this clinical rotation. The CFA rotation would contribute up to 4 hours within the 20 hours required per week for the clinical content. The CFA was considered an outpatient specialty placement, similar to a student spending 4 hours at an asthma clinic, an outpatient neurology clinic, or an outpatient orthopedic clinic. The reasoning for this is that as primary-care providers, these students need a broad base of experience in primary-care settings, and so the majority of clinical hours cannot be specialized.

Ongoing Evaluation

To guarantee that any student involved in a specialized clinical placement, such as the CFA, has sufficient support, the university has four separate mechanisms of oversight. First, each student in the PNP program must meet twice per semester with a site visitor at the clinical location. The site visitor is typically a faculty member of the PNP program and spends time with the student to review his or her experience at the clinical site. Second, every student is in contact with the PNP clinical coordinator, who provides support for any issues that might arise during the course of the clinical placement. Third, the student's preceptor fills out a clinical evaluation tool, detailing how the student is progressing with regard to important skills, such as taking histories, doing physical assessments, and maintaining documentation. In the case of the CFA, the student might not have an opportunity to write prescriptions or perform physical examinations. However, she would gain important experience in collaborative case management and in the care of patients with developmental problems. It is through the preceptor's evaluation that this specific information can be best ascertained. Fourth, the student takes responsibility for self-analysis and maintains a clinical log in which she documents (deidentified) patient care. See Exhibit 17.2 for an excerpt from the student's clinical log.

CASE–CONTINUED

In addition to the usual requirements for evaluation, the student placed at the CFA completed a checklist of nursing activities that she performed on-site. She noted on the checklist that the majority of her time was spent in the company of the physician. She conducted patient assessments and parts of ASD diagnostic tests nearly every clinical day. Nursing actions included: assessing sleep, sensory, and behavioral issues; collecting family histories; referring for medical and genetic evaluations; conducting developmental and ASD screening tests; participating in staff case management meetings; and contributing to plans of care. Additionally, with a longer clinical rotation, there was potential to conduct many other nursing interventions, such as community outreach and parent education, consultation with collaborating professionals, participation in behavioral treatments, and hearing and vision evaluations.

The checklist was used by the clinical faculty to evaluate actual delivery of nursing care during the clinical rotation. The checklist was also used to evaluate how nursing care

(*Continued*)

CASE (Continued)

opportunities might be modified or created for future students (see Exhibit 17.5 for the Checklist of Nursing Activities).

This checklist might be used to collect data on the types and volume of nursing services provided to clients at any site. These data can serve to define nursing care of ASD, to support continuing such clinical rotations, and to justify more focused training of nurses in the integrated care of ASD across service settings (see Exhibit 17.5).

EXHIBIT 17.2

STUDENT NARRATIVE OF ASD CLINICAL EXPERIENCE

I typically arrived at 2:30 p.m. for her 4-hour clinical, but on certain days I would arrive earlier. On days that I arrived early, I would attend various meetings, consultations, or medication follow-ups with her preceptor. The preceptor is the staff psychiatrist at the CFA, so he often has meetings with different therapists about their own Level of Care Assessments (that he must sign off on) or other doctors in consultation about patients they have seen. Beginning at 2:30 p.m., they would review the completed Comprehensive Biopsychosocial Evaluation (CBE) from the prior week and the preceptor would answer any questions that I had, after which they would begin to prepare for the 4:00 p.m. evaluation appointment. To prepare, they would review the intake evaluation paperwork (every child attends an intake evaluation with a therapist before seeing a doctor) and any other prior documentation that the patient has sent in.

By 4:00 p.m. the team would have completed the CBE with one family. The CBE typically lasted about 1.5 to 2 hours, during which they assessed: reason for the evaluation, strengths of the child, all of the key features of autism (social development, language and communication, behaviors), cognitive skills, fine and gross motor skills, sensory issues, daily living skills, sleep habits, unusual or traumatic events (including abuse), pregnancy and birth history, temperament and developmental milestones, early intervention and school history, behavioral health treatment history, medical history, social history, family history (both psychiatric and medical), involvement with other systems (like DHA, juvenile justice system), any additional records or testing, and their own observations of and interactions with the child. For child observation, they used the framework of a pre-set form which assessed social interactions (i.e. eye to eye gaze, facial expression, body postures, gestures, seeking to share enjoyment, social and emotional reciprocity), communication (i.e. spoken language, conversations, use of language, play appropriate to developmental level), and restricted or stereotyped behaviors, interests and activities.

Toward the end of the evaluation, they would break from the family, form a diagnosis based on the evaluation, and return to the family to go over the diagnosis and recommendations. The family would receive the typed CBE in the mail in about a week. My preceptor and I would then discuss the evaluation and discuss any questions or "shades of gray" that were encountered. I would discuss with my professor ways that I thought nursing services were or could be better used during each clinical encounter.

Currently, the relationship with the UPENN SoN and the CFA is primarily through the PNP program; a logical next development would be to add this as a rotation within Psychiatric-Mental Health Nurse Practitioner Program, in which students can perform in-depth mental health assessments and manage complicated medication regimens. This partnership is still in its infancy. It is evident that the UPENN SoN has identified a valuable educational opportunity that can help nursing students improve their clinical skills in treating ASD in their primary-care practices.

CASE–CONTINUED: RECOMMENDATIONS

Approximately 4 weeks after the rotation was completed, clinical faculty and the student reported their evaluation of the rotation. The student was extremely pleased with the selection of the preceptor and commented that not only was this psychiatrist an excellent clinician but the preceptor genuinely enjoyed the collaborative role with the advanced practice nurse. The student was on-site 1 day per week for a 4-hour rotation.

The clinical encounters were primary for the assessment and diagnosis of a child suspected of having an ASD. Typically, the team (and PNP) saw one patient at each encounter. There was a low volume of patients, but each encounter was highly complex, and the team collected in-depth information. The student received in-depth training in the diagnosis of ASD.

The site was described as an excellent place to gain highly specific knowledge. Both the faculty and student desired exposure to more patients but would not like to trade complexity of care for volume of patients. They suggested that a longer experience might correct for low volume. Both teacher and student commented on the lack of coordination between the services delivered at the autism treatment center and those from primary care. This was described as a conspicuous "disconnect," because there was an obvious and discrete need to connect these services. The parties identified this deficit as an area in which nurses may serve as case managers and unite complementary services.

Faculty and student reported the necessity of making sure the staff from the clinical site would understand the purpose of the rotation and the educational goals of the clinical experience. They must be open to allowing a student to participate in other aspects of ASD care when an unplanned opportunity arises. To do this, all the treatment staff at the ASD site should be educated on the expanded role of nurses in ASD care, the special interests of the student who will be placed at the site, the ideal link between behavior and primary care, and the general skills of PNPs.

Implications of Collaboration

Swiadek (2009) stated that health care in the United States "will continue to have a profound effect on the nursing profession" (p. 19). Caring, as an integral part of the nursing profession will continue to be affected by global, national, and local changes in health care. Swiadek (2009) stated that "the future of the profession demands that nurses reestablish a fundamental philosophy for caring-healing work" (p. 20). By placing nursing students at ASD treatment centers, we will contribute to the professional caring–healing work that goes beyond the ordinary to approach the extraordinary. Clinical care is one aspect of comprehensive health care. Another is the building of a body of knowledge to support expert, evidence-based clinical practice. There are many support networks and other resources available to nurses as they learn how to care for people with ASD (see Exhibit 17.4).

SINGLE-CASE RESEARCH

A diagnosis of ASD is based on a set of inclusion criteria, however every individual with ASD expresses the disorder differently. Each person is unique in the way he or she responds to treatments. When studying the care of people with ASD, every patient is a "subject." Single-case research methods might be the ideal approach for building a body of knowledge in the nursing care of people with ASD and in the evaluation of the outcomes of treatment for complex cases. There are many excellent approaches to studying ASD. This next section will present information about a single-case approach to the study of nursing care of ASD.

When considering all the possible ways in which a researcher can collect information about individuals with ASD, one could imagine a spectrum of sampling strategies with shallow sampling of the largest possible group of individuals at one end, and the completely saturated sampling of a single individual on the other. One example of the latter case is a recent study from the Media Lab at the Massachusetts Institute of Technology, led by Deb Roy, which digitally recorded 200,000 hours of audio and video over the first 2 years of a child's life (Roy, Frank, & Roy, 2009). This massive amount of data yielded some data that can now be generalized to the larger population (Roy et al., 2009). The promise of single-case research is that it can generate insights that would not be apparent when examining an amalgamation of discrete data points from myriad subjects (Barlow, Hersen, & Andrasik, 2006).

Characteristics of Single-Case Research

Single-case research has been a valuable tool in the social and behavioral sciences, neurotherapy, and education (Kennedy, 2005; Sandars, 2009). An early example of single-case research was Broca's clinical observation in 1861 of an individual who had lost the ability to speak intelligibly (Barlow, Nock, & Hersen, 2009). Clinical notes paired with autopsy findings led to the identification of a specific area of the cerebral cortex necessary for speech, a major breakthrough in neuroscience that altered the dogma of the field (Barlow et al., 2009).

By studying the behavior of one subject, the researcher's conclusions are not confounded by variation among individuals, in which the average performance of a group could bury the multitude of factors that lead to various outcomes, which has been described as a major confounding factor in the study of ASD (Barlow et al., 2006). Sharp, Jaquess, Morton, & Herzinger (2010) reported that single-case research was particularly appropriate for the study of treatments of pediatric populations with complex and developmental concerns. It can be implemented in many service settings, such as schools and clinics, as opposed to case-controlled studies. Behavioral disorders, such as selective mutism (Carlson, Kratochwill, & Johnston, 1999), ASD (Ganz, Lashley, & Rispoli, 2010), and self-injurious behavior (Moore, Gilles, McComas, & Symons, 2010) have been studied using this methodology.

In a typical randomized control trial with a large number of subjects, researchers can imply causation by testing whether the presence of a treatment is significantly associated with a given outcome. In contrast, single-case research design is not burdened with the expectation of demonstrating causation. Instead, single-case research asks two questions: (a) Did the subject experience the desired outcome? and (b) Is there any evidence that the outcome is linked to an intervention? The second question remains difficult to address with only a single subject, other approaches might therefore be used to discern correlation between outcome and treatment, including collecting data with dense temporal sampling and documenting the amount of variability at each time point (Backman & Harris, 1999). Groeneweg and colleagues (2006) provided a brief account of some statistical tests that might serve to supplement the visual inspection process used to assess people with developmental disabilities and specifically applied them to single-case research. Nonparametric alternatives to the *t* test and the Kolmogorow-Smirnov tests as most suitable for single-case analyses (Ma, 2006). Future nursing researchers might also consider time-series analyses to enhance overall usefulness of single-case studies (Blumberg, 1984; La Grow & Hamilton, 2001; Tryon, 1982).

Controversy with Single-Subject Research

A controversial issue with single-case research is the blurring of the role of clinician and researcher. During clinical trials using control groups, the research process and in particular, the generation of data, must be bias-free. Clinical care does not have the same restriction, and indeed, a control is never used as a comparison when evaluating the outcomes of treatment. To avoid the blurring of the role of clinician versus researcher, checks are placed to ensure that the patient receives optimal treatment and that the objectivity of the research process is not compromised (Johannessen, Fosstevedt, & Petersen, 1990).

There is a potential benefit to having a clinician double as the researcher that can outweigh the potential cost. A clinician trained in research can systematically track a patient/subject's progress while adjusting the design of the study to account for the needs of the patient (Kazi, 1998). Single-case studies allow researchers to identify the factors important for influencing patient outcomes in a highly personalized way that is consistent with the way clinicians think about the unique characteristics of people with ASD. Smith and colleagues (2006) designed a roadmap for the study of ASD treatment, in which the first phase is hypothesis generating using single-case research, because of its descriptive capacity.

In a clinic such as the CFA, there are many different disciplines working together. The clinician might be the primary investigator, the research team might also consist of behavioral therapists, social workers, nurses, and psychologists. When synthesizing the findings of multiple single-case research studies, it is important to account for variation between observers. There are several methods for reducing interobserver variability. Researchers can standardize the terms they use to describe the treatment by clinicians and the behaviors of the patients and ensure that data is collected in the same way using instruments with acceptable psychometric properties. Many instruments have been standardized for use in clinical and research populations. A principal method for reducing interobserver variability is intensive training of all individuals participating in the research, which should include postobservation analysis. In summary, the debate in the ASD field regarding the importance of balancing clinical judgment with rigorous scientific data might be informed by the pursuit of single-case research.

Approach to the Analysis of Single-Case Research

Single-case research is often dismissed as being less scientifically rigorous than other forms of research. Case-control, case-cohort, and clinical trials, are favored due to their reliance on measures of statistical significance. Statistical significance can be achieved along with clinical significance if one considers a different understanding of sample size as referring to the number of subjects, as well as to the number of observations (points of data collection for each subject). The approach to analysis of data in single-case research might be different from that used in studies that are controlled. One will need to ask the question "Does the treatment work for *this* patient?" rather than "Does the treatment work for the *average* patient" (Franklin, Allison, & Gorman, 1996)? Some confounding factors that loom large in this field are serial dependency, cyclicity, and statistical power (Franklin et al., 1996).

Single-Case Studies in Nursing Science

For nursing practice, single-case research offers the opportunity of advancing clinical expertise by better understanding factors that result in successful patient outcomes. The paradigm of single-case research necessitates retrospection to identify critical points in care, a skill that the nursing professional is already well trained to do. Because single-case research has had its most important successes in behavioral research, such as education and social work, this design is particularly well suited for patients with ASD, for whom behavioral outcomes are the primary measure of successful treatment. An advanced practice nurse working at an ASD treatment center has experience conducting and evaluating research. He or she may review and recommend a list of assessment tools for use in single-case research.

Nursing care for patients with ASD occurs over a lifetime. Clinical interventions might occur during periods of rapid developmental change. The large degree of individual variability within these periods might seriously undermine an attempt to make a generalization about an entire group based on averaging data. Examining individual cases preserves the ability to observe learned changes in behavior (Millard, 1998) and preserve the clinical value of findings.

Single-case research can best be used by clinicians who have extensive knowledge of their own patients through long-term care and collaboration with the patients' families and other team members (e.g., social workers, teachers), as is ideally the case with care providers of children with ASD, who often have complicated care regimens. These clinicians might be best able to take published, single-case research and determine if, and how, it applies to their own patient. In this way, single-case research might be carried out by the same clinicians who are the primary consumers of the research.

SPECIAL ISSUES IN THE EXPANDED ROLE OF NURSING CARE FOR ASD

Nursing care of ASD is novel and innovative. We are carving out a role for the profession, labeling our services, and defining our role. Full integration of nursing into the care of this special population will take time. Other health care providers, including behavioral therapists, developmental pediatricians, psychiatrists, and occupational therapists will need to understand the contributions of nurses to the team. A main issue faced by all service providers is the fair, appropriate, and timely compensation for services. If services are "bundled" such that comprehensive care is paid for by "visit" rather than by "treatment," a nurse might be easily integrated with the full team of professionals. If not, nursing care delivered specifically by a nurse practitioner or clinical specialist must be documented and compensated by direct payer or by public or private insurance provider. Payment for the services of an nurse practitioner vary across states in the United States.

Reimbursement for Nursing Activities

At this time in Pennsylvania, nurse practitioners must work in collaboration with a physician. The collaborating partner must maintain a signed agreement that details the scope and elements of the collaboration. Furthermore, a prescriptive authority collaborative agreement is needed for nurse practitioners who have licensure to prescribe medication. If specified in a collaborative agreement, nurse practitioners might perform an extensive set of duties as outlined by each state's Scope-of-Practice Regulations for Nurse Practitioners (Council of State Boards of Nursing, 2008). For example, in the United States, when this chapter was written, there were differences in requirements across states. Thirteen of 50 states and the District of Columbia had no requirements for practice for nurse practitioner. Eight among

50 states required collaborative agreements to prescribe medication. Twenty-five states (including Pennsylvania) required collaborative agreements to diagnose, treat, and prescribe (Fairman et al., 2011). Specific data were not available for the remaining four states.

ASD-related Services in Pennsylvania

The General Assembly of Pennsylvania's House Bill Number 1150 (2007), Act 62 (section 635.2) (Commonwealth of Pennsylvania, 2008) was enacted to ensure coverage of services for individuals under 21 years of age for a maximum benefit of $36,000 per year. This includes diagnostic assessment and treatments related to ASD, with no limit on the number of visits to ASD service providers. Individuals covered by Act 62 are those who are covered under employer group health insurance policies that have more than 50 employees (not self-insured), those who are on medical assistance, and those covered by Pennsylvania's Children's Health Insurance Program. The maximum benefit of $36,000 per year applies to the private health insurance companies and is further applied to the Pennsylvania Department of Public Welfare for individuals enrolled in the Medical Assistance Program. Moreover, at the time this chapter was written, Act 62 required that the Pennsylvania Department of Public Welfare (PDPW) cover the costs of individuals whose coverage exceeds $36,000 per year (Commonwealth of Pennsylvania, 2008).

This act is limited with respect to comprehensive care. The language does not reflect that people with ASD might have medical problems that are directly associated with the diagnosis of ASD, such as seizures or eating disorders. Some medical problems might intensify the behavioral problems. Medical and mental health problems should be treated together. Act 62 does not cover case management services. Furthermore, insurance coverage is not mandated for services that are solely outlined in a person's individualized education program (IEP), which is prepared for his or her special education, but coverable treatment from the IEP can be coordinated with consent of a parent or guardian. (See Table 17.1 for service details of Act 62, the Autism Insurance Act of Pennsylvania).

Role of Behavior Specialist Nurses in ASD Care

Act 62 specifies the behavior specialist as one who designs, implements, or evaluates a behavior modification intervention component of a treatment plan, including those based on applied behavioral analysis. The desired outcomes are the improvement of behavior to prevent loss of attained skill or function, skill acquisition, and the reduction of problematic behavior. Forward-thinking nurse educators can aim to prepare a cohort of advanced practice nurses to become qualified and licensed to deliver behavioral treatments. This extension of the advanced practice nurse's role is an ideal way to provide comprehensive and coordinated care. A nurse can oversee primary care. By having the behavior specialist's role fulfilled by a nurse, the complicated network of services can be streamlined. See Exhibit 17.3 for qualifications of licensure as required by the State Board of Medicine in conjunction with the Department of Public Welfare, as outlined in Act 62.

Intellectual Property Rights

Intellectual property rights protect innovations and their authors (Hing & Back, 2009). Innovations and the development of new ideas are crucial to space the progress of evidence-based nursing practice. The main types of intellectual property are copyrights, patents, trademarks, and design registration (Shemdoe, 2009). The type that would apply to the development of

TABLE 17.1 ■ Service Details of Act 62, the Autism Insurance Act of Pennsylvania.

Services covered	Definition of services	Providers eligible for reimbursement	Monetary source	Maximum benefit	Reference to nurses
Diagnostic services	Assessments, evaluations, or tests to diagnose whether an individual has an ASD	Physician, physician assistant, psychologist, or certified registered nurse practitioner	Insurer (up to $36,000 after which PDPW covers costs)	$36,000/year	Certified registered nurse practitioners
Treatment plan development	N/A	Physician or psychologist	Insurer (up to $36,000 after which PDPW covers costs)	$36,000/year	None
Prescribe, order, and provide treatment (inclusive of services below)	N/A	Physician, physician assistant, psychologist, or certified registered nurse practitioner	Insurer (up to $36,000 after which PDPW covers costs)	$36,000/year	Certified registered nurse practitioners
Pharmacy care	Prescription of medications Prescription/ ordering of evaluation or test in order to determine the need or effectiveness of such medications	Physician, physician assistant, or certified registered nurse practitioner	Insurer (up to $36,000 after which PDPW covers costs)	$36,000/year	Certified registered nurse practitioner
Psychiatric care	Direct or consultative services	Physician who specializes in psychiatry	Insurer (up to $36,000 after which PDPW covers costs)	$36,000/year	None
Psychological care	Direct or consultative services	Psychologist	Insurer (up to $36,000 after which PDPW covers costs)	$36,000/year	None
Rehabilitative care (including ABA)	Services or treatment programs that produce socially significant improvements in human behavior or prevent loss of attained skill or function	Licensed or certified behavior specialist	Insurer (up to $36,000 after which PDPW covers costs)	$36,000/year	None
Therapeutic care	Direct services	Speech–language pathologists, occupational therapists, or physical therapists	Insurer (up to $36,000 after which PDPW covers costs)	$36,000/year	None

EXHIBIT 17.3

Qualifications for Licensure of Behavioral Specialist by the Board of Medicine in Conjunction with the Department of Public Health, as Outlined in Act 62, the Autism Insurance Act of Pennsylvania

Requirements

- Is of good moral character
- Holds a Master's degree or higher degree from board-approved, accredited college or university with a major course of study in school, clinical or counseling psychology, special education, social work, speech therapy, occupational therapy or another related field.
- Has at least one year experience involving functional behavioral assessments, including the development and implementation of behavioral supports or treatment plans
- Has completed 1,000 hours in direct clinical experience with individuals who have behavioral challenges,

OR

- Has completed 1,000 hours in a related field with individuals with ASD.
- Has completed relevant training programs including:
    - Professional ethics
    - Autism-specific training
    - Assessments training
    - Instructional strategies and best practices
    - Crisis intervention
    - Comorbidity and medications
    - Family collaboration and addressing specific skill deficits training

Exclusions

- Conviction of a felony under "The Controlled Substance, Drug, Device, and Cosmetics Act,"

OR

- Conviction of an offense under the laws of another jurisdiction which, if committed in this Commonwealth, would be a felony under "The Controlled Substance, Drug, Device, and Cosmetics Act."*

*The above ban can be nullified if at least 10 years have passed from the date of conviction, if the applicant has made significant progress in personal rehabilitation since the conviction, or if the applicant otherwise satisfies the qualifications contained in or authorized by this section.

products related to the nursing care of people with ASD are copyrights, which protect creative materials, such as educational programs, instructional materials, and research instruments. When developing innovative and unique approaches to care, there is the possibility that instructional or other materials can be commercially developed, copyrighted, or otherwise protected for the owner. Commercialization transforms knowledge into products and

EXHIBIT 17.4

National, Regional, and Selected Local Support Networks and Organizations

United States

Autism Society of America

7910 Woodmont Avenue, Suite 300
Bethesda, MD 20814
301-657-0881; 800-328-8476
www.autism-society.org

National resource with local state chapters under the umbrella as well.

National Institutes of Health Autism Research Activities

National Institutes of Health (NIH)
9000 Rockville Pike
Bethesda, MD 20892
www.nimh.NIH.gov/health/topics/autism-spectrum-disorders-pervasive-developmental-disorders/nih-initiatives/index.shtml

There is also an extensive listing of sites under www.nih.gov with multiple sites for autism in the various branches.
www.nimh.nih.gov/healthinformation/autismmenu.cfm

Centers for Disease Control and Prevention

1600 Clifton Road
Atlanta, GA 30333
800-311-3435
www.cdc.gov
www.cdc.gov/old/science/iso/concerns/mmr_autism_factsheet.htm (for information on the MMR vaccine and autism)

Organization for Autism Research (OAR)

www.researchautism.org

This is another excellent research-support charity and information source for both physicians and parents.

Autism Speaks

2 Park Avenue, 11th Floor
New York, NY 10016
212-252-8676
www.autismspeaks.org

This site is a great resource for information and links to research, national organizations, and also physicians. This is one of the unifying autism resource sites.

(*Continued*)

EXHIBIT 17.4 (Continued)

Southwest Autism Research and Resource Center (SARRC)

300 N 18th Street
Phoenix, AZ 85006
602-340-8717
www.autismcenter.org

Interdisciplinary Council on Developmental and Learning Disorders (ICDL)
4938 Hampton Lane, Suite 800
Bethesda, MD 20814
301-656-2667
www.icdl.com

Stanley Greenspan's organization for autistic spectrum and educational treatment suggestions for behavioral programs.

Treatment and Education of Autistic and Related Communication Handicapped Children (TEACCH)

www.teacch.com

American Academy of Pediatrics

www.aap.org

American Academy of Child and Adolescent Psychiatry

www.aacap.org

Child Neurology Society

www.childneurologysociety.org

National Fragile X Foundation

www.nfxf.org

International Rett Syndrome Association

www.rettsyndrome.org

Online Asperger's Syndrome Information and Support (O.A.S.I.S.)

www.aspergersyndrome.org

Charity Foundations

LADDERS:

Massachusetts General Program for research in autism under Margaret Bauman
www.ladders.org

(Continued)

EXHIBIT 17.4 (Continued)

Doug Flutie Jr. Foundation

Football player with autistic son started charity.
www.dougflutie.org

Dan Marino Foundation

Serving greater Miami and other places as well, started by famous quarterback Dan Marino.
www.danmarinofoundation.org

CANADA

Autism Society of Canada

P.O. Box 635
Fredericton, New Brunswick
Canada E3B 5B4
506-363-8815
www.autismsocietycanada.ca

EXHIBIT 17.5

Student Placement at the Center for Autism Checklist of On-Site Nursing Activities

DATE:______________________ Time: ______________________

Rate the performance of the following nursing actions during each visit to the site. While at the site how often did you:

NURSING ACTION/INTERVENTION	Never	1 time	2–3 times	More than 3
Observation/assessment				
Medical/behavioral chart review				
Vital signs				
Health history				
Family health history				
Family educational needs assessment				
Physical assessment				
Behavioral assessments				
Assess medical comorbidities				
Assess sleep, sensory, and activity issues				
Nutritional assessment				
Family/environment assessment				
Three generation family pedigree				

(*Continued*)

EXHIBIT 17.5 (Continued)

Developmental screening				
ASD screening				
Hearing and vision evaluations				
Monitor reactions to meds				
Monitor side effects of meds				
Monitor response to treatments				
Environmental/home assessment				
Observe evaluation/ASD diagnosis				
Assist with evaluation/ASD diagnosis				
Critique behavioral sessions				
Therapeutic interaction				
Participate in parent interviews/meetings				
Instruct parents/screening				
Instruct parents/milestones				
Instruct parents/medical monitoring				
Instruct parents/behavior therapy				
Community education and outreach on ASD				
Consult with external care providers				
Stress management for family				
Provide sex education for teens				
Collaborate with staff on health issues				
Participate in staff case management meeting				
Contribute to individual plan of care				
Medical/nursing plan of care				
Prevention Specify:				
Treatment Specify:				
Follow-up Specify:				
Child behavioral plan of care				
Prevention Specify:				
Treatment Specify:				
Educational Specify:				
Family plan of care				
Prevention Specify:				
Treatment Specify:				
Educational Specify:				
Delivery/services				
Medication administration				

(*Continued*)

EXHIBIT 17.5 (Continued)

Respiratory treatments				
Care documentation				
Provide first aid				
Assist with hygiene				
Design nutritional plan of care				
Care for disorders related to ASD				
Motor milestone delays (fine or gross)				
Seizures/staring spells				
Gastrointestinal				
Asthma/respiratory				
Diet and nutrition				
Exercise and physical activity				
Behavioral analysis				
Family education/training in ABA				
Odd responses to sensory stimuli				
Aggression/destructiveness				
Impulsivity/hyperactivity				
Extreme fearfulness or fearlessness				
Self-injurious behaviors				
ADVANCED PRACTICE ACTIONS				
Referral for medical evaluations				
Referral to ophthalmologist				
Referral to audiologist				
Referral to psychiatrist				
Home visits for follow–up				
Manage medical comorbidities				
Glucose monitoring and injections				
Administer asthma treatments				
Design comprehensive plans of care				
Symptom management				
Administer behavioral interventions				
Administer sensory integration therapy				
Establish protocols: health issues				
Prescribe laboratory tests				
Venipuncture				
Medicate and manage meds				
Conduct screening clinics in community				

(*Continued*)

EXHIBIT 17.5 (Continued)

Adolescent transition planning				
Conduct parent support groups				
Conduct sibling classes				
Decision-making support for parents				
Coordinate elements of care				
Collaborate in team care				
Stress management for families				
Communicate with family on medical issues				
Community/group activities				
Other:				
Interaction with staff:				

service. A copyright protects original works of authorship embodied in a tangible medium of expression, usually for the life of the author plus 70 years. In particular, it provides an exclusive right to copy or distribute. Materials that are designed for nursing care of the ASD population are in demand and generally not available. When on-site with students, the clinical instructor might explore with the students existing means of care delivery utilized at the site and, as part of their clinical experience, encourage students to research innovative ways of caring for clients at that site. Faculty might learn how to adapt instructional materials for a unique population of patients and work closely with staff and family to optimize the benefits for all. Students should take credit for their work by placing their name, year, and the name of their nursing institution and the year on any printed materials and copyright this material when possible.

SUMMARY

Partnerships between academic institutions and clinical treatment centers create intellectual venues in which best-practices, collaborative health care can be conducted. Patients and families will benefit from such partnerships as the collaborators bring new perspectives to the design and delivery of care. They may become the sources of rich evidence-based data for evaluating treatment outcomes. As we look toward the future of the nursing care of people with ASD, we might keep in mind these general and worthy objectives:

1. Provide research training in an integrated, interdisciplinary partnership that links research to policy and practice;
2. Develop capacity to engage in partnership research that contributes to sustainability;
3. Educate researchers, clinicians, policy makers, and community leaders to create evidence for best-practice nursing care; and
4. Develop and disseminate curriculum materials for use regionally, nationally, and internationally on the expanded role of nurses in ASD care.

According to Frank and Smith (2000), complicated power dynamics are always present and need to be acknowledged during the process of developing partnerships. These may include power differences related to personal characteristics or organizational characteristics, such as resources and institutional reputations (Frankish, Kwan, Larsen, Ratner, & Wharf-Higgins, 2002). Academic institutions and health services have historically been hierarchically structured, but separate in their hierarchy. Moreover, communities may distrust research (Cheadle et al., 1997) of any kind or simply not understand the value of nursing services to their community.

Partnerships are complex and their success relies on a shared commitment to complementary roles and contributions. Despite these complexities, partnerships can be pioneers in promoting the health and well-being of unique patient populations, such as people with ASD.

REFERENCES

American Nurses Credentialing Center. (2005). Nursing case management. Retrieved from http://nursingworld.org/anncc/certification/certs/specialty.html

Backman, C. L., & Harris, S. R. (1999). Case studies, single-subject research and N of 1 randomized trials: Comparisons and contrasts. *American Journal of Physical Medicine and Rehabilitation, 78*, 170–176.

Barlow, D., Hersen, M., & Andrasik, F. (2006). *Single-case experimental designs* (3 ed.). New York: Pearson.

Barlow, D., Nock, M., & Hersen, M. (2009). *Single-case experimental designs: Strategies for studying behavior for change* (3 ed.). New York: Pearson.

Baron-Cohen, S. S., Wheelwright, S., Cox, A., Baird, G., Charman, T., Swettenham, J., . . . Doehring, P. (2000). Early identification of autism by the CHecklist for Autism in Toddlers (CHAT). *Journal of the Royal Society of Medicine, 93*(10), 521–525.

Berument, S. K., Rutter, M., Lord, C., Pickles, A., & Bailey, (1999). Autism screening questionnaire: Diagnostic validity. *British Journal of Psychiatry, 175*, 444–451.

Bevis, E., & Watson, J. (2000). *Toward a caring curriculum. A new pedagogy for nursing*. Sudbury, MA: Jones & Bartlett.

Blumberg, C. J. (1984). Comments on "A simplified time-series analysis for evaluating treatment interventions." *Journal of Applied Behavioral Analysis, 17*, 539–542.

Carlson, J. S., Kratochwill, T. R., & Johnston, H. F. (1999). Sertraline treatment of 5 children diagnosed with selective mutism: A single-case research trial. *Journal of Child & Adolescent Psychopharmacology, 9*(4), 293–306.

Center for Autism. (2011). Our history. Available at http://www.thecenterforautism.org/about-us/our-history.

Cheadle, A., Berry, W., Wagner, E., Fawcett, S., Green, L., Moss, D., . . . Woods, I. (1997). Conference report: Community-based health promotion—State of the art and recommendations for the future. *American Journal of Preventive Medicine, 13*(4), 240–243.

Commonwealth of Pennsylvania. (2008) Act 62 of 2008 (9 July). Retrieved from http://www.legis.state.pa.us/cfdocs/billinfo/billinfo.cfm?syear=2007&sind=0&body=H&type=B&BN=1150

Council of State Boards of Nursing. (2008) *APRN model act/rules and regulations*. Available at http://www.ncsbn.org/APRN_leg_language_approved_0_08.pdf.

de Cordova, P., Collins, S., Peppard, L., Currie, L., Hughes, R., Walsh, M., & Stone, P. (2008). Implementing evidence-based nursing with nursing students and clinicians: Uniting the strengths. *Applied Nursing Research, 21*, 242–245.

Fairman, J. A., Rowe, J. W., Hassmiller, S., & Shalala, D. E. (2011). Broadening the scope of nursing practice. *New England Journal of Medicine, 364*(3), 193–196.

Fawcett, J. (2000). *Analysis and evaluation of contemporary nursing knowledge: Nursing models and theories.* Philadelphia, PA: F. A. Davis.

Frank, F., & Smith, A. (2000). *The partnerships handbook.* Canada: Minister of Public Works and Government Services.

Frankish, J., Kwan, B., Larsen, C., Ratner, P., & Wharf-Higgins, J. (2002). Challenges of community participation in health-system decision making. *Social Science & Medicine, 54*(10), 1471–1480.

Franklin, R. D., Allison, D. B., & Gorman, B. S. (1996). *Design and analysis of single-case research.* Hillsdale, NJ: Lawrence Erlbaum Associates.

Ganz, J. B., Lashley, E., & Rispoli, M. J. (2010). Non-responsiveness to intervention: Children with autism spectrum disorders who do not rapidly respond to communication interventions. *Developmental Neurorehabilitation, 13*(6), 399–407.

Groeneweg, J., Iancioni, G., Bosco, A, Singh, N. N., O'Reilly, M. F., & Sigafoos, J. (2006). A brief account of statistical tests for single-case research with persons with developmental disabilities. *Perceptual and Motor Skills, 103*, 947–950.

Hing, C. B., & Back, D. L. (2009). A review of intellectual property rights in biotechnology. *Surgeon, 7*(4), 228–231.

Horst, L., Werner, R. R., & Werner, C. L. (2000). Case management for children and families. *Journal of Child and Family Nursing, 3*(1), 5–15.

Johannessen, T., Fosstvedt, D., & Petersen, H. (1990). Statistical aspects of controlled single-subject trials. *Family Practice, 7*, 325–328.

Kazi, M. A. F. (1998). *Single-case evaluation by social workers: Evaluative research in social work.* Surrey, UK: Ashgate Publishing.

Kennedy, K. (2005). *Single case designs for educational research.* New York: Allyn & Bacon.

La Grow, S., & Hamilton, C. (2001). The use of single-case experimental designs to evaluate nursing interventions for individual clients. *Australian Journal of Advanced Nursing, 18*(2), 39–42.

Laurant, M., Reeves, D., Hermens, R., Braspenning, J., Grol, R., & Sibbald, B. (2005). Substitution of doctors by nurses in primary care. *Cochrane Database Systematic Review, 2*(CD001271).

Ling, C. (1999). *Case management.* Englewood, CO: Skidmore-Roth.

Ma, H. H. (2006). An alternative method for quantitative synthesis of single-subject research. *Behavioral Modification, 30*, 598–617.

McCance, T., McKenna, H., & Boore, J. (1999). Caring: Theoretical perspectives of relevance to nursing. *Journal of Advanced Nursing, 30*, 1388–1395.

Merriam-Webster (1983). *Merriam-Webster's Ninth New Collegiate Dictionary.* Springfield, MA: Author.

Millard, S. K. (1998). The value of single-case research. *International Journal of Language & Communication Disorders, 33*(suppl), 370–373.

Missal, B., Schafer, B., Halm, M., & Schaffer, M. (2010). A university and health care organization partnership to prepare nurses for evidence-based practice. *Journal of Nursing Education, 49*, 456–461.

Moore, T. R., Gilles, E., McComas, J. J., & Symons, F. J. (2010). Functional analysis and treatment of self-injurious behaviour in a young child with traumatic brain injury. *Brain Injury, 24*(12), 1511–1518.

Naylor, M., & Keating, S. A. (2008). Transitional care. *American Journal of Nursing, 108*(suppl 9), 58–63.

Noddings, N. (1984). *Caring, a feminine approach to ethics & moral education.* Berkeley, CA: University of California Press.

Noddings, N. (1988). An ethic of caring and its implications for instructional arrangements. *American Journal of Education, 96*, 215–229.

Oliver, C. J. (2003). Triage of the autistic spectrum child utilizing the congruence of case management concepts and Orem's Nursing Theories. *Lippincott's Case Management, 8*(2), 66–82.

Pinto-Martin, J., Souders, M., Giarelli, E., & Levy, S. (2005). The role of nurses in screening for Autism Spectrum Disorder in pediatric primary care. *Journal of Pediatric Nursing, 20*, 163–169.

Porter-O'Grady, T. (2000). Visions for the 21st century: New horizons, new health care. *Nursing Administration Quarterly, 25*, 30–38.

Roy, B. C., Frank, M. C., & Roy, D. (2009). *Exploring word learning in a high-density longitudinal corpus.* Proceedings of the 31st Annual Meeting of the Cognitive Science Society, July 29–August 1, Amsterdam, Netherlands.

Sandars, J. (2009). Single-case research: An underused approach for medical educational research. *Education for Primary Care, 20*(1), 8–9.

Sharp, W. G., Jaquess, D. L., Morton, J. F., & Herzinger, C. V. (2010). Pediatric feeding disorders: A quantitative synthesis of treatment outcomes. *Clinical Child & Family Psychology Review, 13*(4), 348–365.

Shemdoe, G. S. (2009). Introduction to intellectual property rights for investigators in health research and institutional intellectual property policy. *Acta Tropica, 112S*, S80–S83.

Smith, T., Scahill, L., Dawson, G., Guthrie, D., Lord, C., Odom, S., Rogers, S., & Wagner, A. (2006). Designing research studies on psychosocial interventions in Autism. *Journal of Autism & Developmental Disorders, 37*(2), 354–366.

Swiadek, J. (2009). The impact of healthcare issues on the future of the nursing profession: The resulting increased influence of community-based and public health nursing. *Nursing Forum, 44*, 19–23.

Tryon, W. W. (1982). A simplified time-series analysis for evaluating treatment interventions. *Journal of Applied Behavioral Analysis, 15*, 423–429.

White, P., & Hall, M. E. (2006). Mapping the literature on case management nursing. *Journal of the Medical Library Association, 94*(2), E99–E106.

Yamamoto, L., & Lucey, C. (2005). Case management "within the walls": A glimpse into the future. *Critical Care Nursing, 28*(2), 162–178.

Legal Issues and Implications for Nursing Care of Autism Spectrum Disorder in the United States 18

Pamela Holtzclaw Williams and Lorri Unumb

Diverse nursing roles interface with the legal and policy landscape while caring for persons living with ASD, their family, and extended community. Just as best nursing practices consider and incorporate a scientific evidence base, they must also consider and incorporate knowledge of the legal and policy environment. For example, nurse clinicians and school nurses must stay informed to maintain competency in their roles of assessing and supporting access to care for the individual, family, or community challenged by existing health insurance and social services-related laws and policies (Strunk, 2009). The advanced practice nurse works within explicit professional competency expectations in advocacy roles that require knowledge of legal and policy issues wherein their patients must leverage policy-changing strategies (Mucklan, 2007). The nurse-scientist working with persons living with ASD and their community shapes relevant health policy through nursing research, by building sound evidence bases for health policy decisions (Hinshaw & Grady, 2011).

In this chapter, we identify and describe key legal and policy issues relevant to health care interactions of people living with ASD with which the diverse nursing roles interface. The discussion aims to inform, and thus support, the provision of best practices within various nursing roles. We have organized the policy discussion under three major frameworks in which nurses might identify autistic patients' problems: (1) access to care, (2) risk factors for autism, and (3) capacity to interact with health care delivery or research. Recent evidence suggests that persons with ASD are significantly at risk for having unmet specialty and therapy care needs, (Chiri & Warfield, 2011). In part one, we address the laws and policies relevant to equitable access to care, such as health insurance laws, the Patient Protection and Affordable Care Act, and the Mental Health Parity Act. This section includes descriptions of key laws that address access to care and dimensions of need for the individual with the diagnosis and his or her family and community. The causative factors of autism are poorly understood; therefore, policies of prevention and control of risks are minimal. In part two, we address policies regarding risk factors for autism. A sustained public concern that vaccines have a causative relationship to autism led to a policy program is discussed. In part three, we address the policies related to the decisional capacity of the person living with autism to participate in his or her own care or research to improve it. This includes a discussion of guardianship and public policy frameworks that "protect" the person living with autism from decisional burdens.

PART ONE: AUTISM AND ACCESS TO CARE

Historically, individuals with autism spectrum disorder (ASD) have had difficulty obtaining meaningful health insurance coverage. Particularly, access to health insurance has been limited in two primary ways: (a) insurance was altogether unattainable, as insurers simply refused to write a policy on an individual or family member with autism, or (b) individuals could obtain a policy, but the policy failed to cover the treatments most commonly prescribed for autism.

Over the past two decades, there have been sporadic lawsuits aimed at remedying this situation that produced minimal large-scale results. However, large-scale results can be anticipated through an emerging national movement toward health insurance legislation for individuals with autism. Since 2007, more than one-half of the states have enacted legislation requiring meaningful health insurance coverage for autism (Autism Speaks, 2011).

In the context of access to care, the term "meaningful" is germane to health insurance coverage for traditionally prescribed and empirically validated treatments, including the most commonly prescribed and proven useful protocol, applied behavior analysis (ABA) therapy (Cohen, Amerine-Dickens, & Smith, 2006; Lovaas, 1987; McEachin, Tristram Smith, & Lovaas, 1993). Unfortunately, intensive treatment is expensive and thus, in the absence of insurance coverage, is not available to many people in the autism population. Most of the autism insurance laws that have been enacted around the country contain similar features (Autism Speaks, 2011; Unumb & Unumb, 2011). These features are listed in Exhibit 18.1.

Unfortunately, many of the laws also contain arbitrary limitations on benefits, such as age limitations or annual dollar limits on the amount of treatment that is available. For example, Missouri's law limits the amount of ABA therapy that must be covered to $40,000 per year. Florida limits coverage to individuals under age 18 years. Some of these limitations may be subject to challenge under federal laws, such as the Patient Protection and Affordable Care Act, (2009), and the Paul Wellstone and Pete Domenici Mental Health Parity and Addiction Equity Act of 2008, (U.S. Department of Health and Human Services [DHHS], 2010). These are discussed in the following subsections.

EXHIBIT 18.1

Features of Autism Insurance Laws

- Coverage for screening, diagnosis, and treatment of autism.
- Prohibiting insurers from refusing to issue a policy, or refusing to renew a policy, because an individual has been diagnosed with, or has received treatment for, autism.
- Prohibiting denials on the basis that treatment is "nonrestorative" or "habilitative" in nature.
- Particular treatments that must be covered are listed:
    - Psychiatric care
    - Psychological care
    - Pharmaceutical care
    - Therapeutic care (speech, occupational, and physical therapies), and
    - Behavioral health treatment, including applied behavior analysis

Debate over Autism Insurance Laws

The passage of autism health insurance laws involved considerable debate in state legislatures about the fiscal impact of mandating such coverage. As with any legislation creating a new "mandate" (a requirement that a particular benefit be covered by insurance), advocacy groups debated whether the benefit of providing access to treatment for individuals with autism outweighed costs. One such advocacy group, the Council for Affordable Health Insurance (CAHI), explained mandates generally and their economic impact. This organization notes that while mandates make health insurance more comprehensive, they also make it more expensive, because mandates require insurers to pay for care consumers previously funded out of their own pockets. The CAHI estimated that mandated benefits currently increase the cost of basic health coverage from a little less than 20% to more than 50%, depending on the state and its mandates. Mandating benefits has been compared to saying to someone in the market for a new car, if you cannot afford an expensive car, loaded with options, then you have to walk. Having that most expensive car would be nice, as would having a health insurance policy that covers everything one might want. However, drivers with less money can find many other affordable car options; whereas, when the price of health insurance soars, few other options exist (CAHI, 2011).

Laws in 50 States

The CAHI document examined the laws in all 50 states plus the District of Columbia and estimated the percentage impact on insurance premiums of a particular mandated service or treatment. For example, the report indicated that mandated coverage for in vitro fertilization increases overall premiums by 3% to 5%. Mandated prescription drug benefits increased premiums by 5% to 10%. The CAHI 2007 report indicated that mandated autism benefits increased premiums by less than 1%, and the 2010 report indicated an increase of 1% to 3% (CAHI, 2011).

Compared to the relatively small increase in costs associated with autism coverage, the increase in benefit to society is immense. A study by the Harvard School of Public Health estimated the incremental societal cost of autism at $3.2 million per person over a lifetime (Ganz, 2007). This cost can be reduced dramatically, or even eliminated, with appropriate intervention, which, for most families, is available only with health insurance coverage.

Refer to Appendix 18.1 for an example of an autism insurance mandate. This Arkansas law is fairly representative of the laws that were enacted between 2007 and 2011. For example, it (a) covers ABA therapy and other common treatments; (b) includes a dollar cap and age cap on coverage; (c) ensures that health insurance coverage does not negatively impact educational services under the Individuals with Disabilities Education Act; and (d) permits insurers to use normal mechanisms of utilization review in handling claims (see Appendix 18.1).

Autism and Access to Care: Patient Protection and Affordable Care Act

In March 2010, Congress passed the Patient Protection and Affordable Care Act (2009), and shortly thereafter the Health Care and Education Reconciliation Act of 2010. Together, these acts became known as the "Affordable Care Act" and represented a major overhaul of the health insurance system in America.

Several provisions of the Affordable Care Act have potential implications on health insurance coverage for autism. Most significant among these provisions is the part of the law that requires insurers to offer certain benefits in health plans offered through "exchanges." An exchange is a marketplace in which people can comparison shop for price and the benefits they want, much like that used for most other products one might purchase.

For health plans offered through exchanges, the federal government set minimum coverage requirements. These minimum coverage requirements are known as the "essential benefits." Within the Affordable Care Act, Congress defined a list of ten essential benefits that must be included. These are listed in Exhibit 18.2.

The DHHS, with help from the Institute of Medicine, is currently working to define the items and services that must be included within each of the 10 categories of the essential benefits package. Congress charged the DHHS with ensuring that the scope of the essential health benefits is "equal to the scope of benefits provided under a typical employer plan" (Patient Protection and Affordable Care Act, 2009). To inform this determination, the DHHS is tasked with conducting "a survey of employer-sponsored coverage to determine the benefits typically covered by employers."

In defining the essential health benefits, the DHHS is required to ensure that essential health benefits reflect an appropriate balance among various categories, so that benefits are not unduly weighted toward any category of services. The benefits must take into account the health care needs of diverse segments of the population, including women, children, persons with disabilities, and other groups, and not make coverage decisions, determine reimbursement rates, establish incentive programs, or design benefits in ways that discriminate against individuals because of their age, disability, or expected length of life.

Other provisions specify that health benefits established as essential not be subject to denial to individuals against their wishes on the basis of the individual's age or expected length of life or of the individual's present or predicted disability, degree of medical dependency, or quality of life. Finally, the provisions must be periodically reviewed and a summary report presented to the U.S. Congressional oversight committee (Patient Protection

EXHIBIT 18.2

Essential Benefits of the Affordable Care Act

1. Ambulatory patient services
2. Emergency services
3. Hospitalization
4. Maternity and newborn care
5. Mental health and substance use disorder services, including *behavioral health treatment*
6. Prescription drugs
7. Rehabilitative and habilitative services and devices
8. Laboratory services
9. Preventive and wellness services and chronic disease management
10. Pediatric services, including oral and vision care

EXHIBIT 18.3

CONTENT OF REQUIRED REPORT TO CONGRESS AND THE PUBLIC

- An assessment of whether enrollees are facing any difficulty accessing needed services for reasons of coverage or cost
- An assessment of whether the essential health benefits need to be modified or updated to account for changes in medical evidence or scientific advancement;
- Information on how the essential health benefits will be modified to address any such gaps in access or changes in the evidence base
- An assessment of the potential of additional or expanded benefits to increase costs and the interactions between the addition or expansion of benefits and reductions in existing benefits to meet certain actuarial limitations

and Affordable Care Act, 2009). See Exhibit 18.3 for a list of the essential contents of the report to Congress.

Large health plans, such as self-funded Employee Retirement Income Security Act (U.S. Congress, 2009) plans and large fully funded groups, are *not* affected by the essential benefits package. It affects only the plans under the exchanges and some individual and small group health plans.

Perhaps the other provision of the Affordable Care Act that is most relevant to the autism community is the provision barring certain annual and lifetime dollar limits. In a subtitle called Immediate Improvements in Health Care Coverage for All Americans, the law prohibits lifetime limits on the dollar value of benefits for any participant or beneficiary and unreasonable annual limits on the dollar value of benefits for any participant or beneficiary (Patient Protection and Affordable Care Act, 2009). However, this prohibition is not to be interpreted to prevent a group health plan or health insurance coverage that is not required to provide essential health benefits from placing annual or lifetime per beneficiary limits on specific covered benefits to the extent that such limits are otherwise permitted under federal or state law.

Autism and Access to Care: Mental Health Parity

Prior to the autism insurance reform movement that began in 2007, some states required insurers to cover autism by including autism within their state mental health parity (MHP) laws. With limited exceptions, however, the laws were largely not effective for those with autism, because they did not require coverage of the most commonly prescribed treatment protocols.

The U.S. Congress also made efforts to secure appropriate mental health benefits for insured individuals across the country. In 1996, Congress enacted the Mental Health Parity Act, which required that annual or lifetime dollar limits on mental health benefits be no lower than any dollar limits for medical and surgical benefits offered by a group health plan (U.S. DHHS, 2011). The Mental Health Parity Act requirements applied beginning in 1998 and had an original sunset provision of September 30, 2001. The U.S. Congress extended the Mental Health Parity Act several times (U.S. Department of Labor, n.d).

The 1996 Mental Health Parity Act offered limited protections. Although insurers had to provide equal annual or lifetime dollar limits for mental health benefits, they could still impose a maximum number of provider visits and caps on the number of days an insurer would cover for inpatient psychiatric hospitalizations. Furthermore, the Mental Health Parity Act did not cover substance abuse or chemical dependency.

To address these deficiencies, in 2008, through a rider on the Troubled Asset Relief Program, Congress enacted the Paul Wellstone and Pete Domenici Mental Health Parity and Addiction Equity Act of 2008 (U.S. DHHS, 2010; American Psychological Association, 2008).

The Wellstone Act, effective as of October 3, 2009, generally requires that group health plans and group health insurers treat mental health and substance abuse disorders the same as medical and surgical benefits with respect to lifetime coverage limitations, annual limits, financial requirements, treatment limitations, and the use of out-of-network providers. Although health plans and group health insurers need not cover any mental health or substance abuse disorders, if they do, they must do so equally. The term "financial requirement" includes deductibles, copayments, coinsurance, and out-of-pocket maximums.

A "treatment limitation" includes the limits on the frequency of treatment, number of visits, dates of coverage, or other similar limits on the scope or duration of the treatment. It can be expressed numerically (quantitative treatment limitations) or not numerically (non-quantitative treatment limitations; U.S. Department of Labor, 2010).

Quantitative treatment limitations include day limits, visit limits, and frequency of treatment limits. Nonquantitative treatment limitations include medical management standards; prescription drug formulary design; standards for provider admission to participate in a network; determination of usual, customary, and reasonable amounts; requirements for using lower therapies before the plan will cover more expensive therapies (known as fail-first policies or step therapy protocols); and conditioning benefits on completion of a course of treatment (U.S. Department of Labor, 2010).

On its face, the Wellstone Act does not make clear whether autism is a mental health condition and whether ABA is a mental health benefit. The Wellstone Act defines "mental health benefits" as those benefits with respect to services for mental health conditions, as defined under the terms of the plan and in accordance with applicable federal and state law.

The regulations implementing the Wellstone Act established that group health plans cannot arbitrarily define a mental health condition. The regulations define "mental health benefits" as defined under the terms of the plan and in accordance with applicable federal and state law (U.S. Department of Labor, 2008). Any condition defined by the plan as a mental health condition (or not) must be consistent with generally recognized independent standards of current medical practice. It then provides examples of such standards to include the most recent version of the *Diagnostic and Statistical Manual of Mental Disorders* (*DSM*; APA, 2000), the most recent version of the International Classification of Disease (ICD), or state guidelines. The preamble to the Wellstone regulations further explains that generally recognized, independent standards of current medical practice do not imply that there is a national standard.

Clarifying the Issue: Is Autism a Mental Health Condition?

Considering all of the above sources, is autism a mental health condition? As noted, the Wellstone Act itself does not answer this question. However, there is evidence in the legislative history of the Wellstone Act that the writers intended to include autism, and the law's House Report uses autism as an example of a mental illness. Additionally, the preamble to the Wellstone regulations mentions autism as an example of a mental disorder that costs employees a large amount in lost earnings. It states that mental disorders cost employees at least $193 billion annually in lost earnings alone, a staggering number that probably is a conservative estimate, because it did not include the costs associated with people in hospitals and prisons and included very few participants with autism, schizophrenia, and other chronic illnesses that are known to greatly affect a person's ability to work (U.S. DHHS, 2010). The explicit references to "autism" as an example of a mental illness/mental health disorder suggest that Congress intended to include autism in the Wellstone Act.

Parity Laws in the United States

As noted, other sources of applicable law are state mental health parity (MHP) laws. Forty-nine states have enacted MHP laws. Nine states explicitly include autism in their MHP laws. Sixteen states implicitly include autism in their state MHP. These states define mental illness by referring to the most recent versions of the *DSM* and/or ICD. Connecticut, Rhode Island, and Washington refer to the *DSM*, and also explicitly exclude a list of disorders not including autism. Minnesota's MHP law defines "mental illness" as an organic disorder of the brain that is listed in the clinical manual of the ICD and its code ranges from 290.0 to 302.99 or 306.0 to 316.0 or the corresponding ICD-9 code. Autism's code in the ICD is 299 (APA, 2000), therefore, it is implicitly included in Minnesota's definition. Nebraska refers to the ICD and then explicitly includes "biological disorder[s] of the brain that substantially limit the life activities of the person with the serious mental illness" (Neb. Rev. Stat. §44-792). New York explicitly includes autism under the category of a "serious emotional disturbance" but not as a "biologically based mental illness." North Carolina provides its own definition of mental illness, but uses the *DSM*'s definition of mental disorders, with the exception of those coded as "V" codes (N.C. Gen. Stat. §58-3-220). In addition, seven states explicitly exclude autism in their MHP laws (Colo. Rev. Stat. §10-16-104; Haw. Rev. Stat. §431M-1; Ind. Code 12-7-2-130; La. Rev. Stat.Ann. §22:1043; Or. Rev. Stat. 743A-168; Tenn. Code Ann. §33-1-101; Utah Code Ann. §31A-22-625).

Each state has different specifications on whether autism and other developmental disorders are considered mental health conditions (see Table 18.1). The laws can be complicated and confusing, especially to parents and guardians who continually advocate for their affected family members. Nurses should be aware of the differences across states with regard to determining eligibility to services.

What is the significance of this complex web of state MHP laws? As long as autism is considered a mental health condition under applicable federal and state law, the protections of the Wellstone Act apply to prevent the application of disparate financial requirements and treatment limitations. This may affect the dollar and age limits that have been enacted in state autism insurance mandates such as those discussed above.

AUTISM AND ACCESS TO CARE: IMPLICATIONS FOR DIVERSE ROLES IN NURSING

Across the world, the social movement advocating increased access to care for autism is gaining momentum (Caruso, 2010). The movement provides collaborative opportunity for

TABLE 18.1 ■ Mental Health Parity (MHP) Laws in the United States[a]

Inclusion/exclusion	States
• Nine states *explicitly include* autism in their MHP laws.	• California, Illinois, Iowa, Maine, Massachusetts, Montana, New Hampshire, New Jersey, and Virginia.
• Sixteen states *implicitly include* autism in their state MHP.	• Alabama, Arkansas, Connecticut, Florida, Georgia, Kansas, Kentucky, Minnesota, Mississippi, Missouri, Nebraska, New York, North Carolina, Rhode Island, Vermont, and Washington.
• Seven states *explicitly exclude* autism in their MHP laws.	• Colorado, Hawaii, Indiana, Louisiana, Oregon, Tennessee, and Utah.
• Ten states list mental illness that they cover and the list does not include autism.	• Delaware, Idaho, Nevada, Ohio, Oklahoma, Pennsylvania, South Carolina, South Dakota, Texas, and West Virginia.
• Seven states have MHP laws, but the statutes *are not clear as to whether autism would be classified* as a mental health condition or not.	• Alaska, Arizona, Maryland, Michigan, New Mexico, North Dakota, and Wisconsin.
• One state has no mental health parity law.	• Wyoming

[a]$N = 50$ states.

nursing care and advocacy roles to directly or indirectly participate at the local, state, and federal levels, depending on the particular policy strategy. Nurse collaborations assist by providing evidence and articulating expert opinions regarding the need for access to care (Chiri & Warfield, 2011). Exercising the nurse-advocate role may include providing expert opinion testimony and position statements and communicating directly with lobbyists and elected officials. Nurses can contribute as advocates from diverse employment perspectives, such as the school, community health, or clinical setting nurse. Visibility of nurses at policy-making sessions that address access of care for the autism community is a way to support policy development.

The nurse–scientist role can contribute to policies regarding access to care by application of research methods that quantify and describe the health care disparities of persons with autism and the impact of legislative reform on quality of life and access to care. Developing scientific programs of research then becomes the bridge for successful policy advocacy. For example, nurse advocates now have an emerging evidence base to advocate to state legislators that health insurance coverage for autism care does not translate into unreasonable financial consequences to premiums (Bouder, Spielman, & Mandell, 2009).

Assisting Families

While families wait for public policies to facilitate access to care, they often look to the educational system to fill voids in health insurance coverage for behavioral and adaptive training and health care support (Caruso, 2010; Holland, 2010). This can place heightened responsibilities on the school nurse's role caring for school-age children with autism (Bellando & Lopez, 2009; Minchella & Preti, 2011).

The financial burden as a stressor and influence on the health of affected individuals and their family members cannot be understated. Nursing interventions indirectly respond to policy shortcomings by addressing the efforts of individuals and families to cope with lack of access to care and financial stressors from inadequate health insurance coverage (Twoy, Connolly, & Novak, 2007).

On a case-by-case basis, the nurse must evaluate the impact on family finances and access to care caused by the patient's health insurance coverage as applied under relevant state laws. As with all health care expenses, where the cost of care is prohibitive for a family's household income. This will restrict nursing referral for specialized options. In those states in which there has been minimal health insurance reform for the autism community to gain access to coverage for care, the school, community health, and clinical nursing networks can collaborate to promote policies that increase and efficiently use existing community services supported by nonprofits and taxpayers. For example, for communities with access to Easter Seals services for autism, nurses from diverse employment perspectives can explore how they can professionally support provision of care through nonprofit organizations' service for autism at various ages (Easter Seals, 2011).

Nurses might refer clients and their families to peer or parent support organizations that are motivated to empower families with self-advocacy skills to gain leverage in educational, legal, research, and health policy systems (Bartley, 2006; Couper, 2004; Hall & Graff, 2011). See Exhibit 18.4.

EXHIBIT 18.4

Description of Autism Speaks—Example of an Advocacy Organization in the United States

Autism Speaks is North America's largest autism science and advocacy organization. Since its inception in 2005, Autism Speaks has made enormous strides, committing over $160 million to research and developing innovative new resources for families. The organization is dedicated to funding research into the causes, prevention, treatment, and eventual cure for autism; increasing awareness of autism spectrum disorders; and advocating for the needs of individuals with autism and their families.

In addition to funding research, Autism Speaks has created resources and programs including the Autism Speaks Autism Treatment Network, Autism Speaks' Autism Genetic Resource Exchange, and several other scientific and clinical programs. Notable awareness initiatives include the establishment of the annual United Nations-sanctioned World Autism Awareness Day on April 2, which Autism Speaks celebrates through its Light it Up Blue initiative. Also, Autism Speaks, award-winning "Learn the Signs" campaign with the Ad Council has received over $286 million in donated media. Autism Speaks' family resources include the Autism Video Glossary, a 100-Day Kit for newly-diagnosed families, a School Community Tool Kit, and a community grant program. Autism Speaks has played a critical role in securing federal legislation to advance the government's response to autism, and has successfully advocated for state insurance reform to cover behavioral treatments. Each year *Walk Now for Autism Speaks* events are held in more than 80 cities across North America. To learn more about Autism Speaks, please visit www.autismspeaks.org. (October 2011)

Source: Reprinted with permission from Autism Speaks.

Leverage may be gained by nurse-driven research into quantifying the cost benefit of providing childhood interventions that promote maximum cognitive and behavioral functioning, which in turn can reduce costs of services and support for the individual and family as the child advances into adulthood. Gaps in health insurance coverage and access to care create additional costs to communities and are areas in which nursing research can inform and shape health policy. Nursing research is needed to contribute to the growing evidence base that establishes how existing health insurance policy laws contribute to lack of access to care and disparities in health care access in the autism community (Chiri & Warfield, 2011; Kogan et al., 2008).

PART TWO: PUBLIC POLICY ADDRESSING RISKS FOR AUTISM—VACCINE COURT

Over the past few decades, Congress has enacted several laws regulating vaccines. In 1986, pursuant to Congressional directive, the DHHS created a National Vaccine Program to achieve optimal prevention of human infectious diseases through immunization and to achieve optimal prevention against adverse reactions to vaccines. Congress also established the National Vaccine Advisory Committee (U.S. DHHS, 1987) with members to include individuals who were engaged in vaccine research or the manufacture of vaccines or who were physicians, members of parent organizations concerned with immunizations, or representatives of state or local public health organizations. The National Vaccine Advisory Committee was charged with studying and recommending ways to encourage the availability of an adequate supply of safe and effective vaccination products in the United States, as well as recommending research priorities and other measures to enhance the safety and efficacy of vaccines.

In 1988, Congress established the National Vaccine Injury Compensation Program, which is commonly referred to as "vaccine court" (U.S. DHHS, 1988). The program allows people who suffered injury as a result of compulsory childhood vaccines to petition the federal government for monetary damages. A special office within the Court of Federal Claims decides the claims.

The idea behind the National Vaccine Injury Compensation Program was to create a no-fault system, in which claimants need not prove negligence, failure to warn, or other tort elements. Instead, claimants must prove only that a covered vaccine caused injury. The program was designed to resolve a perceived crisis that threatened the continued availability of childhood vaccines nationwide. In mandating that vaccine injury claims be considered first under the Vaccine Injury Compensation Program, the statute was intended to reduce lawsuits against physicians and manufacturers, while providing those claiming vaccine injuries a reduced burden of proof (see: http://www.uscfc.uscourts.gov).

As in any product liability case, the initial question for decision in a vaccine case is causation. There are two ways to prove causation. The Vaccine Injury Compensation Program contains a Vaccine Injury Table, which is designed to minimize difficulties petitioners face in proving that their injury resulted from a vaccine. The Vaccine Injury Table lists certain injuries and conditions that, if found to occur within a prescribed period of time following vaccination, create a rebuttable presumption of causation. In such "on-Table" cases, petitioners do not need to provide proof of actual causation. For example, if a petitioner proves that her child received a diphtheria–pertussis–tetanus (DPT) vaccine and that the child suffered an encephalopathy (brain injury) within 3 days thereafter, causation is presumed. If the petitioner can demonstrate the receipt of one of the listed vaccines but claims that some medical condition other than those listed in the statute resulted, or that a listed condition occurred outside the statutory time frame, the petitioner may still pursue a claim but must establish "actual causation." The act's legislative history instructs that evidence in the form of scientific studies or expert medical testimony is needed to demonstrate causation.

For a successful claimant, the Vaccine Injury Compensation Program provides compensation for past and future medical expenses, rehabilitation, therapies, special education expenses, equipment, and placement. For pain and suffering, the Vaccine Injury Compensation Program provides a maximum of $250,000. The Vaccine Injury Compensation Program also provides compensation for lost earnings. The Vaccine Injury Compensation Program provides a $250,000 award for a vaccine-related death.

As of March 1, 2010, cases filed in the Vaccine Injury Compensation Program numbered 13,330, of which 5,617 were autism cases. Of the total, 7,397 had been adjudicated, with 2,409 being compensated; 5,933 cases remained pending (www.hrsa.gov/vaccinecompensation). Most of the pending claims involved autism; those petitioners asked that the Special Masters defer proceedings on their claims until rulings in the "autism test cases" became final (U.S. Court of Federal Claims, 2011).

In the test cases, the petitioners, families of individuals with autism, alleged that certain childhood vaccinations might be causing or contributing to an apparent increase in the diagnosis of ASD. Specifically, the petitioners alleged that cases of autism, or neurodevelopmental disorders similar to autism, may be caused by measles–mumps–rubella (MMR) vaccinations; by the thimerosal ingredient contained in certain DPT, Diphtheria–Pertussis–Tetanus (DPT), hepatitis B, and *Haemophilus influenzae* type b (Hib) vaccinations; or by a combination of the vaccine and thimerosol.

Resolving the Petitions

Because of the large number of autism cases filed in Vaccine Court, a Steering Committee was assembled to strategically pursue the cases. Initially, the Petitioners' Steering Committee planned to advance three different theories of causation in an Omnibus Autism Proceeding. The Office of Special Masters assigned three Special Masters to resolve the autism cases. The Office of Special Masters instructed the Petitioners' Steering Committee to designate three "test cases" for each of the three theories, for a total of nine test cases. The two theories of "general causation" were designated by the Petitioners' Steering Committee: (a) that MMR vaccines and thimerosal-containing vaccines can combine to cause autism; and (b) that thimerosal-containing vaccines can alone cause autism.

During 2007, hearings were conducted in three test cases representing the first general causation theory. Specifically, in June of 2007, Special Master George Hastings presided over *Cedillo v. HHS*, No. 98-916V; in October of 2007 Special Master Patricia Campbell-Smith presided over *Hazlehurst v. HHS*, No. 03-654V; and in November of 2007 Special Master Denise Vowell presided over *Snyder v. HHS*, No. 01-162V.

The evidentiary record for the three cases remained open for some time past the evidentiary hearings. For example, after one of the cases, parties listened to the digital recording of the proceedings and made numerous corrections to the nearly 3,000-page transcript. The parties also filed nearly 500 pages of posthearing briefs. Finally, after the Petitioners' Steering Committee exhausted their efforts to obtain information from similar litigation conducted in Great Britain, the records were closed in the three cases in late 2008.

With the closing of the evidentiary records, the Special Masters began deciding their respective cases. Regarding all three cases, in addition to the 5,000 pages of transcript and the 700-plus pages of posthearing briefs, the records in these three cases contain 939 medical articles, whereas a typical vaccine case presents about 10. Among the three cases, 50 expert reports were filed and 28 experts testified.

The Special Masters issued multi-hundred-page decisions in the three test cases on February 12, 2009, and each of the Special Masters ruled against the petitioners. A Special Master's ruling is appealable to a Judge of the Court of Federal Claims under an "arbitrary and capricious" standard, with further review available before the Court of Appeals for the Federal Circuit and ultimately before the U.S. Supreme Court.

The evidentiary hearings in the three "test cases" for the second theory of causation—whether thimerosal-containing vaccines alone can cause autism—were conducted in May and July of 2008, and decisions were issued on March 12, 2010. Similar decisions were reached by three separate judges.

In *King v. HHS*, No. 03-589V, after studying the evidence Special Master Hastings wrote that the petitioners failed to demonstrate a causal link between the patients' autism and Thimerosol containing vaccines. "In this case, the evidence advanced by the petitioners has fallen far short of demonstrating such a link" (US Court of Federal Claims, 2010, pp. 1–2).

In *Mead v. HHS*, No. 03-215V, Special Master Campbell-Smith wrote that the theory of vaccine-related causation was also scientifically unsupported and the special master could not find the sequence of cause and effect. "Having failed to satisfy their burden of proof under the articulated legal standard, the petitioners did not prevail on their claim of vaccine-related causation" (U.S. Court of Federal Claims, 2010, pp. 1–2).

In *Dwyer v. HHS*, No. 03-1202V, Special Master Vowell wrote that petitioners "have not demonstrated by a preponderance of the evidence that Colin's condition was either caused or significantly aggravated by his vaccinations. Thus, they have failed to establish entitlement to compensation and the petition for compensation is therefore denied" (U.S. Court of Federal Claims, 2010, p. 23).

The petitioners in *King, Mead*, and *Dwyer* did not seek review in the Court of Federal Claims; as such, the judgments became final on April 14, 2010.

Implications of Vaccine Court for Nursing

Nurses providing care for autism patients and their families or communities must stay informed regarding the evidence base for vaccinations' relationship to autism and current status of the legal environment (McGuinness & Lewis, 2010; Rhodes, 2009). Maintaining community connections to facilitate referrals to expertise in handling claims will enhance nursing care for patients wanting to explore this option. Community health nurses must understand the issues and evidence base surrounding the benefit versus risks of childhood vaccinations in the context of autism. Since a significant portion of childhood vaccinations are administered in the community health setting, the community health nurse needs to be able to guide parents through vaccination decisions. The implication of the establishment of a "vaccine court" is a heightened awareness of parents that vaccinations can come with public health risks. This heightened awareness can be anticipated to cause a greater demand for education and counseling of parents in the vaccination process.

Protocols for counseling families that are concerned their child's autism is related to a past vaccination must integrate best practices that consider the best interests of the child as a priority. Again, competence in referrals for investigation and exploration of these concerns are part of best practices. Nurses might also need to participate in developing local public health policy guidelines for reporting patient concerns of suspected vaccination-related autism. Nursing research can contribute to exploring potential causative factors including, but not limited to, vaccination exposures in order to unravel a better understanding of the etiological factors of autism. A strong evidence base for causative factors—whether they are genetic or environmental or a combination of both—is greatly needed to inform policy development in the future.

PART THREE: POLICIES ADDRESSING PROTECTION, SUPPORT, AND DECISIONAL CAPACITY

The wide spectrum of ASD conditions leads to a broad and eclectic spectrum of life-planning legal issues that will arise over an individual's lifetime. Planning by the patient and his/her family or extended support system should include consideration of the individual's decisional capacity and level of other cognitive functioning. For example, some individuals diagnosed with ASD will be able to work and provide for their own support, at least in part, perhaps through subsidized wage or sheltered work environments. This option may invoke the need to exercise protections under the Americans with Disabilities Act (U.S. Congress, 1990). Other individuals with ASD will need lifetime 24-hour health care and a public resource to pay for this care. Whatever the individual's situation, paying for the care and support of an individual with ASD should be addressed for the long term, with an eye toward a plan to fund this care for life.

A critical period to address, specifically, in considering this type of life planning is when a child with autism turns 18 years of age. In most states, 18 is the age of majority, and thus, a child turning 18 becomes a legal adult literally overnight. Many legal issues may come into play at age 18 years.

Guardianship and Conservatorship

When a child reaches the age of majority, in most states, by law that child becomes a legal adult and has the right to make his or her own medical treatment decisions. An 18-year-old is solely legally responsible for providing consent for all medical treatments. Necessary medical treatment generally will not be provided without the informed consent of the 18-year-old.

This issue is often of primary concern to parents of an 18-year-old with ASD if the child is simply not capable of making decisions about, understanding, or articulating what is in his or her medical best interests. If a doctor or parent feels a child is not able to understand the risks and benefits of medical treatment and cannot make informed medical decisions, a legal guardian must be appointed for that purpose.

Guardianship

A "guardianship" is a state-specific legal process, and the law and language regarding guardians are different in every state. Many states have enacted guardianship procedures similar to the provisions in the Uniform Guardianship and Protective Proceedings Act 1997 (National Conferences of Commissioners on Uniform State Laws, 1997) but many variations among the states exist, and a practitioner must be careful to consider the relevant state's guardianship law. Typically, a parent seeking a guardianship must petition the appropriate state court; then a guardian *ad litem* or attorney is appointed for the "proposed protected person," and a due process hearing is held with required evidence from physician examiners and a lay visitor.

Conservatorship

A "conservatorship" is similar in many ways to a guardianship, but a conservatorship concerns the managing of income, property, or assets for an allegedly incapacitated person, while a guardianship is focused on an individual's health and life decision making. Petitioners often seek to become a guardian and a conservator at the same time, depending on the individual's circumstances. Specific issues related to guardianship and conservatorship are described in Table 18.2.

Implications of Policies Addressing Protection, Support, and Decisional Capacity for Nursing Practice

Nurses providing direct care to patients with an ASD diagnosis will demonstrate competency by being knowledgeable of legal options, such as guardianship, that may be relevant during the transition period of advancing to adulthood. The patient and the family will be well served by guidance in assessing the patient's capacity to participate in his or her own health care interactions. Nurse assessment skills can contribute greatly to the family dynamics involved. For patients with levels of decisional capacity or cognitive function that are relatively high within the autistic patient community, the transition to legal adulthood may create conflict between family members regarding the level of protection versus empowerment appropriate.

Nursing and clinical research is needed to develop an evidence base for best practices in assessing health care decisional capacity in adult patients with autism. Research is emerging regarding decisional capacity to consent to treatment and health care–related research. For example, recent evidence showed that adults with autism can attain research consent capacity scores comparable to those of comparison subjects with average cognitive function. This evidence suggests a future direction for nursing research: exploration of consent methods that address patients' individual cognitive differences and adapt to deficits in language, memory, and attention, thus empowering persons with autism to participate in research that can inform best clinical practices (Fisher, Cea, Davidson, & Fried, 2006; Fisher & Oransky, 2008).

Nursing as a profession has been implicitly called to action by the social movement to support the autistic community (Caruso, 2010). The goal of collaboration is to develop best practice nursing care to ensure protection of the rights of people with ASD who require medical care (Caruso, 2010; Fisher & Oransky, 2008). Automatic assumptions that an autism diagnosis equates to lack of capacity for adults with autism to make health care decisions are not appropriate. All nursing roles must stay informed regarding emerging research approaches and findings that support health care delivery and research exploration of ways to empower autistic community members to directly participate in addressing their needs (Fisher et al., 2006; Fisher & Oransky, 2008; Nicolaidis et al., 2011).

TABLE 18.2 Circumstances Related to Guardianship and Conservatorship

Case	Description	Qualification
Social Security Disability/SSI Cessation	• A child with ASD may qualify for disability benefits from birth to age 18 under the Social Security Administration's (SSA) Supplemental Security Income (SSI) program. • A child's condition is reviewed when he or she turns 18, and the benefits may be ceased if SSA determines the individual is no longer legally disabled (these are commonly called "cessation" cases). • The cessation rate for individuals with ASD is quite high, and thus, an individual with ASD should prepare for and anticipate appealing a disability cessation determination right when the individual turns age 18.	To qualify for Social Security Disability or SSI: • A person needs to show they are unable to perform a substantial gainful activity. This can be a burden on an individual with ASD, who is without organized medical records and documented ASD assessments and consistent ASD diagnoses. • Reviews and cessations at age 18 can also often trigger what are called "overpayment" cases, in which SSA determines the individual has been receiving more benefits than they are entitled to receive (and thus, have been "overpaid"), thereby adding further financial pressure right as the individual enters legal adulthood
Child support extensions, modifications, and deviations	• As with guardianships, child support is a matter of state law, and there are variations in child support law among the 50 states, but generally a parent's legal obligation to provide support to a child ends when that child turns age 18. • All states, however, allow for exceptions to this general rule, and one common exception is cases in which there are extraordinary medical, psychological, or educational expenses that will clearly continue past the child's 18th birthday (a child support extension). • An individual with an ASD may well present a strong case for extending the parental obligation to support past the age of 18 and, perhaps, permanently.	Even before the child's turning 18 becomes an issue • Child support calculations can and should be altered by a child's ASD. • All states' child support calculation systems (routinely referred to as "the guidelines") allow for a deviation from the otherwise standard guidelines in cases of extraordinary medical, psychological, or educational expenses, and this may well apply to most individuals with ASD. • Previously ordered child support may well be subject to a child support modification, as the expenses for ASD treatment and care fluctuate through the years depending on availability of insurance or Medicaid coverage, needs of the individual, etc.

From Unumb & Unumb (2011, p. 546).

SUMMARY

Clinical and school nursing roles that interface with persons living with autism require diligence in integrating knowledge from the emerging scientific evidence base to develop best practices within the current legal and policy landscape. Where the clinical and school nurse is competent to incorporate new, scientific-based interventions into practice, an additional factor is whether the legal or policy landscape will underwrite its expense or mandate patient access. Nurses with advocacy roles must maintain competency and keep current to assure appropriate patient access to competent care. Open lines of communication and collaboration among school, clinical, and community health nurses and nursing advocates, such as nurse-lobbyists, nursing professional organization leaders, and nurse-legislators can influence policy. Nursing collaborations among the diverse roles must focus on policies that address access to care, public health risks of autism, and empowering the autistic community to participate directly in improving the health care system.

Where the scientific evidence base is bare, nursing research must collaborate with the network of other nursing roles to promote competence and disseminate new findings in the evidence base for best practices (Minchella & Preti, 2011). An emerging approach to research that informs autism policy is referred to as community-based participatory research. It relies on partnerships with the autistic community. This approach proposes that persons living with autism are partners in setting the research agenda to inform policy (Nicolaidis et al., 2011). Engagement of autistic community stakeholders in research roles other than the passive role of "subject" is a nursing research strategy that promises to more effectively shape equitable health-related laws and policies (Hinshaw & Grady, 2011). Nurse-scientists will want to follow the implications and funded initiatives that may result from the Combating Autism Act of 2006 (Stokstad, 2007; U.S. Congress, 2006).

Nursing advocacy is also an important part of the policy landscape. This advocacy may be shaped by individual nurses employed as legislators or lobbyists or as advisors to public policy agencies. Nursing professional organizations also function in the nurse-advocate role by issuing position statements on various public health laws. All nurse-advocate roles working with individuals, families, or the community living with autism must monitor policy development, litigation, and the court system's resolution of claims against vaccine administration (Stewart, 2009), and schools, insurance, health care, and employers for disability discrimination (Van Wieren, Reid, & McMahon, 2008).

The momentum of the social movement to support persons living with autism will stay fast if nurses join other professionals. There is reason to anticipate meaningful change in the legal and policy landscape. This will call for diligence on the part of all nurses to maintain competence and integrate knowledge of ASD with their practice.

APPENDIX 18.1

Arkansas 2011 House Bill 1315

Coverage for autism spectrum disorders required – Definitions.

(a) As used in this section:

1. "Applied behavior analysis," means the design, implementation, and evaluation of environmental modifications by a board-certified behavior analyst using behavioral stimuli and consequences to produce socially significant improvement in human behavior, including the use of direct observation, measurement, and functional analysis of the relationship between environment and behavior;
2. "Autism services provider" means a person, entity, or group that provides diagnostic evaluations and treatment of ASDs, including licensed physicians, licensed psychiatrists, licensed speech therapists, licensed occupational therapists, licensed physical therapists, licensed psychologists, and board-certified behavior analysts;
3. "Autism spectrum disorder" means any of the pervasive developmental disorders as defined by the most recent edition of the "Diagnostic and Statistical Manual of Mental Disorders", including:
   (A) Autistic disorder;
   (B) Asperger's disorder; and
   (C) Pervasive developmental disorder not otherwise specified;
4. "Board-certified behavior analyst" means an individual certified by the nationally accredited Behavior Analyst Certification Board, a nationally accredited nongovernmental agency that certifies individuals who have completed academic, examination, training, and supervision requirements in applied behavior analysis;
5. (A) "Diagnosis" means medically necessary assessment, evaluations, or tests to diagnose whether or not an individual has an autism spectrum disorder.
   (B) Diagnostic evaluations do not need to be completed concurrently to diagnosis autism spectrum disorder;
6. "Evidence-based treatment" means treatment subject to research that applies rigorous, systematic, and objective procedures to obtain valid knowledge relevant to autism spectrum disorders;
7. (A) "Health benefit plan" means any group or blanket plan, policy, or contract for health care services issued or delivered in this state by health care insurers, including indemnity and managed care plans and the plans providing health benefits to state and public school employees under § 21-5-401 et seq., but excluding individual major medical plans, and plans providing health care services under Arkansas Constitution, Article 5, § 32, the Workers' Compensation Law, § 11-9-101 et seq., and the Public Employee Workers' Compensation Act, § 21-5-601 et seq.
   (B) "Health benefit plan" does not include an accident only, specified disease, hospital indemnity, Medicare supplement, long-term care, disability income, or other limited benefit health insurance policy;

8. "Health care insurer" means any insurance company, hospital and medical service corporation, or health maintenance organization issuing or delivering health benefit plans in this state and subject to any of the following laws:
   (A) The insurance laws of this state;
   (B) Section 23-75-101 et seq., pertaining to hospital and medical service corporations; and
   (C) Section 23-76-101 et seq., pertaining to health maintenance organizations;
9. "Medically necessary" means reasonably expected to do the following:
   (A) Prevent the onset of an illness, condition, injury, or disability;
   (B) Reduce or ameliorate the physical, mental, or developmental effects of an illness, condition, injury, or disability; or
   (C) Assist to achieve or maintain maximum functional capacity in performing daily activities, taking into account both the functional capacity of the individual and the functional capacities that are appropriate for individuals of the same age;
10. "Pharmacy care" means medications prescribed by a licensed physician and any health-related services deemed medically necessary to determine the need or effectiveness of the medications;
11. "Psychiatric care" means direct or consultative services provided by a psychiatrist licensed in the state in which the psychiatrist practices;
12. "Psychological care" means direct or consultative services provided by a psychologist licensed in the state in which the psychologist practices;
13. "Therapeutic care" means services provided by licensed speech therapists, occupational therapists, or physical therapists; and
14. "Treatment" includes:
   (A) The following care prescribed, provided, or ordered for a specific individual diagnosed with an autism spectrum disorder by a licensed physician or a licensed psychologist who determines the care to be medically necessary and evidence-based including without limitation:
      (i) Applied behavior analysis when provided by or supervised by a Board Certified Behavior Analyst;
      (ii) Pharmacy care;
      (iii) Psychiatric care;
      (iv) Psychological care;
      (v) Therapeutic care; and
      (vi) Equipment determined necessary to provide evidence-based treatment; and
   (B) Any care for an individual with autism spectrum disorder that is determined by a licensed physician to be:
      (i) Medically necessary; and
      (ii) Evidence-based.

(b) To the extent that the diagnosis and treatment of autism spectrum disorders are not already covered by a health benefit plan, coverage under this section shall be included in a health benefit plan that is delivered, executed, issued, amended, adjusted, or renewed in this state on or after October 1, 2011.

(c) Applied behavior analysis services shall:

1. Have an annual limitation of fifty thousand dollars ($50,000); and
2. Be limited to children under eighteen (18) years of age.

(d) 1. The coverage required by this section is not subject to:

(A) Any limits on the number of visits an individual may make to an autism services provider; or

(B) Dollar limits, deductibles, or coinsurance provisions that are less favorable to an insured than the dollar limits, deductibles, or coinsurance provisions that apply to a physical illness generally under a health benefit plan.

2. The coverage may be subject to other general exclusions and limitations of the health insurance plan, including without limitation coordination of benefits, participating provider requirements, restrictions on services provided by family or household members, and utilization review of health care services including review of medical necessity, case management, and other managed care provisions.

(e) This section does not limit benefits that are otherwise available to an individual under a health benefit plan.

(f) Coverage for treatment under this section shall not be denied on the basis that the treatment is habilitative in nature.

(g) 1. If an individual is receiving treatment for an autism spectrum disorder, an insurer shall not request a review of the medical necessity of the treatment for autism spectrum disorder to a greater extent than it does for other illnesses covered in the policy.

2. The cost of obtaining the review shall be borne by the insurer.

(h) 1. This section shall not be construed as affecting any obligation to provide services to an individual under an individualized family service plan, an individualized education program under the Individuals with Disabilities Education Act, or an individualized service plan.

2. In accordance with the Individuals with Disabilities Education Act, nothing in this section relieves an insurer from an otherwise valid obligation to provide or to pay for services provided to an individual with a disability.

(i) On and after January 1, 2014:

1. To the extent that this section requires benefits that exceed the essential health benefits specified under section 1302(b) of the Patient Protection and Affordable Care Act, Pub. L. No. 111-148, as amended, the specific benefits that exceed the specified essential health benefits shall not be required of a health benefit plan when the plan is offered by a health care insurer in this state through the state medical exchange; and
2. This section continues to apply to plans offered outside the state medical exchange.

REFERENCES

American Psychiatric Association. (2000). *Diagnostic and statistical manual of mental disorders* (4 ed., text revision). Washington, DC: American Psychiatric Association.

American Psychological Association. (2008). *The Wellstone-Domenici Mental Health Parity Act frequently asked questions.* Retrieved from http://apapracticecentral.org/update/2009/11-23/wellstone-domenici.pdf

Autism Speaks. (2011). *Autism Speaks state autism insurance reform initiatives.* Retrieved from http://www.autism-votes.org/site/c.frKNI3PCImE/b.3909861/k.B9DF/State_Initiatives.htm

Bartley, J. J. (2006). An update on autism: Science, gender, and the law. *Gender and Medicine, 3*(2), 73–78. doi: S1550-8579(06)80197-X [pii]

Bellando, J., & Lopez, M. (2009). The school nurse's role in treatment of the student with autism spectrum disorders. *Journal of Specialists in Pediatric Nursing, 14*(3), 173–182. doi: JSPN195 [pii]

Bouder, J. N., Spielman, S., & Mandell, D. S. (2009). Brief report: Quantifying the impact of autism coverage on private insurance premiums. *Journal of Autism & Developmental Disorders, 39*(6), 953–957. doi: 10.1007/s10803-009-0701-z

Caruso, D. (2010). Autism in the U.S.: Social movement and legal change. *American Journal of Law and Medicine, 36*(4), 483–539.

Chiri, G., & Warfield, M. (2011). Unmet need and problems accessing core health care services for children with autism spectrum disorder. *Maternal and Child Health Journal,* 1–11. doi: 10.1007/s10995-011-0833-6.

Cohen, H., Amerine-Dickens, M., & Smith, T. (2006). Early intensive behavioral treatment: Replication of the UCLA model in a community setting. *Journal of Developmental & Behavioral Pediatrics, 27*(suppl 2), S145–S155.

Couper, J. (2004). Who should pay for intensive behavioural intervention in autism? A parent's view. *Journal of Paediatric and Child Health, 40*(9–10), 559–561. doi: 10.1111/j.1440-1754.2004.00464.x JPC464 [pii]

Council for Affordable Health Insurance. (2011). *Health insurance mandates in the states, 2010.* Retrieved from http://www.cahi.org/cahi_contents/resources/pdf/MandatesintheStates2010.pdf).

Easter Seals. (2011). *Autism services: Services for people with autism spectrum disorder.* Retrieved July 31, 2011, from http://www.easterseals.com/site/PageServer?pagename=ntlc8_autism_service

Fisher, C. B., Cea, C. D., Davidson, P. W., & Fried, A. L. (2006). Capacity of persons with mental retardation to consent to participate in randomized clinical trials. *American Journal of Psychiatry, 163*(10), 1813–1820. doi: 163/10/1813 [pii] 10.1176/appi.ajp.163.10.1813

Fisher, C. B., & Oransky, M. (2008). Informed consent to psychotherapy: Protecting the dignity and respecting the autonomy of patients. *Journal of Clinical Psychology, 64*(5), 576–588. doi: 10.1002/jclp.20472

Ganz, M. L. (2007). The lifetime distribution of the incremental societal costs of autism. *Archives of Pediatric and Adolescent Medicine, 161*(4), 343–349.

Hall, H. R., & Graff, J. C. (2011). The relationships among adaptive behaviors of children with autism, family support, parenting stress, and coping. *Issues in Comprehensive Pediatric Nursing, 34*(1), 4–25. doi: doi:10.3109/01460862.2011.555270

Health Care and Education Reconciliation Act. (2010). Pub.L. 111-152, 124 Stat. 1029. Retrieved from http://thomas.loc.gov/cgi-bin/query/z?c111:H.R.4872

Hinshaw, A., & Grady, P. (Eds.). (2011). *Shaping health policy through nursing research.* New York: Springer Publishing.

Holland, C. (2010). Note: Autism, insurance, and the idea: A comprehensive legal framework. *Cornell Law Review, 95*, 1253–1282.

Kogan, M. D., Strickland, B. B., Blumberg, S. J., Singh, G. K., Perrin, J. M., & van Dyck, P. C. (2008). A national profile of the health care experiences and family impact of autism spectrum disorder among children in the United States, 2005. *Pediatrics, 122*(6), e1149–e1158. doi: 10.1542/peds.2008-1057

Lovaas, O. I. (1987). Behavioral treatment and normal educational and intellectual functioning in young autistic children, *Journal of Consulting in Clinical Psychology, 55*(1), 3–9.

McEachin, J., Smith, T., & Lovaas, O. I. (1993). Long-term outcome for children with autism who received early intensive behavioral treatment. *American Journal of Mental Retardation, 97*(4), 359–372; discussion 373–391.

McGuinness, T. M., & Lewis, S. (2010). Update on autism and vaccines. *Journal of Psychosocial Nursing and Mental Health Services, 48*(6), 15–18. doi: 10.3928/02793695-20100506-02

Minchella, L., & Preti, L. (2011). Autism spectrum disorder: Clinical considerations for the school nurse. *NASN School Nurse, 26*(3), 143–145.

Mucklan, J. (2007). Influencing policy development: The whirling dervish of the autism in-home program. *Journal of Pediatric Nursing, 22*(3), 223–230. doi: doi:10.1016/j.pedn.2007.03.001

National Conference of Commissioners on Uniform State Laws. (1997). Uniform guardianship and protective proceedings act of 1997. Available at http://www.law.upenn.edu/bll/archives/ulc/fnact99/1990s/ugppa97.htm

Nicolaidis, C., Raymaker, D., McDonald, K., Dern, S., Ashkenazy, E., Boisclair, C., . . . Baggs, A. (2011). Collaboration strategies in nontraditional community-based participatory research partnerships: Lessons from an academic-community partnership with autistic self-advocates. *Progressive Community Health Partnership, 5*(2), 143–150. doi: S1557055X11200068 [pii] 10.1353/cpr.2011.0022

Patient Protection and Affordable Care Act. (2009). P.L. 111-148, HR 3590. Retrieved from http://democrats.senate.gov/pdfs/reform/patient-protection-affordable-care-act-as-passed.pdf

Rhodes, A. M. (2009). Autism and the courts. *Journal of Specialists in Pediatric Nursing, 14*(3), 215–216. doi: JSPN202 [pii]10.1111/j.1744-6155.2009.00202.x

Stewart, A. M. (2009). When vaccine injury claims go to court. *New England Journal of Medicine, 360*(24), 2498–2500. doi: doi:10.1056/NEJMp0902316

Stokstad, E. (2007). New autism law focuses on patients, environment. *Science, 315*(5808), 27. doi: 10.1126/science.315.5808.27a

Strunk, J. A. (2009). School nurses' knowledge of autism spectrum disorders. *Journal of School Nursing, 25*(6), 445–452. doi: 1059840509348221 [pii] 10.1177/1059840509348221

Twoy, R., Connolly, P. M., & Novak, J. M. (2007). Coping strategies used by parents of children with autism. *Journal of the American Academy of Nurse Practitioners, 19*(5), 251–260. doi: JAAN222 [pii] 10.1111/j.1745-7599.2007.00222.x

Unumb, L. S., & Unumb, D. R. (2011). *Autism and the law: Cases, statutes, and materials.* Durham, NC: Carolina Academic Press.

U.S. Congress. (1990). Americans with Disabilities Act of 1990, 42 U.S.C. #12101 et seq. Accessed March 3, 2012 at http://www.ada.gov/

U.S. Congress. (1990). Individuals with Disabilities Education Act (IDEA). Accessed March 1, 2012 at http://idea.ed.gov/

U.S. Congress. (2006). Combating Autism Act of 2006. Available at http://georgewbush-whitehouse.archives.gov/news/releases/2006/12/20061219-3.html

U.S. Congress. (2009). Employee Retirement Income Act (ERISA). Available at http://aging.senate.gov/crs/pension7.pdf

U.S. Court of Federal Claims. (2010a). King v. HHS, No. 03-589V. Available at http://www.uscfc.uscourts.gov/sites/default/files/Hastings.King%20Decision.pdf

U.S. Court of Federal Claims. (2010b). Dwyer v. HHS, No. 03-1202V. Available at http://www.uscfc.uscourts.gov/sites/default/files/Vowell.Dwyer.FINAL.pdf

U.S. Court of Federal Claims. (2010c). Mead v. HHS, No. 03-215V. Available at http://www.uscfc.uscourts.gov/sites/default/files/Campbell-Smith%20Mead%20Autism%20Decision.pdf

U.S. Court of Federal Claims. (2011). *Omnibus Autism Proceeding Vaccine Program/Office of Special Masters Omnibus Autism Proceeding*. Retrieved from http://www.uscfc.uscourts.gov/omnibus-autism-proceeding.

U.S. Department of Health and Human Services. (1987). *National Vaccine Advisory Committee (NVAC).* Retrieved from http://www.hhs.gov/nvpo/nvac/

U.S. Department of Health and Human Services. (1988). *National Vaccine Injury Compensation Program (VICP).* Retrieved from http://www.hrsa.gov/vaccinecompensation/

U.S. Department of Health and Human Services. (2010). Interim final rules under the Paul Wellstone and Pete Domenici Mental Health Parity and Addiction Equity Act of 2008. *Federal Register, Rules and Regulations. 75*, (21) (Tuesday, February 2). Retrieved from http://edocket.access.gpo.gov/2010/pdf/2010-

U.S. Department of Health and Human Services. (2011). *The Mental Health Parity and Addiction Equity Act.* Retrieved from http://www.cms.gov/HealthInsReformforConsume/04_TheMentalHealthParityAct.asp

U.S. Department of Labor. (n.d.). *Fact sheet: The Mental Health Parity Act.* Retrieved from http://www.dol.gov/ebsa/newsroom/fsmhparity.html#).

Van Wieren, T. A., Reid, C. A., & McMahon, B. T. (2008). Workplace discrimination and autism spectrum - disorders: The National EEOC Americans with Disabilities Act Research project. *Work, 31*(3), 299–308.

Discussion Questions

V

CHAPTER 17

1. Write a vision statement for an ideal nursing practice partnership for autism spectrum disorder (ASD) care.
2. Analyze a present practice environment for barriers to comprehensive nursing care of patients with ASD.
3. Select a practice area (e.g., emergency department, same-day surgery, labor and delivery) and propose ways the nursing staff might employ or consult with a behaviorist who specializes in ASD care.
4. Discuss the application of the Nursing Code of Ethics to the care of individuals with ASD.
5. Consider your nursing practice area and discuss ways the nursing staff might collaborate with a regional or local autism treatment center.
6. What is your recommendation on best-practices, long-term care of an aging population of individuals with autism.
7. Discuss the impact of a person's diagnosis with ASD on the immediate and extended family.
8. Create a list of questions that you would pose to an autism diagnostic/treatment center to evaluate their knowledge of the role nursing might play in the delivery or expansion of services.

CHAPTER 18

1. Investigate and describe the process of obtaining a copyright on material you created for ASD care in your area. Are institutional approvals needed and if so, from whom? How long will the process take? What legal documents are required, if any?
2. Identify three ASD diagnostic/treatment centers in your city or region and describe potential learning opportunities available there for bachelor's- and master's-level nursing students.
3. Create a set of questions for use in your practice setting to determining the guardianship status of a new patient who has been admitted for care.
4. Present your opinion on the issue of allocation of resources for ASD services in an era of increased prevalence and reduced revenue.
5. Discuss how the policies that will be relevant to nursing care may change as the person with the ASD diagnosis advances in age from early childhood to adult.

6. Describe how the nurse can directly influence the legal landscape at the local, state, and federal levels.
7. Consider the referrals the nurse must make to support a patient's navigation of existing laws and policies that frame his or her access to care. What other disciplines and expertise should be represented in the nurse's community resource referrals?
8. Discuss the factors a nurse will consider in assessing decisional capacity of an adult diagnosed with ASD for treatment consent. What factors must be considered for a research informed-consent process?

Glossary

Accommodations Changes in how a test is administered that do not substantially alter what the test measures, including changes in presentation format, response format, test setting, or test timing. They help to provide equal opportunity to demonstrate knowledge.

Advanced practice registered nurse (APRN) An umbrella term appropriate for a licensed registered nurse prepared at the graduate-degree level as a clinical nurse specialist, nurse anesthetist, nurse-midwife, or nurse practitioner.

Americans with Disabilities Act (ADA) The U.S. law that ensures rights of persons with disabilities with regard to employment and other issues. It was enacted to prohibit discrimination based on disability.

Anhedonia The inability to take pleasure in activities that are normally enjoyable.

Anticipatory guidance Providing in-advance information to parents or caregivers about children's pending growth and developmental changes, including safety and health concerns, communication and motor skills, nutritional needs, and social–emotional considerations.

Antipsychotic medication Drugs typically used for psychosis or schizophrenia. Atypical antipsychotic medications may be used to treat behavioral symptoms in ASD; these medications include Risperdal (risperidone), Zyprexa (olanzapine), Seroquel (quetiapine); Geodon (ziprasidone), Abilify (aripiprazole), and Clozaril (clozapine).

Aphasia The complete or partial loss of ability to use or understand language.

Applied behavioral analysis (ABA) An intensive educational behavioral therapy, also called Lovaas therapy (after the initiator Dr. Ivan Lovaas). It uses a series of trials ("discrete trials") to shape desired behavior or response. Skills are broken down into small components and taught to the child through a system of reinforcement. Applied behavioral analysis currently has a strong research base of evidence of effectiveness for people with autism. Examples of ABA interventions include positive behavioral supports, reinforcement, shaping, fading, and chaining behaviors.

Apraxia A disorder consisting of a partial or total incapacity to execute purposeful movements, without impairment of muscular power and coordination. The person has difficulty sequencing movement. Apraxia may be specific to speech.

Asperger's disorder (or syndrome) Form of high-functioning autism that may present with superior or normal IQ, later diagnosis, and more fluent language. It may be subtle in differences from high-functioning autism in degree of certain auditory-processing issues, spelling, and problems with background stimulation.

Assistive technology device An item, piece of equipment, or product used to maintain or improve the functional capacity of a child with a disability.

Autism Diagnostic Observation Schedule (ADOS) The test considered to be the current gold standard for diagnosing ASD and, along with information from parents, should be incorporated into a child's comprehensive evaluation.

Autonomy Self-determination of the individual.

Basis skills Skills in subjects such as reading, writing, spelling, and mathematics.

Behavior intervention plan A plan of positive behavioral interventions in the individualized educational program of a child whose behaviors interfere with his/her learning, or that of others.

Beneficence Intention to do what is best for others to whom fiduciary responsibility is owed.

Brain-derived neurotrophic factor (BDNF) A neuronal growth stimulant that may be produced as a result of stress to the nervous system or may be needed to prevent impairment to the nervous system. It may be impaired in Rett syndrome (*see also* Rett syndrome).

Casein Protein found in milk, used in forming the basis of cheese and as a food additive.

Case management A professional care role incorporating comprehensive assessment of client and family needs, advocacy, referral to appropriate resources and services, and coordination of services; it is especially focused on communication among clients, service providers, and payers, such as insurance companies.

Chelation A treatment that binds positive metal ions with agents that chemically help remove them from tissues in the body. These drugs may also bond important useful metals or positive ions, such as calcium and iron.

Child find Requirement that states ensure all children with disabilities are identified, located, and evaluated, and determine which children are receiving special education and related services.

Childhood disintegrative disorder A disorder in which development begins normally in all areas, physical and mental. At some point between 2 and 10 years of age, the child loses previously developed skills. The child may lose social and language skills and other functions, including bowel and bladder control.

Chorionic villus sampling (CVS) Prenatal genetic testing typically done between 10 and 13 weeks after the pregnant woman's last menstrual period. The procedure involves extracting a sample of fetal cells from fetal chorionic villi using either a transcervical or transabdominal aspiration under ultrasound to diagnose an array of genetic disorders.

Chromosome 15 duplication syndrome A rare chromosomal disorder. Symptoms may be similar to Prader-Willi and Angelman syndromes and range from cases with no signs of disease to variable combinations of skeletal, neurological, gastrointestinal, psychological, and other abnormalities in association with developmental delay.

Client The term client is used throughout the text to reflect the recipient of nursing care that includes individuals, families, communities, and populations. In the education setting, the "client" includes students being taught, and in research, the "client" includes participants in the research setting.

Competency An observable, performance-based, measurable outcome that indicates the achievement of a particular knowledge component or application or demonstration of a psychomotor behavior or skill.

Compulsions Deliberate repetitive behaviors that follow specific rules pertaining to cleaning, checking, or counting. In young children, restricted patterns of interest may be early signs of compulsions.

Cytomegalovirus (CMV) A common virus of the herpes family. May be asymptomatic in healthy people but may be serious in people with an impaired immune system. Infection in utero may cause serious developmental disorders.

Declarative language Used to communicate what the mind is producing. It is what is most common in conversation, whereas imperative language is used to ask questions, make commands, or give instructions.

Developmental disorder Refers to several disorders that affect normal development. May affect single areas of development (specific developmental disorder) or several (pervasive developmental disorder; *see also*: Pervasive developmental disorders).

Developmental individual difference relationship (DIR) Therapy, also known as Floortime, that seeks to move the child toward increasingly complex interactions through mutually shared engagement. *See also* Floortime.

Developmental milestones Skills or behaviors that most children can do by a certain age; tracking these skills enables parents and professionals to monitor learning, behavior, and development. While each child develops differently, delays in reaching developmental milestones may be a red flag for greater concern.

Developmental pediatrician A medical doctor who is board-accredited and has received subspecialty training in developmental–behavioral pediatrics.

Diagnostic and Statistical Manual of Mental Disorders (DSM) The official system for classification of psychological and psychiatric disorders published by the American Psychiatric Association. It is periodically reviewed and updated or revised based on emerging research findings.

Disability In Section 504 and ADA, defined as impairment that substantially affects one or more major life activities, Also used to denote an individual who has a record of having such impairment or is regarded as having such an impairment. *See also* ADA; Section 504.

Discrete trial teaching (DTT) A technique incorporating principles of ABA, including positive reinforcement, but not in itself ABA. It is used to teach behaviors in a one-to-one setting. Concepts are broken down into small (discrete) parts.

Duty-based ethics Adherence to a set of moral principles applied in all situations.

Dyspraxia The brain's inability to plan muscle movements and carry them out. In speech therapeutics, this term may be used to describe apraxia (*see also* Apraxia).

Early intervention (EI) A state-funded program designed to identify and treat developmental problems or other disabilities as early as possible. Eligibility for EI is from birth to 3 years of age.

Echolalia Repeating words or phrases heard previously, either immediately after hearing the word or phrase, or much later. Delayed echolalia occurs days or weeks later. Functional echolalia is using quoted phrases in a way that has shared meaning, for example, saying "carry you" to ask to be carried.

Expressive labeling The communication of a name for an object or person (*see* Expressive language).

Expressive language Communication of intentions, desires, or ideas to others, through speech or printed words. It includes gestures, signing, use of a communication board, and other forms of expression.

Extended school year (ESY) Means that services are provided during breaks from school, such as during the summer vacation, for students who experience substantial regression in skills during breaks.

Family Educational Rights and Privacy Act (FERPA) Statute about confidentiality and access to education records.

Floortime A developmental intervention for children with autism involving meeting a child at his current developmental level, and building upon a particular set of strengths.

Fragile X A genetic disorder that shares many of the characteristics of autism. Individuals with autistic features may be evaluated for co-occurring Fragile X disorder.

Free appropriate education (FAPE) Education must be provided to all children ages 3 to 21 at public expense.

Functional performance Refers to activities and skills that are not academic or related to a child's academic achievement as measured on achievement tests.

Functional play When an object is used for its appropriate purpose, like rolling a toy car or truck.

Gastroesophageal reflux Returns the stomach contents back up into the esophagus, which frequently causes heartburn due to irritation of the esophagus by stomach acid.

Genetic predisposition A genetic factor that alters an individual's chance(s) of developing a disease or condition.

Genetics Study of individual genes and their impact on relatively rare single-gene disorders.

Genetic testing Genetic testing is the use of a laboratory test to look for genetic variations associated with a disease (For further information, see: http://www.genome.gov/glossary/index.cfm?id=88). Genetic testing may also be used for other purposes (e.g., pharmacogenomics, paternity identification, ancestry identification, and forensics).

Genomics Study of a subset or all the genes in the human genome together, including their interactions with one another, the environment, and other psychosocial and cultural factors.

Genotype The genetic makeup of an organism or group of organisms with reference to a single trait, set of traits, or an entire complex of traits.

Gestures Hand and head movements used to signal to someone else, such as a give-me motion, reaching, waving, pointing, or head shaking. They convey information or express emotions without the use of words.

Global developmental delay A diagnosis in children younger than 5 years of age characterized by delay in two or more developmental domains, sometimes associated with *intellectual disability*.

Gluten A protein present in wheat, rye, and barley.

Guardian *ad litem* Person appointed by the court to represent the rights of minors.

Hyperlexia The ability to read at an early age. To be hyperlexic, a child does not need to understand what he or she is reading.

Hyperresponsiveness, hypersensitivity *See* Sensory defensiveness.

Hyporesponsiveness, hyposensitivity Abnormal insensitivity to sensory input. A child who appears to be deaf, whose hearing is normal, is underreactive. A child who is underreactive to sensory input may have a high tolerance to pain, may be clumsy or sensation-seeking and may act aggressively.

Hypotonia A term that means low muscle tone.

Incidental teaching Teaches a child new skills while in their home or community, in natural context, or "in the moment" to help make sense of what they learn during formal instruction and to generalize new skills.

Inclusion Involves educating all children in regular classrooms, regardless of degree or severity of disability. Effective inclusion takes place with a planned system of training and supports; involves collaboration of a multidisciplinary team, including regular and special educators.

Individual family service plan (IFSP) Developed by a multidisciplinary team, including the family as a primary participant. Describes child's level of development in all areas: family resources, priorities, and concerns; services to be received; and the frequency, intensity, and method of delivery of services. Must state natural environments in which services will occur.

Individual health plan Plan of school-nursing care management incorporated into a student's IEP.

Individualized education plan (IEP) Identifies student's specific learning expectations, how a school will address them with appropriate services, and methods to review progress. For students 16 years of age and older, must contain plan to transition to postsecondary education or the workplace or to help the student live as independently as possible in the community.

Individuals with Disabilities Education Act of 2004 (IDEA) The U.S. law mandating the free and public education of all persons with disabilities between ages 3 and 21.

Infectious agents Organisms that cause infection; can be viruses, bacteria, fungi, or parasites.

Intellectual disability Describes a person with limitations in mental functioning that cause them to develop more slowly than a typical child. They may take longer to learn to speak, walk, and take care of personal needs, such as dressing or eating, and are likely to have trouble learning in school. May be mild or severe.

Joint attention The process of sharing one's experience of observing an object or event by following gaze or pointing gestures. Critical for social development, language acquisition, and cognitive development. Impairment in joint attention is a core deficit of ASD.

Karyotype Analysis of the number and type of chromosomes in an individual. If the person is a male the karyotype is 46 xy. This is a normal male karyotype.

Least-restrictive environment (LRE) Setting that least restricts opportunities for children with disabilities to be with peers without disabilities. The law mandates that every child with a disability be educated in a least-restrictive environment.

Lesch-Nyham syndrome A genetically inherited disease with intellectual disability, speech delay, and self-mutilation behaviors, such as biting hands, arms, and lips, or hitting oneself. Blood tests show elevated serum uric acid levels.

Limbic system The emotional center of the brain.

Mainstreaming A school environment in which special-needs students are expected to participate in existing regular education classes. This is compared to an inclusive program in which participation in the regular classroom may be partial or part-time (e.g., student might attend separate classes for academic subjects and join all students for physical education and lunch).

Maternal rubella A mild, highly contagious virus (also known as German measles) that crosses the placenta from an infected mother and leads to major developmental defects in a developing fetus.

Melatonin A hormone produced by pineal gland, involved in regulating sleeping and waking cycles. Sometimes a synthetic form is given for chronic insomnia. Consult with the child's physician before giving melatonin; it is not recommended for all patients with sleep problems.

Mental retardation See Intellectual Disability.

Modified Checklist of Autism in Toddlers (MCHAT) A screening tool for identifying young children who may be referred to a specialist for further evaluation and possible ASD diagnosis.

Motor deficits Physical skills that a person cannot perform or has difficulty performing.

Motor function (or motor skills) The ability to move and control movements.

Neurocutaneous disorders Genetic disorders leading to abnormal growth of tumors. These usually first appear as skin lesions, like birthmarks, but may eventually lead to tumors affecting the central nervous system and other parts of the body.

Neurologist Refers to a doctor specializing in medical problems associated with the nervous system, specifically the brain and spinal cord.

Neurotransmitter Brain chemicals that act as messengers that transmit or activate a neuronal action in the central or peripheral nervous system.

Nonfunctional routines Specified, sequential, and repeated actions or behaviors that a person engages in, such as lining up toys in a certain order each time instead of playing with them. People with ASD may follow routines that appear to be senseless but that may have significance to them.

Nonmaleficence The intention to avoid harm to others.

Nonverbal behaviors Things done to convey information or express emotions without words, including eye gaze, facial expressions, body postures, and gestures.

Obsessions Persistent and intrusive repetitive thoughts. Preoccupations with specific kinds of objects or actions may be an early sign of obsessions.

Obstructive sleep apnea Breathing disorder interrupting breathing during sleep in which airflow cannot flow through the nose or mouth, although efforts to breathe continue. Throat collapses during sleep, causing snorting and gasping for breath. May cause daytime sleepiness. May increase risk of hypertension and heart problems.

Occupational therapist A trained professional who helps the affected person become more independent in his or her activities of daily living. This is done by adapting the environment to eliminate obstacles and by teaching specific self-help skills to the person.

Occupational therapy Assists development of fine motor skills that aid in daily living. May focus on sensory issues, coordination of movement, balance, and self-help skills, such as dressing, eating with a fork, or grooming. May address visual perception and hand–eye coordination.

Operant conditioning The modification of behavior through positive and/or negative reinforcement.

Orientation and mobility services Includes services to the visually impaired.

Pedigree A graphic illustration of a family health history using standardized symbols.

Perseveration Repetitive movement or speech or sticking to one idea or task in a compulsive manner.

Pervasive developmental disorder—not otherwise specified (PDD-NOS) A category of PDD referring to children who have significant problems with communication and play and some difficulty interacting with others, but are too social for diagnosis of autism.

Pervasive developmental disorders (PDD) A group of conditions involving delays in development of many basic skills, including ability to socialize with others, to communicate, and to use imagination. Includes autism, Asperger's syndrome, childhood disintegrative disorder, Rett syndrome, and pervasive development disorder—not otherwise specified. *See also* entries for these conditions.

Petit mal seizure *See* Seizure, absence.

Phenotype The visible characteristics of an organism resulting from the interaction between its genetic makeup and the environment.

Phenylketonuria (PKU) A metabolic disorder involving deficiency of the enzyme phenylalanine hydroxylase, which leads to harmful buildup of phenylalanine in the body. Symptoms range from mild to severe. May cause mental retardation.

Physical therapist A trained professional who designs and implements physical therapy programs and who may work within a hospital or clinic, in a school, or as an independent practitioner.

Physical therapy Uses specially designed exercises and equipment to help patients regain or improve their physical abilities.

Pica Persistent eating or mouthing of nonnutritive substances for at least 1 month when behavior is developmentally inappropriate (older than 18–24 months). Substances may include items such as clay, dirt, sand, stones, pebbles, hair, feces, lead, laundry starch, vinyl gloves, plastic, erasers, ice, fingernails, paper, paint chips, coal, chalk, wood, plaster, light bulbs, needles, string, cigarette butts, wire, and burnt matches.

Picture exchange communication system (PECS) An alternative communication system using picture symbols. It is taught in phases, starting with a simple exchange of symbol for desired item. Individuals learn to use picture symbols to construct complete sentences, initiate communication, and answer questions.

Pivotal response treatment (PRT) Therapeutic teaching method using incidental teaching opportunities to target and modify key behaviors related to communication, behavior, and social skills.

Polypharmacy Polypharmacy means "many drugs" and refers to problems that can occur when a patient is taking more medications than are actually needed. It is a particular concern for older adults, who make up 13% of the population but account for almost 30% of all prescribed drugs. Polypharmacy is most common in people with multiple medical conditions.

Prevalence The current number of people in a given population who have a specific diagnosis at a specified point in time.

Proprioception The receiving of stimuli originating in muscles, tendons, and other internal tissues.

Pro se Representing oneself without assistance of legal counsel.

Prosody The rhythm and melody of spoken language expressed through rate, pitch, stress, inflection, or intonation. Some children with ASD have unusual intonation (flat, monotonous, stiff, or "singsongy") without emphasis on the important words.

Psychiatrist A doctor specializing in prevention, diagnosis, and treatment of mental illness. Has received additional training and completed a supervised residency in specialty. May have additional training in specialty, such as child psychiatry or neuropsychiatry. Can prescribe medication, which psychologists cannot do.

Psychologist A professional who diagnoses and treats diseases of the brain, emotional disturbance, and behavior problems. May have a master's degree (MA) or doctorate (PhD) in psychology. May have other qualifications, including board certification and additional training in a specific type of therapy.

Reasonable accommodation Adoption of a facility or program that can be accomplished without undue administrative or financial burden.

Receptive labeling *See* Receptive language.

Receptive language The ability to comprehend words and sentences. Begins as early as birth and increases with each stage in development. By 12 months, a child begins to understand words and responds to his or her name and may respond to familiar words in context. By 18 to 20 months, a child identifies familiar people by looking when the person is named (e.g., Where's Mommy?), gives familiar objects when they are named (e.g., Where's the ball?), and points to a few body parts (e.g., Where's your nose?). These skills commonly emerge slightly ahead of expressive language skills.

Rehabilitation Act of 1973 Civil rights statute designed to protect individuals with disabilities from discrimination; purposes are to maximize employment, economic self-sufficiency, independence, and inclusion and integration into society.

Rehabilitative counseling services Includes career development, preparation for employment, and vocational rehabilitation services funded under the Rehabilitation Act of 1973.

Reinforcement, reinforce Any object or event following a response that increases or maintains the rate of responding. A positive reinforcer may be produced by, or be added, after a response.

Relationship development intervention (RDI) A therapeutic teaching method based on building intelligence competencies of social connection—such as referencing, emotion sharing, coregulation, and experience sharing—that normally develop in infancy and early childhood.

Respite care Temporary, short-term care provided to individuals with disabilities, delivered in the home for a few short hours or in an alternate licensed setting for an extended period of time. Respite care allows caregivers to take a break in order to relieve and prevent stress and fatigue.

Rett syndrome A very rare disorder in which the patient has symptoms associated with PDD, along with problems with physical development. They generally lose many motor or movement skills—such as walking and use of hands—and develop poor coordination. The condition has been linked to a defect on the X chromosome, so it almost always affects girls.

Scintillation perfusion computerized tomography (SPECT) Measures blood flow and therefore crudely shows metabolism or areas of increased or decreased metabolism or related blood flow. This can also show areas of microvascular blood flow changes when there are inflammatory changes in the brain.

Screening tests Assessment or testing used to identify individuals at high risk for a disorder; results are then confirmed or ruled out by diagnostic testing. Screens involve some trade-off between sensitivity (ability to differentiate those who do not have the disorder) and specificity (ability to identify those who have the disorder).

Section 504 Section 504 of the Rehabilitation Act protects individuals with disabilities from discrimination due to disability by recipients of federal financial assistance.

Seizure Refers to uncontrolled electrical activity in the brain, which may produce a physical convulsion, minor physical signs, thought disturbances, or a combination of symptoms.

Seizure, absence Seizure that takes the form of a staring spell. Person suddenly seems "absent" or has a brief loss of awareness. May be accompanied by blinking or mouth twitching. Absence seizures have a very characteristic appearance on electroencephalogram. Also called a petit mal seizure.

Seizure, atonic Seizure in which a person loses muscle tone and strength and, unless supported, falls down. "Atonic" means lack of muscle tone and strength.

Seizure, subclinical (electrographic seizures) Seizures that are visible on the electroencephalogram, but do now manifest as observable symptoms in the affected person. Electroencephalography often detects subclinical seizures during sleep.

Seizure, tonic-clonic Seizures involving two phases: the tonic phase, in which the body becomes rigid, and the clonic phase, in which uncontrolled jerking occurs. May be preceded by aura and are often followed by headache, confusion, and sleep. May last for seconds or continue for several minutes.

Self-regulation and self-control Related, but not the same. Self-regulation refers to both conscious and unconscious processes that have an impact on self-control, but regulatory activities take place more or less constantly to allow us to participate in society, work, and family life. Self-control is a conscious activity.

Self-stimulating behaviors or "stimming" (stim) Example of stimming may include rocking, flapping of hands, or humming. For a person with autism, a stim may serve as a regulatory function to calm down, increase concentration, or shut out an overwhelming sound.

Sensory defensiveness A tendency, outside the norm, to react negatively or with alarm to sensory input that is generally considered harmless or nonirritating to others. Also called hypersensitivity.

Sensory input *See* Sensory stimulus.

Sensory integration The way the brain processes sensory stimulation or sensation from the body and then translates that information into specific, planned, coordinated motor activity.

Sensory integration dysfunction A neurological disorder causing difficulties processing information from the five classic senses (vision, hearing, touch, smell, and taste), sense of movement (vestibular system), and positional sense (proprioception). Sensory information is sensed normally, but perceived abnormally. May be a disorder on its own or with other neurological conditions.

Sensory integration therapy Used to improve ability to use incoming sensory information appropriately and encourage tolerance of a variety of sensory inputs.

Sensory stimulus An internal (e.g., heart rate, temperature) or external (e.g., sights, sounds, tastes, smells, touch, and balance) agent, action, or condition that elicits physiological or psychological response. Response depends on ability to regulate and understand stimuli and adjust emotions to demands of surroundings.

Sleep hygiene A set of practices, habits, and environmental factors critically important for sound sleep, such as minimizing noise, light, and temperature extremes and avoiding naps and caffeine.

Smith-Lemli-Opitz syndrome Genetic disorder with low cholesterol levels and autistic features, certain dysmorphic facial features, and usually, subnormal mental ability.

Social reciprocity Back-and-forth flow of social interaction. How behavior of one person influences and is influenced by behavior of another and vice versa.

Social stories Simple stories that describe social events and situations that are difficult for a child with a PDD to understand. For example, a social story might be written about birthday parties, if a child appears to have a difficult time understanding what is expected of him or her or how he or she is supposed to behave at a birthday party.

Social worker A trained specialist in the social, emotional, and financial needs of families and patients. Social workers often help families and patients obtain the services they have been prescribed.

Special education Specially designed instruction, at no cost to families, to meet unique needs of child with a disability, including instruction conducted in the classroom, in the home, in hospitals and institutions, and in other settings, and instruction in physical education.

Speech and language therapist, speech language pathologist Specializes in human communication. The focus is on communication, not speech, to increase a child's ability to impact and understand his or her environment.

Speech and languagc therapy Tasked with the goal of improving an individual's ability to communicate, which includes verbal and nonverbal communication. The treatment is specific to the individual's need.

Spoken language (also referred to as expressive and receptive language) Use of verbal behavior, or speech, to communicate thoughts, ideas, and feelings with others. Involves learning many levels of rules—combining sounds to make words, using conventional meanings of words, combining words into sentences, and using words and sentences in following rules of conversation.

Stereotyped behavior Refers to an abnormal or excessive repetition of an action carried out in the same way over time. May include repetitive movements or posturing of the body or objects.

Stereotyped pattern of interest, restricted pattern of interest Refers to a pattern of preoccupation with a narrow range of interests and activities. Stim or self-stimulation behaviors that stimulate one's senses. Some stims may serve a regulatory function (calming, increasing concentration, or shutting out an overwhelming sound). *See also* Self-stimulating behaviors or "stimming"

Subclinical seizure *See* Seizure, subclinical.

Symbolic play In which children pretend to do things and to be something or someone else. Typically develops between the ages of 2 and 3 years. Also called make-believe or pretend play.

Syndrome A set of signs and symptoms that collectively define or characterize a disease, disorder, or condition.

Tactile defensiveness A strong negative response to a sensation that would not ordinarily be upsetting, such as touching something sticky or gooey or the feeling of soft foods in the mouth. It is specific to touch.

Teleology Ethical decision-making framework based on anticipated outcomes of actions.

Teratogen Agent or factor that damages an embryo or fetus during the developmental period. Teratogens can include environmental contaminants, drugs, and infectious agents, and may cause congenital malformations or death.

Thalidomide A sedative and hypnotic drug that has been the cause of malformation of infants born to mothers using it during pregnancy. Thalidomide acts as an angiogenesis inhibitor and can inhibit bone formation. Currently used to treat certain types of cancer.

Training and Education of Autistic and Related Communication Handicapped Children (TEACCH) A therapeutic approach broadly based on the idea that individuals with autism more effectively use and understand visual cues.

Tonic-clonic seizure *See* Seizure, tonic-clonic.

Tuberous sclerosis A neurocutaneous disorder characterized by mental retardation, seizures, skin lesions, and intracranial lesions. An autosomal dominant disorder that occurs in 1 in 7,000 births.

Typical development (or healthy development) Describes physical, mental, and social development of a child who is acquiring or achieving skills according to the expected time frame. A child developing in a healthy way pays attention to voices, faces, and actions of others, shows and shares pleasure during interactions, and engages in verbal and nonverbal back-and-forth communication.

Valproate, valproic acid An antiepileptic drug used to treat epilepsy, migraines, and bipolar disorder. It is given orally or by injection. Associated with high rate of serious adverse events, including major congenital abnormalities and fetal death with in utero exposure.

Verbal behavior A method of ABA for teaching children with autism, based on B. F. Skinner's description of the system of language.

Vestibular system Refers to the body's system for maintaining equilibrium.

Virtue-based ethic Ethical decisions derive from internal motivations and values.

Wernicke's area Receptive speech area in the posterior temporal parietal region.

X- linked Diseases associated with the X chromosome.

Index